AF352884

Childhood Obesity: Nutrition and Lifestyle Determinants, Prevention and Management

Childhood Obesity: Nutrition and Lifestyle Determinants, Prevention and Management

Editors

Dr. Odysseas Androutsos
Prof. Dr. Evangelia Charmandari

MDPI • Basel • Beijing • Wuhan • Barcelona • Belgrade • Manchester • Tokyo • Cluj • Tianjin

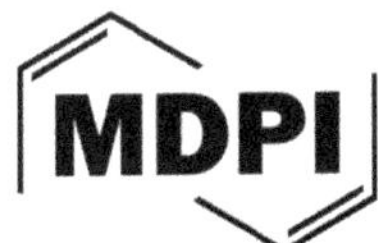

Editors
Dr. Odysseas Androutsos
Laboratory of Clinical Nutrition and Dietetics,
Department of Nutrition and Dietetics,
School of Physical Education,
Sport Science and Dietetics,
University of Thessaly
Greece

Prof. Dr. Evangelia Charmandari
Division of Endocrinology, Metabolism and
Diabetes, First Department of Pediatrics,
National and Kapodistrian University of
Athens Medical School, 'Aghia Sophia'
Children's Hospital
Greece

Editorial Office
MDPI
St. Alban-Anlage 66
4052 Basel, Switzerland

This is a reprint of articles from the Special Issue published online in the open access journal *Nutrients* (ISSN 2072-6643) (available at: https://www.mdpi.com/journal/nutrients/special_issues/Childhood_Obesity_Nutrition_and_Lifestyle_Determinants_Prevention_and_Management).

For citation purposes, cite each article independently as indicated on the article page online and as indicated below:

LastName, A.A.; LastName, B.B.; LastName, C.C. Article Title. *Journal Name* **Year**, *Volume Number*, Page Range.

ISBN 978-3-0365-5093-0 (Hbk)
ISBN 978-3-0365-5094-7 (PDF)

© 2022 by the authors. Articles in this book are Open Access and distributed under the Creative Commons Attribution (CC BY) license, which allows users to download, copy and build upon published articles, as long as the author and publisher are properly credited, which ensures maximum dissemination and a wider impact of our publications.

The book as a whole is distributed by MDPI under the terms and conditions of the Creative Commons license CC BY-NC-ND.

Contents

About the Editors

Dr. Odysseas Androutsos

Dr. Odysseas Androutsos is an Associate Professor of Clinical Nutrition and Dietetics at the Department of Nutrition-Dietetics, University of Thessaly. He has published 113 scientific papers in peer-reviewed journals and more than 100 oral or poster presentations in national and international scientific conferences. Since 2008, he has participated as the Principal Investigator, Project Manager or Member of research groups in national and international research programmes. Dr. Androutsos is a member of the Editorial Board and a reviewer in several scientific journals and in international conferences, books and research proposals. He has provided support as an external Scientific Consultant by the Ministry of Health of Malta and the National Institute of Health of Estonia in the implementation of research programmes for the prevention of childhood obesity. His scientific work has received national and international awards, such as the "John M. Kinney Award" for one of his scientific papers in the field of Pediatric Nutrition in 2019. He is an elected member of the ESDN Obesity of EFAD.

https://sciprofiles.com/profile/1102034

Prof. Dr. Evangelia Charmandari

Prof. Dr. Evangelia Charmandari is a Professor of Pediatrics—Pediatric and Adolescent Endocrinology at the National and Kapodistrian University of Athens Medical School, and Scientific Supervisor of the Division of Endocrinology and Metabolism, Center for Clinical, Experimental Surgery and Translational Research, Biomedical Research Foundation of the Academy of Athens, Athens, Greece. She is also the Director of the MSc Program entitled 'General Pediatrics and Pediatric Subspecialties: Clinical Practice and Research', the Chair of the ESPE Clinical Practice Committee and a Member of the ENDO-ERN Steering Committee.

Professor Charmandari's research work has focused on the hypothalamic–pituitary–adrenal axis' physiology, pathophysiology and its disorders; the molecular mechanisms of glucocorticoid receptor action; growth disorders; and childhood obesity.

She has more than 400 publications in SCI journals, books, and international conference proceedings (impact factor: 700; citations: 9200; h-index: 46; i10-index: 90). She was awarded the 'Henning Andersen Prize' of the European Society of Pediatric Endocrinology and received several awards of the Hellenic Endocrine Society, Hellenic Society of Adolescent Medicine and Health Care Business Awards. She has been an invited speaker in more than 250 national and international meetings. Finally, she has attracted approximately EUR 3.2m worth of research funding.

https://sciprofiles.com/profile/1134274

Preface to "Childhood Obesity: Nutrition and Lifestyle Determinants, Prevention and Management"

The prevalence of obesity has significantly increased over the last four decades worldwide. Obesity is associated with an increased prevalence of cardiometabolic disorders across the lifespan. The etiology of obesity has been attributed to demographic, socioeconomic, behavioral (e.g., unhealthy nutrition and low levels of physical activity), prenatal, perinatal, and clinical risk factors. However, their exact role, interplay, and mechanisms implicated in this process remain unclear. The trends of childhood obesity call for actions regarding the prevention and management of this disease early in life.

The Special Issue "Childhood Obesity: Nutrition and Lifestyle Determinants, Prevention and Management" of the journal *Nutrients* has collected original articles and reviews to advance the current knowledge on the role of lifestyle behaviors in the development of overweight and obesity, provide evidence about the nutritional habits of overweight and obese children and adolescents, and describe novel approaches for the screening, prevention, and management of obesity in youth. Towards achieving these goals, twenty articles were published in this Special Issue, and their main results are presented in the following paragraphs.

The studies by Sarintohe et al. and Thamrin et al. present new data regarding the prevalence of obesity in Indonesia [1,2]. Sarintohe et al. focused on adolescents (n = 411) attending private schools in Indonesia. According to the results, 36.3% of the participants were overweight, with the prevalence being significantly higher in boys compared to girls (47% vs. 24%), in urban compared to suburban areas (40.3% vs. 30.4%) and in adolescents who reported previous dieting at least once compared to those who never followed a restrictive diet plan (49.8% vs. 23.1%). Interestingly, boys living in urban areas were at higher risk of being overweight, suggesting that this specific group may need to be prioritized in future obesity-prevention measures. Similarly, Thamrin et al. showed that the prevalence of obesity was high in all the island clusters of Indonesia, which were included in their study. Different distributions of determinants of obesity were also recorded in these areas, highlighting the need for tailoring the policies and interventions to tackle the rising trends of obesity, accordingly.

Two more cross-sectional studies focused on the impact of the COVID-19 pandemic on children's and adolescents' lifestyle behaviors, well-being and body weight [3,4]. The COVEAT study by Androutsos et al. was conducted during the first lockdown implemented in Greece in April–May 2020 and examined its influence on 397 children's and adolescents' body weights and lifestyle behaviors. As expected, physical activity levels decreased, while sleep duration and screen time increased. Regarding the dietary behavior, children's and adolescents' consumption of fruit, fresh fruit juices, vegetables, dairy products, pasta, sweets, total snacks and breakfast increased. By contrast, fast-food consumption decreased. More than 1 out of 3 participants increased their body weight during the 2-month home confinement, which may be attributable to their increased consumption of certain foods/snacks and decreased level of physical activity. Similarly, the study by Morres et al. conducted a web-based survey with 950 adolescents during the second lockdown period implemented in Greece (November 2020–January 2021). This study showed that participants' quality of life was below the WHO threshold for possible depressive symptoms. In addition, low levels of physical activity and eating behavior scores were recorded. Overall, the studies by Androutsos et al. and Morres et al. highlighted the negative impact of the COVID-19 lockdown measures on children's and adolescents' lifestyles, well-being and body weights, indicating a need to support healthy lifestyles in potential future lockdowns and similar circumstances of home confinement.

The studies by Usheva et al. and Hampson et al. shed more light on the determinants of obesity in early life [5–7]. More specifically, Usheva et al. examined the role of breastfeeding and complementary feeding in a large-scale European cohort (ToyBox-study). In total, 7554 children from six European countries (Belgium, Bulgaria, Germany, Greece, Poland and Spain) were included in the statistical analyses. The percentage of families who adhered to the WHO recommendation of exclusive breastfeeding for 6 months was particularly low (6.3%), while about half of the children breastfed for 4–6 months, thus indicating a need for public health actions to support breastfeeding in Europe. Moreover, the results of the two studies by Usheva et al. did not identify any significant association between breastfeeding or the timing of solid food introduction and obesity at preschool age, after adjusting for several potential confounders. Hampson et al. conducted a longitudinal study, using data from the "Southern California Mother's Milk Study", to investigate the impact of infant formulas made with added corn-syrup solids on Hispanic children's eating behavior. At 2 years of follow-up, the consumption of this type of formula led to the development of greater food fussiness and reduced enjoyment of food compared to the observations recorded in breastfed children.

Guivarch et al. conducted a longitudinal study using data from the "EDEN mother-child cohort" to explore the determinants of obesity in toddlerhood [8]. More specifically, the authors examined the associations between an infant's appetite (at months 4, 8, 12 and 24 of life) and genetic susceptibility to obesity with parental feeding practices. The study showed that the genetic susceptibility to obesity was not associated with parental feeding practices. Furthermore, the infant's appetite was associated with restrictive feeding, while the parents of boys with high appetite in infancy more frequently used food to regulate their children's emotions. Considering that parental feeding practices comprise a key determinant for children's nutritional intakes and, consequently, their weight status, future obesity-prevention interventions should aim to improve them, possibly by targeting parents' perceptions of their children's appetites.

The narrative review by Mahmood et al. examined the associations of parents' dietary behavior and practices with their children's dietary behavior [9]. In total, 83 studies with data from 2–13-year-old children were included in this review and produced important results that are expected to be considered for future dietary interventions in youth. First, family meals seem to play a crucial role for modeling the dietary behavior of parents and their children, since it provides the time and opportunity to interact and exert control wherever needed. Secondly, parental encouragement and the avoidance of excessive pressure and restrictions against food consumption may support healthy eating and set a basis for the prevention of overconsumption and excessive weight gain in childhood and adolescence.

The cross-sectional study by Tani et al. included a sample of 5257 children aged 9–14 from Japan and examined whether the cooking skills of caregivers could influence children's dietary intakes and weight status [10]. The results showed that caregivers with poor cooking skills cooked less frequently at home and that their children were less likely to consume vegetables frequently, and they were at high risk for being obese. These findings indicate a need to improve cooking skills as a strategy to promote healthy eating and prevent childhood obesity.

The aforementioned risk factors, along with other risk factors previously described in the scientific literature, contribute to the development of excessive weight gain and childhood obesity. The detrimental effect of obesity on health is largely attributed to the excessive body fat. The study by Orsso et al. aimed to describe the developmental trajectories of adipose tissue from intrauterine life to adolescence, and highlight the determinants of adiposity [11]. Different developmental phases were associated with different changes in body composition. The intrauterine factors influencing the development of adipose tissue included maternal health, maternal nutrition, exposure to toxins and genetic predisposition, while in infancy, feeding practices and the gut microbiome played significant roles. In puberty, sexual dimorphism in hormone secretion comprised the key determinant of adiposity and was accompanied by other risk factors, such as dietary behavior, the gut microbiome and immune cell function.

The short-term, negative effects of obesity on children's health are well-known. The study by Zapata et al. aimed to describe the potential effect of obesity on Caucasian children's and adolescents' resting energy expenditure (REE) [12]. Both the REE and body composition of the participants were assessed using gold-standard techniques (i.e., indirect calorimetry and air-displacement plethysmography, respectively). According to the results of this study, REE was not influenced by obesity in children and adolescents after adjusting for fat-free mass (FFM). Another interesting finding was that this association remained insignificant in 8–10-year-old children, although a positive correlation between serum leptin and REE/FFM was recorded. These observations may be useful in the estimation of children's and adolescents' energy requirements, as well as in understanding of the impact of obesity on individuals' health.

Previous studies have suggested that certain anthropometric indices widely used in clinical practice, such as the body mass index (BMI), are not sensitive enough for identifying children at high risk for developing cardiometabolic disorders. Therefore, the study by Chin et al. used data from the "Adolescent Nutrition and Health Survey" in Taiwan and the "Multilevel Risk Profiles for Adolescent Metabolic Syndrome Study" to test adipose indices that could identify adolescents with metabolic syndrome [13]. Only body-fat- and lipid-enhanced adiposity indicators could identify adolescents with metabolic syndrome, while the waist circumference in males and abdominal volume index in females could be used to identify risk for metabolic syndrome in the transition from adolescence to adulthood.

This Special Issue also includes four intervention studies, which focused on the prevention or treatment of childhood obesity [14–17]. Zhu et al. implemented a school-based intervention to decrease the consumption of sugar-sweetened beverages (SSBs) among children and adolescents from China. The intervention was designed based on the ecological model, targeted multiple levels for behavioral change (individuals, families, peers and school) and was implemented over 1 year by teachers in collaboration with public health doctors at the local community health centers. The authors recorded significant reductions in both the frequency and the quantity of SSBs consumed in the intervention compared to the control group, especially in the elementary schools and in boys. Furthermore, the study by Lubrecht et al. examined the effectiveness of a lifestyle intervention in children aged 2–18 years with severe obesity. More specifically, the authors adopted a longitudinal design to compare the effects of a standardized intervention between younger children (2–12 years old) and adolescents (13–18 years old) over a period of 2 years. The intervention was delivered by a multidisciplinary team, consisting of pediatricians, dieticians, psychologists, pedagogues, physical activity coaches and nurses, and included a personalized approach based on the children's/adolescents' characteristics and needs. The findings showed that the BMI z-scores tended to decrease more in children compared to in adolescents over time. The intervention led to significant improvements in participants' cardiometabolic indices (e.g., lipid profiles, the levels of glucose metabolism indices, and alanine aminotransferase), indicating that lifestyle modifications in severe obesity can produce clinically significant improvements in children's/adolescents' weight status and health. The study by Hawkins et al. implemented the "Healthy Schoolhouse 2.0 program" in elementary schools in Washington, DC, USA, over a 5-year period. This study was specifically designed to provide equitable access to the intervention for the participants and aimed to increase their nutrition literacy. During follow-up, an increase in students' nutrition knowledge scores was observed in the intervention group, especially among students whose teachers delivered three nutrition lessons compared to those who implemented fewer. Finally, Jones et al. present the design of a novel dietary intervention (RCT) in women with gestational diabetes, which aims to prevent obesity among their offspring by the age of 3 years. This intervention will restrict energy intake through women's diets, using a whole-diet replacement, and the results are expected from 2026 onwards.

The review of Motevalli et al. introduced an "Etiology-Based Personalized Intervention Strategy Targeting Childhood Obesity" (EPISTCO) model, which provides a guide to healthcare professionals (HCPs) working with children to better understand the determinants of childhood obesity and then deliver tailormade interventions according to children's and adolescents' personalized characteristics and needs [18]. In this context, several biological, behavioral and environmental factors are assessed, and the individual's barriers and facilitators for the adoption of healthy lifestyle behaviors are identified. The novelty of this model is that it includes a four-step, multicomponent intervention, which foresees the personalization of the whole process by the multidisciplinary team of HCPs, thus potentially increasing the effectiveness of the intervention.

The systematic review by Leme et al. focused on obesity-prevention strategies in adolescence and compared the effectiveness of two types of interventions: those targeting energy balance (decreasing energy intake and/or increasing energy expenditure) and those aiming to reduce disordered eating behaviors to promote a positive food and eating relationship [19]. Both types of studies demonstrated poor clinical outcomes, with the interventions focusing on energy balance failing to support adolescents in maintaining the positive changes in their lifestyle behaviors and weight status achieved during their implementation, while the second group of interventions were not effective in reducing weight over time. Considering that the interventions aiming to reduce disordered eating behaviors were effective in reducing adolescents' body dissatisfaction, dieting and weight-control behaviors, the authors suggested that new studies in this field needed to be considered and designed accordingly to achieve weight loss.

Another study by Flores-Ramírez et al. reviewed the combined effects of L-citrulline supplementation and aerobic training on vascular function in different age groups [20]. The findings of this study provide evidence to support the implementation of moderate-to-high-intensity interventions (duration: 12–32 weeks) for improving indices of vascular function and cardiovascular risk factors. Moreover, L-citrulline supplementation seems to be effective in improving children's and adults' nitric-oxide levels and the bioavailability of L-citrulline, which plays a pivotal role in nitrogen homeostasis and improves various cardiovascular risk factors in adults (especially in those with obesity). Given these results, the authors suggested that new interventions aiming to examine the combined effects of L-citrulline supplementation and aerobic training on the vascular function of children and/or young adults living with obesity and/or impaired metabolic profiles are needed to address the negative impact of obesity on health in the early stages of life.

In conclusion, the results of the studies included in the Special Issue "Childhood Obesity: Nutrition and Lifestyle Determinants, Prevention and Management" of the journal Nutrients show high rates of childhood obesity; provide new insights regarding the use of novel methods in identifying impaired cardiometabolic profiles in children with obesity, as well as on the role and interplay of its determinants; and present new interventions and models for the prevention or treatment of obesity in children and adolescents. With the hope that this new evidence will open new horizons in the field of childhood obesity and will further improve the healthcare process in pediatric health, the Guest Editors would like to thank all the contributors for the publication of this Special Issue.

References

1. Sarintohe, E.; Larsen, J.K.; Burk, W.J.; Vink, J.M. The Prevalence of Overweight Status among Early Adolescents from Private Schools in Indonesia: Sex-Specific Patterns Determined by School Urbanization Level. *Nutrients* **2022**, *14*, 1001.

2. Thamrin, S.A.; Arsyad, D.S.; Kuswanto, H.; Lawi, A.; Arundhana, A.I. Obesity Risk-Factor Variation Based on Island Clusters: A Secondary Analysis of Indonesian Basic Health Research 2018. *Nutrients* **2022**, *14*, 971.

3. Androutsos, O.; Perperidi, M.; Georgiou, C.; Chouliaras, G. Lifestyle Changes and Determinants of Children's and Adolescents' Body Weight Increase during the First COVID-19 Lockdown in Greece: The COV-EAT Study. *Nutrients* **2021**, *13*, 930.

4. Morres, I.D.; Galanis, E.; Hatzigeorgiadis, A.; Androutsos, O.; Theodorakis, Y. Physical Activity, Sedentariness, Eating Behaviour and Well-Being during a COVID-19 Lockdown Period in Greek Adolescents. *Nutrients* **2021**, *13*, 1449.

5. Usheva, N.; Galcheva, S.; Cardon, G.; De Craemer, M.; Androutsos, O.; Kotowska, A.; Socha, P.; Koletzko, B.V.; Moreno, L.A.; Iotova, V.; et al. Complementary Feeding and Overweight in European Preschoolers: The ToyBox-Study. *Nutrients* **2021**, *13*, 1199.

6. Usheva, N.; Lateva, M.; Galcheva, S.; Koletzko, B.V.; Cardon, G.; De Craemer, M.; Androutsos, O.; Kotowska, A.; Socha, P.; Moreno, L.A.; et al. Breastfeeding and Overweight in European Preschoolers: The ToyBox Study. *Nutrients* **2021**, *13*, 2880.

7. Hampson, H.E.; Jones, R.B.; Berger, P.K.; Plows, J.F.; Schmidt, K.A.; Alderete, T.L.; Goran, M.I. Adverse Effects of Infant Formula Made with Corn-Syrup Solids on the Development of Eating Behaviors in Hispanic Children. *Nutrients* **2022**, *14*, 1115.

8. Guivarch, C.; Charles, M.A.; Forhan, A.; Ong, K.K.; Heude, B.; de Lauzon-Guillain, B. Associations between Children's Genetic Susceptibility to Obesity, Infant's Appetite and Parental Feeding Practices in Toddlerhood. *Nutrients* **2021**, *13*, 1468.

9. Mahmood, L.; Flores-Barrantes, P.; Moreno, L.A.; Manios, Y.; Gonzalez-Gil, E.M. The Influence of Parental Dietary Behaviors and Practices on Children's Eating Habits. *Nutrients* **2021**, *13*, 1138.

10. Tani, Y.; Isumi, A.; Doi, S.; Fujiwara, T. Associations of Caregiver Cooking Skills with Child Dietary Behaviors and Weight Status: Results from the A-CHILD Study. *Nutrients* **2021**, *13*, 4549.

11. Orsso, C.E.; Colin-Ramirez, E.; Field, C.J.; Madsen, K.L.; Prado, C.M.; Haqq, A.M. Adipose Tissue Development and Expansion from the Womb to Adolescence: An Overview. *Nutrients* **2020**, *12*, 2735.

12. Karina Zapata, J.; Catalán, V.; Rodríguez, A.; Ramírez, B.; Silva, C.; Escalada, J.; Salvador, J.; Calamita, G.; Cristina Azcona-Sanjulian, M.; Frühbeck, G.; et al. Resting Energy Expenditure Is Not Altered in Children and Adolescents with Obesity. Effect of Age and Gender and Association with Serum Leptin Levels. *Nutrients* **2021**, *13*, 1216.

13. Chin, Y.T.; Lin, W.T.; Wu, P.W.; Tsai, S.; Lee, C.Y.; Seal, D.W.; Chen, T.; Huang, H.L.; Lee, C.H. Characteristic-Grouped Adiposity Indicators for Identifying Metabolic Syndrome in Adolescents: Develop and Valid Risk Screening Tools Using Dual Population. *Nutrients* **2020**, *12*, 3165.

14. Zhu, Z.; Luo, C.; Qu, S.; Wei, X.; Feng, J.; Zhang, S.; Wang, Y.; Su, J. Effects of School-Based Interventions on Reducing Sugar-Sweetened Beverage Consumption among Chinese Children and Adolescents. *Nutrients* **2021**, *13*, 1862.

15. Lubrecht, K.G.H.; Hesselink, J.W.; Winkens, M.L.; Van Dielen, B.; Vreugdenhil, F.M.H.; Van De Pas, K.G.H.; Lubrecht, J.W.; Hesselink, M.L.; Winkens, B.; Van Dielen, F.M.H.; et al. The Effect of a Multidisciplinary Lifestyle Intervention on Health Parameters in Children versus Adolescents with Severe Obesity. *Nutrients* **2022**, *14*, 1795.

16. Hawkins, M.; Belson, S.I.; McClave, R.; Kohls, L.; Little, S.; Snelling, A. Healthy Schoolhouse 2.0

Health Promotion Intervention to Reduce Childhood Obesity in Washington, DC: A Feasibility Study. *Nutrients* **2021**, *13*, 2935.

17. Jones, D.; De, E.; Rolfe, L.; Rennie, K.L.; Oude Griep, L.M.; Kusinski, L.C.; Hughes, D.J.; Brage, S.; Ong, K.K.; Beardsall, K.; et al. Antenatal Determinants of Childhood Obesity in High-Risk Offspring: Protocol for the DiGest Follow-Up Study. *Nutrients* **2021**, *13*, 1156.

18. Motevalli, M.; Drenowatz, C.; Tanous, D.R.; Khan, N.A.; Wirnitzer, K. Management of Childhood Obesity—Time to Shift from Generalized to Personalized Intervention Strategies. *Nutrients* **2021**, *13*, 1200.

19. Leme, A.C.B.; Haines, J.; Tang, L.; Dunker, K.L.L.; Philippi, S.T.; Fisberg, M.; Ferrari, G.L.; Fisberg, R.M. Impact of Strategies for Preventing Obesity and Risk Factors for Eating Disorders among Adolescents: A Systematic Review. *Nutrients* **2020**, *12*, 3134.

20. Flores-Ramírez, A.G.; Tovar-Villegas, V.I.; Maharaj, A.; Garay-Sevilla, M.E.; Figueroa, A. Effects of L-Citrulline Supplementation and Aerobic Training on Vascular Function in Individuals with Obesity across the Lifespan. *Nutrients* **2021**, *13*, 2991.

Dr. Odysseas Androutsos and Prof. Dr. Evangelia Charmandari

Editors

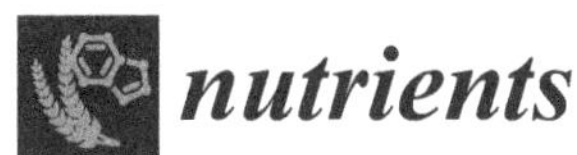

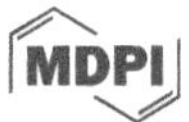

Review

Adipose Tissue Development and Expansion from the Womb to Adolescence: An Overview

Camila E. Orsso [1], Eloisa Colin-Ramirez [2], Catherine J. Field [1], Karen L. Madsen [3], Carla M. Prado [1] and Andrea M. Haqq [4,*]

[1] Department of Agricultural, Food and Nutritional Science, University of Alberta, Edmonton, AB T6G 2E1, Canada; orsso@ualberta.ca (C.E.O.); cjfield@ualberta.ca (C.J.F.); carla.prado@ualberta.ca (C.M.P.)

[2] Department of Pediatrics, University of Alberta, Edmonton, AB T6G 2E1, Canada; eloisa@ualberta.ca

[3] Department of Medicine, University of Alberta, Edmonton, AB T6G 2C2, Canada; karen.madsen@ualberta.ca

[4] Department of Pediatrics and Department of Agricultural, Food and Nutritional Science, University of Alberta, Edmonton, AB T6G 2R7, Canada

* Correspondence: haqq@ualberta.ca; Tel.: +1-780-492-0015

Received: 12 August 2020; Accepted: 2 September 2020; Published: 8 September 2020

Abstract: Prevalence rates of pediatric obesity continue to rise worldwide. Adipose tissue (AT) development and expansion initiate in the fetus and extend throughout the lifespan. This paper presents an overview of the AT developmental trajectories from the intrauterine period to adolescence; factors determining adiposity expansion are also discussed. The greatest fetal increases in AT were observed in the third pregnancy trimester, with growing evidence suggesting that maternal health and nutrition, toxin exposure, and genetic defects impact AT development. From birth up to six months, healthy term newborns experience steep increases in AT; but a subsequent reduction in AT is observed during infancy. Important determinants of AT in infancy identified in this review included feeding practices and factors shaping the gut microbiome. Low AT accrual rates are maintained up to puberty onset, at which time, the pattern of adiposity expansion becomes sex dependent. As girls experience rapid increases and boys experience decreases in AT, sexual dimorphism in hormone secretion can be considered the main contributor for changes. Eating patterns/behaviors and interactions between dietary components, gut microbiome, and immune cells also influence AT expansion. Despite the plasticity of this tissue, substantial evidence supports that adiposity at birth and infancy highly influences its levels across subsequent life stages. Thus, a unique window of opportunity for the prevention and/or slowing down of the predisposition toward obesity, exists from pregnancy through childhood.

Keywords: adipose tissue; obesity; children; adolescence; development

---

1. Introduction

Prevalence rates of childhood obesity continue to rise worldwide. Analysis of data pooled from studies conducted between 1975 and 2016 revealed a 4.9% and 6.9% global increase in the prevalence of obesity among girls and boys aged 5–19 years, respectively [1]. Although the etiology of obesity is multifactorial, it can be simply defined as excess of body fat (or adiposity) [2]. Adipose tissue (AT) is one of the largest organs in the body and provides protection and support for other organs and acts as an endocrine tissue [3]. Recent research has shown the existence of varied AT subtypes, but only the brown and white AT have been extensively characterized in humans [3,4]. Although both AT types are important for energy homeostasis, they differ considerably given their characteristic distribution, lipid composition, and cytokine profiles (Table 1) [3,4]. Notably, the thermogenic role of brown AT contributes to insulin sensitivity and increased energy expenditure [5]. On the other hand, excess of white AT has been associated with metabolic dysfunction, reduced cardiorespiratory fitness, and psychological disorders during childhood [6–8]. White AT is generally classified as subcutaneous AT (SAT) or visceral AT (VAT); the latter is found in distinct depots (e.g., omental, epicardial, pericardial) and composed of heterogeneous cell types depending on the depot, conferring them specific metabolic signatures and capacity for development and expansion [9–11].

Adipose tissue development is a dynamic process. The first adipose cells, also called adipocytes, appear during the intrauterine period and continue to develop and expand throughout life [12]. Although AT accretion in each stage of development follows a general pattern that is specific to that stage, studies have shown that adiposity in prenatal life and infancy tracks into childhood and then into adulthood [13–17]. Several components have been shown to contribute to healthy (or unhealthy) AT growth, including genetic factors as well as prenatal and postnatal exposure to dietary, lifestyle, and environmental factors. Thus, there has been an extensive effort to develop effective preventive and treatment strategies targeting these determinants of AT expansion. In this narrative review, we describe the trajectories of AT development from the intrauterine period to late adolescence and examine the role of prenatal and postnatal factors that have been identified to contribute to its development and expansion. Articles discussed here were identified through a literature search in PubMed from its conception until August 2020. The search strategy consisted of a combination of keywords related to the following concepts: AT development and expansion, life stages, fetal programming, breastfeeding, environmental exposures, genetics, dietary intake, gut microbiome, and physical activity/exercise. Here, we focus on white AT (at the tissue level), as it is the largest component of total fat mass (FM; at the molecular level) and it has been extensively characterized in the pediatric population; specifically, about 80% of AT is FM [18].

Table 1. Key differences in morphology, distribution, and primary function between white and brown adipose tissues.

	White Adipose Tissue [3,19]	Brown Adipose Tissue [20]
Morphology	• Large unilocular lipid droplets: 95% of cell volume is composed of triglycerides • Adipocytes with sparse mitochondrial population • *UCP1* is not expressed	• Small lipid droplets (multilocular) • Dense network of mitochondria and vasculature in adipocytes • High basal levels of the mitochondrial *UCP1*
Distribution	• Found in subcutaneous and visceral adipose tissues and ectopic depots • Distribution varies across age, sex, nutritional status, and metabolic health	• Infants: interscapular and perirenal regions • Adults: cervical, supraclavicular, axillary, and suprarenal regions • Infants have greater amounts than adults • Individuals with obesity have lower quantity than those of normal weight
Primary function	• Energy homeostasis: store lipids and release energy in form of free fatty acids and glycerol • Endocrine: secretion of hormones, pro-inflammatory cytokines • Mechanical: protect organs against external mechanical stress, prevent heat loss (insulator)	• Cold-induced thermogenesis: produce heat via the action of *UCP1* • Energy expenditure

Abbreviation: *UCP1*: uncoupling protein 1.

2. Adipose Tissue Development

The development and expansion of AT, with consequent increases in total body fat, are dynamic processes that begin in the second trimester of gestation and extend throughout life (Figure 1) [12]. These processes involve either enlargement of adipocyte cells by augmented lipid storage (i.e., hypertrophy) or increases in the number of adipocytes (i.e., hyperplasia) within a lobule through differentiated progenitor or mesenchymal cells [21]. Sun et al. further classify the AT expansion into healthy and unhealthy processes [22]. The first classification is related to the formation of small new adipocytes that are adequately vascularized and minimal inflammation is present [22].

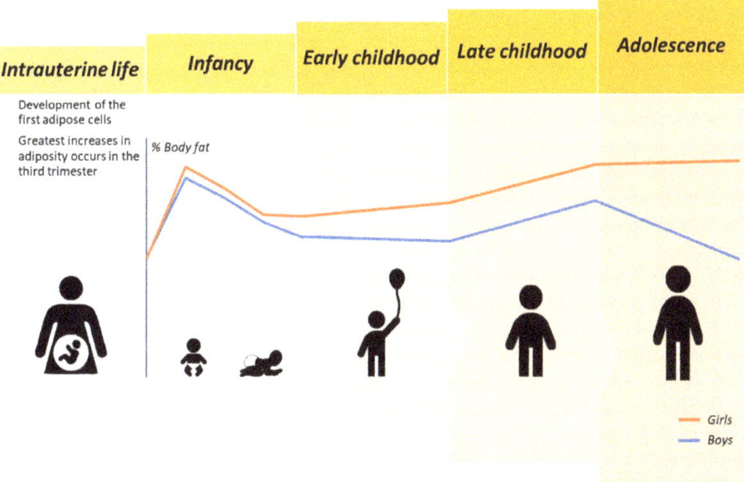

Figure 1. Schema representing the developmental trajectories of body fat from intrauterine life to adolescence in healthy girls and boys. Note that although the lines depicting percent body fat in girls and boys were plotted based on reference data from Fomon et al. [23] and Ellis [24], we did not intend to provide values for this body compartment as it can vary depending on the body composition technique used, race/ethnicity, and other factors. Herein, we intended to present an overview of the general expansion patterns of adiposity stratified by sex.

On the other hand, unhealthy expansion is often observed in individuals with obesity under a persistent positive energy balance [11,22]. In these individuals, there is a rapid increase of pre-existing adipocyte size in SAT due to greater lipid accumulation. With inadequate angiogenesis, the tissue is prone to hypoxia and adipocyte dysfunction. Because there is a limit for lipid storage in adipocytes, adipocyte hypertrophy is followed by hyperplasia, or leakage of lipids to other tissues (e.g., liver and muscle), and consequent de novo lipogenesis and lipotoxicity [11,22]. According to Sethi et al., the degree of toxicity will depend on the extent and duration of positive energy supply, effectiveness of lipid transport and storage mechanisms, and organ oxidative capacity [25]. In contrast to this "limited adiposity expandability" hypothesis, a recent study demonstrated that greater turnover of triglycerides and mature adipocytes in abdominal and gluteal SAT of adolescents girls with obesity may determine the accumulation of fat in the liver and metabolic dysfunction in this population [26]. Another hypothesis is that a persistent positive energy balance affects the secretion of adipokines (e.g., leptin, adiponectin, tumor necrosis factor alpha (TNF-α), interleukin-6 (IL-6)), with implications for glucose homeostasis and lipid metabolism and flux [25]. Further sections will discuss the trajectories of both healthy and unhealthy AT expansion throughout growth stages as well as the evidence regarding factors potentially contributing to AT in each specific life stage (Figure 2).

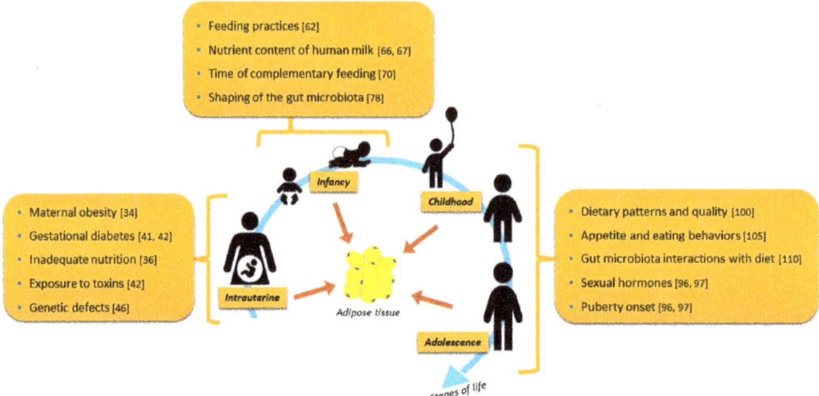

Figure 2. Summary of factors discussed in this review that potentially contribute to adipose tissue development and expansion in the early stages of life.

2.1. Intrauterine Adipose Tissue Accrual

Histological analysis of buccal fat pads from human fetuses revealed that intrauterine AT development occurs in five different stages, with an overlap in stages 2 to 4 [27]. The first stage, at 14 weeks, is marked by an outgrowth of loose connective tissue. Right after (stage 2 at 14.5 weeks), there is an early vascularization of the tissue. Stage 3 is characterized by the onset of mesenchymal cell growth at 19 weeks; although several studies have shown a mesodermal origin of these growth cells, recent investigation using mouse models suggests that mesenchymal cells associated with head AT formation originate from neural crest cells [28]. The first adipocytes appear in stage 4, and at 28 weeks (stage 5), fat lobules are formed and can be distinguished from other structures. Despite the later development of adipocytes, findings from molecular body composition analysis estimated a lipid accretion rate of 7.8 g/day at earlier stages (24–28 weeks) and increases up to 19.8 g/day at 36–40 weeks [29]. There is extremely limited knowledge on intrauterine AT accrual in the third trimester of pregnancy due to the inability of current techniques to assess body composition [30]. Using magnetic resonance imaging (MRI), one study reported increases of 2.5 mm in the truncal AT thickness of fetuses from weeks 29 to 39–40 of gestational age [31].

2.1.1. Health and Nutrition during Pregnancy as Determinants of Adipose Tissue

Prenatal maternal health and nutritional status have been shown to contribute to obesity development during childhood and adolescence [32,33]. Findings from a large study including 1173 mother–child pairs (mostly Caucasians) demonstrated that maternal obesity during early pregnancy was associated with a 0.63 standard deviation increase in body mass index (BMI) z-score ($p = 0.006$) and a 11.5% increase in sum of skinfold thickness ($p < 0.001$) in children at 6 years old (adjusted analysis for maternal covariates) [34]. More specifically, VAT thickness (measured by ultrasound) in the first trimester explained the variations in newborn birth weight centile to the greatest extent compared to SAT and BMI ($R^2 = 15.8\%$, $p = 0.002$) [35]. Interestingly, maternal diet quality (assessed by the Healthy Eating Index—2015) during pregnancy and lactation was positively associated with infant percent body fat (%BF) and FM (in kg, by air-displacement plethysmography (ADP)) at 6 months of age [36]. Furthermore, although it is clear that an imbalance between ω-6 and ω-3 polyunsaturated fatty acids intake during pregnancy affects children's neurocognitive development [37], the effects of prenatal ω-3 polyunsaturated fatty acid supplementation on children's obesity risk and AT expansion remain to be confirmed [38].

Increasing maternal blood glucose concentrations have been associated with adverse pregnancy outcomes. The relationships between maternal glucose metabolism (assessed by oral glucose tolerance test (OGTT) and glycated hemoglobin) during pregnancy and children's %BF at 10 to 14 years were evaluated by Lowe Jr. et al. [39]. After adjusting for confounders (e.g., child's sexual maturation, adiposity, and maternal variables), the authors found that the odds ratio (OR) for having high %BF (>85th percentile for age and sex; measured by ADP) during childhood and adolescence ranged from 1.14 to 1.18 for maternal glucose markers, all $p < 0.05$ [39]. Other studies also indicated that exposure to gestational diabetes during fetal growth may impact children's adiposity [40,41].

2.1.2. Effects of Intrauterine Exposure to Toxins on Adipose Tissue Development

Maternal exposure to toxins and endocrine disrupting chemicals, such as bisphenol A that is found in plastics, has been shown to affect fetal AT development [42]. Bisphenol A appears to cross the placenta, and researchers have quantified human exposure in several body fluids, including breast milk, umbilical cord blood, and amniotic fluid. Although several animal studies confirm prenatal exposure to bisphenol A and its effects on health through the peroxisome proliferator-activated receptors pathways (see Shafei et al., for a detailed description on the mechanism), epidemiological studies have not been conducted to investigate the implication of bisphenol A in adiposity development in humans [43]. The effects of prenatal exposure to smoking and air pollution on infant adiposity and body weight have been Start evaluated in the Healthy study [44,45]. Infants born from mothers who were active smokers or exposed to second-hand smoke during gestation had lower birth weight and FM (by ADP) than non-exposed infants [44]. Furthermore, researchers found positive associations between ozone in the third trimester of pregnancy and infant adiposity at the five-month follow-up, although the average of air pollutants was considered low [45].

2.1.3. Genetic Defects

Structural changes in genes including deletions, variations, or mutations in proteins responsible for encoding proteins related to metabolism and appetite regulation can lead to genetic forms of obesity [46]. These genetic variants can be inherited in an autosomal or x-linked pattern, and there are currently three classifications for genetic obesity: monogenic, syndromic, and polygenic obesity [46]. Monogenic non-syndromic obesity results from a single-gene mutation associated with increased appetite (i.e., hyperphagia), early onset severe obesity, and endocrine dysfunction in some patients [47]. Several single-gene mutations have been identified, including dysfunctions in the leptin (*LEP*) gene and its receptor (*LEPR*) or regulator (*SH2B* adaptor protein 1 (*SH2B1*)), proopiomelanocortin (*POMC*) gene, and melanocortin 4 receptor (*MC4R*) [47]. Syndromic obesity results from single- or multiple-gene mutations but differs from the other two by the characteristic cognitive delay, dysmorphic features, extreme hyperphagia, organ-specific abnormalities, and other characteristics of hypothalamic dysfunction [48]. More recently, analysis of whole-exome sequencing data from a large cohort of children with severe early onset of obesity revealed variants in the pleckstrin homology domain interacting protein (PHIP) that were associated with obesity, either in the presence or absence of developmental delay [49]. Using in vitro analysis, the authors further demonstrated that variants in the nuclear PHIP suppressed the transcription of the *POMC* gene, which may contribute to hyperphagia [49]. On the other hand, polygenic obesity is characterized by multiple-gene dysfunction that results in obesity due to their interaction with the environment [50]. Importantly, polygenes enclose one allele that is susceptible to higher and another to lower body weight. More than 100 polygenes associate with body weight regulation have been described as a result of the implementation of genome-wide association studies. It is not our intent to describe the clinical features of these genetic forms of obesity; thus, we refer the readers to the recent reviews cited above.

2.2. Postnatal and Infant Adipose Tissue Accrual

Soon after birth, newborns lose body weight due to changes in hydration of fat-free mass (FFM), but not FM [51], as an adaptation to extrauterine life. Fat mass development is marked by steep increases from birth up to 6 months of age and a subsequent reduction in the rate of FM accrual in healthy term boys and girls, as assessed by multicompartment model [52]. In fact, %BF accrual during infancy also differs between term and preterm newborns. Preterm infants at term-corrected age (i.e., chronologic age adjusted for gestational age) had higher %BF (14.8% ± 4.4% by ADP) than term infants (8.6% ± 3.71%, $p < 0.0001$) [53]. Similar findings using ADP were reported by Ramel et al. in a longitudinal analysis; preterm infants with appropriate size for gestational age (AGA) at term-corrected age had higher %BF than term infants (17.8% vs. 15.2%, $p < 0.0001$), but these differences disappeared in measures obtained at 3 to 4 months (27.7% vs. 23.9%, $p = 0.07$) [54]. Regarding the distribution of body fat, Toro-Ramos et al. summarized the findings from several studies reporting infant body composition data and highlight the predominance of SAT rather than VAT in the first months of life [30].

Compared to AGA infants, those infants born small for-gestational age (SGA) were shown to have lower %BF by ADP at term birth [55]. According to Zegher et al., the greater levels of circulating preadipocyte factor 1 (Pref-1) found in SGA than in AGA newborns may partially explain the impaired intrauterine AT development [56], as Pref-1 has a role in suppressing adipocyte differentiation [57]. In contrast, SGA infants experienced subsequent rapid gains in body weight and normalization of %BF by one year, which has been associated with metabolic disturbances [56]. Catch-up in growth was accompanied by thicker carotid intima-media thickness at 1 and 2 years old, and greater pre-peritoneal fat at 2 years old; however, no differences in cardiovascular markers or cardiac morphometry were found [56]. Furthermore, findings from the Generation R Study revealed that children with a growth pattern characterized by negative fetal weight gain, but consecutive increases in weight during infancy, had the greatest VAT volume (by MRI adjusted for height cubed) and liver fat fraction at a mean age of 9.8 years [58]. In order to further investigate the molecular mechanisms underlying the associations between catch-up growth and metabolic disturbances, animal models may be used; it is noteworthy, however, that researchers should interpret the findings in view of the litter sizes, as smaller ones may have greater access to food leading to overfeeding and higher rates of early growth [59].

2.2.1. Associations between Feeding Practices and Adipose Tissue in Infancy

Feeding practices during infancy have been associated with excess adiposity. The benefits of breastfeeding to infant's health have been extensively described in the literature and includes, for example, improved immunity and cognitive development [60,61]. However, there is contradictory evidence on whether breastfeeding influences AT development. One study has shown positive associations between exclusive breastfeeding duration and %BF (by ADP) and SAT (by ultrasound), but not VAT at 3 and 6 months [62]. Comparisons between breastfed and formula-fed healthy newborns from low-risk pregnancies revealed greater %BF (using ADP) at 3 and 6 months in those who were breastfed [63]. In contrast, no differences in %BF or FM (also by ADP) were found between predominantly breastfed and exclusively formula-fed infants at 1, 4, and 7 months of age in another study [64]. Some evidence suggests that feeding practices determine the extent of FM accretion and metabolic disturbances in SGA infants early in life [65]. More specifically, breastfed SGA and AGA infants had similar FM levels (by dual-energy X-ray absorptiometry (DXA)) and greater insulin sensitivity at 12 months, whereas SGA infants fed with a protein-rich infant formula experienced gains in FM and decreases in high-molecular-weight (HMW) adiponectin and elevated levels of insulin-like growth factor 1 (IGF-1) [65].

Indeed, the nutrient content of human milk appears to influence AT development as negative associations between carbohydrate content in human milk and FM or %BF (by ultrasound) have been reported in infants aged 2, 5, 9, and/or 12 months [66]. Differences in human milk fatty acid composition have also been shown to determine adiposity in exclusively breastfed infants [67,68]. For example, %BF (by ADP) increased 4.7% in infants (from the ages of two weeks to four months) for each 1-unit increase in the ω-6 to ω-3 polyunsaturated fatty acids ratio ($p = 0.010$) in human milk [67]. Specifically, human milk samples with a high ratio of ω-6 to ω-3 polyunsaturated fatty acids had greater concentrations of pro-inflammatory cytokines (IL-6 and TNF-α) than samples with medium and low ratios, which stimulated the expression of genes responsible for depositing triacylglycerol in adipose cells [68]. Furthermore, associations between hormones in breast milk and infant adiposity measures have also been investigated; higher levels of leptin and intermediate levels of insulin were found to be associated with lower weight-for-length and BMI z-scores at 4 and 12 months of age, independent of several covariates (i.e., maternal pre-pregnancy BMI, ethnicity, parity, diabetes, smoking, breastfeeding exclusivity at sampling, and lactation stage) [69]. Thus, infants may respond differently to breastfeeding regarding AT development because nutrient and hormone content of human milk, which varies among mothers, can affect this association.

The time of complementary feeding introduction is also a determining factor for adiposity accrual early in life and during childhood. A prospective study has shown that children who were breastfed during infancy and had complementary feeding initiated earlier than 4 months had a greater likelihood of presenting with higher truncal fat (by DXA) in mid-childhood ($\beta = 0.33$ [95% CI, 0.01, 0.65]) and early adolescence ($\beta = 1.20$ [95% CI, 0.33, 2.06]) than breastfed children who had complementary feeding initiated at 4 to 6 months [70]. Similar associations were found in formula-fed children; complementary feeding earlier than 4 months was positively associated with truncal fat at mid-childhood ($\beta = 0.52$ [95% CI, 0.07, 0.97]) and %BF at early adolescence ($\beta = 2.55$ [95% CI, 0.20, 4.91]). Interesting, 82% of the children who received complementary feeding at earlier than 4 months had infant cereals, whereas 30% had fruits, 22% were fed vegetables, and 30% fruit juice [70].

2.2.2. Gut Microbiome

The gut microbiome during the first years of life also plays a role in adiposity development and is influenced by several factors, including mode of delivery, feeding practices, antibiotic and drug use, and environmental exposures [71]. The associations between these factors and risk of obesity development have been evaluated in humans [72–74]. For example, a report from the Canadian Healthy Infant Longitudinal Development (CHILD) birth cohort has shown that infants born by caesarean delivery from mothers with overweight were five times more likely to present as overweight by one year old [73]; this association was mediated by the abundance of organisms from the Lachnospiraceae family, which was high in the infant gut microbiome at 3–4 months old. Additionally, a subset of breastfed infants from the same birth cohort had a lower risk of becoming overweight at 12 months than formula-fed infants; authors also found a negative association between breastfeeding exclusiveness and the abundance of Lachnospiraceae organisms [75]. Regarding antibiotic use, a recent meta-analysis found a small association between antibiotic use during infancy and risk of children becoming overweight or obese (based on weight indices) at older age (OR = 1.05; 95% CI 1.00, 1.11), as previous studies have presented controversial results [74]. Despite these findings, mechanistic studies using germ-free animal models have confirmed the causal role of gut microbiome in the obesity pathogenesis and the associations between Lachnospiraceae family and adiposity development [76–79]. Please see Kincaid et al. for a comprehensive review of the literature discussing the most recent animal and human evidence on the interactions between gut microbiome, early life exposures, and obesity onset [78].

2.3. Adipose Tissue Development in Childhood and Adolescence

There are a limited number of studies evaluating adiposity between the ages of two and five due to limitations of current body composition techniques, including lack of age-specific predictive equations, minimal movement required for exam success, and lack of appropriate devices for small bodies or that can be used in children across all age stages (e.g., ADP is unavailable for children aged two to six years) [80,81]. Using data from reference children, Fomon et al. reported low %BF accrual rates in early childhood, with boys and girls presenting with 19.5% and 20.4% of %BF at 2 years and 14.6% and 16.7% at 5 years, respectively [23]. More recently, Wells et al. reported cross-sectional reference data for adiposity (FM and FM index (FMI)) estimated by isotope dilution from the ages of 6 weeks to 5 years old [82]. However, several studies in populations with varied ethnic origins have reported body composition reference data for late childhood and adolescence, as summarized below.

Using a longitudinal design, McConnell-Nzunga et al. investigated the %BF accrual (by DXA) in Canadians of Caucasian and Asian origins from ages 10 to 18 years [83]. The authors found that those children in the highest %BF centiles (90th and 97th) had greater increases in %BF from 10 to 11 years, but a sharp reduction from 12 to 15 years. In a study on Caucasian children from Southern England, %BF peaked at age 11 years for those in the 50th percentile; after this age, %BF decreased in boys but rose progressively up to 18 years in girls [84]. Comparing %BF between sexes at age 18, girls had 60% more %BF than boys. A similar pattern of %BF accrual was observed in a recent study in Southern Brazilians; although a cross-sectional design was used to acquire data, girls in the 50th percentile had higher %BF with advancing ages. It is interesting to note that the 50th percentile had a flat shape in boys, but the 97th showed a lower FM (kg) from 13 to 16 years, which was again higher with older ages [85]. In summary, although these studies have assessed body composition in children and adolescents of distinct ethnic origins, adiposity accrual appears to follow a similar pattern across ethnicities. With the onset of puberty, adiposity levels decrease in boys along with concurrent FFM increases, while adiposity increases in girls.

Similar to whole-body adiposity accrual, the pattern of adiposity distribution is also sex dependent. For instance, Taylor et al. compared FM in the trunk, waist, and hip lines (measured by DXA) between males and females at different pubertal stages [86]. Sex differences in trunk fat appeared at late puberty (Tanner stages 4–5), with boys having 17% greater trunk fat than girls ($p < 0.001$). Regarding FM at the waistline (i.e., android fat), sexual dimorphisms were observed at all puberty stages (boys having greater fat than girls); on the other hand, girls had greater amount of fat at the hip (i.e., gynoid fat) than boys [86]. Using MRI, a more accurate technique, Shen et al. compared SAT and VAT between sexes; results from regression analysis showed sexual dimorphism in SAT also after entering puberty, with girls having a larger SAT volume than boys [87]. Differences in VAT between sexes were not significant during adolescence but became clearer with advancing age. An ecological explanation for this sexual dimorphism is that with puberty, females need to store energy in SAT for the subsequent period of pregnancy and lactation [88]. We refer the readers to Chang et al. [89] for a recent review on potential factors explaining the sex differences in AT development, expansion, and metabolism.

It is also noteworthy that adolescent pregnancy may affect the patterns of adiposity expansion to support fetal development as well as to prepare the mother for the lactation period [90]. However, there is limited data on maternal body composition during gestation in adolescents or adults due to the changes in uterine contents and total body water that affect the technique's underlying assumptions [90]. In adults, gains in whole-body FM occur throughout pregnancy, as assessed by four-compartment models [91,92], and ADP and quantitative magnetic resonance [93]. Furthermore, pregnant women experience marked increases in thigh and suprailiac skinfolds (which are surrogate measures of subcutaneous AT) during the first six months of gestation but mobilization of these adiposity depots in the last 10–12 weeks of pregnancy to enhance fetal growth [94]. To our knowledge, only one study has compared skinfold thickness between pregnant adolescents and adults across gestation [95]. During the first 28 weeks of gestation, growing adolescents showed small increases in triceps and subscapular skinfolds compared to those adolescents who had already attained peak growth and adults, but no differences between groups were found for skinfold thickness at 28 weeks. Even though this study did not assess lower body adiposity, the authors further showed that growing adolescents continue to deposit adiposity in the trunk and arm after week 28 up to postpartum, whereas mature adolescents and adults experienced decreases in these adiposity depots [95].

2.3.1. Hormonal Influences on Adipose Tissue Expansion among Boys and Girls

Hormonal differences between boys and girls also explain the characteristic sexual dimorphism of whole-body adiposity and its distribution patterns at puberty [96]. The levels of estrogen, a hormone responsible for suppressing appetite and increasing energy expenditure, are higher in females [96]. Besides regulating energy metabolism, estrogen also increases sympathetic tone and downregulates androgen receptors expression in SAT, favoring lipid accumulation in this fat depot in females [97]. It is noteworthy that girls with obesity enter puberty at younger ages than girls with normal weight [98]. The adipokines leptin and adiponectin may play a role in the inverse association between menarche onset and weight status by modulating the hypothalamic–pituitary–gonadal axis [99]. Briefly, leptin activates the hypothalamus through secretion of the hormone kisspeptin to secrete gonadotropin releasing hormone. This hormone then activates the pituitary gland to produce follicle stimulating hormone and luteinizing hormone, resulting in the secretion of estrogen by the ovaries and, consequently, menarche onset. On the other hand, adiponectin inhibits the secretion of gonadotropin releasing hormone and delays puberty onset [99].

2.3.2. Dietary Intake and Interactions with Gut Microbiome

Studies have also investigated the implications of dietary patterns on AT expansion during childhood and adolescence. After following 325 children for four years (age period from 3.8 to 7.8 years old), Wosje et al. observed an association between higher fried-food intake and higher FM (using DXA) after adjusting for several biological and lifestyle covariates [100]. Furthermore, a positive association between glycemic load at 9.6 years old and %BF (by DXA) at 11.7 years old was reported in children at risk of obesity (parents with obesity) [101]. Prospective studies evaluating the associations between diet quality at baseline and FM (by DXA) at follow-up revealed mixed findings. Lower diet quality indices in mid-childhood (8 to 10 years) [102] were associated with greater FM at follow-up (at 10 to 12 years old, respectively). Contrary to these results, Nguyen et al. reported that positive associations between diet quality and BMI were explained by greater FFM index and not %BF or FMI [103]. The different approaches used to calculate the diet quality index may partially justify the heterogeneous findings.

Appetite and eating behaviors have been shown to influence the development of childhood obesity, as regulation of food intake contributes to energy homeostasis. According to Boswell et al., appetite is related to physiological (homeostatic) and psycho-social needs (hedonic), and eating behaviors are the actions during eating events [104]. In the absence of physiological energy needs, consumption of palatable food characterizes the hedonic eating and triggers the release of dopamine in the nucleus accumbens, leading to overeating and consequent obesity [105]. Thus, hedonic eating is driven by the reward of food consumption and not by metabolic need. Eating behaviors are influenced by many factors, including mothers' eating behaviors [106], stress [107], attention-deficit/hyperactivity disorder [108], and eating disorders (e.g., binge eating and lack of control over eating) [109].

Expansion of AT can also occur during childhood and adolescence as a result of the interactions between dietary components, gut microbiome, and immune cells [110]. A diet low in fermentable fibers is particularly associated with suboptimal production of short-chain fatty acids by the gut microbiome, limiting the beneficial secretion of anorexigenic hormones, anti-inflammatory cytokines, and mucin on the protective intestinal mucus layer [111–113]. Furthermore, a high-fat diet has been shown to promote metabolic endotoxemia, which can lead to increases in AT, inflammation as well as diabetes [114]. Regarding microbiome composition, children with obesity presented with a lower abundance of the beneficial bacteria *Akkermansia muciniphila* [115] (known to promote barrier integrity) and enriched *Bacteroides eggerthii* [116] and *Bacteroides fragilis* [117] (positively associated with adiposity and inflammation). Moreover, negative associations between adiposity indices and the abundance of *A. muciniphila* have been consistently reported in the pediatric population and in animal studies [118,119]. Indeed, an elegant study by Everard et al. demonstrated that treatment with isolated and viable *A. muciniphila* restored the intestinal mucus layer, reduced inflammation, and decreased the ratio of FM/lean mass in mice with diet-induced obesity; one of the proposed mechanisms was through increases in circulating endocannabinoids [119].

2.3.3. Physical Activity

Children with obesity generally report lower moderate-to-vigorous physical activity (MVPA) [120] and greater time spent in sedentary behaviors [121], which have been associated with greater adiposity measures [122]. As several randomized controlled trials (RCTs) investigating the effects of exercise on

%BF, FM, or AT in healthy children across weight status have been published to date, pooled analyses of their findings were made possible through meta-analyses [123–125]. For example, García-Hermoso et al. reported an effect of a supervised exercise intervention on reducing body fat in children with either healthy weight or overweight/obese, independent of mode and intensity [123]. It is noteworthy, however, that most of the included studies have combined exercise with additional interventions (i.e., dietary counseling and environmental changes), concealing the direct effect of exercise on adiposity measures. Another recent meta-analysis including RCTs of exercise-only interventions with a duration ≥4 weeks in children with overweight or obesity compared the effects of exercise mode on FM and %BF [124]. Pooled data analysis revealed that combining aerobic and strength exercises resulted in the greatest reductions of adiposity measures, although aerobic exercise alone also reduced adiposity compared to control arms. Moreover, supervised exercise alone was shown to promote reductions in both VAT and SAT in children with overweight or obesity [125].

Even though the meta-analyses discussed above reported positive effects of exercise on adiposity measures, some studies did not observe changes in this body compartment after exercise interventions [126,127]. For instance, a 12-week high-intensity interval training combined with dietary counseling did not result in changes in FM or %BF (by DXA) and abdominal VAT and SAT (by MRI) as observed in children with obesity aged 7 to 16 years old [126]. As one of the proposed pathways for lipolysis is through the release of growth hormone, the authors suggested that the reduced growth hormone levels and catecholamine responses to acute exercise can be associated with a disadvantage in reduction of adiposity in children with obesity [126]. Another explanation for the lack of positive exercise effects on adiposity resides in the constrained model of energy expenditure proposed by Pontzer [128]. According to the author, the human body compensates for the increases in energy expenditure through exercise by reducing the energy expended in non-physical-activity metabolic activity; therefore, a negative energy balance that results in adiposity changes is unlikely to occur. More recent studies in the adult population have shown that increases in dietary intake accompanied by exercise initiation is a mechanism often observed that contributes to compensation [129,130]. In adolescents with obesity, energy intake ad libitum was greater at the end of long-term exercise programs (≥12 weeks) compared to baseline, with compensation being a characteristic of restrained eaters [131,132]. Additionally, the timing of exercise in relation to meal also appears to influence prospective food consumption in adolescents with obesity; although no significant differences were found in ad libitum total energy intake after 60 or 180 min from an exercise session (30 min), exercising closer to lunch time (60 min) led to a reduction of 170 kcal in energy intake [133].

Studies investigating the effects of school- and community-based programs, with a physical activity component, on childhood obesity prevention have been conducted worldwide. To summarize previous research, a systematic review evaluated adiposity-related outcomes from interventions of different designs and found that most of the school-based programs that were RCTs showed improvements on these outcomes [134]. However, community-based programs have yielded mixed findings [134]. After reporting null results on anthropometric indices of adiposity from a two-school-year, community-based healthy lifestyle program conducted in four Spanish cities (children aged 8–10 years), Gómez et al. discussed the limitations that could have contributed to the findings [135]. According to the authors, the young age of participants, length of follow-up, intervention components, and inability to change the environment and current policies were determinant factors that should be addressed in future investigations [135].

3. Associations between Adipose Tissue in Childhood and Adulthood

There is evidence that the amount of adiposity at birth and during the first year of life determines its levels in childhood, albeit only a few studies have investigated longitudinal adiposity changes using body composition methods [14–17]. As an example, Admassu et al. explored the associations between FM (assessed by ADP) at term birth and at 4 years of age in healthy Ethiopians [17]. For every increase of 1 kg in FM at birth, there was a 1.17 kg/m^2 rise in FMI at 4 years old. In addition, FM accrual in the first four months was positively associated with FMI at 4 years ($\beta = 0.30$; 95% CI $= 0.12, 0.47$), after controlling for several sociodemographic and parental covariates [17]. Regarding the tracking of adiposity from childhood to adulthood, a 20-year longitudinal follow-up study showed that whole-body and trunk FM z-scores (by DXA) early in life (entry age 8–15 years) were predictors of these body compartments by the age of 28 years [136].

Studies examining AT samples obtained from biopsies have been conducted to elucidate adipocyte development and expansion during infancy, childhood, and adulthood [137,138]. In a cross-sectional study, infants showed increases in cell size to an adult level from ages 6 months to one year, with reductions between one and two years [137]. Researchers were able to stratify the analysis by weight categories only after age of two year, and it was noted that cell size was greater in children with obesity compared to that in children without obesity. In children of normal weight, adult levels for adipocyte size were reached at 11 to 13 years old; however, cell size in children with obesity was similar to that of adults at age two. Regarding adipocyte cell number, increases were found throughout childhood and adolescence for children with obesity; but those children of normal weight had differences in cell number only after 10 years old [137]. Longitudinal analysis of AT samples confirms a similar pattern of adiposity accrual in cell size and number across infancy and childhood [137]. Furthermore, Spalding et al. compared results from a study in childhood and adolescence with data obtained in adults (aged 20 years and older) and observed no further increases in the number of adipocytes during adulthood [139]. Differences in adipocyte morphology and metabolism also exist across AT depots [9]. In this context, Tarabra et al. reported that adipocytes from omental AT samples were smaller but had a greater lipolytic activity than abdominal SAT in adolescent girls (16–22 years old) with severe obesity [140].

Although adults with obesity showed a greater amount of AT cells than those of normal weight, the number of cells remained similar to that observed at younger ages [21]. More recently, research using in vivo analysis has shown that adipocyte cells can undergo a process called de novo adipogeneses (i.e., adipocyte turnover) contributing to obesity onset [141]. Once adulthood is reached, there is also a pattern that is specific to weight status with regards to adipocyte turnover (death of adipocytes and generation of new cells). For example, although there seems to be no differences in the death rate of adipocytes across weight status, adults with obesity had 2.6 times the number of adipocytes generated per year than adults with normal weight [139].

These findings, however, should be interpreted with caution due to the technical limitations of AT biopsy and analysis, anatomic sampling location, and interindividual variability [9,142,143]. In fact, Laforest et al. compared the diameter of adipocytes from abdominal SAT of adult women using three distinct techniques (i.e., collagenase digestion, osmium tetroxide fixation, and histological analysis) and found different results between these approaches [143]. Using counting methods, previous studies have estimated the percentage of adipocytes in AT ranging from ~15% to ~93%, as reviewed by Lenz et al. [9]. Furthermore, it has been suggested that the lipid droplet may not be completely apparent in AT cross-sectional slices, which can limit the findings from counting methods [9,144]. Techniques considered of superior accuracy have been used in more recent research [9,142]. For instance, Glastonbury et al. demonstrated, through analysis of RNA-Seq-based gene expression profile, a median percentage of 62% adipocytes for lower-leg AT samples obtained by surgical incision (Genotype-Tissue Expression project) and 82% for abdominal AT samples by punch biopsies (Twins UK study) in adults [142]. Another study employed a combination of whole-tissue microarray and RNA-Seq-based gene expression profile to evaluate adipocyte content in different AT depots, and showed that SAT has the greatest proportion of adipocytes (74%) followed by omental AT (~66%) [9]. To move forward, standardization of biopsy techniques and biobanking of samples of larger cohorts with at least different biologic characteristics (age, sex, ethnicity, and weight status) are necessary.

In individuals with obesity, the expansion of AT also occurs with concomitant accumulation of AT macrophages (specifically, M1 macrophages) and consequent secretion of pro-inflammatory cytokines. To our knowledge, although longitudinal studies have not yet been conducted in humans to evaluate whether macrophage infiltration early in life determines adiposity inflammation in adulthood, there is some evidence that the unhealthy AT expansion takes place across the lifespan. For instance, TNF-α expression in macrophages was greater in cord blood samples from neonates born of mothers with obesity than that in those born of mother without obesity [145]. Furthermore, children with obesity had greater number of macrophages infiltrated in AT compared to that of their lean peers ($p < 0.001$); however, macrophage number was not correlated with serum levels of high-sensitivity c-reactive protein (hs-CRP) nor IL-6 and TNF-α (serum levels and AT expression) [138]. Among adolescents with obesity, those with higher proportions of VAT to total abdominal obesity had also greater AT macrophage infiltration and expression of genes related to the inflammasome containing leucine-rich containing family, pyrin domain containing 3 (*NLRP3*), which are responsible for mediating pro-inflammatory responses [146]. Moreover, the expression of AT macrophages in both SAT and VAT was positively associated with adiposity measures in adults [147,148]. It is noteworthy that the macrophage profile appears to be AT depot specific [9,149,150]. To our knowledge, only one study compared SAT and omental AT in adolescent girls with severe obesity; although the differences were not statistically significant, omental AT had a smaller infiltration of CD68+ cells than abdominal SAT ($p = 0.09$) [140]. Moreover, a greater infiltration of macrophages (CD8+ and CD4+ T cells) in epicardial and pericardial AT were found in samples from patients with coronary artery disease and congenital heart disease [9]. Given the pro-inflammatory profile of epicardial and pericardial AT, several studies have investigated their roles on chronic diseases, such as diabetes [151] and cardiovascular diseases [152].

Further cues concerning the etiology of obesity and its related metabolic comorbidities are available from studies investigating monozygotic twins discordant for body weight, in which the influences of intrauterine, genetic, biological (i.e., sex, age, and race/ethnicity), and environmental factors can be ruled out [153,154]. These studies have shown twin pairs clustering into groups of distinct metabolic profiles, despite the marked differences in whole-body adiposity within the pairs. Specifically, some twin pairs were metabolically healthy, whereas others had only the co-twin with obesity presenting with concurrent metabolic dysfunction (e.g., fatty liver, insulin resistance). Furthermore, biopsies of abdominal SAT revealed a unique metabolic signature in the co-twins with obesity and metabolically unhealthy, characterized by downregulation of mitochondrial oxidative pathways and upregulation of inflammatory pathways [153,154]. Larger adipocyte size was also observed in the co-twin with obesity compared to the leaner co-twin [153] and in those with metabolic dysfunction [154]. Thus, these findings suggest that factors other than genetics and early life programming of AT may determine obesity and related metabolic comorbidities at adulthood, but previous weight-discordant twin studies have not been powered to determine these factors.

4. Conclusions and Perspectives

This narrative review discussed the trajectories of AT development from the prenatal period up to adolescence and identified potential factors determining AT expansion (Figures 1 and 2). We identified that studies assessing developmental trajectories of this body compartment in early childhood (especially from ages 2 to 5 years) are extremely limited. Further research is needed to determine body composition techniques that, when used solely, are accurate and capable of depicting changes in adiposity across the lifespan. Indeed, with this gap in research filled, body composition reference data will be available in multiethnic populations with a varied weight status, contributing to a better understanding of the healthy and unhealthy trajectories of adiposity development. Future longitudinal studies should also evaluate the distribution of AT into distinct SAT and VAT depots throughout childhood and adolescence. Despite these limitations, our work supports the argument that the interval between pregnancy to childhood provides a unique window of opportunity for the prevention of obesity and related comorbidities. Once high levels of adiposity are set, the negative effects of adiposity become noticeable. Thus, these preventive strategies should focus on ensuring adequate maternal nutrition and reduced exposure to toxins for a healthy pregnancy as well as targeting feeding/eating practices and behaviors and gut microbiome composition in infancy and childhood.

Author Contributions: Conceptualization, C.E.O., C.M.P., and A.M.H.; literature search, C.E.O.; writing—original draft preparation, C.E.O.; writing—review and editing, C.E.O., E.C.-R., C.J.F., K.L.M., C.M.P., and A.M.H. All authors have read and agreed to the published version of the manuscript.

Funding: This work has been funded by the generous support of the Stollery Children's Hospital Foundation through the Women and Children's Health Research Institute (RES0040520). C.E.O. is supported by the Alberta Diabetes Institute and is a recipient of the 2018 Alberta SPOR Graduate Studentship in Patient-Oriented Research, which is jointly funded by Alberta Innovates and the Canadian Institutes of Health Research. C.M.P. is supported by a Canadian Institutes of Health Research New Investigator Salary Award, a Campus Alberta Innovates Program, and a Canadian Foundation for Innovation John R. Evans Leaders Fund (Project # 34115).

Conflicts of Interest: The authors declare no conflict of interest. A.M.H. has received grant funding from Rhythm pharmaceuticals and Levo therapeutics outside of the submitted work. The funders had no role in the design of the study; in the collection, analyses, or interpretation of data; in the writing of the manuscript; or in the decision to publish the results.

References

1. NCD Risk Factor Collaboration (NCD-RisC). Worldwide trends in body-mass index, underweight, overweight, and obesity from 1975 to 2016: A pooled analysis of 2416 population-based measurement studies in 128·9 million children, adolescents, and adults. *Lancet* **2017**, *390*, 2627–2642. [CrossRef]

2. Kumar, S.; Kelly, A.S. Review of childhood obesity: From epidemiology, etiology, and comorbidities to clinical assessment and treatment. *Mayo Clin. Proc.* **2017**, *92*, 251–265. [CrossRef] [PubMed]

3. Heinonen, S.; Jokinen, R.; Rissanen, A.; Pietiläinen, K.H. White adipose tissue mitochondrial metabolism in health and in obesity. *Obes. Rev.* **2019**, *21*, 1–23. [CrossRef] [PubMed]

4. Min, S.Y.; Desai, A.; Yang, Z.; Sharma, A.; DeSouza, T.; Genga, R.M.; Kucukural, A.; Lifshitz, L.M.; Nielsen, S.; Scheele, C.; et al. Diverse repertoire of human adipocyte subtypes develops from transcriptionally distinct mesenchymal progenitor cells. *Proc. Natl. Acad. Sci. USA* **2019**, *116*, 17970–17979. [CrossRef]

5. Virtanen, K.A.; Lidell, M.E.; Orava, J.; Heglind, M.; Westergren, R.; Niemi, T.; Taittonen, M.; Laine, J.; Savisto, N.J.; Enerbäck, S.; et al. Functional brown adipose tissue in healthy adults. *N. Engl. J. Med.* **2009**, *360*, 1518–1525. [CrossRef]

6. Kindler, J.M.; Lobene, A.J.; Vogel, K.A.; Martin, B.R.; McCabe, L.D.; Peacock, M.; Warden, S.J.; McCabe, G.P.; Weaver, C.M. Adiposity, insulin resistance, and bone mass in children and adolescents. *J. Clin. Endocrinol. Metab.* **2018**, *104*, 892–899. [CrossRef]

7. Lee, S.J.; Arslanian, S.A. Cardiorespiratory fitness and abdominal adiposity in youth. *Eur. J. Clin. Nutr.* **2007**, *61*, 561–565. [CrossRef]

8. Schvey, N.A.; Marwitz, S.E.; Mi, S.J.; Galescu, O.A.; Broadney, M.M.; Young-Hyman, D.; Brady, S.M.; Reynolds, J.C.; Tanofsky-Kraff, M.; Yanovski, S.Z.; et al. Weight-based teasing is associated with gain in BMI and fat mass among children and adolescents at-risk for obesity: A longitudinal study. *Pediatr. Obes.* **2019**, *14*, 1–14. [CrossRef]

9. Lenz, M.; Arts, I.C.; Peeters, R.L.; de Kok, T.M.; Ertaylan, G. Adipose tissue in health and disease through the lens of its building blocks. *Sci. Rep.* **2020**, *10*, 1–4. [CrossRef]

10. Cleal, L.; Aldea, T.; Chau, Y.Y. Fifty shades of white: Understanding heterogeneity in white adipose stem cells. *Adipocyte* **2017**, *6*, 205–216. [CrossRef]

11. Haylett, W.L.; Ferris, W.F. Adipocyte–progenitor cell communication that influences adipogenesis. *Cell Mol. Life Sci.* **2020**, *77*, 115–128. [CrossRef]

12. Laharrague, P.; Casteilla, L. The emergence of adipocytes. In *Adipose Tissue Development: From Animal Models to Clinical Conditions*; Levy-Marchal, C., Pénicaud, L., Eds.; Karger Medical and Scientific Publishers: Basel, Switzerland, 2010; Volume 19, pp. 21–30.

13. Hao, G.; Wang, X.; Treiber, F.A.; Harshfield, G.; Kapuku, G.; Su, S. Body mass index trajectories in childhood is predictive of cardiovascular risk: Results from the 23-year longitudinal Georgia Stress and Heart study. *Int. J. Obes.* **2018**, *42*, 923–925. [CrossRef] [PubMed]

14. Koontz, M.B.; Gunzler, D.D.; Presley, L.; Catalano, P.M. Longitudinal changes in infant body composition: Association with childhood obesity. *Pediatr. Obes.* **2014**, *9*, e141–e144. [CrossRef] [PubMed]

15. Ong, K.K.; Emmett, P.; Northstone, K.; Golding, J.; Rogers, I.; Ness, A.R.; Wells, J.C.; Dunger, D.B. Infancy weight gain predicts childhood body fat and age at menarche in girls. *J. Clin. Endocrinol. Metab.* **2009**, *94*, 1527–1532. [CrossRef] [PubMed]

16. Chomtho, S.; Wells, J.C.; Williams, J.E.; Davies, P.S.; Lucas, A.; Fewtrell, M.S. Infant growth and later body composition: Evidence from the 4-component model. *Am. J. Clin. Nutr.* **2008**, *87*, 1776–1784. [CrossRef] [PubMed]

17. Admassu, B.; Ritz, C.; Wells, J.C.; Girma, T.; Andersen, G.S.; Belachew, T.; Owino, V.; Michaelsen, K.F.; Abera, M.; Wibaek, R.; et al. Accretion of fat-free mass rather than fat mass in infancy is positively associated with linear growth in childhood. *J. Nutr.* **2018**, *148*, 607–615. [CrossRef] [PubMed]

18. Shen, W.; St-Onge, M.; Wang, Z.; Heymsfield, S. Study of body composition: An overview. In *Human Body Composition*, 2nd ed.; Heymsfield, S., Lohman, T., Wang, Z., Going, S., Eds.; Human Kinetics: Champaign, IL, USA, 2005; pp. 3–14.

19. Lee, M.J.; Wu, Y.; Fried, S.K. Adipose tissue heterogeneity: Implication of depot differences in adipose tissue for obesity complications. *Mol. Aspects Med.* **2013**, *34*, 1–11. [CrossRef]

20. Jung, S.M.; Sanchez-Gurmaches, J.; Guertin, D.A. Brown adipose tissue development and metabolism. In *Brown Adipose Tissue*; Springer: Cham, Switzerland, 2018; pp. 3–36.

21. Lecoutre, S.; Petrus, P.; Rydén, M.; Breton, C. Transgenerational epigenetic mechanisms in adipose tissue development. *Trends Endocrinol. Metab.* **2018**, *29*, 675–685. [CrossRef]

22. Sun, K.; Kusminski, C.M.; Scherer, P.E. Adipose tissue remodeling and obesity. *J. Clin. Investig.* **2011**, *121*, 2094–2101. [CrossRef]

23. Fomon, S.J.; Haschke, F.; Ziegler, E.E.; Nelson, S.E. Body composition of reference children from birth to age 10 years. *Am. J. Clin. Nutr.* **1982**, *35*, 1169–1175. [CrossRef]

24. Ellis, K.J. Human body composition: In vivo methods. *Physiol. Rev.* **2000**, *80*, 649–680. [CrossRef] [PubMed]

25. Sethi, J.K.; Vidal-Puig, A.J. Thematic review series: Adipocyte biology. Adipose tissue function and plasticity orchestrate nutritional adaptation. *J. Lipid Res.* **2007**, *48*, 1253–1262. [PubMed]

26. Nouws, J.; Fitch, M.; Mata, M.; Santoro, N.; Galuppo, B.; Kursawe, R.; Narayan, D.; Vash-Margita, A.; Pierpont, B.; Shulman, G.I.; et al. Altered in vivo lipid fluxes and cell dynamics in subcutaneous adipose tissues are associated with the unfavorable pattern of fat distribution in obese adolescent girls. *Diabetes* **2019**, *68*, 1168–1177. [CrossRef] [PubMed]

27. Poissonnet, C.M.; Burdi, A.R.; Bookstein, F.L. Growth and development of human adipose tissue during early gestation. *Early Hum. Dev.* **1983**, *8*, 1–11. [CrossRef]

28. Billon, N.; Monteiro, M.C.; Dani, C. Developmental origin of adipocytes: New insights into a pending question. *Biol. Cell* **2008**, *100*, 563–575. [CrossRef]

29. Ziegler, E.E.; O'donnell, A.M.; Nelson, S.E.; Fomon, S.J. Body composition of the reference fetus. *Growth* **1976**, *40*, 329–341.

30. Toro-Ramos, T.; Paley, C.; Pi-Sunyer, F.X.; Gallagher, D. Body composition during fetal development and infancy through the age of 5 years. *Eur. J. Clin. Nutr.* **2015**, *69*, 1279–1289. [CrossRef]

31. Berger-Kulemann, V.; Brugger, P.C.; Reisegger, M.; Klein, K.; Hachemian, N.; Koelblinger, C.; Weber, M.; Prayer, D. Quantification of the subcutaneous fat layer with MRI in fetuses of healthy mothers with no underlying metabolic disease vs. fetuses of diabetic and obese mothers. *J. Perinat. Med.* **2012**, *40*, 179–184.

32. Kwon, E.J.; Kim, Y.J. What is fetal programming?: A lifetime health is under the control of in utero health. *Obs. Gynecol. Sci.* **2017**, *60*, 506–519. [CrossRef]

33. Harding, J.; Johnston, B. Nutrition and fetal growth. *Reprod. Fertil. Dev.* **1995**, *7*, 539–547. [CrossRef]

34. Dalrymple, K.V.; Thompson, J.M.; Begum, S.; Godfrey, K.M.; Poston, L.; Seed, P.T.; McCowan, L.M.; Wall, C.; Shelling, A.; North, R.; et al. Relationships of maternal body mass index and plasma biomarkers with childhood body mass index and adiposity at 6 years: The Children of SCOPE study. *Pediatr. Obes.* **2019**, *14*, 1–12. [CrossRef] [PubMed]

35. Jarvie, E.M.; Stewart, F.M.; Ramsay, J.E.; Brown, E.A.; Meyer, B.J.; Olivecrona, G.; Griffin, B.A.; Freeman, D.J. Maternal adipose tissue expansion, a missing link in the prediction of birth weight centile. *J. Clin. Endocrinol. Metab.* **2020**, *105*, e814–e825. [CrossRef] [PubMed]

36. Tahir, M.J.; Haapala, J.L.; Foster, L.P.; Duncan, K.M.; Teague, A.M.; Kharbanda, E.O.; McGovern, P.M.; Whitaker, K.M.; Rasmussen, K.M.; Fields, D.A.; et al. Higher maternal diet quality during pregnancy and lactation is associated with lower infant weight-for-length, body fat percent, and fat mass in early postnatal life. *Nutrients* **2019**, *11*, 632. [CrossRef] [PubMed]

37. Shrestha, N.; Sleep, S.L.; Cuffe, J.S.; Holland, O.J.; Perkins, A.V.; Yau, S.Y.; McAinch, A.J.; Hryciw, D.H. Role of omega-6 and omega-3 fatty acids in fetal programming. *Clin. Exp. Pharmacol. Physiol.* **2020**, *47*, 907–915. [CrossRef]

38. Vahdaninia, M.; Mackenzie, H.; Dean, T.; Helps, S. The effectiveness of ω-3 polyunsaturated fatty acid interventions during pregnancy on obesity measures in the offspring: An up-to-date systematic review and meta-analysis. *Eur. J. Nutr.* **2019**, *58*, 2597–2613. [CrossRef]

39. Lowe, W.L., Jr.; Lowe, L.P.; Kuang, A.; Catalano, P.M.; Nodzenski, M.; Talbot, O.; Tam, W.H.; Sacks, D.A.; McCance, D.; Linder, B.; et al. Maternal glucose levels during pregnancy and childhood adiposity in the Hyperglycemia and Adverse Pregnancy Outcome Follow-up Study. *Diabetologia* **2019**, *62*, 598–610. [CrossRef]

40. Hockett, C.W.; Harrall, K.K.; Moore, B.F.; Starling, A.P.; Bellatorre, A.; Sauder, K.A.; Perng, W.; Scherzinger, A.; Garg, K.; Ringham, B.M.; et al. Persistent effects of in utero overnutrition on offspring adiposity: The Exploring Perinatal Outcomes among Children (EPOCH) study. *Diabetologia* **2019**, *62*, 2017–2024. [CrossRef]

41. Wang, J.; Pan, L.; Liu, E.; Liu, H.; Liu, J.; Wang, S.; Guo, J.; Li, N.; Zhang, C.; Hu, G. Gestational diabetes and offspring's growth from birth to 6 years old. *Int. J. Obes.* **2019**, *43*, 663–672. [CrossRef]

42. Hoepner, L.A. Bisphenol A: A narrative review of prenatal exposure effects on adipogenesis and childhood obesity via peroxisome proliferator-activated receptor gamma. *Environ. Res.* **2019**, *173*, 54–68. [CrossRef]

43. Shafei, A.E.; Nabih, E.S.; Shehata, K.A.; Abd Elfatah, E.S.; Sanad, A.B.; Marey, M.Y.; Hammouda, A.A.; Mohammed, M.M.; Mostafa, R.; Ali, M.A. Prenatal exposure to endocrine disruptors and reprogramming of adipogenesis: An early-life risk factor for childhood obesity. *Child. Obes.* **2018**, *14*, 18–25. [CrossRef]

44. Moore, B.F.; Starling, A.P.; Magzamen, S.; Harrod, C.S.; Allshouse, W.B.; Adgate, J.L.; Ringham, B.M.; Glueck, D.H.; Dabelea, D. Fetal exposure to maternal active and secondhand smoking with offspring early-life growth in the Healthy Start study. *Int. J. Obes.* **2019**, *43*, 652–662. [CrossRef] [PubMed]

45. Starling, A.P.; Moore, B.F.; Thomas, D.S.K.; Peel, J.L.; Zhang, W.; Adgate, J.L.; Magzamen, S.; Martenies, S.E.; Allshouse, W.B.; Dabelea, D. Prenatal exposure to traffic and ambient air pollution and infant weight and adiposity: The Healthy Start study. *Environ. Res.* **2020**, *8*, 109130. [CrossRef] [PubMed]

46. Pigeyre, M.; Yazdi, F.T.; Kaur, Y.; Meyre, D. Recent progress in genetics, epigenetics and metagenomics unveils the pathophysiology of human obesity. *Clin. Sci.* **2016**, *130*, 943–986. [CrossRef] [PubMed]

47. Pigeyere, M.; Meyre, D. Monogenic obesity. In *Pediatric Obesity: Etiology, Pathogenesis and Treatment*, 2nd ed.; Freemark, M.S., Ed.; Springer International Publishing: New York, NY, USA, 2018; pp. 135–152.

48. Irizarry, K.A.; Haqq, A.M. Syndromic obesity. In *Pediatric Obesity: Etiology, Pathogenesis and Treatment*, 2nd ed.; Freemark, M.S., Ed.; Springer International Publishing: New York, NY, USA, 2018; pp. 153–182.

49. Marenne, G.; Hendricks, A.E.; Perdikari, A.; Bounds, R.; Payne, F.; Keogh, J.M.; Lelliott, C.J.; Henning, E.; Pathan, S.; Ashford, S.; et al. Exome sequencing identifies genes and gene sets contributing to severe childhood obesity, linking PHIP variants to repressed POMC transcription. *Cell Metab.* **2020**, *31*, 1107–1119. [CrossRef]

50. Hinney, A.; Giuranna, J. Polygenic obesity. In *Pediatric Obesity: Etiology, Pathogenesis and Treatment*, 2nd ed.; Freemark, M.S., Ed.; Springer International Publishing: New York, NY, USA, 2018; pp. 183–204.

51. Moulton, C.R. Age and chemical development in mammals. *J. Biol. Chem.* **1923**, *57*, 79–97.

52. Griffin, I.J.; Cooke, R.J. Development of whole body adiposity in preterm infants. *Early Hum. Dev.* **2012**, *88*, S19–S24. [CrossRef]

53. Roggero, P.; Giannì, M.L.; Amato, O.; Orsi, A.; Piemontese, P.; Morlacchi, L.; Mosca, F. Is term newborn body composition being achieved postnatally in preterm infants? *Early Hum. Dev.* **2009**, *85*, 349–352. [CrossRef]

54. Ramel, S.E.; Gray, H.L.; Ode, K.L.; Younge, N.; Georgieff, M.K.; Demerath, E.W. Body composition changes in preterm infants following hospital discharge: Comparison with term infants. *J. Pediatr. Gastroenterol. Nutr.* **2011**, *53*, 333–338. [CrossRef]

55. Sebastiani, G.; García-Beltran, C.; Pie, S.; Guerra, A.; López-Bermejo, A.; de Toledo, J.S.; de Zegher, F.; Rosés, F.; Ibáñez, L. The sequence of prenatal growth restraint and postnatal catch-up growth: Normal heart but thicker intima-media and more pre-peritoneal fat in late infancy. *Pediatr. Obes.* **2019**, *14*, e12476. [CrossRef]

56. De Zegher, F.; Díaz, M.; Sebastiani, G.; Martín-Ancel, A.; Sánchez-Infantes, D.; López-Bermejo, A.; Ibáñez, L. Abundance of circulating preadipocyte factor 1 in early life. *Diabetes Care* **2012**, *35*, 848–849. [CrossRef]

57. Wang, Y.; Kim, K.A.; Kim, J.H.; Sul, H.S. Pref-1, a preadipocyte secreted factor that inhibits adipogenesis. *J. Nutr.* **2006**, *136*, 2953–2956. [CrossRef] [PubMed]

58. Vogelezang, S.; Santos, S.; Toemen, L.; Oei, E.H.; Felix, J.F.; Jaddoe, V.W. Associations of fetal and infant weight change with general, visceral, and organ adiposity at school age. *JAMA Netw. Open* **2019**, *2*, e192843. [CrossRef] [PubMed]

59. Parra-Vargas, M.; Ramon-Krauel, M.; Lerin, C.; Jimenez-Chillaron, J.C. Size does matter: Litter size strongly determines adult metabolism in rodents. *Cell Metab.* **2020**, *32*, 334–340. [CrossRef] [PubMed]

60. Victora, C.G.; Bahl, R.; Barros, A.J.; França, G.V.; Horton, S.; Krasevec, J.; Murch, S.; Sankar, M.J.; Walker, N.; Rollins, N.C. The Lancet Breastfeeding Series Group. Breastfeeding in the 21st century: Epidemiology, mechanisms, and lifelong effect. *Lancet* **2016**, *387*, 475–490. [CrossRef]

61. Rollins, N.C.; Bhandari, N.; Hajeebhoy, N.; Horton, S.; Lutter, C.K.; Martines, J.C.; Piwoz, E.G.; Richter, L.M.; Victora, C.G. The Lancet Breastfeeding Series Group. Why invest, and what it will take to improve breastfeeding practices? *Lancet* **2016**, *387*, 491–504. [CrossRef]

62. Breij, L.M.; Abrahamse-Berkeveld, M.; Acton, D.; Rolfe, E.D.; Ong, K.K.; Hokken-Koelega, A.C. Impact of early infant growth, duration of breastfeeding and maternal factors on total body fat mass and visceral fat at 3 and 6 months of age. *Ann. Nutr. Metab.* **2017**, *71*, 203–210. [CrossRef]

63. Rodríguez-Cano, A.M.; Mier-Cabrera, J.; Allegre-Dávalos, A.L.; Muñoz-Manrique, C.; Perichart-Perera, O. Higher fat mass and fat mass accretion during the first six months of life in exclusively breastfed infants. *Pediatr. Res.* **2020**, *87*, 588–594. [CrossRef]

64. Bell, K.A.; Wagner, C.L.; Feldman, H.A.; Shypailo, R.J.; Belfort, M.B. Associations of infant feeding with trajectories of body composition and growth. *Am. J. Clin. Nutr.* **2017**, *106*, 491–498. [CrossRef]

65. De Zegher, F.; Sebastiani, G.; Diaz, M.; Gómez-Roig, M.D.; López-Bermejo, A.; Ibáñez, L. Breast-feeding vs formula-feeding for infants born small-for-gestational-age: Divergent effects on fat mass and on circulating IGF-I and high-molecular-weight adiponectin in late infancy. *J. Clin. Endocrinol. Metab.* **2013**, *98*, 1242–1247. [CrossRef]

66. Gridneva, Z.; Rea, A.; Tie, W.J.; Lai, C.T.; Kugananthan, S.; Ward, L.C.; Murray, K.; Hartmann, P.E.; Geddes, D.T. Carbohydrates in human milk and body composition of term infants during the first 12 months of lactation. *Nutrients* **2019**, *11*, 1472. [CrossRef]

67. Rudolph, M.C.; Young, B.E.; Lemas, D.J.; Palmer, C.E.; Hernandez, T.L.; Barbour, L.A.; Friedman, J.E.; Krebs, N.F.; MacLean, P.S. Early infant adipose deposition is positively associated with the n-6 to n-3 fatty acid ratio in human milk independent of maternal BMI. *Int. J. Obes.* **2017**, *41*, 510–517. [CrossRef] [PubMed]

68. Vaidya, H.; Cheema, S.K. Breastmilk with a high omega-6 to omega-3 fatty acid ratio induced cellular events similar to insulin resistance and obesity in 3T3-L1 adipocytes. *Pediatric. Obes.* **2018**, *13*, 285–291. [CrossRef] [PubMed]

69. Chan, D.; Goruk, S.; Becker, A.B.; Subbarao, P.; Mandhane, P.J.; Turvey, S.E.; Lefebvre, D.; Sears, M.R.; Field, C.J.; Azad, M.B. Adiponectin, leptin and insulin in breast milk: Associations with maternal characteristics and infant body composition in the first year of life. *Int. J. Obes. (Lond.)* **2018**, *42*, 36–43. [CrossRef] [PubMed]

70. Gingras, V.; Aris, I.M.; Rifas-Shiman, S.L.; Switkowski, K.M.; Oken, E.; Hivert, M.F. Timing of complementary feeding introduction and adiposity throughout childhood. *Pediatrics* **2019**, *144*, e20191320. [CrossRef] [PubMed]

71. Bäckhed, F.; Roswall, J.; Peng, Y.; Feng, Q.; Jia, H.; Kovatcheva-Datchary, P.; Li, Y.; Xia, Y.; Xie, H.; Zhong, H.; et al. Dynamics and stabilization of the human gut microbiome during the first year of life. *Cell Host Microbe* **2015**, *17*, 690–703. [CrossRef]

72. Mueller, N.T.; Whyatt, R.; Hoepner, L.; Oberfield, S.; Dominguez-Bello, M.G.; Widen, E.M.; Hassoun, A.; Perera, F.; Rundle, A. Prenatal exposure to antibiotics, cesarean section and risk of childhood obesity. *Int. J. Obes.* **2015**, *39*, 665–670. [CrossRef]

73. Tun, H.M.; Bridgman, S.L.; Chari, R.; Field, C.J.; Guttman, D.S.; Becker, A.B.; Mandhane, P.J.; Turvey, S.E.; Subbarao, P.; Sears, M.R.; et al. Roles of birth mode and infant gut microbiota in intergenerational transmission of overweight and obesity from mother to offspring. *JAMA Pediatr.* **2018**, *172*, 368–377. [CrossRef]

74. Miller, S.A.; Wu, R.K.S.; Oremus, M. The association between antibiotic use in infancy and childhood overweight or obesity: A systematic review and meta-analysis. *Obes. Rev.* **2018**, *19*, 1463–1475. [CrossRef]

75. Forbes, J.D.; Azad, M.B.; Vehling, L.; Tun, H.M.; Konya, T.B.; Guttman, D.S.; Field, C.J.; Lefebvre, D.; Sears, M.R.; Becker, A.B.; et al. Association of exposure to formula in the hospital and subsequent infant feeding practices with gut microbiota and risk of overweight in the first year of life. *JAMA Pediatr.* **2018**, *172*, e181161. [CrossRef]

76. Caesar, R.; Tremaroli, V.; Kovatcheva-Datchary, P.; Cani, P.D.; Bäckhed, F. Crosstalk between gut microbiota and dietary lipids aggravates WAT inflammation through TLR signaling. *Cell Metab.* **2015**, *22*, 658–668. [CrossRef]

77. Cho, I.; Yamanishi, S.; Cox, L.; Methe, B.A.; Zavadil, J.; Li, K.; Gao, Z.; Mahana, D.; Raju, K.; Teitler, I.; et al. Antibiotics in early life alter the murine colonic microbiome and adiposity. *Nature* **2012**, *488*, 621–626. [CrossRef] [PubMed]

78. Kincaid, H.J.; Nagpal, R.; Yadav, H. Microbiome-immune-metabolic axis in the epidemic of childhood obesity: Evidence and opportunities. *Obes. Rev.* **2020**, *21*, e12963. [CrossRef] [PubMed]

79. Soderborg, T.K.; Clark, S.E.; Mulligan, C.E.; Janssen, R.C.; Babcock, L.; Ir, D.; Young, B.; Krebs, N.; Lemas, D.J.; Johnson, L.K.; et al. The gut microbiota in infants of obese mothers increases inflammation and susceptibility to NAFLD. *Nat. Commun.* **2018**, *9*, 1–2. [CrossRef]

80. Gallagher, D.; Andres, A.; Fields, D.A.; Evans, W.J.; Kuczmarski, R.; Lowe, W.L., Jr.; Lumeng, J.C.; Oken, E.; Shepherd, J.A.; Sun, S.; et al. Body composition measurements from birth through 5 years: Challenges, gaps, and existing & emerging technologies-A National Institutes of Health workshop. *Obes. Rev.* **2020**, *21*, e13033. [PubMed]

81. Orsso, C.E.; Silva, M.I.; Gonzalez, M.C.; Rubin, D.A.; Heymsfield, S.B.; Prado, C.M.; Haqq, A.M. Assessment of body composition in pediatric overweight and obesity: A systematic review of the reliability and validity of common techniques. *Obes. Rev.* **2020**, *21*, e13041. [CrossRef] [PubMed]

82. Wells, J.C.; Davies, P.S.; Fewtrell, M.S.; Cole, T.J. Body composition reference charts for UK infants and children aged 6 weeks to 5 years based on measurement of total body water by isotope dilution. *Eur. J. Clin. Nutr.* **2020**, *74*, 141–148. [CrossRef]

83. McConnell-Nzunga, J.; Naylor, P.J.; Macdonald, H.M.; Rhodes, R.E.; Hofer, S.M.; McKay, H.A. Body fat accrual trajectories for a sample of Asian-Canadian and Caucasian-Canadian children and youth: A longitudinal DXA-based study. *Pediatr. Obes.* **2020**, *15*, e12570. [CrossRef]

84. McCarthy, H.D.; Cole, T.J.; Fry, T.; Jebb, S.A.; Prentice, A.M. Body fat reference curves for children. *Int. J. Obes.* **2006**, *30*, 598–602. [CrossRef]

85. Ripka, W.L.; Orsso, C.E.; Haqq, A.M.; Luz, T.G.; Prado, C.M.; Ulbricht, L. Lean mass reference curves in adolescents using dual-energy x-ray absorptiometry (DXA). *PLoS ONE* **2020**, *15*, e0228646. [CrossRef]

86. Taylor, R.W.; Grant, A.M.; Williams, S.M.; Goulding, A. Sex differences in regional body fat distribution from pre- to postpuberty. *Obesity* **2010**, *18*, 1410–1416. [CrossRef]

87. Shen, W.; Punyanitya, M.; Silva, A.M.; Chen, J.; Gallagher, D.; Sardinha, L.B.; Allison, D.B.; Heymsfield, S.B. Sexual dimorphism of adipose tissue distribution across the lifespan: A cross-sectional whole-body magnetic resonance imaging study. *Nutr. Metab. (Lond.)* **2009**, *6*, 1–9. [CrossRef] [PubMed]

88. Kaplan, H.S.; Lancaster, J.B. An evolutionary and ecological analysis of human fertility, mating patterns, and parental investment. In *Offspring: Human Fertility Behavior in Biodemographic Perspective Panel*; Wachter, K., Bulatao, R., Eds.; National Academy of Sciences: Washington, DC, USA, 2003; pp. 170–223.

89. Chang, E.; Varghese, M.; Singer, K. Gender and sex differences in adipose tissue. *Curr. Diabetes Rep.* **2018**, *18*, 69. [CrossRef]

90. Widen, E.M.; Gallagher, D. Body composition changes in pregnancy: Measurement, predictors and outcomes. *Eur. J. Clin. Nutr.* **2014**, *68*, 643–652. [CrossRef] [PubMed]

91. Kopp-Hoolihan, L.E.; Van Loan, M.D.; Wong, W.W.; King, J.C. Fat mass deposition during pregnancy using a four-component model. *J. Appl. Physiol.* **1999**, *87*, 196–202. [CrossRef] [PubMed]

92. Lederman, S.A.; Paxton, A.; Heymsfield, S.B.; Wang, J.; Thornton, J.; Pierson, R.N., Jr. Body fat and water changes during pregnancy in women with different body weight and weight gain. *Obstet. Gynecol.* **1997**, *90*, 483–488. [CrossRef]

93. Bosaeus, M.; Andersson-Hall, U.; Andersson, L.; Karlsson, T.; Ellegård, L.; Holmäng, A. Body composition during pregnancy: Longitudinal changes and method comparisons. *Reprod. Sci.* **2020**, *28*, 1–3. [CrossRef] [PubMed]

94. Lassek, W.D.; Gaulin, S.J. Changes in body fat distribution in relation to parity in American women: A covert form of maternal depletion. *Am. J. Phys. Anthropol.* **2006**, *131*, 295–302. [CrossRef]

95. Scholl, T.O.; Hediger, M.L.; Schall, J.I.; Khoo, C.S.; Fischer, R.L. Maternal growth during pregnancy and the competition for nutrients. *Am. J. Clin. Nutr.* **1994**, *60*, 183–188. [CrossRef]

96. Palmer, B.F.; Clegg, D.J. The sexual dimorphism of obesity. *Mol. Cell Endocrinol.* **2015**, *15*, 113–119. [CrossRef]

97. Brown, L.; Clegg, D. Central effects of estradiol in the regulation of adiposity. *J. Steroid Biochem. Mol. Biol.* **2010**, *122*, 65–73. [CrossRef]

98. Currie, C.; Ahluwalia, N.; Godeau, E.; Gabhainn, S.N.; Due, P.; Currie, D.B. Is obesity at individual and national level associated with lower age at menarche? Evidence from 34 countries in the health behaviour in school-aged children study. *J. Adolesc. Health* **2012**, *50*, 621–626. [CrossRef] [PubMed]

99. Nieuwenhuis, D.; Pujol-Gualdo, N.; Arnoldussen, I.A.; Kiliaan, A.J. Adipokines: A gear shift in puberty. *Obes. Rev.* **2020**, *21*, e13005. [CrossRef] [PubMed]

100. Wosje, K.S.; Khoury, P.R.; Claytor, R.P.; Copeland, K.A.; Hornung, R.W.; Daniels, S.R.; Kalkwarf, H.J. Dietary patterns associated with fat and bone mass in young children. *Am. J. Clin. Nutr.* **2010**, *92*, 294–303. [CrossRef] [PubMed]

101. Suissa, K.; Benedetti, A.; Henderson, M.; Gray-Donald, K.; Paradis, G. Effects of dietary glycemic index and load on children's cardiovascular risk factors. *Ann. Epidemiol.* **2019**, *40*, 1–7. [CrossRef] [PubMed]

102. Setayeshgar, S.; Maximova, K.; Ekwaru, J.P.; Gray-Donald, K.; Henderson, M.; Paradis, G.; Tremblay, A.; Veugelers, P. Diet quality as measured by the Diet Quality Index-International is associated with prospective changes in body fat among Canadian children. *Public Health Nutr.* **2017**, *20*, 456–463. [CrossRef]

103. Nguyen-Rodriguez, S.T.; Gallo, L.C.; Isasi, C.R.; Buxton, O.M.; Thomas, K.S.; Sotres-Alvarez, D.; Redline, S.; Castañeda, S.F.; Carnethon, M.R.; Daviglus, M.L.; et al. Adiposity, depression symptoms and inflammation in Hispanic/Latino youth: Results from HCHS/SOL youth. *Ann. Behav. Med.* **2020**, *54*, 529–534. [CrossRef]

104. Boswell, N.; Byrne, R.; Davies, P.S.W. Aetiology of eating behaviours: A possible mechanism to understand obesity development in early childhood. *Neurosci. Biobehav. Rev.* **2018**, *95*, 438–448. [CrossRef]

105. Appelhans, B.M. Neurobehavioral inhibition of reward-driven feeding: Implications for dieting and obesity. *Obesity* **2009**, *17*, 640–647. [CrossRef]

106. Campbell, K.J.; Crawford, D.A.; Salmon, J.; Carver, A.; Garnett, S.P.; Baur, L.A. Associations between the home food environment and obesity-promoting eating behaviors in adolescence. *Obesity* **2007**, *15*, 719–730. [CrossRef]

107. Hill, D.C.; Moss, R.H.; Sykes-Muskett, B.; Conner, M.; O'Connor, D.B. Stress and eating behaviors in children and adolescents: Systematic review and meta-analysis. *Appetite* **2018**, *123*, 14–22. [CrossRef]

108. Fuemmeler, B.F.; Sheng, Y.; Schechter, J.C.; Do, E.; Zucker, N.; Majors, A.; Maguire, R.; Murphy, S.K.; Hoyo, C.; Kollins, S.H. Associations between attention deficit hyperactivity disorder symptoms and eating behaviors in early childhood. *Pediatr. Obes.* **2020**, *15*, e12631. [CrossRef] [PubMed]

109. He, J.; Cai, Z.; Fan, X. Prevalence of binge and loss of control eating among children and adolescents with overweight and obesity: An exploratory meta-analysis. *Int. J. Eat. Disord.* **2017**, *50*, 91–103. [CrossRef] [PubMed]

110. Nicolucci, A.C.; Hume, M.P.; Martínez, I.; Mayengbam, S.; Walter, J.; Reimer, R.A. Prebiotics reduce body fat and alter intestinal microbiota in children who are overweight or with obesity. *Gastroenterology* **2017**, *153*, 711–722. [CrossRef] [PubMed]

111. Chambers, E.S.; Viardot, A.; Psichas, A.; Morrison, D.J.; Murphy, K.G.; Zac-Varghese, S.E.; MacDougall, K.; Preston, T.; Tedford, C.; Finlayson, G.S.; et al. Effects of targeted delivery of propionate to the human colon on appetite regulation, body weight maintenance and adiposity in overweight adults. *Gut* **2015**, *64*, 1744–1754. [CrossRef] [PubMed]

112. Larraufie, P.; Martin-Gallausiaux, C.; Lapaque, N.; Dore, J.; Gribble, F.M.; Reimann, F.; Blottiere, H.M. SCFAs strongly stimulate PYY production in human enteroendocrine cells. *Sci. Rep.* **2018**, *8*, 74. [CrossRef]

113. Willemsen, L.E.; Koetsier, M.A.; Van Deventer, S.J.; Van Tol, E.A. Short chain fatty acids stimulate epithelial mucin 2 expression through differential effects on prostaglandin E(1) and E(2) production by intestinal myofibroblasts. *Gut* **2003**, *52*, 1442–1447. [CrossRef]

114. Cani, P.D.; Amar, J.; Iglesias, M.A.; Poggi, M.; Knauf, C.; Bastelica, D.; Neyrinck, A.M.; Fava, F.; Tuohy, K.M.; Chabo, C.; et al. Metabolic endotoxemia initiates obesity and insulin resistance. *Diabetes* **2007**, *56*, 1232–1242. [CrossRef]

115. Borgo, F.; Verduci, E.; Riva, A.; Lassandro, C.; Riva, E.; Morace, G.; Borghi, E. Relative abundance in bacterial and fungal gut microbes in obese children: A case control study. *Child. Obes.* **2017**, *13*, 78–84. [CrossRef]

116. López-Contreras, B.E.; Morán-Ramos, S.; Villarruel-Vázquez, R.; Macías-Kauffer, L.; Villamil-Ramírez, H.; León-Mimila, P.; Vega-Badillo, J.; Sánchez-Muñoz, F.; Llanos-Moreno, L.E.; Canizalez-Román, A.; et al. Composition of gut microbiota in obese and normal-weight Mexican school-age children and its association with metabolic traits. *Pediatr. Obes.* **2018**, *13*, 381–388. [CrossRef]

117. Indiani, C.M.; Rizzardi, K.F.; Castelo, P.M.; Ferraz, L.F.; Darrieux, M.; Parisotto, T.M. Childhood obesity and Firmicutes/Bacteroidetes ratio in the gut microbiota: A systematic review. *Child. Obes.* **2018**, *14*, 501–509. [CrossRef]

118. Mbakwa, C.A.; Hermes, G.D.; Penders, J.; Savelkoul, P.H.; Thijs, C.; Dagnelie, P.C.; Mommers, M.; Zoetendal, E.G.; Smidt, H.; Arts, I.C. Gut microbiota and body weight in school-aged children: The KOALA birth cohort study. *Obesity* **2018**, *26*, 1767–1776. [CrossRef] [PubMed]

119. Everard, A.; Belzer, C.; Geurts, L.; Ouwerkerk, J.P.; Druart, C.; Bindels, L.B.; Guiot, Y.; Derrien, M.; Muccioli, G.G.; Delzenne, N.M.; et al. Cross-talk between Akkermansia muciniphila and intestinal epithelium controls diet-induced obesity. *Proc. Natl. Acad. Sci. USA* **2013**, *110*, 9066–9071. [CrossRef] [PubMed]

120. Adamo, K.B.; Colley, R.C.; Hadjiyannakis, S.; Goldfield, G.S. Physical activity and sedentary behavior in obese youth. *J. Pediatr.* **2015**, *166*, 1270–1275. [CrossRef]

121. Herman, K.M.; Sabiston, C.M.; Mathieu, M.E.; Tremblay, A.; Paradis, G. Sedentary behavior in a cohort of 8- to 10-year-old children at elevated risk of obesity. *Prev. Med. (Baltim)* **2014**, *60*, 115–120. [CrossRef] [PubMed]

122. Wiersma, R.; Haverkamp, B.F.; van Beek, J.H.; Riemersma, A.M.; Boezen, H.M.; Smidt, N.; Corpeleijn, E.; Hartman, E. Unravelling the association between accelerometer-derived physical activity and adiposity among preschool children: A systematic review and meta-analyses. *Obes. Rev.* **2020**, *21*, e12936. [CrossRef] [PubMed]

123. García-Hermoso, A.; Alonso-Martinez, A.M.; Ramírez-Vélez, R.; Izquierdo, M. Effects of exercise intervention on health-related physical fitness and blood pressure in preschool children: A systematic review and meta-analysis of randomized controlled trials. *Sports Med.* **2020**, *50*, 187–203. [CrossRef]

124. Kelley, G.A.; Kelley, K.S.; Pate, R.R. Exercise and adiposity in overweight and obese children and adolescents: A systematic review with network meta-analysis of randomised trials. *BMJ Open* **2019**, *9*. [CrossRef]

125. González-Ruiz, K.; Ramirez-Velez, R.; Correa-Bautista, J.E.; Peterson, M.D.; García-Hermoso, A. The effects of exercise on abdominal fat and liver enzymes in pediatric obesity: A systematic review and meta-analysis. *Child Obes.* **2017**, *13*, 272–282. [CrossRef]

126. Dias, K.A.; Ingul, C.B.; Tjønna, A.E.; Keating, S.E.; Gomersall, S.R.; Follestad, T.; Hosseini, M.S.; Hollekim-Strand, S.M.; Ro, T.B.; Haram, M.; et al. Effect of high-intensity interval training on fitness, fat mass and cardiometabolic biomarkers in children with obesity: A randomised controlled trial. *Sport Med.* **2018**, *48*, 733–746. [CrossRef]

127. Hay, J.; Wittmeier, K.; MacIntosh, A.; Wicklow, B.; Duhamel, T.; Sellers, E.; Dean, H.; Ready, E.; Berard, L.; Kriellaars, D.; et al. Physical activity intensity and type 2 diabetes risk in overweight youth: A randomized trial. *Int. J. Obes. (Lond.)* **2016**, *40*, 607–614. [CrossRef]

128. Pontzer, H. Constrained total energy expenditure and the evolutionary biology of energy balance. *Exerc. Sport Sci. Rev.* **2015**, *43*, 110–116. [CrossRef] [PubMed]

129. Martin, C.K.; Johnson, W.D.; Myers, C.A.; Apolzan, J.W.; Earnest, C.P.; Thomas, D.M.; Rood, J.C.; Johannsen, N.M.; Tudor-Locke, C.; Harris, M.; et al. Effect of different doses of supervised exercise on food intake, metabolism, and non-exercise physical activity: The E-MECHANIC randomized controlled trial. *Am. J. Clin. Nutr.* **2019**, *110*, 583–592. [CrossRef] [PubMed]

130. Riou, M.È.; Jomphe-Tremblay, S.; Lamothe, G.; Finlayson, G.S.; Blundell, J.E.; Décarie-Spain, L.; Gagnon, J.C.; Doucet, É. Energy compensation following a supervised exercise intervention in women living with overweight/obesity is accompanied by an early and sustained decrease in non-structured physical activity. *Front. Physiol.* **2019**, *10*, 1–12. [CrossRef] [PubMed]

131. Thivel, D.; Julian, V.; Miguet, M.; Pereira, B.; Beaulieu, K.; Finlayson, G.; Richard, R.; Duclos, M. Introducing eccentric cycling during a multidisciplinary weight loss intervention might prevent adolescents with obesity from increasing their food intake. The TEXTOO study. *Physiol. Behav.* **2020**, *214*, 112744. [CrossRef] [PubMed]

132. Miguet, M.; Fearnbach, N.S.; Metz, L.; Khammassi, M.; Julian, V.; Cardenoux, C.; Pereira, B.; Boirie, Y.; Duclos, M.; Thivel, D. Effect of HIIT versus MICT on body composition and energy intake in dietary restrained and unrestrained adolescents with obesity. *Appl. Physiol. Nutr. Metab.* **2020**, *45*, 437–445. [CrossRef]

133. Fillon, A.; Mathieu, M.E.; Masurier, J.; Roche, J.; Miguet, M.; Khammassi, M.; Finlayson, G.; Beaulieu, K.; Pereira, B.; Duclos, M.; et al. Effect of exercise-meal timing on energy intake, appetite and food reward in adolescents with obesity: The TIMEX study. *Appetite* **2020**, *146*, 104506. [CrossRef]

134. Bleich, S.N.; Vercammen, K.A.; Zatz, L.Y.; Frelier, J.M.; Ebbeling, C.B.; Peeters, A. Interventions to prevent global childhood overweight and obesity: A systematic review. *Lancet Diabetes Endocrinol.* **2018**, *6*, 332–346. [CrossRef]

135. Gómez, S.F.; Esteve, R.C.; Subirana, I.; Serra-Majem, L.; Torrent, M.F.; Homs, C.; Bawaked, R.A.; Estrada, L.; Fíto, M.; Schröder, H. Effect of a community-based childhood obesity intervention program on changes in anthropometric variables, incidence of obesity, and lifestyle choices in Spanish children aged 8 to 10 years. *Eur. J. Pediatr.* **2018**, *177*, 1531–1539. [CrossRef]

136. Barbour-Tuck, E.; Erlandson, M.; Muhajarine, N.; Foulds, H.; Baxter-Jones, A. Influence of childhood and adolescent fat development on fat mass accrual during emerging adulthood: A 20-year longitudinal study. *Obesity* **2018**, *26*, 613–620. [CrossRef]

137. Knittle, J.L.; Timmers, K.; Ginsberg-Fellner, F.; Brown, R.E.; Katz, D.P. The growth of adipose tissue in children and adolescents: Cross-sectional and longitudinal studies of adipose cell number and size. *J. Clin. Investig.* **1979**, *63*, 239–246. [CrossRef]

138. Landgraf, K.; Rockstroh, D.; Wagner, I.V.; Weise, S.; Tauscher, R.; Schwartze, J.T.; Löffler, D.; Bühligen, U.; Wojan, M.; Till, H.; et al. Evidence of early alterations in adipose tissue biology and function and its association with obesity-related inflammation and insulin resistance in children. *Diabetes* **2015**, *64*, 1249–1261. [CrossRef]

139. Spalding, K.L.; Arner, E.; Westermark, P.O.; Bernard, S.; Buchholz, B.A.; Bergmann, O.; Blomqvist, L.; Hoffstedt, J.; Näslund, E.; Britton, T.; et al. Dynamics of fat cell turnover in humans. *Nature* **2008**, *453*, 783–787. [CrossRef] [PubMed]

140. Tarabra, E.; Nouws, J.; Vash-Margita, A.; Nadzam, G.S.; Goldberg, R.; Van Name, M.; Pierpont, B.; Knight, J.R.; Shulman, G.I.; Caprio, S. The omentum of obese girls harbors small adipocytes and browning transcripts. *JCI Insight* **2020**, *5*, e135448. [CrossRef] [PubMed]

141. Jeffery, E.; Church, C.D.; Holtrup, B.; Colman, L.; Rodeheffer, M.S. Rapid depot-specific activation of adipocyte precursor cells at the onset of obesity. *Nat. Cell Biol.* **2015**, *17*, 376–385. [CrossRef] [PubMed]

142. Glastonbury, C.A.; Alves, A.C.; Moustafa, J.S.; Small, K.S. Cell-type heterogeneity in adipose tissue is associated with complex traits and reveals disease-relevant cell-specific eQTLs. *Am. J. Hum. Genet.* **2019**, *104*, 1013–1024. [CrossRef]

143. Laforest, S.; Michaud, A.; Paris, G.; Pelletier, M.; Vidal, H.; Géloën, A.; Tchernof, A. Comparative analysis of three human adipocyte size measurement methods and their relevance for cardiometabolic risk. *Obesity* **2017**, *25*, 122–131. [CrossRef]

144. Lenz, M.; Roumans, N.J.; Vink, R.G.; van Baak, M.A.; Mariman, E.C.; Arts, I.C.; de Kok, T.M.; Ertaylan, G. Estimating real cell size distribution from cross-section microscopy imaging. *Bioinformatics* **2016**, *32*, i396–i404. [CrossRef]

145. Cifuentes-Zúñiga, F.; Arroyo-Jousse, V.; Soto-Carrasco, G.; Casanello, P.; Uauy, R.; Krause, B.J.; Castro-Rodríguez, J.A. IL-10 expression in macrophages from neonates born from obese mothers is suppressed by IL-4 and LPS/INFγ. *J. Cell Physiol.* **2017**, *232*, 3693–3701. [CrossRef]

146. Kursawe, R.; Dixit, V.D.; Scherer, P.E.; Santoro, N.; Narayan, D.; Gordillo, R.; Giannini, C.; Lopez, X.; Pierpont, B.; Nouws, J.; et al. A role of the inflammasome in the low storage capacity of the abdominal subcutaneous adipose tissue in obese adolescents. *Diabetes* **2016**, *65*, 610–618. [CrossRef]

147. Michaud, A.; Drolet, R.; Noël, S.; Paris, G.; Tchernof, A. Visceral fat accumulation is an indicator of adipose tissue macrophage infiltration in women. *Metabolism* **2012**, *61*, 689–698. [CrossRef]

148. Klimcakova, E.; Roussel, B.; Kovacova, Z.; Kovacikova, M.; Siklova-Vitkova, M.; Combes, M.; Hejnova, J.; Decaunes, P.; Maoret, J.J.; Vedral, T.; et al. Macrophage gene expression is related to obesity and the metabolic syndrome in human subcutaneous fat as well as in visceral fat. *Diabetologia* **2011**, *54*, 876–887. [CrossRef] [PubMed]

149. Hardy, O.T.; Perugini, R.A.; Nicoloro, S.M.; Gallagher-Dorval, K.; Puri, V.; Straubhaar, J.; Czech, M.P. Body mass index-independent inflammation in omental adipose tissue associated with insulin resistance in morbid obesity. *Surg. Obes. Relat. Dis.* **2011**, *7*, 60–67. [CrossRef] [PubMed]

150. Girón-Ulloa, A.; González-Domínguez, E.; Klimek, R.S.; Patiño-Martínez, E.; Vargas-Ayala, G.; Segovia-Gamboa, N.C.; Campos-Peña, V.; Rodríguez-Arellano, M.E.; Meraz-Ríos, M.A.; Campos-Campos, S.F.; et al. Specific macrophage subsets accumulate in human subcutaneous and omental fat depots during obesity. *Immunol. Cell Biol.* **2020**. [CrossRef] [PubMed]
151. Christensen, R.H.; von Scholten, B.J.; Lehrskov, L.L.; Rossing, P.; Jørgensen, P.G. Epicardial adipose tissue: An emerging biomarker of cardiovascular complications in type 2 diabetes? *Ther. Adv. Endocrinol. Metab.* **2020**, *11*, 1–16. [CrossRef]
152. Villasante Fricke, A.C.; Iacobellis, G. Epicardial adipose tissue: Clinical biomarker of cardio-metabolic risk. *Int. J. Mol. Sci.* **2019**, *20*, 5989. [CrossRef]
153. Naukkarinen, J.; Heinonen, S.; Hakkarainen, A.; Lundbom, J.; Vuolteenaho, K.; Saarinen, L.; Hautaniemi, S.; Rodriguez, A.; Frühbeck, G.; Pajunen, P.; et al. Characterising metabolically healthy obesity in weight-discordant monozygotic twins. *Diabetologia* **2014**, *57*, 167–176. [CrossRef]
154. Muniandy, M.; Heinonen, S.; Yki-Järvinen, H.; Hakkarainen, A.; Lundbom, J.; Lundbom, N.; Kaprio, J.; Rissanen, A.; Ollikainen, M.; Pietiläinen, K.H. Gene expression profile of subcutaneous adipose tissue in BMI-discordant monozygotic twin pairs unravels molecular and clinical changes associated with sub-types of obesity. *Int. J. Obes. (Lond.)* **2017**, *41*, 1176–1184. [CrossRef]

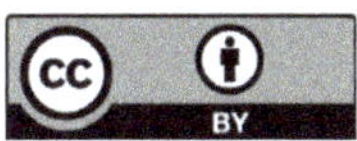

© 2020 by the authors. Licensee MDPI, Basel, Switzerland. This article is an open access article distributed under the terms and conditions of the Creative Commons Attribution (CC BY) license (http://creativecommons.org/licenses/by/4.0/).

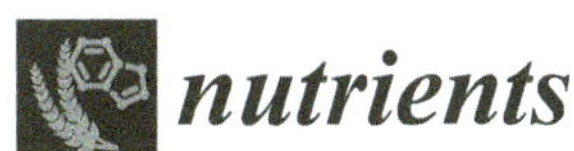 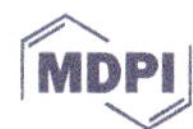

Review

Impact of Strategies for Preventing Obesity and Risk Factors for Eating Disorders among Adolescents: A Systematic Review

Ana Carolina B. Leme [1,2,*], Jess Haines [2], Lisa Tang [2], Karin L. L. Dunker [3], Sonia T. Philippi [1], Mauro Fisberg [4,5], Gerson L. Ferrari [6] and Regina M. Fisberg [1]

[1] Department of Nutrition, School of Public Health, University of São Paulo, São Paulo 01246-904, Brazil; soniatphilippi@gmail.com (S.T.P.); regina.fisberg@gmail.com (R.M.F.)

[2] Family Relations and Applied Nutrition, University of Guelph, Guelph, ON N1G 2W1, Canada; jhaines@uoguelph.ca (J.H.); lisa.tang@uoguelph.ca (L.T.)

[3] Department of Psychiatric, Federal University of São Paulo, São Paulo 04038-000, Brazil; kdunker00@yahoo.com.br

[4] Nutrition and Feeding Difficulties Excellence Center, PENSI Institute, Sabará Children's Hospital, São Paulo 01228-200, Brazil; mauro.fisberg@gmail.com

[5] Department of Pediatrics, Escola Paulista, Federal University of São Paulo, São Paulo 04023-062, Brazil

[6] Laboratorio de Ciencias de la Actividad Física, el Deporte y la Salud, Facultad de Ciencias Médicas, Universidad de Santiago de Chile, Santiago 8320000, Chile; gersonferrari08@yahoo.com.br

* Correspondence: acarol.leme@gmail.com

Received: 12 August 2020; Accepted: 9 October 2020; Published: 14 October 2020

Abstract: An effective behavior change program is the first line of prevention for youth obesity. However, effectiveness in prevention of adolescent obesity requires several approaches, with special attention paid to disordered eating behaviors and psychological support, among other environmental factors. The aim of this systematic review is to compare the impact of two types of obesity prevention programs, inclusive of behavior change components, on weight outcomes. "Energy-balance" studies are aimed at reducing calories from high-energy sources and increasing physical activity (PA) levels, while "shared risk factors for obesity and eating disorders" focus on reducing disordered eating behaviors to promote a positive food and eating relationship. A systematic search of ProQuest, PubMed, PsycInfo, SciELO, and Web of Science identified 8825 articles. Thirty-five studies were included in the review, of which 20 regarded "energy-balance" and 15 "shared risk factors for obesity and eating disorders". "Energy-balance" studies were unable to support maintenance weight status, diet, and PA. "Shared risk factors for obesity and eating disorders" programs also did not result in significant differences in weight status over time. However, the majority of "shared risk factors for obesity and eating disorders" studies demonstrated reduced body dissatisfaction, dieting, and weight-control behaviors. Research is needed to examine how a shared risk factor approach can address both obesity and eating disorders.

Keywords: obesity; eating disorders; adolescents; prevention programs; systematic review

---

1. Introduction

Pediatric obesity is a well-accepted major public health concern [1]. The World Health Organization (WHO) defines pediatric obesity as a body mass index (BMI) at or above the 95th percentile among children and adolescents of the same age and sex, often measured on BMI growth charts [2]. The global age-standardized prevalence of obesity increased more than 5% for girls and almost 8% for boys over the last 40 years [2]. Causes and effects of obesity are complex and multifaceted, and obesity is associated with increased risk of these chronic conditions, such as cardiovascular diseases, type II diabetes, and certain types of cancer. However, children with obesity experience weight stigmatization, defined as the societal devaluing of an individual because of their body size [3], which often manifests in childhood as weight-based teasing and bullying [3].

Due to this stigmatization, obesity in youth has been shown to be a risk factor for psychopathology, which may manifest itself through body dissatisfaction, shape and weight concerns, and dieting and eating disorder behaviors, such as binge eating and purging [4,5]. Research has also shown that obesity in youth is associated with sneaking and hoarding food, eating when not hungry, and feelings of self-consciousness or embarrassment when eating in front of others [6,7]. Although disordered eating behaviors and eating disorders both encompass a broad array of dimensional maladaptive cognitions and behaviors relating to eating and weight, they differ in their diagnosis. The term "eating disorder" refers to a psychiatric disorder and include the following four categories: anorexia nervosa (AN), bulimia nervosa (BN), binge eating disorder (BED), and avoidant restrictive food intake disorder (ARFID) [8]. Those individuals who do not meet the specific diagnostic criteria of an eating disorder may fall into the category of a weight-related disorder, which includes disordered eating behaviors [9]. Thus, research exists to support the assessment of obesity-related problems should include disordered eating as disordered eating behaviors and obesity have similar risk factors, such as body dissatisfaction and weight control behaviors [4,10]. Eating disorders are more prevalent among those with obesity [4]. Indeed, overweight adolescents have up to five times higher odds of developing eating disorders than normal weight youth [11,12].

Prevention programs that include diet, physical activity (PA), and/or sedentary behavior components are currently the first line of prevention for obesity in adolescent youth [6]. However, focusing on diet and PA may increase the risk for eating disorders. In this approach, individuals should decrease their caloric intake and increase their levels of PA, which may encourage them to diet. Evidence has shown that the majority of individuals with eating disorders reported that they started to diet before they initiated their disordered eating behaviors [4]. The WHO Commission on Ending Childhood Obesity report [13] suggest a multi-component approach that includes comprehensive lifestyle weight-management support for youth who have an unhealthy weight status as part of a universal youth healthcare plan. Multidisciplinary prevention programs do not have a specific definition. However, the WHO report [13] noted that a comprehensive prevention plan should include psychosocial and family support in addition to common components such as nutrition and PA or sedentary behavior change. Indeed, obesity prevention programs that predominantly focus on energy-balance approaches, including diet (e.g., avoiding or choosing certain food sources) and PA (e.g., to "burn" calories), have proven to not be effective over a long period of time and may lead to an increase in the risk for disordered eating behaviors [14].

"Energy-balance" programs have a starting point on outcomes of weight gain resulting in increased caloric intake and/or decreased energy expenditure. The major components targeted are sources and amounts of foods and beverages, while energy expenditure is mainly guided by PA and metabolic rates [15]. On the other hand, "shared risk for obesity and eating disorders" programs focused on maintaining a positive relationship between food and weight through a more mindful approach in order to promote sustainable lifestyle changes [16,17].

Thus, it is important to examine the implications of the aforementioned strategies and their impact on disordered eating risk factors and obesity prevention among adolescent youth in order to build a more sustainable approach through the integration of diet and PA components with psychosocial support. Previous systematic reviews and meta-analyses [6,18] have assessed the impact of obesity treatment on eating disorders in overweight or obese children and adolescents. However, there is a gap in the literature examining the impact of obesity prevention programs among youth on risk factors for disordered eating. Thus, the aims of this systematic review are to (1) compare the impact of "energy-balance" and "shared risk factor for obesity and eating disorders" prevention programs on weight outcome changes; and (2) if the eating disorder risk factors were improved in the "shared risk factor for obesity and eating disorders" programs.

2. Methods

The protocol for this systematic review was registered with PROSPERO (CRD 42017076547) [10], accessible at https://www.crd.york.ac.uk/prospero/, and has been reported according to Preferred Reporting Items for Systematic Reviews and Meta-Analyses (PRISMA) guidelines [19].

2.1. Data Sources and Search Strategy

A systematic search of the published literature up to February 2020 was undertaken using five electronic databases, namely, PsycINFO, ProQuest, PubMed, SciElo (Scientific Electronic Library Online), and Web of Science. The following structured search strings were used: Adolescents OR Children OR Girls OR Boys OR Prevention OR Intervention AND Obesity OR Overweight OR Weight-Related Disorders OR Disordered Eating. Relevant truncations and adjacencies were used to enhance results by allowing variations of the search terms. The search was limited to studies in adolescents. Hand searching of reference lists was conducted to identify studies that may have been missed. Records were downloaded to EndNote X9.2 and duplicates removed. Records were first assessed by title and abstract and then full text. All records were assessed for inclusion based on the defined criteria. Any uncertainties regarding the inclusion of a study were resolved through discussion among A.L. and K.D. or. R.F.

2.2. Eligibility Criteria

All studies were assessed according to the following inclusion and exclusion criteria summarized according to PICO framework (Participants, Intervention Comparison, and Outcome):

Participants: Studies were eligible if they included adolescents, aged 10–19 years, as defined by the WHO [20], and inclusive of all weight statuses. Adolescents must have participated in either of the two obesity prevention programs focused on (i) energy-balance approaches (targeting diet and PA); or (ii) shared risk factors for obesity and eating disorders. All participants were eligible if they participated at the beginning of each intervention type. Participants with a pre-existing disease, an organic cause for obesity and eating disorders, or on medication that could affect weight were excluded.

Intervention: Energy-balance interventions were defined as an approach to improve diet (e.g., energy, fat, sugar, sodium, and fruit and vegetables intake), increase (moderate-to-vigorous) PA, and reduce screen-time with the intent to increase energy expenditure [21]. Shared risk factors for obesity and eating disorders programs were described as an approach to promote a positive relationship with weight and diet, through an improvement in the following factors that may have relevance for body image concerns: dieting, media use, body image, weight-control behaviors (e.g., use of food substitutes, diet pills, and diuretics), and maladaptive responses to weight-based teasing. These factors were selected on the basis that they are both amenable to change and suitable for addressing within prevention programs for youth [4]. Assessment of weight-related programs were obtained through the adolescents' weight status, as well as dietary, physical activity, and sedentary behavior questionnaires. The eating disorder (ED) risk factors were obtained through a variety of different psychometric questionnaires.

Comparison: Different study designs (i.e., randomized controlled trials, non-randomized controlled trials, quasi-experimental control trials, and pre-post uncontrolled studies with no comparison group) were included in this review.

Outcome: The key outcome of interest was the impact of obesity prevention programs on disordered eating behaviors in adolescents. The outcomes assessed were related to body or shape satisfaction, weight-control behaviors, weight-teasing and/or diet intake (measured via reports), and PA levels. A secondary outcome was the impact of the programs on adolescent weight outcomes expressed as Body Mass Index (BMI), the BMI z-score (BMIz).

Excluded studies focused on the treatment of individuals with overweight or obesity. Interventions relating to the treatment of EDs or psychological morbidity were also excluded, as were studies treating secondary or syndromic causes of obesity. Search data were not time limited. No exclusion criteria were placed on intervention duration, length of follow-up, or date, but this review was limited to studies published in the English, Portuguese, and Spanish languages.

2.3. Data Extraction

Data were independently extracted from eligible studies by one reviewer and cross-checked for accuracy by a second reviewer. The extracted data included sample characteristics, intervention setting, intensity and design, type of studies, tools used to assess outcome measurement, and pre-, post-intervention and/or follow-up data for both types of approaches.

2.4. Data Synthesis

Due to the heterogeneity of the study population's characteristics and programs features (i.e., length of treatment, outcomes measured, and timing of assessment), it was not possible to perform a meta-analysis. A narrative summary of the findings was conducted.

2.5. Quality Assessment and Risk of Bias

Study quality was assessed using a designed appraisal tool developed by Cochrane: Version 2 of the Cochrane Risk-of-Bias tool for randomized trials (RoB 2) [22] and Risk-Of-Bias In Non-Randomized Studies (ROBINS-I tool) [23]. Individual component quality rankings, including the risk of bias measures, are included in Figure 1. Component and overall quality ratings were scored as "low risk", "moderate", or "high" for the RoB 2; and as "low risk", "moderate", and "serious" for the ROBINS-I [22,23].

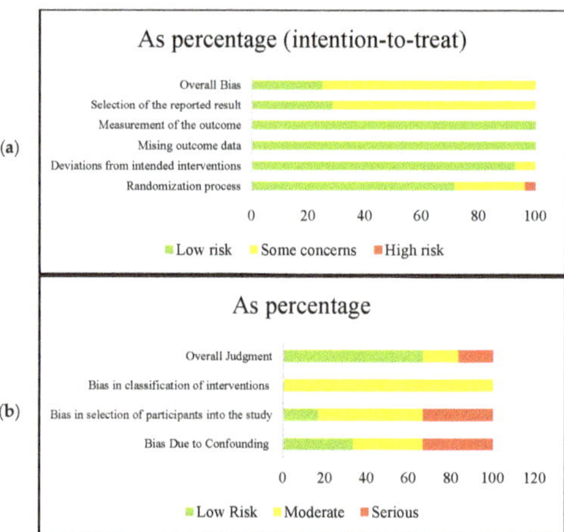

Figure 1. Risk of bias for randomized controlled trials (*n* = 27) (**a**) and non-randomized controlled trials (**b**). Based on the revised Cochrane Risk-of-Bias tools for randomized controlled trials (ROB-2) and non-randomized controlled trials (ROBINS-1) (*n* = 6).

3. Results

3.1. Overview of Studies

A flowchart summarizing the study selection procedure is presented in Figure 2. Electronic searches returned 8825 records. To begin, duplicates (*n* = 4106) were removed. Secondly, a total of 4629 studies were screened by titles and abstracts. Finally, 211 studies were further excluded after reading through the full text. Of the excluded studies, 83 targeted children (≤10 years old) or adults (≥20 years old), 101 included non-healthy individuals (e.g., obese, eating disorders, or other health conditions), and in 28 studies an intervention was not considered. The remaining 35 studies met the inclusion criteria and were therefore eligible and included in this review. A total of 20 studies were energy-balance intervention studies, and 15 studies regarded a shared risk obesity and eating disorders program.

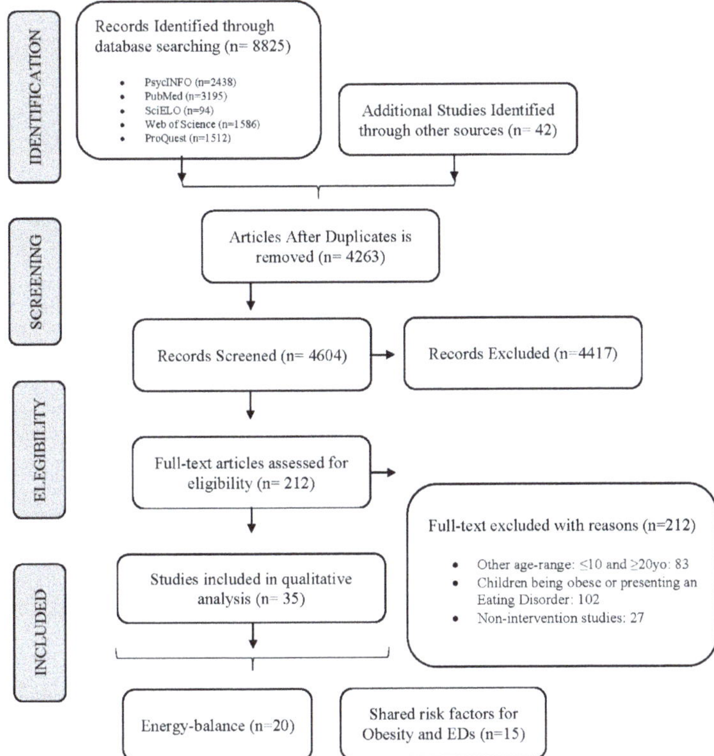

Figure 2. Flowchart showing the process of article selection.

Data abstraction revealed 15 programs that had multiple publications; these included protocols, additional cohorts, further follow-up timepoints, different outcome measures, or other secondary analysis. Thus, for reporting and analysis, studies were grouped by program cohort. Any uncertainties regarding appropriate program cohort for categorization were resolved through discussion.

3.2. Study Characteristics

The characteristics of the selected studies are reported in Table 1 and divided by intervention types: "energy-balance" and "shared risk factors for obesity and eating disorders" programs. All studies were published between 2005 and 2019.

Overall, twelve studies (33.3%) were conducted in the U.S., five studies (14.7%) were conducted in Australia and other countries in Occania [24–28], and three studies (8.8%) in Brazil [5,29,30] and in Spain [31–33]. Other studies included countries within Europe [34–38] and Asia [39–41], Canada [42], Mexico [43], and Israel [44]. Programs were evaluated as controlled trials ($n = 31$, 91.2%), randomized controlled trials ($n = 23$, 67.6%), quasi-experimental ($n = 7$, 20.5%), non-randomized ($n = 2$, 5.8%), and as interrupted time series without a comparison group ($n = 3$, 8.8%).

3.2.1. Energy-Balance Programs

For the energy-balance programs, 20 studies were found [24,25,30,32,34,37–41,44–50]; of these, five studies were conducted in the USA [45–47,49,50], six in Europe [32,34,35,37,38], four in Australia [24–27], three in Asia [39,40,44], and one in Brazil [30] and in Tonga [41]. When considering the study design, 13 studies were randomized controlled trials (RCT) [25–27,30,36–38,40,45–47,49–51], four were quasi-experimental trials [24,34,39,41], and one non-randomized controlled trial [44]. Two studies were one-group pre- and post-test assessments [32,50]. The sample size for the energy-balance programs ranged from 51 [46] to 3638 [35] and the mean age was 12.7 ± 1.8 years old. Two targeted only females [26,46] and one only males [25]. Eight studies reported following a theoretical basis, with six studies following the Social Cognitive Theory [25–27,45,47,49], and two the Self-Determination Theory [25,45]. Although not reporting a theoretical framework, 10 [24–27,35–37,41,44,47] combined educational techniques with changes in the environment.

3.2.2. Shared Risk Factors for Obesity and Eating Disorders Programs

With regards to the "shared risk factors for obesity and eating disorders" programs, fifteen studies were included in this systematic review [5,28,29,31,33,42,43,51–58]. Seven studies were conducted in the USA [51,52,54,56–58], two in Spain [31,33] and in Brazil [5,29], and one in Australia [28], Canada [42], and Mexico [43]. The programs included nine RCT [5,29,51,53–58], three quasi-experimental trials [31,33,43], one non-RCT [42], and one one-group pre- and post-test assessment [52]. The sample size ranged from 27 [52] to 1451 [56] adolescents participating in the shared risk factors for obesity and eating disorders program, with 15.1 ± 2.6 years old as the mean age of the participants. Six targeted only females [5,29,31,43,51,52,57]. From a theoretical approach, five was based on Social Cognitive Theory [5,29,33,51,55] and eight combined educational techniques with changes in the environment [5,29,31,42,51,56–58]. This was followed by focusing on approaches to reduce the risk for eating disorders, such as Media Literacy [28,31,33], Dissonance Behavioral Intervention [31,52], and Interpersonal Therapy [58].

3.3. The Studies' Techniques

3.3.1. Energy-Balance Programs

The majority ($n = 13$, 65%) of the energy-balance programs used schools as the main settings for integrating diet and PA for promoting behavioral changes [24–27,32,34,37–39,41,44,45,50], 3 (15%) use the home setting [30,47,50], and two (10%) developed a web-based platform to deliver the intervention [40,46]. Some programs, which used schools as the main setting, combined multiple components to deliver the intervention, such as combining weekly text messages and other mobile device technology (e.g., developing an app) [25,26], or integrating the family context (e.g., parents newsletters, homework, and booklets) [26,34,50].

3.3.2. Shared Risk Factors for Obesity and Eating Disorders Programs

From the fourteen studies that have shared risk factors for obesity and eating disorders as the program approach, thirteen (92.3%) were conducted at school or university [5,28,29,31,33,42,43, 51–54,56,57], and one was delivered through an internet-based platform [55]. Some of the school programs focused only on psychotherapy sessions to promote a healthy relationship with body and food [28,33,42,43,52,54,58], while others ($n = 6$, 42.8%) [5,29,31,51,56,57] focused on both the psychotherapy sessions and other components to help achieve a sustainable diet and PA behaviors through their life course. Other components included weekly text messages, cooking classes, enhanced physical education classes, and healthy lunches and morning snacks at school time. Two studies [29,51] used individual counseling techniques to promote intrinsic motivational for behavior change via the motivational interview technique.

3.4. The Studies' Assessment Tools

3.4.1. Energy-Balance Programs

Weight status was assessed in all the energy balance studies. Some of these studies (*n* = 13, 65.0%) [25–27,30,36–39,41,44,49,50] combined other measurements to assess anthropometric outcomes, such as body fat percentage, waist circumference, and/or waist-to-hip ratio. Dietary intake was assessed with either food frequency questionnaires [25–27,30,44] or 24 h recalls [34,45,46,49]. Those studies that utilized 24 h recalls used at least two records to estimate participants' usual intake. For those studies that measured PA, some used questionnaires [24,30,34,39,45], while others used objective measurements such as accelerometers [25–27,49] or pedometers [34]. Some studies (*n* = 6, 30.0%) evaluated the youth's physical fitness (e.g., cardiovascular, flexibility, muscular, strength, and agility) [25,27,36,39, 45,50]. Five studies (25.0%) evaluated sedentary behaviors, with a particular focus on screen-time questionnaires [24–26,37,46]. Four studies (20.0%) [24,34,39,44] assessed nutrition and PA knowledge gained through the program, and four studies assessed other mental health outcomes (e.g., health-related quality of life, depressive symptomatology, or disordered eating components) [24,34,35,47]. Studies that assessed mental health outcomes were not identified as a shared risk factors for obesity and eating disorders program as they did not target these components on the intervention but rather used this as an indicator of inclusionary/exclusionary criteria of participants, and as a secondary outcome of the intervention. Three studies (15.0%) [37,39,50] used biomarkers, such as plasma glucose and lipids, as an outcome of diet and PA behavior change. Finally, two studies (10.0%) [38,47] targeted the pre-adolescent age group (10–12 years old).

3.4.2. Shared Risk Factors for Obesity and Eating Disorders Programs

For the shared risk factors for obesity and eating disorders program, all of these studies evaluated participant weight status through the use of BMI. Five studies (35.7%) [5,51,54,57,58] combined this measure with other anthropometric measures, including waist circumference and % body fat (measured using DEXA, bioimpedance, or skinfolds). Seven studies (50.0%) evaluated diet intake through validated and reproduced food frequency questionnaires [5,52,54] and others through 24 h recalls [28,51,56,57]. Those studies that used a 24 h recall only collected data from one-day of diet intake. PA was assessed by seven studies: five studies [5,51,52,56,57] used at least a 3-day recall to assess the PA of the participants, while the remaining studies [28,43,54] used a validated and reproduced questionnaire (e.g., International Physical Activity Questionnaire (IPAQ) [59] and the Paffenbarg Activity Questionnaire [60]).

Measures used to evaluate the shared risk factors for obesity and eating disorders are shown in Table 1 along with the study characteristics. Ten studies (71.4%) [28,31,33,42,52,54,55,58,61] used validated and reliable measurements that are used to assess eating disorders, including the "Eating Disorder Diagnostic Screening (EDDS)" [62], "Eating Disorder Questionnaire with Instruction (EDQ-I)" [63,64], "Difficulties in Emotion Regulation Scale (DERS)" [65], "Sociocultural Attitudes Towards Appearance Scale (SATAQ)" [66], and "Perceptions Of Teasing Scale (POTS)" [67], or used measures to assess emotion regulation and positive and negative effects through the "Dutch Restrained Eating Scale (DERS)" [68] and "Positive and Negative Scale—Revised (PANAS-X)" [69]. The purpose of these scales is to evaluate the occurrence of eating disorder symptoms, disordered eating behaviors, body shape and weight satisfaction, and weight-teasing by family and friends/peers. The other five studies (35.7%) [5,42,51,56,57] assessed these measures through questionnaires used in previous surveillance studies, specifically the "Youth Risk Behavioral Surveillance System Survey (YRBSSS)" and "Project EAT". These questionnaires assessed the risk for disordered eating behaviors, including dieting, weight control behaviors, binge eating, weight-teasing, and body/weight/shape concern.

Table 1. Characteristics of the included studies, assessments, and outcomes of the intervention strategies.

Studies	Intervention Name (Country)	Study Design	Sample Characteristics	Strategy and Techniques
		Shared Risk Factors for Obesity and Eating Disorders Programs		
Simpson et al. 2019 [52]	INSPIRE (USA)	One-group pre-post-design	27 female adolescents (M = 18.6 ± SD 1.01 years old)	Dissonance-based intervention + healthy weight + dialectical behavioral therapy.
Leme et al., 2019 [5]	Healthy Habits, Healthy Girls—Brazil (Brazil)	Randomized controlled trial with post- and 6-month	253 adolescent girls (M = 16.1 ± SE 0.1 years old); 142 in intervention group	Social Cognitive Theory. Achieve sustainable diet and physical activity behaviors, and decrease risk factors for eating disorders.
Castillo et al. 2019 [43]	No intervention name (Mexico)	Three-arm quasi experimental study with post and 3-month follow-up	361 adolescent girls (M = 19.78 ± 2.06 years old); 133 in experimental group; 105 in control skills group and 123 non-intervention group	Cognitive Dissonance and Constructivist Approach. Raise awareness to beauty standards and perpetuated by the mass media. Increase physical activity and healthy eating. Improve self-esteem, build positive self-concept, and reduce extreme perfectionism, and resolve conflicts.
Lenz and Claudino et al. 2018 [29]	Adaption of the US New Moves (Brazil)	Randomized Controlled trial with post- and 6-month follow-up.	270 adolescent girls (M = 13.4 ± 0.64 years old) with 139 in intervention group.	Social Cognitive Theory. Address issues related to female adolescents to promote health.
Shomaker et al. 2017 [58]	No intervention name (USA)	Randomized Controlled trial with post-intervention, 6 month and 1-year follow-up	29 pre-adolescents (M = 11.7 ± 1.6 years old) with 15 in intervention group.	Family-Based Interpersonal Therapy. Psycho-education on interpersonal model of loss of control-eating and general skill-building applied to improve communication, increase support, and resolve conflict between parent and child.
Sánchez-Carracedo et al. 2016 [31]	The MABIC Project (Spain)	Non-randomized controlled trial with post- and 1-year follow-up.	565 adolescent girls (M= 13.8 ± 0.5 years old) with 152 in intervention group.	Social Cognitive Theory, Media Literacy Education Approach, and Cognitive Dissonance Theory. Increase knowledge through sessions of the practical and relevant aspects of foods.
Wilksch et al. 2015 [28]	No intervention name (Australia)	Four-arm randomized controlled trial with post, intervention, 6-month and 12-month follow-up.	1316 adolescents (M = 13.21 ± 0.68 years old) with 269 in media smart, 347 in life smart and 225 HELPP group.	Principles of media internalization (Media Smart group). Principles that health is more than weight (Life Smart group). Principles of eating disorder risk factors of internalization of social appearance ideals and comparisons. Evidence principles of being interactive, avoiding psychoeducation on weight-related concerns and with multiple sessions.

Table 1. *Cont.*

Studies	Intervention Name (Country)	Study Design	Sample Characteristics	Strategy and Techniques
		Shared Risk Factors for Obesity and Eating Disorders Programs		
Stice et al. 2013 [54]	Healthy Weight 2 (USA)	Randomized controlled trial post-, 6 month, 1-year and 2-year follow-up.	398 young adults (M = 18.4, 17–20 years old) with 192 in intervention group.	Healthy weight approach to reduce eating disorders and obesity. Nutrition science principles for health behavior changes.
Franko et al. 2013 [55]	BodyMojo (USA)	Randomized controlled trial with 4–6 weeks and 3-month follow-up.	65 boys (M = 15.4 ± 1.4 years old) and 113 girls (M = 15.2 ± 0.3 years old), randomized in classes.	Socio-Cognitive Theory, Health Belief Model, Theory of Planned Behavior, Transtheoretical Model. Internet-based program for health behavior change through technology and social engagement, offering a personalized experience, goal setting, and interactive games and videos.
Gonzalez et al. 2011 [33]	No intervention name (Spain)	Three arms quasi-experimental design with post-intervention, 6 and 30-month follow-up.	443 adolescents (M = 13.5 ± 0.4 years old) with 143 media literacy and 99 media literacy and nutrition.	Social Cognitive Theory. Focus on media literacy to increase nutrition awareness. Interactive format, sessions, and new activism and media literacy components. Critical thinking and promotion of health and well-being to develop resilience for sociocultural messages.
Neumark-Sztainer et al. 2010 [51]	New Moves (USA)	Randomized controlled trial with post and 9-month follow-up.	356 adolescent girls (M = 15.8 ± 1.2 years old) with 182 in intervention group.	Social Cognitive Theory and Transtheoretical Model. Socio-environmental, personal, and behavioral factors for changes in diet, physical activity, and weight-control behaviors.
Stock et al. 2007 [42]	Healthy Bodies (Canada)	Prospective pilot study with post-intervention.	199 adolescents (4th to 7th grade) with 128 in intervention group.	Prescribed learning outcomes from the British Columbia Minister of Health. 3 main components of healthy living: be physical activity, eat healthy, and positive body image. 21 lessons over the study school year.
Austin et al. 2007 [56]	The 5-2-1 go! (USA)	Randomized controlled trial with post intervention.	1451 adolescents (6th and 7th grade) with 614 in intervention group.	Learning outcomes from previous trial (Planet Girls). Multiple modules in schools to address nutrition and physical activity in various domains: nutrition services, physical education, and policies and environment.
Austin et al. 2005 [57]	Planet Health (USA)	Randomized controlled trial with post-and 21-month follow-up.	480 adolescent girls (M = 11.5 ± 0.7 years old) with 254 in intervention group	Social Cognitive Theory. Interdisciplinary curriculum with materials integrated in major subject areas and physical education classes via grade- and subject appropriate skills and competencies.

Table 1. *Cont.*

Studies	Intervention Name (Country)	Study Design	Sample Characteristics	Strategy and Techniques
		Energy-Balance Programs		
Sgambato et al. 2019 [30]	PAAPPAS—"Parents, Students, Community Health Agents and teachers for Healthy Eating" (Brazil)	Randomized controlled trial with post-interventions	2447 adolescents (M = 11.5 ± 1.4 years old) with 1290 in intervention group.	Family Health System. Reduce weight gain at school and home environments.
Aperman-Itzhak et al. 2018 [44]	No intervention name (Israel)	Controlled, non-randomized and non-blinded trial with post-intervention	373 adolescents (10–12 years old) with 187 in intervention group.	Program developed by a registered dietitian and cardiologist. Promote healthy eating and physical activity, integrating the head of the local council stakeholders and school teachers
Yang et al. 2017 [39]	No intervention name (South Korea)	Quasi-experimental trial with 1-year follow-up	768 adolescents (M = 11.0 ± 1.5 years old) with 418 in intervention group.	Based on pre-intervention results + personalized suggestions for improving physical strength and dietary intake. School-based interventions with continuation in the community.
Rerksuppaphol and Rerksuppaphol 2017 [40]	No intervention name (Thailand)	Randomized controlled trial with post-intervention.	217 adolescents (M = 10.7 ± 3.1 years old) with 111 in intervention group.	Internet-based obesity program. Information on health nutrition, food habits, and physical activity included in text and graphics. Participants collect their weight and height and interpreted their weight status.
Malakellis et al. 2017 [24]	It's Your Move—ACT IYM (Australia)	Quasi-experimental trial with 2-year follow-up.	880 adolescents (12–16 years old) with 628 in intervention group.	ANGELO framework—identify and prioritize key determinants, considering gaps in knowledge community capacity, culturally specific needs, and current health promotion. Changes in school and community-based environment.
Ardic and Erdogan 2017 [34]	COPE Healthy lifestyles teen program (Turkey)	Quasi-experimental trial with post and 12-month follow-up.	100 adolescents (M = 12.8 ± 0.8 years old) with 50 in intervention group.	Adaptation of US study (COPE). Cognitive behavioral skill building. Educational information for healthy lifestyle.
Lubans et al. 2016 [25]	ATLAS Boys (Australia)	Randomized controlled trial with post, 8- and 18-month follow-up.	361 adolescent boys (M = 12.7 ± 0.5 years old) with 181 in intervention group.	Self-Determination and Social Cognitive Theory. Increase autonomy, competence, and relatedness to improve autonomous motivation for leisure time physical activity and school sports.
Fulkerson et al. 2015 [47]	Home Plus (USA)	Randomized controlled trial with 12- and 21-month follow-up.	149 families (children M = 10.3 ± 1.4 and; parents M = 41.6 ± 7.6 years old) with 74 families in intervention group.	Social Cognitive Theory and Social Ecological Model. Family changes on planning, frequency, and healthiness of family meals and snacks (limiting meals related to screen-time).

Table 1. *Cont.*

Studies	Intervention Name (Country)	Study Design	Sample Characteristics	Strategy and Techniques
		Energy-Balance Programs		
Lazorick et al. 2015 [45]	MATCH (USA)	Randomized controlled trial with post-intervention follow-up.	362 adolescents (M = 13.1 ± 0.5 years old) with 189 in intervention group.	Social Cognitive Theory and Self-Determination Theory. Education and behavioral curriculum (school). Lessons delivered in sequence of a planned manner, repeated key concepts, and applied enhance skills for healthy choices.
González-Jiménez et al. 2014 [32]	No intervention name (Spain)	One group, pre post-test design	91 adolescents (15–17 years old)	Knowledge education program to reduce weight gain. Three workshops on healthy eating. Activities during physical education classes
Grydeland et al. 2014 [38]	HEIA Study (Norway)	Randomized controlled trial with 2-month follow-up	1485 adolescents (M = 11.2 ± 0.3 years old) with 465 in intervention group.	Social Ecological Framework. Multiple components for health promotion to increase awareness and physical activity, and reduce screen-time.
Nollen et al. 2014 [46]	No intervention name (USA)	Randomized controlled trial with post, 8-week and 12-week follow-up.	51 adolescent girls (M = 11.3 ± 1.6 years old) with 26 in intervention group.	Mobile technology with four-week 3 modules: to improve fruit and vegetable and sugar-sweetened beverages intake and screen-time.
Dewar et al. 2013 [26]	NEAT Girls (Australia)	Randomized controlled trial with 12- and 24-month follow-up.	357 adolescent girls (M = 13.2 ± 0.5 years old) with 178 in intervention group. 3538 adolescents	Social Cognitive Theory. Range of strategies to promote lifestyle and lifetime physical activity, improve diet intake, and reduce time on screens.
Bonsergent et al. 2013 [35]	PRALIMAP trial (France)	Randomized Controlled trial with mid- and post-intervention follow-up.	(M = 15.6 ± 0.7 years old) with 1949 in education strategy and 1589 in non-education strategy. Education was divided in environmental with 1029 and non-environmental with 920 individuals. Non-education divided in environmental with 699 and non-environmental with 890 individuals.	Personal skills were used for educational strategy, detection of weight-related problems, and proposing a care model for a screening strategy and favorable and supportive environment for environmental strategy. * Screening = non-education
Lubans et al. 2011 [27]	Physical Activity Leaders—PAL (Australia)	Randomized controlled trial with 3- and 6-month follow-up.	100 adolescents (M = 14.3 ± 0.6 years old) with 50 in intervention group.	Social Cognitive Theory. Promotion of lifestyle and lifetime activities.

Table 1. *Cont.*

Studies	Intervention Name (Country)	Study Design	Sample Characteristics	Strategy and Techniques
Energy-Balance Programs				
Jansen et al. 2011 [36]	Lekker Fit (Enjoy being fit) (The Netherlands)	Randomized controlled trial with post-intervention.	1236 adolescents (M = 10.8 ± 1.0 years old) with 583 in intervention group.	Theory of Planned Behavior. ANGELO framework (identify and prioritize environmental determinants). Intervention targeted individual behaviors, school policies, and curriculum.
Fotu et al. 2011 [41]	Ma'alahi Youth Project (Tonga)	Quasi-experimental design with 3-year follow-up	1712 adolescents (M = 14.8 ± 1.9 years old) with 897 in intervention group.	Develop on communities the capacity to build on their own promotion for a healthy lifestyle. Social marketing approaches, community capacity building, and grass-roots activities.
Chen et al. 2011 [49]	WEB ABC study (USA)	Randomized controlled trial with 2-, 6- and 8-month follow-up	63 adolescents (M = 12.5 ± 3.2 years old) with 27 in intervention group	Transtheoretical Model and Social Cognitive Theory. Web-based program to enhance diet and physical activity self-efficacy, ease comprehension, and use problem solving skills.
Simon et al. 2008 [37]	No intervention name (France)	Randomized controlled trial with post and 4-year follow-up.	954 adolescents (M = 11.6 ± 0.6 years old) with 475 in intervention group	Multilevel theory-based. Provide environment institutional conditions to promote health use knowledge and skills acquired. Changes attitudes towards health and social support from parents and educators.
Shaw-Peri et al. 2007 [50]	NEEMA (USA)	One-group with pre-post design.	269 adolescents (M = 10.5 ± 0.7 years old)	Based on the learning outcomes of a previous study reporting increased risk for diabetes type 2. Changes in social structures to promote physical activity, fiber intake, and reduce saturated fat, sugar, and sedentary time.

3.5. Outcomes

The focus of this review was to assess the impact of obesity prevention programs on improving disordered eating behaviors and maintaining a healthy weight status among adolescents by comparing the types of interventions: energy-balance and shared risk factors for obesity and eating disorders programs (Table 2).

3.5.1. Energy-Balance Programs

Ten studies [24,26,27,32,35,37–39,44,50,70] showed small improvements on youth weight status as measured by BMI, the BMI z-scores, or percent prevalence for being overweight/obese. A reduction was observed by a difference between groups (intervention vs. control) of at least 0.1 kg/m^2, or by a 1.7% decrease on the prevalence of being overweight/obese from baseline to post-intervention/follow-up assessments. Five studies [25,26,34,40] did not find any significant effects on weight status change, while three studies [30,36,41] showed an increase in weight status change. For example, one study showed a large increase in overweight and obesity prevalence (10.1% and 12.6%) [41], and another study [30] showed a small increase in BMI of 0.2 kg/m^2 for the intervention group and a decrease in % of body fat. Interestingly, a study conducted by Fulkerson et al. [47] found that although they found no significant treatment group differences in BMI z-scores post-intervention, a post-hoc stratification by pubertal onset indicated pre-pubescent youth had significantly lower BMI z-scores than their control group counterparts (ß = 0.08, 95%CI 0.01, 0.34).

Four studies (20.0%) [26,30,41,45] did not find significant differences in diet outcomes after the intervention, which included the reduction of total energy intake and improvement on the intake of certain food groups (e.g., fruit and vegetables). However, five studies (25.0%) [25,27,34,46,49] showed an improvement in the intake of sugar-sweetened beverages, as well as fruit and vegetables. Sgambato et al. [30] did not find any significant differences when evaluating diet intake using a food frequency questionnaire; however, analyses of 30% of the sample that used a 24 h recall showed a significant decrease in the intake of fruit juice (△ = −0.42 ± 0.18 serving/day) compared to the control group.

PA level was improved in four studies (20.0%) [30,34,37,49] with an average of +12.5 min/week. Two studies conducted by Lubans et al., one targeting only boys [25] and the other both sexes [27], found an improvement in physical fitness (i.e., muscular fitness and resistance training) despite finding no significant effect on PA level. The remaining four studies [26,32,45,46] found no significant effect on PA level. Shawn-Peri et al. [50] found that large classes and short physical education periods are major challenges when implementing programs. Sedentary behaviors or screen-time were improved in three studies [25,26,37]. Dewar et al. [26] showed improvement in screen-time behaviors at immediate post-intervention (after 12 months from the baseline), but at follow-up (after 24 months) found no significant differences. An average of the significant difference was −30.7 min/day.

Three studies [34,44,49] evaluated the participants' knowledge of nutrition and PA, and found significant improvements in their knowledge. Three studies [39,49,50] assessed the biological markers to verify the improvements in lifestyle behaviors, including blood pressure and fasting capillary plasma. Significant results were found among male participants with a higher BMI and older adolescents.

Table 2. Findings from the intervention studies.

Author, Publication Year	Assessment at Follow-Up	Summary of Main Results
Shared Risk Factors for Obesity and Eating Disorders Studies		
Simpson et al. 2019 [52]	Eating disorders symptoms/Body shape satisfaction. Emotion regulation. Positive/negative affect. Weight status. Diet intake. Physical activity.	↓eating pathology, eating satisfaction, thin-ideal internalization, restrained eating, negative affect, emotion dysregulation. ↓ fat intake. No significant increase in BMI. Acceptable and feasible.
Leme et al. 2019 [5]	Body and shape satisfaction. Weight-control behaviors. Weight stigma. Social cognitive aspects of diet and PA. Diet intake. Physical activity. Weight status.	No significant decrease in BMI. Increase in waist circumference. Week and weekends decrease time on screens. Weekends increase vegetables intake. Social support and strategies were improved. Unhealthy weight was increased (favoring intervention group).
Castillo et al. 2019 [43]	Body and weight image. Risk factors for eating disorders. Emotion regulation. Sex-specific image concerns. Physical Activity. Weight status.	Male students did not present any significant effect. Girls improved significant for thin-ideal internalization and disordered eating attitudes.
Dunker and Claudino 2018 [29]	Body image. Emotional regulations. Weight status.	No significant results for any eating disorders risk factors. Participants' low adherence in the program.
Shomaker et al. 2017 [58]	Weight status and body fat. Risk factors for eating disorders. Emotional regulation. Positive/negative affect.	Intervention was feasible and acceptable. Benefits to social interactions and eating. Family-based interpersonal therapy improved depression and anxiety, and loss of control compared to health education (control). Family-based interpersonal therapy reduced disordered eating attitudes. No significant differences in BMI
Sanchez-Carracedo et al. 2016 [31]	Risk for eating disorders. Body image concern. Emotional regulations. Weight status and body fat. Diet intake. Physical activity.	Media Smart and HELPP were less concerned about their shape and weight compared to control girls. Media Smart and control had less eating concerns and pressure than HELPP girls. Media Smart and HELPP benefitted from media internalization compared to control boys. Media Smart had more physical activity than HELPP and control participants. Media Smart had less time spent on screens than control participants.

Table 2. *Cont.*

Author, Publication Year	Assessment at Follow-Up	Summary of Main Results
	Shared Risk Factors for Obesity and Eating Disorders Studies	
Wilksch et al. 2015 [28]	Weight status Risk for eating disorders. Body image concern. Emotional regulations. Weight status and body fat. Diet intake. Physical activity.	Intervention group reduced body dissatisfaction and eating disorders symptoms. No effects for BMI, depressive symptoms, dieting, energy intake, and physical activity.
Stice et al. 2013 [54]	Risk factors for eating disorders. Body image concern. Emotion regulation.	Intervention decreased body image concerns compared to control girls (but not sustained over a 3-month follow-up). Among boys there were no significant differences between intervention and control groups.
Franko et al. 2013 [55]	Weight status. Risk factors for eating disorders. Body image concern.	Prevention presented lower risk factors for eating disorders and body image concern than the control group.
Gonzalez et al. 2011 [33]	Weight status and body fat %. Physical activity. Diet intake. Body image concern. Weight control behaviors. Social cognitive aspects of health.	No significant differences in BMI. Improvement in screen-time, diet intake, weight-control behaviors, and body image. Friends, teachers and family support for diet and physical activity behaviors.
Neumark-Sztainer et al. 2010 [51]	Weight status. Cardiovascular markers. Physical fitness. Knowledge on behavior and attitudes towards health behaviors. Emotional regulation. Body image concern. Risk for eating disorders.	BMI and weight decreased. Improvement in health knowledge: body image, eating disorders risk factors, physical activity and diet. Increase in systolic blood pressure.
Stock et al. 2007 [42]	Weight control behaviors. Diet intake. Physical activity. Weight status and body fat %.	Girls reported less weight-control behaviors after intervention. No significant differences for boys.
Austin et al. 2007 [56]	Weight control behaviors. Diet intake. Physical activity. Weight status and body fat %.	Girls reported less purging and using diet pills to control weight from both intervention and control groups.

Table 2. *Cont.*

Author, Publication Year	Assessment at Follow-Up	Summary of Main Results
Shared Risk Factors for Obesity and Eating Disorders Studies		
Austin et al. 2005 [57]	Eating disorders symptoms/Body shape satisfaction. Emotion regulation. Positive/negative affect. Weight status. Diet intake. Physical activity.	↓eating pathology, eating satisfaction, thin-ideal internalization, restrained eating, negative affect, emotion dysregulation. ↓ fat intake. No significant increase in BMI. Acceptable and feasible.
Energy-Balance Programs		
Sgambato et al. 2019 [30]	Diet intake. Physical Activity. Health knowledge, attitudes and behaviors. Weight status and body fat %.	Weight status increased in the intervention group. Small decrease in body fat %. No significant differences on daily frequency intake of foods. Physical activity increased in the intervention group. 30% of the sample was analyzed using a 24 h Recall and significantly decrease fruit juice in the intervention group.
Aperman-Itzhak et al. 2018 [44]	Weight status, waist circumference, and body fat %. Blood pressure. Physical fitness. Health behaviors: physical activity, sleep, and diet intake. Nutrition knowledge. Body image. Emotion regulations. Parents' obesity social-determinants aspects.	Overweight and obesity decreased only in the intervention group. Religious children have increased risk for being overweight. Knowledge improved in the intervention and control groups.
Yang et al. 2017 [39]	Weight status, body fat %. Blood pressure. Physical fitness.	No significant difference in overweight incidence between the intervention and control groups. Intervention decreased BMI, height, body fat %, and increased muscular fitness compared to the control group. Blood pressure was significantly reduced, mainly in those with higher BMI, boys, and older children. Physical fitness was improved. Normal weight boys and younger individuals showed better weight-related outcomes.
Rerksuppaphol and Rerksuppaphol 2017 [40]	Weight status.	Control showed an increased in overweight and BMI compared to the intervention group.
Malakellis et al. 2017 [24]	Weight status. Health knowledge, attitudes and behaviors. Environment perceptions (home, school, and neighborhood). Emotional regulations.	Two of three intervention schools decreased the prevalence of overweight.

Table 2. *Cont.*

Author, Publication Year	Assessment at Follow-Up	Summary of Main Results
Energy-Balance Programs		
Ardic and Erdocan 2017 [34]	Weight status. Physical activity (daily steps). Diet and water intake. Nutrition and physical activity knowledge. Emotional regulations.	Intervention group improve diet, physical activity, and stress management. Increased number of daily steps/weeks, fruit and vegetables, and water intake. Knowledge about nutrition and physical activity was improved. Anxiety levels and BMI were reduced, but effects were not significant.
Lubans et al. 2016 [25]	Weight status and waist circumference. Physical activity and sedentary behaviors. Sugar-sweetened beverages intake. Muscular fitness and resistance training skills. School sports motivation regulation.	No significant effect for BMI, waist circumference, and body fat %. No significant effect for physical activity. Screen-time, sugar-sweetened beverages, muscular fitness, and resistance training were improved.
Lazorick et al. 2015 [45]	Weight status. Physical fitness. Diet intake. Physical activity and sedentary behaviors. Sleep behaviors.	MATCH significant decreased BMI compared to the control group. Subgroup analysis showed decreased among overweight and obese participants. Lifestyle behaviors were not significant.
Fulkerson et al. 2015 [47]	Weight status. Pubertal development scale. Family dinner frequency.	No significant difference in BMI; but promising reduction in excess weight gain. Subgroup analysis showed that pre-pubescent children showed lower BMI in the intervention group.
Gonzalez-Jimenez et al. 2014 [32]	Weight status, waist circumference, and waist-to-hip ratio. Pubertal category scores	Weight status was improved. Significant results for diet intake. No significant results for physical activity.
Nollen et al. 2014 [46]	Home availability of fruit and vegetables, sugar-sweetened beverages, and screen devices. Diet intake. Screen-time behaviors.	Mobile technology used the program about 63% of days compared to the control girls. Non-significant increase in fruit and vegetables and decrease in sugar-sweetened beverage intake. No significant differences for BMI and screen-time use.
Dewar et al. 2013 [26]	Weight status and body fat %. Physical activity and sedentary behaviors. Diet intake.	Non-significant effect on the decrease for BMI and body fat % between the intervention and control groups. Screen-time was significantly reduced. No significant effect for physical activity, diet intake, and self-esteem.
Bonsergent et al. 2013 [35]	Weight status. Emotional regulations. Risk factors for eating disorders.	Screening improved the BMI and decreased the overweight incidence compared to the non-screening strategy. Education and environment strategies were less effective.

Table 2. *Cont.*

Author, Publication Year	Assessment at Follow-Up	Summary of Main Results
Energy-Balance Programs		
Lubans et al. 2011 [27]	Weight status, body fat %, and waist circumference. Physical fitness. Physical activity. Fruit and vegetables, sugar-sweetened beverages, and water intake.	Significant effect in BMI and body fat %. No significant effect for waist circumference, muscular fitness, and physical activity. Adolescents reported less intake on sugar-sweetened beverages after intervention.
Jansen et al. 2011 [36]	Weight status and waist circumference. Physical fitness.	Overweight increased at both the intervention and control groups. No significant effects for BMI.
Fotu et al. 2011 [41]	Weight status and body fat %. Diet intake. Physical activity.	Increased in overweight prevalence. Intervention group decrease body fat %. Diet and physical activity were not improved.
Chen et al. 2011 [49]	Weight status and waist-to-hip ratio. Blood pressure. Diet and physical activity knowledge and self-efficacy. Diet intake. Physical activity.	Waist-to-hip ratio and diastolic blood pressure were decreased. Fruit and vegetables intake, and physical activity were improved. Nutrition and physical activity knowledge improved.
Grydeland et al. 2014 [38]	Weight status, waist circumference, and waist-to-hip circumference.	Effects on BMI only for girls. Beneficial effect for BMI in participants with high educated parents. Negative effects for waist-to-hip ratio in participants with low educated parents. No significant for waist circumference and weight status.
Simon et al. 2008 [37]	Weight status. Physical activity. Plasma lipids.	Intervention lower increased in BMI than control groups. Intervention better effect on non-overweight students. Non-significant differences in overweight students. Intervention improved supervised PA, screen-time, and HDL-c.
Shaw-Peri et al. 2007 [51]	Weight status and % body fat. Plasma glucose.	Fitness laps, fasting glucose, and % body fat improved by the end of the study.

3.5.2. Shared Risk Factors for Obesity and Eating Disorders Programs

All 14 studies showed no significant effects on weight status post-intervention. Two programs [42,52] showed an increase in BMI and weight from post-intervention to follow-up. This increase in BMI ranged from 0.2 to 0.4 kg/m^2, reflecting on average increase of 2.9 kg. Leme et al. [5], although not finding significant results for BMI, found that results favored the intervention group ($\Delta = -0.26$ kg/m^2), with a lower increase in waist circumference for both groups. Female participants with high levels of anxiety demonstrated stabilization in adiposity (% body fat). Moderation analyses also indicated a stronger BMI effect for youths with initially elevated symptoms of eating disorders and higher initial BMI scores [54,55], as well as for weaker eating disorder symptoms and body image dissatisfaction [54].

Six studies [28,33,51,52,56,57] also found a reduction in several risk factors that were sustained at follow-up; specifically, eating pathology, appearance satisfaction, a thin ideal, negative affect, and emotion dysregulation. Two studies [43,55] that targeted both sexes found an interaction effect for time and group in thin idealization, but disordered eating attitudes/behaviors for females only. Leme et al. [5] and Sanchez-Carracedo et al. [31] found that results for eating disorder risk factors were in the opposite hypothesis direction, including results for appearance attitudes, eating disorders symptoms, and unhealthy weight control behaviors (e.g., skipped meals, eating very little, and fasting).

Leme et al. [5], Simpson et al. [52], and Neumark-Sztainer et al. [51] were the only studies that assessed the dietary intake, PA, and sedentary behaviors of the participants. These two studies showed an improvement in healthy eating and PA. Both showed that social support, particularly for the family, was improved after intervention along with other socio-cognitive aspects. For example, behavioral strategies for healthy eating, such as preparing meals or snacks with little fat or sugar.

4. Discussion

This systematic review filled a gap in the literature by assessing the impact of obesity prevention programs, with behavior change components, on weight outcomes in adolescents. Diet intervention, as either a primary goal or combined with PA, has emerged as a promising component in youth obesity prevention programs. In order to assess the impact of these programs, two approaches were compared: "energy-balance" and "shared risk factors for obesity and eating disorders". This systematic review highlights the specific differences in the program components and outcomes that goes above and beyond simply using BMI or other anthropometric measurement as the primary outcome. This review demonstrates better anthropometric outcome measures in the "energy-balance" programs that include PA components, such as enhanced physical education classes and encouragement of behavior change activities immediately post-intervention. Upon examination of interventional studies, PA seems to be moderately to highly effective in improving body composition, especially with improving resistance exercise [25,27,50] and increasing lean mass [71]. However, a posteriori effect on BMI and body weight may not be affected by PA. In line with previous work [71], several intervention studies were unable to prove success at long-term follow-up with PA outcomes. This may be explained by the approach used in these interventions, specifically educational and behavioral, which did not produce sustainable results. As shown in the risk of bias, a meta-analysis of reviews [71] has found low methodological quality of the studies included in the meta-analysis, a high level of heterogeneity, a limited number of studies available, mixed populations of overweight and non-overweight adolescents, as well as inadequate description of the interventions.

4.1. Combining Diet and Physical Activity Components to Promote Sustainable Lifestyle Behaviors

Numerous programs have been evaluated in the literature; however, the most effective strategy remains to be developed. Studies that have diet as a primary component have not been shown to be sustainable over time. The combination of diet and PA was shown to be a more effective tool against preventing youth obesity than diet alone. Schools were the most common setting where these interventions were implemented. Alternatively, results derived from combining PA or a diet with a secondary component like education and/or changes in the environment, such as policies focused on food canteens and the school curriculum, were associated with smaller effect sizes or even non-significant results [71]. When integrating diet and PA via mindfulness-based approaches seem to be more effective in preventing eating disorder risk factors, such as body image concerns and weight-control behaviors, and as consequence would help maintain a healthy weight status and well-being [72].

4.2. Maintaining Healthy Weight through Preventing Eating Disorders Risk Factors

Population-based interventions designed to maintain a healthy weight status that focused on shared risk factors for obesity and eating disorders have been a focus of attention in the general adolescent literature over the past few years [4,10,73,74]. However, few studies have been designed to reduce the burden of these shared risk factors. Indeed, results of at least some of the prevention programs suggest that weight status should not be the main outcome when considering obesity management strategies. This is because some of the disordered eating factors, mainly dieting, can lead to unsustainable dietary practices, which can lead to unhealthy weight gain or eating disorders [4]. Tanofsky-Kraff et al. [53], via exploratory post-hoc analyses, suggested evaluating the baseline social-adjustment problems (as an index for mental health problems) [75] and anxiety as moderators of the group effect on weight gain. This study revealed that adolescents with more psychosocial difficulties initially had the most benefit with intervention programs using interpersonal techniques compared to health education techniques. Moreover, both social functioning and anxiety moderate the intervention outcomes for depressed adolescents [76], as youths with a worse baseline psychosocial functioning experience the greatest improvements in depressive symptoms if they received interpersonal interventions targeting the shared risk factors as opposed to conventional approaches. Therefore, social adjustment and anxiety are important components for weight-related prevention trials and should directly focus on improving interpersonal functioning and negative mood states.

4.3. Other Factors That May Be Associated with an Increased Risk for Eating Disorders and Obesity, Which May Be the Target for Behavioral Interventions

Despite an overall improvement in the disordered eating risk factors, such as body satisfaction, unhealthy weight control behaviors, and teasing, two studies [5,31] identified an increased risk for these factors at follow-up, and female adolescents tend to have a less favorable impact on these risk factors than male participants. One study reported an increased risk for skipping meals, eating too little, and fasting at 6-month follow-up [5]. Similarly, a Spanish quasi-experimental trial [31] found that, post-intervention, a drive for thinness, being negatively affected, and self-esteem were in the hypothesized direction, but socio-attitudes towards appearance and eating disorder symptoms were in the opposite direction to what was hypothesized. All outcomes were non-significant. It is uncertain if these findings differ from the typical rate of development of eating disorders or obesity that are seen within obesity prevention trials targeting adolescents, and especially adolescent girls. Nevertheless, the early signs and symptoms of these shared risk factors in adolescents attempting to lose weight may be missed, particularly when the focus is on weight loss or the adolescent remains within or above a healthy weight status [18]. These findings support previous recommendations [77] that interventionists, public health policy makers, and other behavior-change researchers should monitor for the development of or exacerbation of these combined risk factors during weight-related prevention programs.

4.4. Caution When Targeting Other Modifiable and Non-Modifiable Risk Factors for Weight-Prevention Programs

Research suggests that attitudes towards individuals with obesity may be reduced through the provision of non-modifiable risk factors for these specific concerns [78]. Considering this, studies that focused on causes and risk factors for obesity and eating disorders identified in this review, as well as other corroborating reviews [73,79,80], showed that biological and genetic factors played a minor role in the etiology of these shared risk factors when compared with social–cultural factors. This was confirmed in studies that include both public and health professionals [73]. Thus, the published literature seems to indicate an opportunity for change in this respect. Even if successful, prevention programs of this kind presented conflicting ethical questions [81].

4.5. Interventions Should Be Based on Theory and Use of Psychometric Tested Measurements

The findings demonstrated that less than half of the studies with an energy-balance approach was theory-based, with the Social Cognitive Theory (SCT) [82,83] being the most used. A review suggest that interventions aimed at changing health behaviors in adolescents should target the key constructs of the theories [84]. For example, the core construct of the SCT is self-efficacy, which is the individual confidence in personal ability to acquire a certain health behavior [85]. Research criterion and findings with adolescents suggested that these constructs are important and reliable mechanisms of dietary and PA behaviors that can be changed when using extant intervention programs. However, given the validity of the theoretical determinants of behavior change in adolescents, it is hard to provide a conclusion. This might be due to the use of less optimal measures of mediators [84]. A product-o-coefficients test may be used to examine potential mechanisms of dietary [86] and physical activity behavior change [87], and this method has been used to identify mediators even if the intervention effects are not significant.

A study that tested the social cognitive mediators of behavior change [86], although none of the action theory results were significant, showed there was a few significant conceptual theory test results; this suggests that the intervention was not successful in changing key dietary and physical activity behaviors, yet the significant conceptual theory test results demonstrated that specific social cognitive constructs predicted behavior change in this trial [86,87]. Hence, findings of this review suggested the need for further good-quality, trial-based evidence, and highlights the importance of these potential mediators in changing health behaviors [88].

4.6. Final Thoughts on Effective Behavioral Change Interventions for Youth

As previously known [4,89], eating disorders and obesity share similar traits, but have not been the focus in the majority of the prevention trials. Further trials combining both fields are needed to clarify the components added to promote a positive food and weight relationship. For example, adding weight-teasing and body image with weight-status measurement are necessary to examine if the "shared risk factors for obesity and eating disorders" programs demonstrate key sustainable lifestyle behaviors from each weight-related component by motivating youth under a social–cognitive approach. Establishing such components would greatly inform a more precise weight-related behavioral-change prevention programs and public health policies.

4.7. Strengths and Limitations

The strength of this systematic review includes the development of a comprehensive search strategy applied in order to fill the literature gap on the impact of weight-related prevention trials, maintenance of a healthy weight status, and decreasing the burden of the shared risk factors for obesity and eating disorders among adolescents. However, there are some limitations of the current review that should be noted. Despite the authors' extensive efforts, including systematic searching of databases and manual searching of literature reference lists, it is possible that studies meeting the inclusion criteria may have been missed. Furthermore, only one author performed title, abstract, and full-text screenings. However, any uncertainties regarding study inclusion were resolved through discussion among three authors. Moreover, although strict inclusion and exclusion criteria were established, the aim of some studies included in this review was not explicitly to measure the influence of weight-related concerns on weight status and other behaviors. Thus, some outcome data was not provided in detail, limiting the conclusions able to be drawn in these instances. This review was also limited by the heterogeneity of the included studies, whereby reporting measures and outcomes were often not consistent. Finally, uncertainties on risk of bias information may be considered as a limitation. Some studies did not provide relevant information on certain sources of bias, such as allocation concealment and blinding of participants, personnel and outcome assessment, an underpowered study, and an analysis not accounting for clustering.

5. Conclusions

In sum, this systematic review showed that energy-balance interventions produced better results on weight outcomes when integrating physical activity associated with changes in school or other community environments. Improved disordered risk factors were seen in the shared risk factors, e.g., weight-control behaviors and shape and weight concerns, especially among overweight adolescents. However, some studies found non-significant effects or even an increased risk of these shared risk factors at the post-intervention stage among adolescent girls, suggesting that a more intensive or targeted approach may be needed for this at-risk group. These findings may suggest that efficacious approaches to support a sustainable weight status, by integrating the risk factors for eating disorders with changes in the environment, could promote healthy lifestyle behaviors, especially regarding diet and physical activity. However, more research is needed to examine how a shared risk factor approach can address both obesity and eating disorders, as well as to identify whether additional support is needed for adolescent girls.

Author Contributions: The review protocol was developed by A.C.B.L. Retrieval and screening of articles for inclusion criteria was undertaken A.C.B.L. with assistance from K.L.L.D. The risk of bias assessment was undertaken by A.C.B.L. and K.L.L.D. Significant revisions were completed by J.H., L.T., R.M.F. Additional revisions were provided by S.T.P., M.F., and G.L.F. All authors have read and agreed to the published version of the manuscript.

Funding: This research was funded by São Paulo State Research Foundation (FAPESP), grant number 2015/20852-7. R.M.F. receives productivity funding from the National Council for Scientific and Technological Development (grant number 402674/2016-2; 301597/207-0). São Paulo State Research Foundation (grant number 2017/23115-9) funded R.M.F. studies.

Conflicts of Interest: The authors declare no conflict of interest.

References

1. Rome, E.S. Obesity prevention and treatment. *Pediatr. Rev.* **2011**, *32*, 363–373. [CrossRef]
2. NCD Risk Factor Collaboration (NCD-RisC). Worldwide trends in body-mass index, underweight, overweight, and obesity from 1975 to 2016: A pooled analysis of 2416 population-based measurement studies in 128.9 million children, adolescents, and adults. *Lancet* **2017**, *390*, 2627–2642. [CrossRef]
3. Pont, S.J.; Puhl, R.; Cook, S.R.; Slusser, W. Stigma experienced by children and adolescents with obesity. *Pediatrics* **2017**, *140*, e20173034. [CrossRef]
4. Haines, J.; Neumark-Sztainer, D. Prevention of obesity and eating disorders: A consideration of shared risk factors. *Health Educ. Res.* **2006**, *21*, 770–782. [CrossRef]
5. Leme, A.C.B.; Philippi, S.T.; Thompson, D.; Nicklas, T.; Baranowski, T. "Healthy habits, healthy girls-Brazil": An obesity prevention program with added focus on eating disorders. *Eat. Weight Disord. EWD* **2019**, *24*, 107–119. [CrossRef]
6. De Giuseppe, R.; Di Napoli, I.; Porri, D.; Cena, H. Pediatric obesity and eating disorders symptoms: The role of the multidisciplinary treatment. A systematic review. *Front. Pediatr.* **2019**, *7*, 123. [CrossRef]
7. Fiechtner, L.; Fonte, M.L.; Castro, I.; Gerber, M.; Horan, C.; Sharifi, M.; Cena, H.; Taveras, E.M. Determinants of binge eating symptoms in children with overweight/obesity. *Child. Obes.* **2018**, *14*, 510–517. [CrossRef]
8. Swanson, S.A.; Crow, S.J.; Le Grange, D.; Swendsen, J.; Merikangas, K.R. Prevalence and correlates of eating disorders in adolescents. Results from the national comorbidity survey replication adolescent supplement. *Arch. Gen. Psychiatry* **2011**, *68*, 714–723. [CrossRef]
9. Murray, S.B.; Griffiths, S.; Mond, J.M. Evolving eating disorder psychopathology: Conceptualising muscularity-oriented disordered eating. *Br. J. Psychiatry* **2016**, *208*, 414–415. [CrossRef]

10. Leme, A.C.B.; Thompson, D.; Lenz Dunker, K.L.; Nicklas, T.; Tucunduva Philippi, S.; Lopez, T.; Vezina-Im, L.A.; Baranowski, T. Obesity and eating disorders in integrative prevention programmes for adolescents: Protocol for a systematic review and meta-analysis. *BMJ Open* **2018**, *8*, e020381. [CrossRef]

11. Evans, E.H.; Adamson, A.J.; Basterfield, L.; Le Couteur, A.; Reilly, J.K.; Reilly, J.J.; Parkinson, K.N. Risk factors for eating disorder symptoms at 12 years of age: A 6-year longitudinal cohort study. *Appetite* **2017**, *108*, 12–20. [CrossRef] [PubMed]

12. Veses, A.M.; Martínez-Gómez, D.; Gómez-Martínez, S.; Vicente-Rodriguez, G.; Castillo, R.; Ortega, F.B.; González-Gross, M.; Calle, M.E.; Veiga, O.L.; Marcos, A. Physical fitness, overweight and the risk of eating disorders in adolescents. The AVENA and AFINOS studies. *Pediatr. Obes.* **2014**, *9*, 1–9. [CrossRef]

13. World Health Organization. *Report of the Commission on Ending Childhood Obesity: Implementation Plan: Executive Summary*; World Health Organization: Geneva, Switzerland, 2017.

14. Rubino, F.; Puhl, R.M.; Cummings, D.E.; Eckel, R.H.; Ryan, D.H.; Mechanick, J.I.; Nadglowski, J.; Ramos Salas, X.; Schauer, P.R.; Twenefour, D.; et al. Joint international consensus statement for ending stigma of obesity. *Nat. Med.* **2020**, *26*, 485–497. [CrossRef]

15. Pegington, M.; French, D.P.; Harvie, M.N. Why young women gain weight: A narrative review of influencing factors and possible solutions. *Obes. Rev. Off. J. Int. Assoc. Study Obes.* **2020**, *21*, e13002. [CrossRef] [PubMed]

16. Neumark-Sztainer, D. Integrating messages from the eating disorders field into obesity prevention. *Adolesc. Med. State Art Rev.* **2012**, *23*, 529–543.

17. Neumark-Sztainer, D.; Levine, M.P.; Paxton, S.J.; Smolak, L.; Piran, N.; Wertheim, E.H. Prevention of body dissatisfaction and disordered eating: What next? *Eat. Disord.* **2006**, *14*, 265–285. [CrossRef]

18. Jebeile, H.; Gow, M.L.; Baur, L.A.; Garnett, S.P.; Paxton, S.J.; Lister, N.B. Treatment of obesity, with a dietary component, and eating disorder risk in children and adolescents: A systematic review with meta-analysis. *Obes Rev.* **2019**, *20*, 1287–1298. [CrossRef]

19. Moher, D.; Liberati, A.; Tetzlaff, J.; Altman, D.G.; The, P.G. Preferred Reporting items for systematic reviews and meta-analyses: The PRISMA statement. *PLoS Med.* **2009**, *6*, e1000097. [CrossRef]

20. World Health Organization (WHO). Health Topics—*Adolescent Health*. Available online: https://www.who.int/health-topics/adolescent-health#tab=tab_1 (accessed on 11 October 2020).

21. Schoenberg, N.E.; Tarasenko, Y.N.; Snell-Rood, C. Are evidence-based, community-engaged energy balance interventions enough for extremely vulnerable populations? *Transl. Behav. Med.* **2018**, *8*, 733–738. [CrossRef]

22. Sterne, J.A.C.; Savović, J.; Page, M.J.; Elbers, R.G.; Blencowe, N.S.; Boutron, I.; Cates, C.J.; Cheng, H.-Y.; Corbett, M.S.; Eldridge, S.M.; et al. RoB 2: A revised tool for assessing risk of bias in randomised trials. *BMJ (Clin. Res. Ed.)* **2019**, *366*, l4898. [CrossRef]

23. Sterne, J.A.C.; Hernán, M.A.; Reeves, B.C.; Savović, J.; Berkman, N.D.; Viswanathan, M.; Henry, D.; Altman, D.G.; Ansari, M.T.; Boutron, I.; et al. ROBINS-I: A tool for assessing risk of bias in non-randomised studies of interventions. *BMJ (Clin. Res. Ed.)* **2016**, *355*, i4919. [CrossRef] [PubMed]

24. Malakellis, M.; Hoare, E.; Sanigorski, A.; Crooks, N.; Allender, S.; Nichols, M.; Swinburn, B.; Chikwendu, C.; Kelly, P.M.; Petersen, S.; et al. School-Based systems change for obesity prevention in adolescents: Outcomes of the Australian capital territory "It's Your Move!". *Aust. N. Z. J. Public Health* **2017**, *41*, 490–496. [CrossRef]

25. Lubans, D.R.; Smith, J.J.; Plotnikoff, R.C.; Dally, K.A.; Okely, A.D.; Salmon, J.; Morgan, P.J. Assessing the sustained impact of a school-based obesity prevention program for adolescent boys: The ATLAS cluster randomized controlled trial. *Int. J. Behav. Nutr. Phys. Act.* **2016**, *13*, 92. [CrossRef]

26. Dewar, D.L.; Morgan, P.J.; Plotnikoff, R.C.; Okely, A.D.; Collins, C.E.; Batterham, M.; Callister, R.; Lubans, D.R. The nutrition and enjoyable activity for teen girls study: A cluster randomized controlled trial. *Am. J. Prev. Med.* **2013**, *45*, 313–317. [CrossRef]

27. Lubans, D.R.; Morgan, P.J.; Aguiar, E.J.; Callister, R. Randomized controlled trial of the physical activity leaders (PALs) program for adolescent boys from disadvantaged secondary schools. *Prev. Med. Int. J. Devoted Pract. Theory* **2011**, *52*, 239–246. [CrossRef]

28. Wilksch, S.M.; Paxton, S.J.; Byrne, S.M.; Austin, S.B.; McLean, S.A.; Thompson, K.M.; Dorairaj, K.; Wade, T.D. Prevention across the spectrum: A randomized controlled trial of three programs to reduce risk factors for both eating disorders and obesity. *Psychol. Med.* **2015**, *45*, 1811–1823. [CrossRef]

29. Lenz Dunker, K.L.; Claudino, A.M. Preventing weight-related problems among adolescent girls: A cluster randomized trial comparing the Brazilian 'New Moves' program versus observation. *Obes. Res. Clin. Pract.* **2018**, *12*, 102–115. [CrossRef]

30. Sgambato, M.R.; Cunha, D.B.; da Silva Nalin Souza, B.; Henriques, V.T.; da Rocha Muniz Rodrigues, R.; Viegas Rego, A.L.; Pereira, R.A.; Yokoo, E.M.; Sichieri, R. Effectiveness of school-home intervention for adolescent obesity prevention: Parallel school-randomized study. *Br. J. Nutr.* **2019**, 1–20. [CrossRef]

31. Sánchez-Carracedo, D.; Fauquet, J.; López-Guimerà, G.; Leiva, D.; Puntí, J.; Trepat, E.; Pàmias, M.; Palao, D. The MABIC project: An effectiveness trial for reducing risk factors for eating disorders. *Behav. Res. Ther.* **2016**, *77*, 23–33. [CrossRef]

32. González-Jiménez, E.; Cañadas, G.R.; Lastra-Caro, A.; Cañadas-De la Fuente, G.A. Efectividad de una intervención educativa sobre nutrición y actividad física en una población de adolescentes: Prevención de factores de riesgos endocrino-metabólicos y cardiovasculares. *Aquichan* **2014**, *14*, 549–559. [CrossRef]

33. Gonzalez, M.; Penelo, E.; Gutierrez, T.; Raich, R.M. Disordered eating prevention programme in schools: A 30-month follow-up. *Eur. Eat. Disord. Rev.* **2011**, *19*, 349–356. [CrossRef]

34. Ardic, A.; Erdogan, S. The effectiveness of the COPE healthy lifestyles TEEN program: A school-based intervention in middle school adolescents with 12-month follow-up. *J. Adv. Nurs.* **2017**, *73*, 1377–1389. [CrossRef]

35. Bonsergent, E.; Agrinier, N.; Thilly, N.; Tessier, S.; Legrand, K.; Lecomte, E.; Aptel, E.; Hercberg, S.; Collin, J.-F.; Briançon, S.; et al. Overweight and obesity prevention for adolescents: A cluster randomized controlled trial in a school setting. *Am. J. Prev. Med.* **2013**, *44*, 30–39. [CrossRef]

36. Jansen, W.; Borsboom, G.; Meima, A.; Joosten-Van Zwanenburg, E.; Mackenbach, J.P.; Raat, H.; Brug, J. Effectiveness of a primary school-based intervention to reduce overweight. *Int. J. Pediatr. Obes.* **2011**, *6*, e70–e77. [CrossRef]

37. Simon, C.; Schweitzer, B.; Oujaa, M.; Wagner, A.; Arveiler, D.; Triby, E.; Copin, N.; Blanc, S.; Platat, C. Successful overweight prevention in adolescents by increasing physical activity: A 4-year randomized controlled intervention. *Int. J. Obes.* **2008**, *32*, 1489–1498. [CrossRef]

38. Grydeland, M.; Bjelland, M.; Anderssen, S.A.; Klepp, K.-I.; Bergh, I.H.; Andersen, L.F.; Ommundsen, Y.; Lien, N. Effects of a 20-month cluster randomised controlled school-based intervention trial on BMI of school-aged boys and girls: The HEIA study. *Br. J. Sport. Med.* **2014**, *48*, 768. [CrossRef]

39. Yang, Y.; Kang, B.; Lee, E.Y.; Yang, H.K.; Kim, H.S.; Lim, S.Y.; Lee, J.H.; Lee, S.S.; Suh, B.K.; Yoon, K.H. Effect of an obesity prevention program focused on motivating environments in childhood: A school-based prospective study. *Int. J. Obes.* **2017**, *41*, 1027–1034. [CrossRef]

40. Rerksuppaphol, L.; Rerksuppaphol, S. Internet based obesity prevention program for Thai school children—A randomized control trial. *J. Clin. Diagn. Res.* **2017**, *11*, SC07–SC11. [CrossRef]

41. Fotu, K.F.; Millar, L.; Mavoa, H.; Kremer, P.; Moodie, M.; Snowdon, W.; Utter, J.; Vivili, P.; Schultz, J.T.; Malakellis, M.; et al. Outcome results for the Ma'alahi Youth Project, a Tongan community-based obesity prevention programme for adolescents. *Obes. Rev.* **2011**, *12*, 41–50. [CrossRef]

42. Stock, S.; Miranda, C.; Evans, S.; Plessis, S.; Ridley, J.; Yeh, S.; Chanoine, J.-P. Healthy buddies: A novel, peer-led health promotion program for the prevention of obesity and eating disorders in children in elementary school. *Pediatrics* **2007**, *120*, e1059–e1068. [CrossRef]

43. Castillo, I.; Solano, S.; Sepulveda, A.R. A controlled study of an integrated prevention program for improving disordered eating and body image among Mexican university students: A 3-month follow-up. *Eur. Eat. Disord. Rev.* **2019**, *27*, 541–556. [CrossRef]

44. Aperman-Itzhak, T.; Yom-Tov, A.; Vered, Z.; Waysberg, R.; Livne, I.; Eilat-Adar, S. School-Based intervention to promote a healthy lifestyle and obesity prevention among fifth- and sixth-grade children. *Am. J. Health Educ.* **2018**, *49*, 289–295. [CrossRef]

45. Lazorick, S.; Fang, X.; Hardison, G.T.; Crawford, Y. Improved body mass index measures following a middle school-based obesity intervention-the MATCH program. *J. Sch. Health* **2015**, *85*, 680–687. [CrossRef]

46. Nollen, N.L.; Mayo, M.S.; Carlson, S.E.; Rapoff, M.A.; Goggin, K.J.; Ellerbeck, E.F. Mobile technology for obesity prevention: A randomized pilot study in racial- and ethnic-minority girls. *Am. J. Prev. Med.* **2014**, *46*, 404–408. [CrossRef]

47. Fulkerson, J.A.; Friend, S.; Flattum, C.; Horning, M.; Draxten, M.; Neumark-Sztainer, D.; Gurvich, O.; Story, M.; Garwick, A.; Kubik, M.Y. Promoting healthful family meals to prevent obesity: HOME Plus, a randomized controlled trial. *Int. J. Behav. Nutr. Phys. Act.* **2015**, *12*, 154. [CrossRef]

48. Smith, J.J.B.; Morgan, P.J.P.; Plotnikoff, R.C.P.; Dally, K.A.P.; Salmon, J.P.; Okely, A.D.P.; Finn, T.L.; Lubans, D.R.P. Smart-Phone obesity prevention trial for adolescent boys in low-income communities: The ATLAS RCT. *Pediatrics* **2014**, *134*. [CrossRef]

49. Chen, J.-L.; Weiss, S.; Heyman, M.B.; Cooper, B.; Lustig, R.H. The efficacy of the web-based childhood obesity prevention program in Chinese American adolescents (Web ABC study). *J. Adolesc. Health* **2011**, *49*, 148–154. [CrossRef]

50. Shaw-Perry, M.; Horner, C.; Treviño, R.P.; Sosa, E.T.; Hernandez, I.; Bhardwaj, A. NEEMA: A school-based diabetes risk prevention program designed for African-American children. *J. Natl. Med. Assoc.* **2007**, *99*, 368–375.

51. Neumark-Sztainer, D.R.; Friend, S.E.; Flattum, C.F.; Hannan, P.J.; Story, M.T.; Bauer, K.W.; Feldman, S.B.; Petrich, C.A. New moves-preventing weight-related problems in adolescent girls a group-randomized study. *Am. J. Prev. Med.* **2010**, *39*, 421–432. [CrossRef]

52. Simpson, C.C.; Burnette, C.B.; Mazzeo, S.E. Integrating eating disorder and weight gain prevention: A pilot and feasibility trial of INSPIRE. *Eat. Weight Disord. EWD* **2019**, 761–775. [CrossRef]

53. Tanofsky-Kraff, M.; Shomaker, L.B.; Wilfley, D.E.; Young, J.F.; Sbrocco, T.; Stephens, M.; Brady, S.M.; Galescu, O.; Demidowich, A.; Olsen, C.H.; et al. Excess weight gain prevention in adolescents: Three-year outcome following a randomized controlled trial. *J. Consult. Clin. Psychol.* **2017**, *85*, 218–227. [CrossRef]

54. Stice, E.; Rohde, P.; Shaw, H.; Marti, C.N. Efficacy trial of a selective prevention program targeting both eating disorders and obesity among female college students: 1- and 2-year follow-up effects. *J. Consult. Clin. Psychol.* **2013**, *81*, 183–189. [CrossRef]

55. Franko, D.L.; Cousineau, T.M.; Rodgers, R.F.; Roehrig, J.P. BodiMojo: Effective Internet-based promotion of positive body image in adolescent girls. *Body Image* **2013**, *10*, 481–488. [CrossRef]

56. Austin, S.B.; Kim, J.; Wiecha, J.; Troped, P.J.; Feldman, H.A.; Peterson, K.E. School-Based overweight preventive intervention lowers incidence of disordered weight-control behaviors in early adolescent girls. *Arch. Pediatr. Adolesc. Med.* **2007**, *161*, 865. [CrossRef]

57. Austin, S.B.; Field, A.E.; Wiecha, J.; Peterson, K.E.; Gortmaker, S.L. The impact of a school-based obesity prevention trial on disordered weight-control behaviors in early adolescent girls. *Arch. Pediatr. Adolesc. Med.* **2005**, *159*, 225–230. [CrossRef]

58. Shomaker, L.B.; Tanofsky-Kraff, M.; Matherne, C.E.; Mehari, R.D.; Olsen, C.H.; Marwitz, S.E.; Bakalar, J.L.; Ranzenhofer, L.M.; Kelly, N.R.; Schvey, N.A.; et al. A randomized, comparative pilot trial of family-based interpersonal psychotherapy for reducing psychosocial symptoms, disordered-eating, and excess weight gain in at-risk preadolescents with loss-of-control-eating. *Int. J. Eat. Disord.* **2017**, *50*, 1084–1094. [CrossRef]

59. Lee, P.H.; Macfarlane, D.J.; Lam, T.H.; Stewart, S.M. Validity of the International Physical Activity Questionnaire Short Form (IPAQ-SF): A systematic review. *Int. J. Behav. Nutr. Phys. Act.* **2011**, *8*, 115. [CrossRef]

60. Simpson, K.; Parker, B.; Capizzi, J.; Thompson, P.; Clarkson, P.; Freedson, P.; Pescatello, L.S. Validity and reliability question 8 of the Paffenbarger Physical Activity Questionnaire among healthy adults. *J. Phys. Act. Health* **2015**, *12*, 116–123. [CrossRef]

61. Trott, M.; Jackson, S.E.; Firth, J.; Jacob, L.; Grabovac, I.; Mistry, A.; Stubbs, B.; Smith, L. A comparative meta-analysis of the prevalence of exercise addiction in adults with and without indicated eating disorders. *Eat. Weight Disord.* **2020**, 1–10. [CrossRef]

62. Stice, E.; Fisher, M.; Martinez, E. Eating disorder diagnostic scale: Additional evidence of reliability and validity. *Psychol. Assess.* **2004**, *16*, 60–71. [CrossRef]

63. Goldfein, J.A.; Devlin, M.J.; Kamenetz, C. Eating Disorder Examination-Questionnaire with and without instruction to assess binge eating in patients with binge eating disorder. *Int. J. Eat. Disord.* **2005**, *37*, 107–111. [CrossRef]

64. Fairburn, C.G.; Beglin, S.J. Assessment of eating disorders: Interview or self-report questionnaire? *Int. J. Eat. Disord.* **1994**, *16*, 363–370.

65. Gratz, K.L.; Roemer, L. Multidimensional assessment of emotion regulation and dysregulation: Development, factor structure, and initial validation of the difficulties in emotion regulation scale. *J. Psychopathol. Behav. Assess.* **2004**, *26*, 41–54. [CrossRef]

66. Thompson, J.K.; van den Berg, P.; Roehrig, M.; Guarda, A.S.; Heinberg, L.J. The sociocultural attitudes towards appearance scale-3 (SATAQ-3): Development and validation. *Int. J. Eat. Disord.* **2004**, *35*, 293–304. [CrossRef] [PubMed]

67. Thompson, J.K.; Cattarin, J.; Fowler, B.; Fisher, E. The Perception of Teasing Scale (POTS): A revision and extension of the Physical Appearance Related Teasing Scale (PARTS). *J. Personal. Assess.* **1995**, *65*, 146–157. [CrossRef] [PubMed]

68. Van Strien, T.; Frijters, J.E.R.; van Staveren, W.A.; Defares, P.B.; Deurenberg, P. The predictive validity of the Dutch Restrained Eating Scale. *Int. J. Eat. Disord.* **1986**, *5*, 747–755. [CrossRef]

69. Watson, D.; Clark, L.A. Affects Separable and Inseparable: On the Hierarchical Arrangement of the Negative Affects. *J. Personal. Soc. Psychol.* **1996**, *62*, 489–505. [CrossRef]

70. Lacey, J.; Lomax, A.J.; McNeil, C.; Marthick, M.; Levy, D.; Kao, S.; Nielsen, T.; Dhillon, H.M. A supportive care intervention for people with metastatic melanoma being treated with immunotherapy: A pilot study assessing feasibility, perceived benefit, and acceptability. *Support. Care Cancer* **2019**, *27*, 1497–1507. [CrossRef]

71. Psaltopoulou, T.; Tzanninis, S.; Ntanasis-Stathopoulos, I.; Panotopoulos, G.; Kostopoulou, M.; Tzanninis, I.G.; Tsagianni, A.; Sergentanis, T.N. Prevention and treatment of childhood and adolescent obesity: A systematic review of meta-analyses. *World J. Pediatr.* **2019**, *15*, 350–381. [CrossRef]

72. Morillo Sarto, H.; Barcelo-Soler, A.; Herrera-Mercadal, P.; Pantilie, B.; Navarro-Gil, M.; Garcia-Campayo, J.; Montero-Marin, J. Efficacy of a mindful-eating programme to reduce emotional eating in patients suffering from overweight or obesity in primary care settings: A cluster-randomised trial protocol. *BMJ Open* **2019**, *9*, e031327. [CrossRef]

73. Bullivant, B.; Rhydderch, S.; Griffiths, S.; Mitchison, D.; Mond, J.M. Eating disorders "mental health literacy": A scoping review. *J. Ment. Health* **2020**, *29*, 336–349. [CrossRef]

74. Philippi, S.T.; Leme, A.C.B. Weight-Teasing: Does body dissatisfaction mediate weight-control behaviors of Brazilian adolescent girls from low-income communities? *Cad. Saude Publica* **2018**, *34*, e00029817. [CrossRef]

75. Rzepa, S.; Weissman, M. Social Adjustment Scale Self-Report (SAS-SR). *Encycl. Qual. Life Well-Being Res.* **2014**, 6017–6021. [CrossRef]

76. Gunlicks-Stoessel, M.; Mufson, L.; Jekal, A.; Turner, J.B. The impact of perceived interpersonal functioning on treatment for adolescent depression: IPT-A versus treatment as usual in school-based health clinics. *J. Consult. Clin. Psychol.* **2010**, *78*, 260–267. [CrossRef]

77. Goldschmidt, A.B.; Aspen, V.P.; Sinton, M.M.; Tanofsky-Kraff, M.; Wilfley, D.E. Disordered eating attitudes and behaviors in overweight youth. *Obesity* **2008**, *16*, 257–264. [CrossRef]

78. Pena-Romero, A.C.; Navas-Carrillo, D.; Marin, F.; Orenes-Pinero, E. The future of nutrition: Nutrigenomics and nutrigenetics in obesity and cardiovascular diseases. *Crit. Rev. Food Sci. Nutr.* **2018**, *58*, 3030–3041. [CrossRef]

79. Hauck, C.; Cook, B.; Ellrott, T. Food addiction, eating addiction and eating disorders. *Proc. Nutr. Soc.* **2020**, *79*, 103–112. [CrossRef]

80. Wu, X.Y.; Yin, W.Q.; Sun, H.W.; Yang, S.X.; Li, X.Y.; Liu, H.Q. The association between disordered eating and health-related quality of life among children and adolescents: A systematic review of population-based studies. *PLoS ONE* **2019**, *14*, e0222777. [CrossRef]

81. Andersson, M.A.; Harkness, S.K. When do biological attributions of mental illness reduce stigma? Using qualitative comparative analysis to contextualize attributions. *Soc. Ment. Health* **2017**, *8*, 175–194. [CrossRef]

82. Bandura, A. *Social Foundations of Thought and Action: A Social Cognitive Theory*; Prentice-Hall, Inc.: Englewood Cliffs, NJ, USA, 1986.

83. Sittig, S.; McGowan, A.; Iyengar, S. Extensive review of persuasive system design categories and principles: Behavioral obesity interventions. *J. Med. Syst.* **2020**, *44*, 128. [CrossRef]

84. Neumark-Sztainer, D.; Story, M.; Hannan, P.J.; Rex, J. New Moves: A school-based obesity prevention program for adolescent girls. *Prev. Med.* **2003**, *37*, 41–51. [CrossRef]

85. Leme, A.C.; Philippi, S.T. Cultural adaptation and psychometric properties of social cognitive scales related to adolescent dietary behaviors. *Cad. Saúde Coletiva* **2014**, *22*, 252–259. [CrossRef]

86. McCabe, B.E.; Plotnikoff, R.C.; Dewar, D.L.; Collins, C.E.; Lubans, D.R. Social cognitive mediators of dietary behavior change in adolescent girls. *Am. J. Health Behav.* **2015**, *39*, 51–61. [CrossRef] [PubMed]

87. Dewar, D.L.; Plotnikoff, R.C.; Morgan, P.J.; Okely, A.D.; Costigan, S.A.; Lubans, D.R. Testing social-cognitive theory to explain physical activity change in adolescent girls from low-income communities. *Res. Q. Exerc. Sport* **2013**, *84*, 483–491. [CrossRef] [PubMed]
88. Cerin, E.; Barnett, A.; Baranowski, T. Testing theories of dietary behavior change in youth using the mediating variable model with intervention programs. *J. Nutr. Educ. Behav.* **2009**, *41*, 309–318. [CrossRef]
89. Irving, L.M.; Neumark-Sztainer, D. Integrating the prevention of eating disorders and obesity: Feasible or futile? *Prev. Med.* **2002**, *34*, 299–309. [CrossRef]

Publisher's Note: MDPI stays neutral with regard to jurisdictional claims in published maps and institutional affiliations.

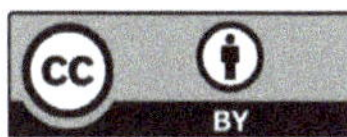

© 2020 by the authors. Licensee MDPI, Basel, Switzerland. This article is an open access article distributed under the terms and conditions of the Creative Commons Attribution (CC BY) license (http://creativecommons.org/licenses/by/4.0/).

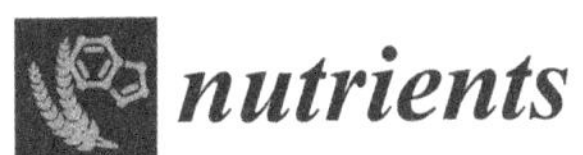 *nutrients*

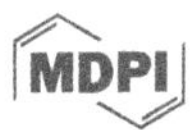

Article

Characteristic-Grouped Adiposity Indicators for Identifying Metabolic Syndrome in Adolescents: Develop and Valid Risk Screening Tools Using Dual Population

Yu-Ting Chin [1], Wei-Ting Lin [1,2], Pei-Wen Wu [1], Sharon Tsai [3], Chun-Ying Lee [4,5], David W. Seal [2], Ted Chen [2], Hsiao-Ling Huang [6] and Chien-Hung Lee [1,7,8,*]

[1] Department of Public Health, College of Health Sciences, Kaohsiung Medical University, Kaohsiung 80708, Taiwan; kiki13336586@gmail.com (Y.-T.C.); wtlin0123@gmail.com (W.-T.L.); catstar1211@gmail.com (P.-W.W.)

[2] Department of Global Community Health and Behavioral Sciences, School of Public Health and Tropical Medicine, Tulane University, New Orleans, LA 70112, USA; dseal@tulane.edu (D.W.S.); tchen@tulane.edu (T.C.)

[3] Department of Laboratory Medicine, Kaohsiung Municipal Siaogang Hospital, Kaohsiung 81267, Taiwan; 870718@kmuh.org.tw

[4] School of Medicine, College of Medicine, Kaohsiung Medical University, Kaohsiung 80708, Taiwan; cying@ms19.hinet.net

[5] Department of Family Medicine, Kaohsiung Medical University Hospital, Kaohsiung Medical University, Kaohsiung 807378, Taiwan

[6] Department of Oral Hygiene, College of Dental Medicine, Kaohsiung Medical University, Kaohsiung 80708, Taiwan; hhuang@kmu.edu.tw

[7] Research Center for Environmental Medicine, Kaohsiung Medical University, Kaohsiung 80708, Taiwan

[8] Department of Medical Research, Kaohsiung Medical University Hospital, Kaohsiung Medical University, Kaohsiung 80756, Taiwan

[*] Correspondence: cnhung@kmu.edu.tw; Tel.: +886-7-312-1101 (ext. 2141); Fax: +886−7−311−0811

Received: 23 August 2020; Accepted: 14 October 2020; Published: 16 October 2020

Abstract: A simple, robust, and characterized adiposity indicator may be appropriate to be used as a risk screening tool for identifying metabolic syndrome (MetS) in adolescents. This study used dual adolescent populations to develop and validate efficient adiposity indicators from 12 characterized candidates for identifying MetS that may occur during the transition from adolescence to young adulthood. Data from the adolescent Nutrition and Health Survey in Taiwan (n = 1920, 12–18 years) and the multilevel Risk Profiles for adolescent MetS study (n = 2727, 12–16 years) were respectively used as training and validation datasets. The diagnostic criteria defined by the International Diabetes Federation for adolescents (IDF-adoMetS) and the Joint Interim Statement for adults (JIS-AdMetS) were employed to evaluate MetS. In the training dataset, principal component analysis converted 12 interrelated obesity indices into bodyfat-, lipid-, and body-shape-enhanced groups, with the first two characteristic-groups having a higher discriminatory capability in identifying IDF-adoMetS and JIS-AdMetS. In the validation dataset, abdominal volume index (AVI) among girls and waist circumference (WC) among boys were respectively validated to have a higher Youden's index (0.740–0.816 and 0.798–0.884) in identifying the two MetS. Every 7.4 and 4.3 positive tests of AVI (cutoff = 13.96) had an accurate IDF-adoMetS and JIS-AdMetS, respectively, and every 32.4 total tests of WC (cutoff = 90.5 cm) had a correct identification for the two MetS. This study stresses the discriminatory capability of bodyfat- and lipid-enhanced adiposity indicators for identifying MetS. AVI and WC were, respectively, supported as a risk screening tool for identifying female and male MetS as adolescents transition to adulthood.

Keywords: adolescent; adiposity indicators; discriminatory capability; metabolic syndrome; obesity; principal component analysis; risk screening tool; Taiwan

---

1. Introduction

Metabolic syndrome (MetS) is a health hazard condition that reflects a constellation of several cardiometabolic risk factors, including excessive abdominal adiposity, high blood pressure and fasting plasma glucose, and abnormal triglyceride and high-density lipoprotein-cholesterol [1]. Longitudina studies have demonstrated that MetS makes adolescents higher susceptible to developing MetS, type 2 diabetes mellitus, and cardiovascular diseases in adult life [2–4]. Because MetS and its risk components occurring in childhood can be restored to normal [5], identifying and treating adolescents with this syndrome through an efficient risk screening implement is an advocated strategy for controlling subsequent adverse disease consequence.

Among 5 components of MetS, 3 cardiometabolic dysfunctions must be determined via blood biochemical examination. Because blood assessment is an invasive and more costly test approach, using it as a universal screening tool for MetS may be less feasible among younger children. Therefore, the development and validation of a simple and robust screening instrument for identifying adolescent MetS is a vital work for pediatric public health.

Anthropometric studies have reported that, compared with entire body fatness measured by body mass index (BMI), regional fat distribution is more associated with metabolic disturbances and cardiovascular health risks [6]. Adiposity investigations into measurement of bodyfat distribution have indicated that body adiposity index (BAI) can directly estimate bodyfat percentage [7]; body roundness index (BRI) is a predictor of the percentages of bodyfat and visceral adipose tissue [8]; waist-to-height ratio (WHtR) acts as a better risk marker for cardiovascular risk and shorter lifespan than BMI [9,10]; abdominal volume index (AVI) can be employed to estimate overall abdominal volume that theoretically comprises intra-abdominal fat and adipose tissue volumes [11]; waist circumference (WC) was a stronger predictor of obesity-related cancers [12]; waist-to-hip ratio (WHR) measures apple- or pear-like body shape [13]; a body shape index (ABSI) expresses the excess risk from high WC adjusted for the effect of BMI [14]; and conicity index (CoI) is a double cone-shaped derived indicator for abdominal obesity that can better predict 10-year cardiovascular risk [15,16]. In insulin and fat function studies, triglyceride-glucose index (TGI) was used as a surrogate for identifying insulin resistance among healthy subjects [17], and visceral adiposity index (VAI) was identified as an indicator of visceral adipose function and insulin sensitivity [18]. Furthermore, lipid accumulation product (LAP) has been recommended as a lipid overaccumulation indicator [19]. Although these adiposity indices were developed from adult populations, they may be appropriate to be used as a risk screening tool for identifying adolescent MetS, given that obesity has been a major risk for adult MetS [20,21].

Adiposity indices created to measure body adiposity, abdominal obesity, body shape, and visceral fat accumulation are a group of interrelated variables that may have a characteristic aggregation. Principal component (PC) analysis is a statistical method that can convert interrelated variables into reduced independent and interpretable PCs with a specific characteristic through multilinear subspace algorithms, and produce a characteristic-weighted combined score for each retained PC [22]. This technique has been used to study the clustering of pediatric cardiometabolic risk factors [23,24], and is an appropriate method to investigate the characteristic groups of adiposity indicators.

In one school-based longitudinal investigation of the alteration of MetS typology, 16.4%, 5.7%, and 1.1% of adolescents were observed to have new incident, unstable/remitted, or persistent MetS, respectively, as adolescents aged into young adulthood [5]. This raises the question of what kind of adiposity indicators can effectively identify MetS for children in school settings using criteria for adolescents and young adults. In the present study, data from the adolescent Nutrition and Health Survey in Taiwan (ado-NAHSIT) was used to develop efficient adiposity indicators from 12 characterized candidates for identifying MetS that may occur during the transition from adolescence to young adulthood. Data from the multilevel Risk Profiles for adolescent Metabolic Syndrome (mRP-aMS) study was employed to validate the accuracy and efficiency of determining MetS for the selected adiposity indicators.

2. Materials and Methods

2.1. Study Participants

The development and validation of adiposity indicators for this study were carried out using 2 sample series of participants. The first sample, obtained from the ado-NAHSIT, was used as a training dataset to derive optimal adiposity indicators for the identification of MetS using the criteria for adolescents and young adults. Two commonly applied diagnosis criteria for the 2 types of MetS were used. The second sample, obtained from the mRP-aMS study, was used as a validation dataset to verify the accuracy and efficiency of determining each MetS for the chosen obesity indicators. All participants and their guardians in the two studies provided a written informed assent and consent. The research protocol for this study was approved by the Institutional Review Board of Kaohsiung Medical University Hospital (IRB No., KMUHIRB-20120103; date of approval, 16 August 2019).

2.2. The Adolescent Nutrition and Health Survey in Taiwan (ado-NAHSIT)

The ado-NAHSIT as a nationwide adolescent survey in Taiwan that used a multistage, geographic area and population density stratified random sampling design to recruit nationally representative samples for investigating the health and nutritional status of adolescents aged 12–18 years during 2010–2011 [25]. Adolescents who had an official student status in the period of 2010–2011 and were enrolled in the public/private junior high schools and senior high/vocational schools in Taiwan were included in the study population; however, the adolescents who were enrolled in extension schools, special schools, and schools for overseas Chinese were excluded in the study population [26]. A comprehensive working group, consisting of trained interviewers, nutritionists, and medical personnel was organized to collect sociodemographic characteristics, dietary patterns, lifestyle factors, physical activity, puberty status, health and disease related information, anthropometry measurements, and clinical biochemical data from study participants. A detailed explanation for data collection, measurements, and laboratory assessments has been given previously [24–27]. Data were preserved for analysis of 1920 adolescents (971 girls and 949 boys) who had complete study variables and clinical parameters used to determine MetS (5 participants were excluded due to no information on sex variable).

2.3. The Multilevel Risk Profiles for Adolescent Metabolic Syndrome (mRP-aMS) Study

The mRP-aMS investigation was a large-scale cross-sectional study that employed a multistage, geographically stratified cluster sampling scheme to recruit representative adolescents for monitoring multilevel risk profiles of MetS in southern Taiwan during 2007–2009 [28–31]. In this study, data were collected about demographic characteristics, dietary patterns, lifestyle factors, physical activity, anthropometry variables, and biochemical data for 2727 adolescents (1399 girls and 1328 boys, response rate: 72.1%), aged 12–16 years [28,29]. All participants were included in the dataset for validating the accuracy of adiposity indicators in identifying MetS.

2.4. Diagnosis of Metabolic Syndrome

The International Diabetes Federation definition of MetS for adolescents aged 10–18 years (IDF-adoMetS) and the Joint Interim Statement for adult MetS (JIS-AdMetS) were respectively employed to determine MetS [20,32]. The 2 definitions correspond to a worldwide consensus for MetS diagnosis in adolescents and young adults. The categorical criteria and discrepancies for each risk component of IDF-adoMetS and JIS-AdMetS—including central obesity, high blood pressure, low high-density lipoprotein cholesterol, increased triglyceride, and elevated fasting plasma glucose—are presented in Supplementary Table S1. The IDF-adoMetS diagnosis requires an adolescent to have central obesity and 2 other abnormal components [32]. The JIS-AdMetS diagnosis requires having >3 any abnormal components [20].

2.5. Single Adiposity Indicators

Body weight, height, WC, and hip circumference was measured according to World Heatlh Organization standards [33]. Adiposity indicators—including BMI, BAI [7], BRI [8], WHR [13], WHtR [10], AVI [11], ABSI [14], CoI [15], TGI [17], VAI [18], and LAP [19]—were calculated using the following formulas:

$$\text{BMI} = \text{Weight (kg)} / \text{Height}^2 (\text{m})$$

$$\text{BAI} = \left[\text{Hip circumference (cm)} / \text{Height}^{1.5} (\text{m})\right] - 18$$

$$\text{BRI} = 364.2 - 365.5 \times \left\{1 - \left[\frac{\text{WC (m)}}{\pi \times \text{Height (m)}}\right]^2\right\}^{1/2}$$

$$\text{WHR} = \text{WC (cm)} / \text{Hip circumference (cm)}$$

$$\text{WHtR} = \text{WC (cm)} / \text{Height (cm)}$$

$$\text{AVI} = \left\{2 \times \text{WC}^2 (\text{cm}) + 0.7 \times \left[\text{WC (cm)} - \text{Hip circumference (cm)}\right]^2\right\} / 1000$$

$$\text{ABSI} = \text{WC (m)} / \left[\text{BMI}^{2/3} \times \text{Height}^{1/2} (\text{m})\right]$$

$$\text{CoI} = \text{WC (m)} / \left[0.109 \times \sqrt{\text{weight (kg)} / \text{height (m)}}\right]$$

$$\text{TGI} = \ln[\text{TG (mg/dL)} \times \text{FPG (mg/dL)} / 2]$$

$$\text{VAI}_{\text{female}} = \left[\frac{\text{WC (cm)}}{36.58 + (1.89 \times \text{BMI})}\right] \times \left[\frac{\text{Triglyceride (mmol/l)}}{0.81}\right] \times \left[\frac{1.52}{\text{HDL (mmol/l)}}\right]$$

$$\text{VAI}_{\text{male}} = \left[\frac{\text{WC (cm)}}{39.68 + (1.88 \times \text{BMI})}\right] \times \left[\frac{\text{Triglyceride (mmol/l)}}{1.03}\right] \times \left[\frac{1.31}{\text{HDL (mmol/l)}}\right]$$

$$\text{LAP}_{\text{female}} = [\text{WC (cm)} - 58] \times \text{Triglyceride (mmol/L)}$$

$$\text{LAP}_{\text{male}} = [\text{WC (cm)} - 65] \times \text{Triglyceride (mmol/L)}$$

To avoid the occurrence of non-positive values in LAP, we assigned the WC values of 59 cm and 66 cm to female and male participants, respectively, who had a negative LAP value [34]. This process does not affect the evaluation of discriminatory ability for this adiposity indicator.

2.6. Combined Adiposity Indicators

The indicators studied are adiposity-based variables that correlate with each other and may have a characteristic clustering. A combined score that additionally weights characterized adiposity indicators may offer a better discriminatory capability in identifying MetS. To investigate this issue, we transformed 12 adiposity indicators into 3 uncorrelated PCs that explained the majority of overall variance using PC analysis, as has been done in previous studies [22,23,35]. The technique of varimax rotation was employed to obtain 3 combined adiposity scores for the 3 PCs. Each combined score is a linear sum of the z-score of each adiposity indicator multiplying its corresponding factor loading. A factor loading represents the weight of an adiposity indicator in the linear sum and measures the correlation between an indicator and a combined score.

2.7. Statistical Analysis

Figure 1 presents a schematic framework of 6 analytic procedures for the development and validation of adiposity indicators using the training and validation datasets. First, the distributions of anthropometric characteristics and adiposity indicators for adolescents in the ado-NAHSIT and mRP-aMS studies were analyzed using means, standard deviations, or percentages. Second, PC analysis was used to determine the retained PCs from 12 adiposity indicators according to the criteria: eigenvalues ≥ 1 or PCs that exceeded the break in the scree plot [22,23]. The first 3 PCs—including PC1, PC2, and PC3—were retained. Because of the clustering, the 12 obesity indices were grouped as bodyfat-, body-shape-, and lipid-enhanced adiposity indicators. Third, partial correlation (pCorr), partial R-square (pR^2), and logistic regression-derived odds ratio (OR) were used to measure the adjusted correlation, contribution, and risk of each adiposity indicator for IDF-adoMetS and JIS-AdMetS, respectively, after controlling for possible confounding effects. Adjusted covariates included study area, age, daily energy intake, physical activity, puberty status, cigarette smoking, and alcohol drinking.

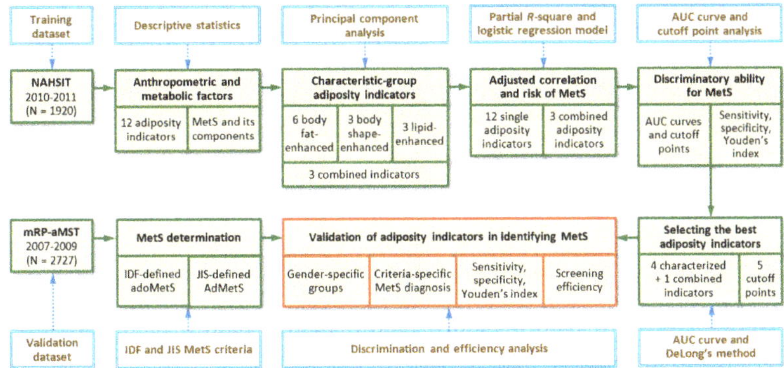

Figure 1. Schematic diagram of data analysis for the development and validation of adiposity indicators in discriminating adolescent metabolic syndrome. MetS, metabolic syndrome; IDF-defined adoMetS, International Diabetes Federation-defined adolescent MetS; JIS-defined AdMetS, Joint Interim Statement for adult MetS; AUC, area under receiver operating characteristic curve.

Fourth, area under receiver operating characteristic curve (AUC) and the sensitivity and specificity of each cutoff point were calculated for each adiposity indicator, and were used to evaluate the discriminatory ability in identifying IDF-adoMetS and JIS-AdMetS. The best cutoff points for each MetS identification were determined by maximizing the Youden's index (YI, i.e., sensitivity+specificity-1). Fifth, the adiposity indicators that have the greatest AUC and/or YI in each characteristic-group and in the PC score group were selected to verify their discriminatory capability in identifying each MetS. We employed DeLong et al.'s non-parametric approach to evaluate the difference of AUCs across the selected adiposity indicators [36]. Lastly, the external discriminatory abilities for the selected indicators in identifying each MetS were verified in the validation dataset for both sexes. Sensitivity, specificity, the number of positive tests per case identified, and total number of tests per case identified were used to evaluate screening efficiency of identifying MetS. All of the data were analyzed using the statistical software Stata version 16 (StataCorp., College Station, TX, USA).

3. Results

Table 1 displays the distribution of anthropometric characteristics, obesity indicators, and MetS, stratified by sex, for adolescents in the ado-NAHSIT and mRP-aMS studies. In both investigations, sex differences in anthropometric parameters and adiposity indicators were notable. The boys had higher levels of WC, systolic blood pressure, and fasting plasma glucose than the girls, whereas the girls had greater levels of high-density lipoprotein cholesterol than the boys. In the ado-NAHSIT study, 2.37% and 4.11% of girls and boys, respectively, had IDF-adoMetS; and 3.30% and 4.53% of girls and boys, respectively, had JIS-AdMetS. In the mRP-aMS investigation, 1.43% and 3.16% of female and male adolescents, respectively, had IDF-adoMetS; and 2.72% and 3.46% of female and male adolescents, respectively, had JIS-AdMetS.

In the training dataset, the principal component analysis (PCA) procedure converted 12 obesity indicators into a comparable PC structure in each sex, with the first 3 PCs explaining 92.4% and 93.8% of the overall variance for girls and boys, respectively (Table 2). Among girls, PC1, PC2, and PC3 scores were respectively more correlated with bodyfat-, body-shape-, and lipid-enhanced adiposity indicators (factor loadings: 0.366–0.419, 0.416–0.656, and 0.417–0.650; total variance explained: 52.7%, 20.7%, and 19.0%, respectively). Among boys, PC1 to PC3 were separately more associated with bodyfat-, lipid-, and body-shape-enhanced obesity indicators (factor loadings: 0.365–0.414, 0.314–0.682, and 0.377–0.767; total variance explained: 59.7%, 17.8%, and 16.3%, respectively).

Table 1. Distributions of anthropometric characteristics, obesity indicators, and metabolic syndrome (MetS) for adolescents in the adolescent Nutrition and Health Survey in Taiwan (ado-NAHSIT) and multilevel Risk Profiles for adolescent Metabolic Syndrome (mRP-aMS) studies.

Variables [1]	ado-NAHSIT			mRP-aMS		
	Girls	Boys	p [2]	Girls	Boys	p [2]
	(n = 971)	(n = 949)	Value	(n = 1399)	(n = 1328)	Value
Age, year	15.13 ± 1.86	15.18 ± 1.85	0.593	13.43 ± 1.02	13.43 ± 1.04	0.934
Weight, Kg	52.60 ± 10.50	62.39 ± 15.64	<0.001	50.92 ± 11.39	57.97 ± 15.84	<0.001
Height, cm	158.18 ± 5.81	168.02 ± 8.37	<0.001	156.20 ± 5.96	162.03 ± 8.85	<0.001
Hip circumference, cm	93.56 ± 7.81	94.13 ± 10.14	0.208	89.98 ± 8.45	91.16 ± 10.52	0.001
Adiposity indicators						
Body mass index	20.97 ± 3.68	21.96 ± 4.71	<0.001	20.79 ± 4.06	21.88 ± 4.92	<0.001
Body adiposity index	29.07 ± 3.79	25.24 ± 4.10	<0.001	28.11 ± 3.98	26.23 ± 4.47	<0.001
Body roundness index	2.97 ± 1.01	2.76 ± 1.28	<0.001	2.46 ± 1.06	2.71 ± 1.32	<0.001
Waist-to-hip ratio	0.80 ± 0.05	0.82 ± 0.04	<0.001	0.77 ± 0.06	0.81 ± 0.07	<0.001
Waist-to-height ratio	0.48 ± 0.05	0.46 ± 0.07	<0.001	0.45 ± 0.06	0.46 ± 0.07	<0.001
Abdominal volume index	11.72 ± 2.80	12.54 ± 3.99	<0.001	10.18 ± 2.88	11.57 ± 3.92	<0.001
A body shape index, 10^{-1}	0.79 ± 0.03	0.77 ± 0.03	<0.001	0.74 ± 0.05	0.75 ± 0.05	<0.001
Conicity index	1.20 ± 0.05	1.17 ± 0.06	<0.001	1.12 ± 0.08	1.15 ± 0.08	<0.001
Triglyceride-glucose index	8.04 ± 0.38	8.07 ± 0.42	0.054	8.03 ± 0.43	8.04 ± 0.48	0.602
Visceral adiposity index	2.52 ± 1.72	1.90 ± 1.33	<0.001	2.38 ± 1.40	1.73 ± 1.14	<0.001
Lipid accumulation product	72.14 ± 67.53	61.23 ± 78.42	0.001	53.38 ± 62.13	53.35 ± 77.21	0.986
Components of MetS						
Waist circumference, cm	75.23 ± 8.71	77.60 ± 12.01	<0.001	69.56 ± 9.72	74.31 ± 12.31	<0.001
Systolic blood pressure, mmHg	98.88 ± 8.71	108.86 ± 10.72	<0.001	106.54 ± 11.52	112.03 ± 13.24	<0.001
Diastolic blood pressure, mmHg	59.70 ± 7.68	60.25 ± 8.15	0.127	64.45 ± 9.02	64.61 ± 10.02	0.668
Triglyceride, mg/dL	71.50 ± 30.18	72.96 ± 34.48	0.327	75.18 ± 33.46	75.40 ± 39.15	0.874
High-density lipoprotein, mg/dL	57.43 ± 12.54	52.02 ± 11.60	<0.001	58.32 ± 13.35	55.79 ± 13.51	<0.001
Fasting plasma glucose, mg/dL	93.41 ± 10.45	96.51 ± 8.78	<0.001	89.55 ± 8.71	92.29 ± 8.32	<0.001
IDF-adoMetS (SE), %	2.37 (0.49)	4.11 (0.64)	0.034	1.43 (0.32)	3.16 (0.48)	0.003
JIS-AdMetS (SE), %	3.30 (0.57)	4.53 (0.68)	0.163	2.72 (0.43)	3.46 (0.50)	0.262

IDF-adoMetS, International Diabetes Federation-defined adolescent MetS; JIS-AdMetS, Joint Interim Statement for adult MetS. [1] Distribution was displayed as mean ± standard deviation or percentage and standard error. [2] p values for sex difference were obtained adjusted for age, except for variable 'age'.

Table 2. Factor loadings and characteristics for the first 3 principal components of obesity indicators in adolescents, stratified by sex, the ado-NAHSIT study.

Variables	Factor Loadings for Girls (n = 971)			Factor Loadings for Boys (n = 949)		
	PC1g	PC2g	PC3g	PC1b	PC2b	PC3b
Adiposity indicators						
Body mass index	0.419	−0.170	−0.004	0.414	−0.019	−0.193
Body adiposity index	0.399	−0.256	−0.062	0.383	−0.037	−0.165
Body roundness index	0.385	0.052	−0.012	0.366	−0.026	0.044
Waist-to-height ratio	0.387	0.056	−0.020	0.367	−0.025	0.046
Abdominal volume index	0.369	0.076	0.001	0.367	−0.003	−0.007
Waist circumference	0.366	0.100	−0.010	0.365	−0.005	0.003
A body shape index	−0.124	0.656	−0.019	−0.081	0.004	0.767
Conicity index	0.135	0.526	−0.027	0.200	−0.008	0.449
Waist-to-hip ratio	0.161	0.416	0.036	0.215	−0.025	0.377
Triglyceride-glucose index	−0.058	−0.048	0.650	−0.034	0.682	−0.004
Visceral adiposity index	−0.005	0.018	0.630	0.003	0.658	0.003
Lipid accumulation product	0.188	0.041	0.417	0.228	0.314	0.012
Eigenvalue	6.319	2.487	2.281	7.168	2.140	1.951
Proportion of variance explained	52.7%	20.7%	19.0%	59.7%	17.8%	16.3%
Cumulative proportion	52.7%	73.4%	92.4%	59.7%	77.6%	93.8%
Factor characteristic of PC score	Bodyfat-enhanced factor	Body-shape enhanced factor	Lipid-enhanced factor	Bodyfat-enhanced factor	Lipid-enhanced factor	Body-shape enhanced factor

PC1g-PC3g, principal components 1 to 3 for girls; PC1b-PC3b, principal components 1 to 3 for boys.

Figure 2 illustrates the covariate-adjusted risks of IDF-adoMetS and JIS-AdMetS associated with single and combined adiposity indicators in the training dataset. Apart from ABSI for the girls, all obesity indicators were associated with a significantly higher risk of developing MetS. Standardized LAP was the strongest risk factor for girls in the IDF-adoMetS and JIS-AdMetS (adjusted OR = 5.5 and 7.9, respectively), while standardized WC was the strongest risk factor for boys in the 2 MetS (adjusted OR = 6.2 and 5.5, respectively).

Table 3 presents the pCorr and pR^2 of single and combined adiposity indicators associated with the number of abnormal IDF-adoMetS and JIS-AdMetS components in ado-NAHSIT participants. For the IDF-adoMetS, AVI, WHR, LAP, and PC1 respectively had the highest pCorr (0.613, 0.443, 0.613, and 0.621 in girls and 0.623, 0.502, 0.648, and 0.622 in boys) in bodyfat-enhanced, body-shape-enhanced, lipid-enhanced, and combined adiposity index groups, after adjusting for the covariates. These obesity indicators separately explained the greatest variability in the number of abnormal IDF-adoMetS components in each group (pR^2, 19.6–38.6% in girls; 25.2–42.1% in boys). Comparable pCorr and pR^2 patterns for these adiposity indicators were observed for the JIS-AdMetS.

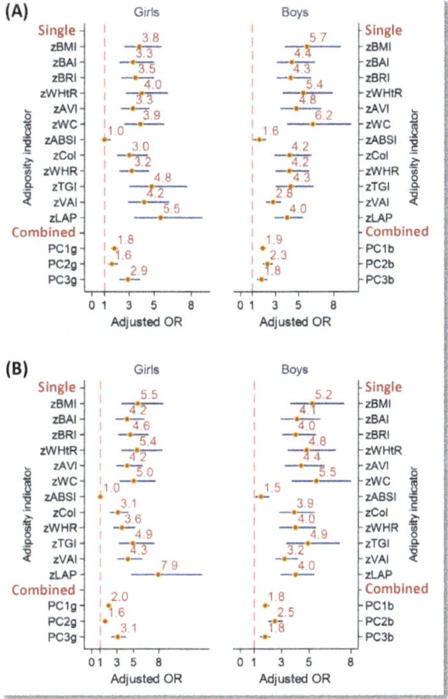

Figure 2. Adjusted odds ratios of IDF-adoMetS (**A**) and JIS-AdMetS (**B**) associated with single and combined adiposity indicators in adolescents, the ado-NAHSIT study. Adjusted ORs were adjusted for study area, age, daily energy intake, physical activity, puberty status, cigarette smoking and alcohol drinking. Adiposity indicators were standardized to a z-score. MetS, metabolic syndrome; OR, odds ratio; IDF-adoMetS, International Diabetes Federation-defined adolescent MetS; JIS-AdMetS, Joint Interim Statement for adult MetS; BMI, body mass index; BAI, body adiposity index; BRI, body roundness index; WHtR, waist-to-height ratio; AVI, abdominal volume index; WC, waist circumference; ABSI, a body shape index; CoI, conicity index; WHR, waist-to-hip ratio; TGI, triglyceride-glucose index; VAI, visceral adiposity index; LAP, lipid accumulation product; PC1g-PC3g, principal component 1 to 3 for girls; PC1b-PC3b, principal component 1 to 3 for boys.

Table 3. Partial correlations of single and combined adiposity indicators with the number of abnormal metabolic syndrome components in adolescents, the ado-NAHSIT study.

Variables	IDF-adoMetS				JIS-AdMetS			
	Girls		Boys		Girls		Boys	
	pCorr [1]	pR^2	pCorr [1]	pR^2	pCorr [1]	pR^2	pCorr [1]	pR^2
Single indicator								
Bodyfat-enhanced group								
Body mass index	0.596 *	35.5%	0.618 *	38.2%	0.601 *	36.2%	0.618 *	38.2%
Body adiposity index	0.471 *	22.2%	0.525 *	27.6%	0.479 *	23.0%	0.525 *	27.6%
Body roundness index	0.606 *	36.7%	0.611 *	37.4%	0.607 *	36.9%	0.611 *	37.4%
Waist-to-height ratio	0.605 *	36.6%	0.601 *	36.2%	0.607 *	36.9%	0.601 *	36.2%
Abdominal volume index	0.613 *	37.6%	0.623 *	38.8%	0.611 *	37.3%	0.623 *	38.8%
Waist circumference	0.612 *	37.5%	0.610 *	37.2%	0.611 *	37.4%	0.610 *	37.2%
Body-shape-enhanced group								
A body shape index	0.022	0.1%	0.127 *	1.6%	0.006	0.0%	0.127 *	1.6%
Conicity index	0.376 *	14.1%	0.471 *	22.2%	0.364 *	13.3%	0.471 *	22.2%
Waist-to-hip ratio	0.443 *	19.6%	0.502 *	25.2%	0.437 *	19.1%	0.502 *	25.2%
Lipid-enhanced group								
Triglyceride-glucose index	0.402 *	16.2%	0.482 *	23.3%	0.414 *	17.1%	0.482 *	23.3%
Visceral adiposity index	0.544 *	29.6%	0.555 *	30.8%	0.565 *	31.9%	0.555 *	30.8%
Lipid accumulation product	0.613 *	37.6%	0.648 *	42.1%	0.606 *	36.7%	0.648 *	42.1%
Combined indicator (score) [2]								
PC1	0.621 *	38.6%	0.622 *	38.7%	0.623 *	38.8%	0.622 *	38.7%
PC2	0.230 *	5.3%	0.558 *	31.1%	0.215 *	4.6%	0.558 *	31.1%
PC3	0.535 *	28.6%	0.254 *	6.5%	0.547 *	29.9%	0.254 *	6.5%

pCorr, partial correlation coefficient; pR^2, partial *R*-square; PC, principal component; *, $p < 0.05$. [1] pCorr and pR^2 were adjusted for study area, age, daily energy intake, physical activity, puberty status, cigarette smoking and alcohol drinking. [2] PC1, PC2, and PC3 were bodyweight-, bodyshape-, and lipid-enhanced factors, respectively, in girls. The corresponding PCs were bodyweight-, lipid-, and bodyshape-enhanced factors, respectively, in boys.

Table 4 presents the discriminatory abilities of adiposity indicators in identification of IDF-adoMetS and JIS-AdMetS among ado-NAHSIT adolescents. For both sexes, AVI/WC, WHR, LAP, and PC1 respectively had the greatest AUC for identifying IDF-adoMetS (0.941/0.941, 0.826, 0.942, and 0.939 among girls; 0.955/0.955, 0.898, 0.956, and 0.953 among boys) in bodyfat-enhanced, body- shape-enhanced, lipid-enhanced, and combined indicator groups. Similar results for these 5 indicators were found for the JIS-AdMetS (0.916/0.916, 0.833, 0.921, and 0.918 among girls; 0.922/0.922, 0.871, 0.938, and 0.922 among boys). YI provided comparable information for the two MetS. Using the AVI cutoff points of 13.96 for girls and 16.57 for boys, respectively, this adiposity indicator revealed a superior discrimination in identifying IDF-adoMetS (sensitivity/specificity: 95.7%/86.7% among girls; 100.0%/88.4% among boys) and JIS-AdMetS (sensitivity/specificity: 93.8%/87.4% among girls and 90.7%/88.3% among boys).

Figure 3 illustrates the differences in AUCs for identifying IDF-adoMetS and JIS-AdMetS across 5 superlative adiposity indicators in the training dataset. The AUCs were compatible across AVI, WC, LAP, and PC1. Nevertheless, all were significantly greater than that for WHR for the 2 MetS across both sexes (all *p*-values $\leq$ 0.028).

Table 5 presents the MetS discriminatory ability for the selected adiposity indicators in mRP-aMS adolescents using the cutoff points determined by the training dataset. Among girls, AVI (0.816) and PC1 (0.826) had the highest YI for identifying IDF-adoMetS and JIS-AdMetS, respectively, and the second highest YI was WC (0.814) and AVI (0.740). Among boys, WC provided the greatest YI for IDF-adoMetS (0.884) and JIS-AdMetS (0.798), and AVI (0.860) and PC1 (0.787) offered the second highest YI for the 2 MetS, respectively. For girls, AVI had a superior identification efficiency in positive test number, in that every 7.4 and 4.3 positive tests of AVI had a correct IDF-adoMetS and JIS-AdMetS identification. For boys, WC had an exceptional detection efficiency in total test number, in that every 32.4 tests of WC had an accurate identification in both MetS.

Table 4. Discriminations of single and combined adiposity indicators in the identification of adolescent metabolic syndrome in the ado-NAHSIT study.

| | IDF-adoMetS | | | | | | | | | | JIS-AdMetS | | | | | | | | | |
| | Girls | | | | | Boys | | | | | Girls | | | | | Boys | | | | |
Variables	AUC	Cutoff Point	Sen. %	Spe. %	YI	AUC	Cutoff Point	Sen. %	Spe. %	YI	AUC	Cutoff Point	Sen. %	Spe. %	YI	AUC	Cutoff Point	Sen. %	Spe. %	YI
Single indicator																				
Bodyfat-enhanced group																				
BMI	0.937 *	23.34	95.7	81.4	0.771	0.954*	27.10	97.4	89.0	0.864	0.913 *	23.34	93.8	82.1	0.759	0.925 *	27.10	88.4	89.0	0.773
BAI	0.841 *	29.94	91.3	65.4	0.567	0.904 *	27.39	97.4	75.8	0.733	0.830 *	31.12	81.3	76.4	0.576	0.876 *	27.39	93.0	75.9	0.690
BRI	0.924 *	3.60	95.7	82.4	0.780	0.943 *	3.60	100.0	82.7	0.827	0.907 *	3.60	93.8	83.1	0.768	0.912 *	3.60	93.0	82.8	0.758
WHtR	0.924 *	0.51	95.7	82.4	0.780	0.943 *	0.51	100.0	82.7	0.827	0.907 *	0.51	93.8	83.1	0.768	0.912 *	0.51	93.0	82.8	0.758
AVI	0.941 *	13.96	95.7	86.7	0.824	0.955 *	16.57	100.0	88.4	0.884	0.916 *	13.96	93.8	87.4	0.812	0.922 *	16.57	90.7	88.3	0.790
WC	0.941 *	82.7	95.7	86.3	0.819	0.955 *	90.5	100.0	88.2	0.882	0.916 *	82.7	93.8	87.0	0.808	0.922 *	90.5	90.7	88.2	0.789
Body-shape-enhanced group																				
ABSI	0.492	0.082	30.4	79.5	0.100	0.632 *	0.076	84.6	44.8	0.295	0.489	0.083	15.6	90.1	0.057	0.614 *	0.076	81.4	44.8	0.262
CoI	0.767 *	1.26	52.2	89.8	0.419	0.896 *	1.22	92.3	83.1	0.754	0.758 *	1.26	53.1	90.2	0.433	0.864*	1.22	86.0	83.1	0.692
WHR	0.826 *	0.82	82.6	70.6	0.532	0.898 *	0.85	92.3	80.0	0.723	0.833 *	0.82	81.3	71.0	0.523	0.871 *	0.85	88.4	80.1	0.685
Lipid-enhanced group																				
TGI	0.849 *	8.55	73.9	92.4	0.663	0.860 *	8.24	87.2	70.4	0.576	0.853 *	8.55	71.9	93.0	0.648	0.872 *	8.40	79.1	80.7	0.598
VAI	0.915 *	4.21	73.9	92.7	0.666	0.877 *	2.60	76.9	82.6	0.596	0.910 *	3.60	78.1	88.4	0.665	0.887 *	2.60	79.1	83.0	0.621
LAP	0.942 *	91.67	95.7	79.3	0.750	0.956 *	93.33	100.0	82.0	0.820	0.921 *	137.87	78.1	93.6	0.717	0.938 *	93.33	97.7	82.2	0.799
Combined indicator [1]																				
PC1 score	0.939 *	1.61	95.7	81.9	0.775	0.953 *	2.54	100.0	86.4	0.864	0.918 *	2.69	87.5	89.8	0.773	0.922 *	2.54	93.0	86.4	0.794
PC2 score	0.669 *	1.56	52.2	85.9	0.380	0.883 *	0.81	79.5	80.8	0.603	0.673 *	1.06	56.3	78.5	0.347	0.893 *	0.81	81.4	81.1	0.625
PC3 score	0.887 *	1.97	73.9	93.7	0.676	0.732 *	0.23	79.5	62.5	0.420	0.887 *	1.42	78.1	90.2	0.683	0.710 *	0.23	74.4	62.5	0.369

IDF-adoMetS, International Diabetes Federation-defined adolescent MetS; JIS-AdMetS, Joint Interim Statement for adult MetS; AUC, area under receiver operating characteristic curve; Sen., sensitivity; Spe., specificity; YI, Youden's index; BMI, body mass index; BAI, body adiposity index; BRI, body roundness index; WHtR, waist-to-height ratio; AVI, abdominal volume index; WC, waist circumference; ABSI, a body shape index; CoI, conicity index; WHR, waist-to-hip ratio; TGI, triglyceride-glucose index; VAI, visceral adiposity index; LAP, lipid accumulation product; PC, principal component. * denotes $p < 0.05$ for a significant discriminatory ability of adiposity indicator using AUC analysis. [1] PC1, PC2, and PC3 were bodyweight-, bodyshape-, and lipid-weighted factors, respectively, in girls, and the corresponding PCs were bodyweight-, lipid-, and bodyshape-weighted factors in boys.

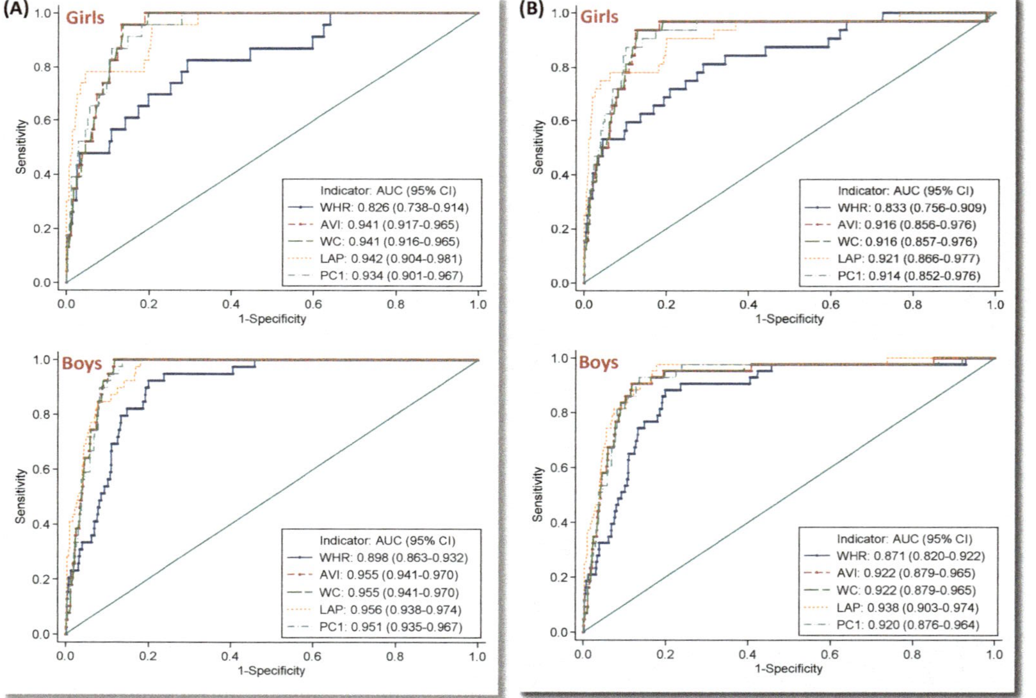

Figure 3. Receiver operating characteristic curves of identifying (**A**) IDF-adoMetS and (**B**) JIS-AdMetS for selected adiposity indicators in girls and boys, the ado-NAHSIT study. The AUCs of identifying IDF-adoMetS for AVI, WC, LAP, and PC1 were significantly higher than that for WHR in girls and boys (all p values ≤ 0.020), and the AUCs of determining JIS-AdMetS for AVI, WC, LAP, and PC1 were also significantly greater than that for WHR in girls and boys (all p values ≤ 0.028). AUC, area under receiver operating characteristic curve; WHR, waist-to-hip ratio; AVI, abdominal volume index; WC, waist circumference; LAP, lipid accumulation product; PC1, principal component 1 (bodyfat-enhanced factor).

Table 5. Discriminations of selected adiposity indicators in the identification of adolescent metabolic syndrome in the validation data in the mRP-aMS study.

Factors	Girls ($n = 1399$)										Boys ($n = 1328$)									
	IDF-adoMetS Proportion = 1.43%					JIS-AdMetS Proportion = 2.72%					IDF-adoMetS Proportion = 3.16%					JIS-AdMetS Proportion = 3.46%				
	AVI	WC	WHR	LAP	PC1	AVI	WC	WHR	LAP	PC1	AVI	WC	WHR	LAP	PC1	AVI	WC	WHR	LAP	PC1
Cutoff point	13.96	82.7	0.82	91.67	1.61	13.96	82.7	0.82	137.87	2.69	16.57	90.5	0.85	93.33	2.54	16.57	90.5	0.85	93.33	2.54
Discrimination																				
Sensitivity (SE), %	90.0 (6.7)	90.0 (6.7)	85.0 (8.0)	85.0 (8.0)	95.0 (4.9)	81.6 (6.3)	81.6 (6.3)	84.2 (5.9)	76.3 (6.9)	92.1 (4.4)	95.2 (3.3)	97.6 (2.4)	95.2 (3.3)	92.9 (4.0)	97.6 (2.4)	87.0 (5.0)	89.1 (4.6)	89.1 (4.6)	93.5 (3.6)	91.3 (4.2)
Specificity (SE), %	91.6 (0.7)	91.4 (0.8)	79.8 (1.1)	85.7 (0.9)	82.2 (1.0)	92.4 (0.7)	92.3 (0.7)	80.7 (1.1)	94.1 (0.6)	90.4 (0.8)	90.7 (0.8)	90.7 (0.8)	75.9 (1.2)	83.4 (1.0)	87.4 (0.9)	90.7 (0.8)	90.7 (0.8)	75.9 (1.2)	83.7 (1.0)	87.4 (0.9)
Youden's index	0.816	0.814	0.648	0.707	0.772	0.740	0.739	0.649	0.704	0.826	0.860	0.884	0.711	0.763	0.850	0.777	0.798	0.650	0.772	0.787
No. of positive test per case identified	7.4	7.6	17.4	12.6	13.9	4.3	4.4	9.2	3.8	4.7	4.0	3.9	8.8	6.5	5.0	4.0	3.9	8.5	5.9	4.8
Total no. of test per case identified	77.7	77.7	82.3	82.3	73.6	45.1	45.1	43.7	48.2	40.0	33.2	32.4	33.2	34.1	32.4	33.2	32.4	32.4	30.9	31.6

IDF-adoMetS, International Diabetes Federation-defined adolescent MetS; JIS-AdMetS, Joint Interim Statement for adult MetS; AVI, abdominal volume index; WC, waist circumference; WHR, waist-to-hip ratio; LAP, lipid accumulation product; PC1, bodyfat-enhanced principal component; SE, standard error.

4. Discussion

Except for the ABSI for girls, the single and combined adiposity indicators investigated were all qualified as a risk marker for IDF-adoMetS and JIS-AdMetS after taking multiple confounding effects into account. In the training dataset, AVI/WC, WHR, LAP, and PC1 were, respectively, the principal adiposity indicators for identifying the 2 MetS among bodyfat-enhanced, body-shape-enhanced, lipid-enhanced, and combined indicator groups for both sexes. In the validation dataset, AVI/WC for IDF-adoMetS and PC1/AVI for JIS-AdMetS among girls, and WC/AVI for IDF-adoMetS and WC/PC1 for JIS-AdMetS among boys were validated to have an excellent discrimination for the identification of MetS.

For the diagnosis of MetS, the IDF-adoMetS criteria (central obesity + 2 other abnormal components) are stricter than that for JIS-AdMetS (any 3 or more abnormal components) [20,32]; thus, the proportions of MetS for IDF-adoMetS in the 2 study samples were both lower than that for JIS-AdMetS (Table 1). Adolescence is an important growth stage that can carry health hazards into young adulthood. Our study examined and validated the accuracy of adiposity indicators for determining IDF-adoMetS and JIS-AdMetS. This method can investigate the possible application for obesity indicators in identifying MetS during the transition from adolescence to young adulthood.

The assessed obesity indicators were derived from mathematical models for abdominal fat and adipose tissue volumes [11,13–15], the measurements of bodyfat and visceral adipose tissue using dual energy X-ray absorptiometry and/or magnetic resonance imaging [7,8], or their association with visceral fat dysfunction, central lipid accumulation, and cardiometabolic risks [9,10,17–19,37]. Nevertheless, their correlations with each other are undiscussed. Our PC analysis indicated that BMI, BAI, BRI, WHtR, AVI, and WC were relatedly clustered in bodyfat-enhanced PC, ABSI, CoI, and WHR in body shape-enhanced PC, and TGI, VAI and LAP in lipid-enhanced PC, respectively. This implies that these adiposity indicators have characteristic aggregation. Additionally, the 3 characterized PC scores were associated with IDF-adoMetS and JIS-AdMetS in a different risk (lipid-enhanced PC score having the highest risk in both MetS, Figure 2) and with abnormal MetS component numbers in a heterogenous correlation (bodyfat-enhanced PC score having the greatest correlation, Table 3) among both sexes. These findings suggest that characteristic-specific adiposity indicators should be separately considered in the valuation of their associations with various health risks given their interrelated nature.

This study revealed that all adiposity indicators (ABSI aside) were positively associated with IDF-adoMetS and JIS-AdMetS risks and their abnormal component numbers among girls and boys, and the associations were statistically independent of potential confounders. Obesity is a vital contributor of adolescent MetS [21,32]. In a meta-analysis, childhood adiposity was verified as a significant predictor for the risks of abnormal carotid intima media thickness and dysglycemia in adulthood [38]. Although specific nutritional intake and lifestyles might be valuable for enhancing the accuracy of MetS screening, the adiposity indictor is still a single, simple, robust, and applicable risk-screening tool for identifying adolescent MetS in the community. Even the selection of an appropriate indicator and its associated cutoff point may depend on sex, age, and ethnic/cultural group. ABSI is an indicator that was created to adjust for the effect of BMI [14]. As observed in this study this index was not substantially associated with the BMI-correlated MetS outcomes.

In the training dataset, we found that bodyfat- and lipid-enhanced adiposity indicators generally had a better discriminating ability for identifying IDF-adoMetS and JIS-AdMetS than did body-shape-enhanced indicators among both sexes (AUCs, 0.830–0.956 vs. 0.489–0.898, Table 4). The AUCs for the superlative adiposity indicators of bodyfat- and lipid-enhanced groups were both significantly higher than that for the body-shape-enhanced group (Figure 3). Brazilian, Chilean, and Spanish investigators have recommended the bodyfat-enhanced indicators WHtR, AVI, and BMI as an excellent screening tool for adolescent MetS [39–42]. Although no adolescent studies have investigated LAP and VAI, one adult study reported that LAP was the most accurate indicator for determining male and female MetS [43]. Obesity is a growing global health problem that increases the risk of multiple physical and mental disorders [44–46]. These results indicate that bodyfat- and lipid-enhanced adiposity indicators should be intensively applied in risk assessments of the association between pediatric obesity and cardiometabolic diseases.

Studies that have evaluated anthropometric indicators for the identification of adolescent MetS in the community have found that AVI and WC for both girls and boys in Spain, BMI/WC for females and WHtR/WC for males in Chile, and WHtR for both sexes in Brazil have an excellent capacity for discriminating MetS [39–41]. However, there was a lack of validation of screening accuracy and efficiency for the indicators in these studies. Using a comparable adolescent population for validation, this investigation demonstrated that AVI/WC for girls and WC/AVI for boys had an excellent discriminating ability for identifying IDF-adoMetS in the community; however, the best indicators in discriminating JIS-AdMetS were PC1/AVI for girls and WC/PC1 for boys. This indicates that the AVI- and WC-included bodyfat-enhanced combined score (PC1) becomes more significant in detecting JIS-AdMetS. Although PC1 was recognized as an excellent adiposity indicator for identifying JIS-AdMetS, it requires intricate calculation. In community practices, our study suggests AVI as a female, and WC as a male, risk screening tool for MetS that can be applied to the transition from adolescence to young adulthood in a Taiwanese population.

In this study, the AVI cutoff points for identifying female IDF-adoMetS and JIS-AdMetS were both 13.96. Evaluated in the validation sample, 90.0% and 81.6% of sensitivity and 91.6% and 92.4% of specificity were observed (YI, 0.816 and 0.740), respectively, for the two MetS. AVI also was recommended as a risk-screening instrument for identifying female IDF-adoMetS in Spanish adolescents; however, the YI of this indicator with cutoff of 10.89 was only 0.70 (sensitivity, 100.0% and specificity, 70.0%) [39]. In our investigation, the WC cutoff points for determining male IDF-adoMetS and JIS-AdMetS were both 90.5 cm, which is close to the abnormal level of central obesity defined for Asian adults (WC $\geq$ 90 cm) [20]. Evaluated in the validation sample, every 32.4 tests of WC were observed to have an accurate IDF-adoMetS and JIS-AdMetS, respectively. In Spain, WC was suggested as an anthropometric discriminator for identifying male IDF-adoMetS, in which the cutoff of 75.0 cm rendered a 0.57 of YI (sensitivity, 100.0% and specificity, 75.0%) [39]. The discriminating abilities of AVI and WC for identifying IDF-adoMetS were confirmed in a southeast Spanish adolescent population [47].

In a clinically established adolescent database, if the blood samples of the participants had not been collected, or blood samples had not been examined for MetS-related variables, an adiposity indicator with very high sensitivity may be used as a tool for discovering adolescent MetS. Furthermore, an adiposity indicator with very high specificity may be employed as an instrument for confirming adolescent MetS. This framework can be applied to clinical settings. However, the appropriate adiposity indicators and their associated cutoff points have to be developed for the study population.

This study had several strengths. First, a large-scale nationally representative sample was used to develop efficient adiposity indicators and the accuracy and efficiency of the selected indicators were validated in another large-scale representative sample. Second, the clustering characteristics of obesity indicators and characterized functions were evaluated and validated. Third, multiple adiposity indicators were concurrently assessed and were used to investigate their discriminating capability for identifying MetS in the transition from adolescence to young adulthood. Fourth, although appropriate adiposity indicators and their cutoff points might vary by study populations, our research methodology and network can be applied to other countries that want to develop their specific obesity indicators. Alternatively, we recognize the limitations of our analyses. First, the recommended adiposity indicators had no causally predictive capability in determining MetS since they were all developed in a cross-sectional nature. Second, the participants used to develop indicators were Taiwanese adolescents, thus our findings may not be directly generalizable to other populations.

5. Conclusions

In cardiometabology, this study uncovered the characteristic cluster of adiposity indicators. Bodyfat- and lipid-enhanced adiposity indicators revealed a higher risk and discriminatory ability for

MetS than did body-shape-enhanced indicators in adolescents. This highlights the consideration of indicator characteristics when evaluating the association between pediatric obesity and cardiometabolic diseases. In public health, the findings from the development and validation procedures support AVI as a female, and WC as a male, risk-screening tool for MetS that can be applied during the transition from adolescence to young adulthood in Taiwan.

Supplementary Materials: The following are available online at http://www.mdpi.com/2072-6643/12/10/3165/s1, Table S1: Criteria of metabolic syndrome (MetS) and its abnormal components (AC) defined by IDF and JIS-Adult.

Author Contributions: Conceptualization, C.-H.L., Y.-T.C. and W.-T.L.; Project Administration, W.-T.L., P.-W.W. and S.T.; Methodology, Y.-T.C. and C.-H.L.; Formal Analysis, Y.-T.C., W.-T.L. and C.-H.L.; Writing—Original Draft, Y.-T.C., W.-T.L. and C.-H.L.; Writing—Review and Editing, Y.-T.C., W.-T.L., C.-Y.L., H.-L.H., T.C., D.W.S. and C.-H.L.; Supervision, C.H.L. All authors have read and agreed to the published version of the manuscript.

Funding: This research was funded by the Taiwan Ministry of Science and Technology (MOST 103-2314-B-037-019-MY3, 106-2314-B-037-021-MY3, and 109-2314-B-037-070-MY3) and partially supported by the grant of the Research Center for Environmental Medicine, Kaohsiung Medical University (KMU-TC108A01) from the Featured Areas Research Center Program within the framework of the Higher Education Sprout Project by the Taiwan Ministry of Education.

Acknowledgments: The ado-NAHSIT survey data were obtained from the Nutrition and Health Survey in Taiwan (NAHSIT) on Junior and Senior High School Students, 2010–2011. This NAHSIT project was sponsored by the Food and Drug Administration, Department of Health, Executive Yuan (99TFDA-FS-408 and 100TFDA-FS-406). This nationwide survey was conducted by the Division of Preventive Medicine and Health Services Research, the Institute of Population Health Sciences of the National Health Research Institutes (NHRI). We thank the director Wen-Harn Pan and all members of the office of Nutrition Survey, the Division of Preventive Medicine and Health Services Research, the Institute of Population Health Sciences of NHRI for providing the dataset. The views expressed here are solely those of the authors.

Conflicts of Interest: The authors declare no conflict of interest.

Abbreviations

ABSI: a body shape index; ado-NAHSIT, nutrition and health survey in Taiwan for adolescents; AUC, area under receiver operating characteristic curve; VI, abdominal volume index; BAI, body adiposity index; BMI, body mass index; BRI, body roundness index; CoI, conicity index; IDF-adoMetS, the International Diabetes Federation-defined criteria for adolescent MetS; JIS-AdMetS, the Joint Interim Statement for adult MetS; LAP, lipid accumulation product; MetS, metabolic syndrome; mRP-aMS, multilevel risk profiles for adolescent metabolic syndrome; OR, odds ratio; PC, principal component; pCorr, partial correlations; pR^2, partial R-square; TGI, triglyceride-glucose index; VAI, visceral adiposity index; WC, waist circumference; WHtR, waist-to-height ratio; WHR, waist-to-hip ratio; YI, Youden's index.

References

1. DeBoer, M.D. Assessing and managing the metabolic syndrome in children and adolescents. *Nutrients* **2019**, *11*, 1788. [CrossRef]

2. Morrison, J.A.; Friedman, L.A.; Gray-McGuire, C. Metabolic syndrome in childhood predicts adult cardiovascular disease 25 years later: The Princeton Lipid Research Clinics Follow-up Study. *Pediatrics* **2007**, *120*, 340–345. [CrossRef]

3. Morrison, J.A.; Friedman, L.A.; Wang, P.; Glueck, C.J. Metabolic syndrome in childhood predicts adult metabolic syndrome and type 2 diabetes mellitus 25 to 30 years later. *J. Pediatr.* **2008**, *152*, 201–206. [CrossRef]

4. DeBoer, M.D.; Gurka, M.J.; Woo, J.G.; Morrison, J.A. Severity of metabolic syndrome as a predictor of cardiovascular disease between childhood and adulthood: The Princeton Lipid Research Cohort Study. *J. Am. Coll. Cardiol.* **2015**, *66*, 755–757. [CrossRef]

5. Stanley, T.L.; Chen, M.L.; Goodman, E. The typology of metabolic syndrome in the transition to adulthood. *J. Clin. Endocrinol. Metab.* **2014**, *99*, 1044–1052. [CrossRef]

6. De Larochelliere, E.; Cote, J.; Gilbert, G.; Bibeau, K.; Ross, M.K.; Dion-Roy, V.; Pibarot, P.; Despres, J.P.; Larose, E. Visceral/epicardial adiposity in nonobese and apparently healthy young adults: Association with the cardiometabolic profile. *Atherosclerosis* **2014**, *234*, 23–29. [CrossRef]

7. Bergman, R.N.; Stefanovski, D.; Buchanan, T.A.; Sumner, A.E.; Reynolds, J.C.; Sebring, N.G.; Xiang, A.H.; Watanabe, R.M. A better index of body adiposity. *Obesity* **2011**, *19*, 1083–1089. [CrossRef]

8.   Thomas, D.M.; Bredlau, C.; Bosy-Westphal, A.; Mueller, M.; Shen, W.; Gallagher, D.; Maeda, Y.; McDougall, A.; Peterson, C.M.; Ravussin, E.; et al. Relationships between body roundness with body fat and visceral adipose tissue emerging from a new geometrical model. *Obesity* **2013**, *21*, 2264–2271. [CrossRef]

9.   Ashwell, M.; Gunn, P.; Gibson, S. Waist-to-height ratio is a better screening tool than waist circumference and BMI for adult cardiometabolic risk factors: Systematic review and meta-analysis. *Obes. Rev.* **2012**, *13*, 275–286. [CrossRef]

10.   Ashwell, M.; Mayhew, L.; Richardson, J.; Rickayzen, B. Waist-to-height ratio is more predictive of years of life lost than body mass index. *PLoS ONE* **2014**, *9*, e103483. [CrossRef]

11.   Guerrero-Romero, F.; Rodriguez-Moran, M. Abdominal volume index. An anthropometry-based index for estimation of obesity is strongly related to impaired glucose tolerance and type 2 diabetes mellitus. *Arch. Med. Res.* **2003**, *34*, 428–432. [CrossRef]

12.   Chadid, S.; Kreger, B.E.; Singer, M.R.; Loring Bradlee, M.; Moore, L.L. Anthropometric measures of body fat and obesity-related cancer risk: Sex-specific differences in Framingham Offspring Study adults. *Int. J. Obes.* **2020**, *44*, 601–608. [CrossRef] [PubMed]

13.   Zhu, Q.; Wang, X.B.; Yao, Y.; Ning, C.X.; Chen, X.P.; Luan, F.X.; Zhao, Y.L. Association between anthropometric measures and cardiovascular disease (CVD) risk factors in Hainan centenarians: Investigation based on the Centenarian's health study. *BMC Cardiovasc. Disord.* **2018**, *18*, 73. [CrossRef] [PubMed]

14.   Krakauer, N.Y.; Krakauer, J.C. A new body shape index predicts mortality hazard independently of body mass index. *PLoS ONE* **2012**, *7*, e39504. [CrossRef]

15.   Valdez, R. A simple model-based index of abdominal adiposity. *J. Clin. Epidemiol.* **1991**, *44*, 955–956. [CrossRef]

16.   Motamed, N.; Perumal, D.; Zamani, F.; Ashrafi, H.; Haghjoo, M.; Saeedian, F.S.; Maadi, M.; Akhavan-Niaki, H.; Rabiee, B.; Asouri, M. Conicity index and waist-to-hip ratio are superior obesity indices in predicting 10-year cardiovascular risk among men and women. *Clin. Cardiol.* **2015**, *38*, 527–534. [CrossRef]

17.   Simental-Mendia, L.E.; Rodriguez-Moran, M.; Guerrero-Romero, F. The product of fasting glucose and triglycerides as surrogate for identifying insulin resistance in apparently healthy subjects. *Metab. Syndr. Relat. Disord.* **2008**, *6*, 299–304. [CrossRef]

18.   Amato, M.C.; Giordano, C.; Galia, M.; Criscimanna, A.; Vitabile, S.; Midiri, M.; Galluzzo, A.; AlkaMeSy Study, G. Visceral adiposity index: A reliable indicator of visceral fat function associated with cardiometabolic risk. *Diabetes Care* **2010**, *33*, 920–922. [CrossRef]

19.   Kahn, H.S. The "lipid accumulation product" performs better than the body mass index for recognizing cardiovascular risk: A population-based comparison. *BMC Cardiovasc. Disord.* **2005**, *5*, 26. [CrossRef]

20.   Alberti, K.G.; Eckel, R.H.; Grundy, S.M.; Zimmet, P.Z.; Cleeman, J.I.; Donato, K.A.; Fruchart, J.C.; James, W.P.; Loria, C.M.; Smith, S.C., Jr. Harmonizing the metabolic syndrome: A joint interim statement of the International Diabetes Federation Task Force on Epidemiology and Prevention; National Heart, Lung, and Blood Institute; American Heart Association; World Heart Federation; International Atherosclerosis Society; and International Association for the Study of Obesity. *Circulation* **2009**, *120*, 1640–1645. [CrossRef]

21.   Niklowitz, P.; Rothermel, J.; Lass, N.; Barth, A.; Reinehr, T. Link between chemerin, central obesity, and parameters of the Metabolic Syndrome: Findings from a longitudinal study in obese children participating in a lifestyle intervention. *Int. J. Obes.* **2018**, *42*, 1743–1752. [CrossRef] [PubMed]

22.   Hsu, F.C.; Kritchevsky, S.B.; Liu, Y.; Kanaya, A.; Newman, A.B.; Perry, S.E.; Visser, M.; Pahor, M.; Harris, T.B.; Nicklas, B.J.; et al. Association between inflammatory components and physical function in the health, aging, and body composition study: A principal component analysis approach. *J. Gerontol. Ser. A Biol. Sci. Med. Sci.* **2009**, *64*, 581–589. [CrossRef] [PubMed]

23.   Lin, W.T.; Lin, P.C.; Lee, C.Y.; Chen, Y.L.; Chan, T.F.; Tsai, S.; Huang, H.L.; Wu, P.W.; Chin, Y.T.; Lin, H.Y.; et al. Effects of insulin resistance on the association between the circulating retinol-binding protein 4 level and clustering of pediatric cardiometabolic risk factors. *Pediatr. Diabetes* **2018**, 611–621. [CrossRef] [PubMed]

24.   Lin, W.T.; Lee, C.Y.; Tsai, S.; Huang, H.L.; Wu, P.W.; Chin, Y.T.; Seal, D.W.; Chen, T.; Chao, Y.Y.; Lee, C.H. Clustering of metabolic risk components and associated lifestyle factors: A nationwide adolescent study in Taiwan. *Nutrients* **2019**, *11*, 584. [CrossRef] [PubMed]

25.   National Health Research Institutes. Nutrition and Health Survey in Taiwan. Available online: https://www.hpa.gov.tw/EngPages/Detail.aspx?nodeid=1077&pid=6201 (accessed on 1 July 2020).

26. National Health Research Institutes. Nutrition and Health Survey in Taiwan, 2010–2011: Study Materials and Methods. Available online: https://www.hpa.gov.tw/Pages/Detail.aspx?nodeid=1774&pid=9996 (accessed on 1 July 2020).

27. Chen, C.M.; Lou, M.F.; Gau, B.S. Prevalence of impaired fasting glucose and analysis of related factors in Taiwanese adolescents. *Pediatr. Diabetes* **2014**, *15*, 220–228. [CrossRef]

28. Lin, W.T.; Huang, H.L.; Huang, M.C.; Chan, T.F.; Ciou, S.Y.; Lee, C.Y.; Chiu, Y.W.; Duh, T.H.; Lin, P.L.; Wang, T.N.; et al. Effects on uric acid, body mass index and blood pressure in adolescents of consuming beverages sweetened with high-fructose corn syrup. *Int. J. Obes.* **2013**, *37*, 532–539. [CrossRef]

29. Chan, T.F.; Lin, W.T.; Huang, H.L.; Lee, C.Y.; Wu, P.W.; Chiu, Y.W.; Huang, C.C.; Tsai, S.; Lin, C.L.; Lee, C.H. Consumption of sugar-sweetened beverages is associated with components of the metabolic syndrome in adolescents. *Nutrients* **2014**, *6*, 2088–2103. [CrossRef]

30. Lin, W.T.; Chan, T.F.; Huang, H.L.; Lee, C.Y.; Tsai, S.; Wu, P.W.; Yang, Y.C.; Wang, T.N.; Lee, C.H. Fructose-rich beverage intake and central adiposity, uric acid, and pediatric insulin resistance. *J. Pediatr.* **2016**, *171*, 90–96.e1. [CrossRef]

31. Lee, C.Y.; Lin, W.T.; Tsai, S.; Hung, Y.C.; Wu, P.W.; Yang, Y.C.; Chan, T.F.; Huang, H.L.; Weng, Y.L.; Chiu, Y.W.; et al. Association of parental overweight and cardiometabolic diseases and pediatric adiposity and lifestyle factors with cardiovascular risk factor clustering in adolescents. *Nutrients* **2016**, *8*, 567. [CrossRef]

32. Zimmet, P.; Alberti, K.G.; Kaufman, F.; Tajima, N.; Silink, M.; Arslanian, S.; Wong, G.; Bennett, P.; Shaw, J.; Caprio, S.; et al. The metabolic syndrome in children and adolescents—An IDF consensus report. *Pediatr. Diabetes* **2007**, *8*, 299–306. [CrossRef]

33. Nishida, C.; Ko, G.T.; Kumanyika, S. Body fat distribution and noncommunicable diseases in populations: Overview of the 2008 WHO Expert Consultation on Waist Circumference and Waist-Hip Ratio. *Eur. J. Clin. Nutr.* **2010**, *64*, 2–5. [CrossRef] [PubMed]

34. Du, T.; Yuan, G.; Zhang, M.; Zhou, X.; Sun, X.; Yu, X. Clinical usefulness of lipid ratios, visceral adiposity indicators, and the triglycerides and glucose index as risk markers of insulin resistance. *Cardiovasc. Diabetol.* **2014**, *13*, 146. [CrossRef] [PubMed]

35. Leal-Witt, M.J.; Ramon-Krauel, M.; Samino, S.; Llobet, M.; Cuadras, D.; Jimenez-Chillaron, J.C.; Yanes, O.; Lerin, C. Untargeted metabolomics identifies a plasma sphingolipid-related signature associated with lifestyle intervention in prepubertal children with obesity. *Int. J. Obes.* **2018**, *42*, 72–78. [CrossRef] [PubMed]

36. DeLong, E.R.; DeLong, D.M.; Clarke-Pearson, D.L. Comparing the areas under two or more correlated receiver operating characteristic curves: A nonparametric approach. *Biometrics* **1988**, *44*, 837–845. [CrossRef] [PubMed]

37. Ofstad, A.P.; Sommer, C.; Birkeland, K.I.; Bjorgaas, M.R.; Gran, J.M.; Gulseth, H.L.; Johansen, O.E. Comparison of the associations between non-traditional and traditional indices of adiposity and cardiovascular mortality: An observational study of one million person-years of follow-up. *Int. J. Obes.* **2019**, *43*, 1082–1092. [CrossRef] [PubMed]

38. Ajala, O.; Mold, F.; Boughton, C.; Cooke, D.; Whyte, M. Childhood predictors of cardiovascular disease in adulthood. A systematic review and meta-analysis. *Obes. Rev.* **2017**, *18*, 1061–1070. [CrossRef]

39. Perona, J.S.; Schmidt Rio-Valle, J.; Ramirez-Velez, R.; Correa-Rodriguez, M.; Fernandez-Aparicio, A.; Gonzalez-Jimenez, E. Waist circumference and abdominal volume index are the strongest anthropometric discriminators of metabolic syndrome in Spanish adolescents. *Eur. J. Clin. Investig.* **2019**, *49*, e13060. [CrossRef]

40. Vasquez, F.; Correa-Burrows, P.; Blanco, E.; Gahagan, S.; Burrows, R. A waist-to-height ratio of 0.54 is a good predictor of metabolic syndrome in 16-year-old male and female adolescents. *Pediatr. Res.* **2019**, *85*, 269–274. [CrossRef]

41. Oliveira, R.G.; Guedes, D.P. Performance of anthropometric indicators as predictors of metabolic syndrome in Brazilian adolescents. *BMC Pediatr.* **2018**, *18*, 33. [CrossRef]

42. Arellano-Ruiz, P.; Garcia-Hermoso, A.; Garcia-Prieto, J.C.; Sanchez-Lopez, M.; Vizcaino, V.M.; Solera-Martinez, M. Predictive ability of waist circumference and waist-to-height ratio for cardiometabolic risk screening among Spanish children. *Nutrients* **2020**, *12*, 415. [CrossRef]

43. Guo, S.X.; Zhang, X.H.; Zhang, J.Y.; He, J.; Yan, Y.Z.; Ma, J.L.; Ma, R.L.; Guo, H.; Mu, L.T.; Li, S.G.; et al. Visceral adiposity and anthropometric indicators as screening tools of metabolic syndrome among low income rural adults in Xinjiang. *Sci. Rep.* **2016**, *6*, 36091. [CrossRef]

44. Haslam, D.W.; James, W.P. Obesity. *Lancet* **2005**, *366*, 1197–1209. [CrossRef]
45. Carsley, S.; Tu, K.; Parkin, P.C.; Pullenayegum, E.; Birken, C.S. Overweight and obesity in preschool aged children and risk of mental health service utilization. *Int. J. Obes.* **2019**, *43*, 1325–1333. [CrossRef] [PubMed]
46. Shen, Y.C.; Kung, S.C.; Chang, E.T.; Hong, Y.L.; Wang, L.Y. The impact of obesity in cognitive and memory dysfunction in obstructive sleep apnea syndrome. *Int. J. Obes.* **2019**, *43*, 355–361. [CrossRef] [PubMed]
47. Perona, J.S.; Schmidt-RioValle, J.; Fernandez-Aparicio, A.; Correa-Rodriguez, M.; Ramirez-Velez, R.; Gonzalez-Jimenez, E. Waist circumference and abdominal volume index can predict metabolic syndrome in adolescents, but only when the criteria of the International Diabetes Federation are employed for the diagnosis. *Nutrients* **2019**, *11*, 1370. [CrossRef] [PubMed]

Publisher's Note: MDPI stays neutral with regard to jurisdictional claims in published maps and institutional affiliations.

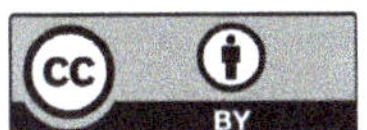

© 2020 by the authors. Licensee MDPI, Basel, Switzerland. This article is an open access article distributed under the terms and conditions of the Creative Commons Attribution (CC BY) license (http://creativecommons.org/licenses/by/4.0/).

nutrients

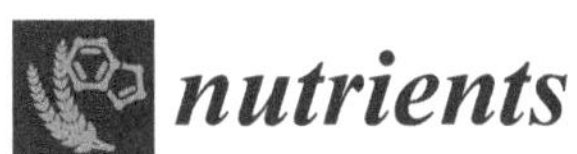

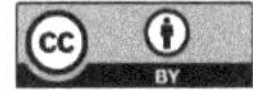

Article

Lifestyle Changes and Determinants of Children's and Adolescents' Body Weight Increase during the First COVID-19 Lockdown in Greece: The COV-EAT Study

Odysseas Androutsos [1,*], Maria Perperidi [1], Christos Georgiou [1] and Giorgos Chouliaras [2]

[1] Department of Nutrition and Dietetics, School of Physical Education, Sport Science and Dietetics, University of Thessaly, 42132 Trikala, Greece; mperper@msn.com (M.P.); cri.georgiou@gmail.com (C.G.)
[2] Second Department of Paediatrics, School of Medicine, National and Kapodistrian University of Athens, 11527 Athens, Greece; georgehouliaras@msn.com
* Correspondence: oandroutsos@uth.gr; Tel.: +30-24310-47108

Abstract: Previous studies showed that the coronavirus disease 2019 (COVID-19) lockdown imposed changes in adults' lifestyle behaviors; however, there is limited information regarding the effects on youth. The COV-EAT study aimed to report changes in children's and adolescents' lifestyle habits during the first COVID-19 lockdown and explore potential associations between changes of participants' lifestyle behaviors and body weight. An online survey among 397 children/adolescents and their parents across 63 municipalities in Greece was conducted in April–May 2020. Parents self-reported changes of their children's lifestyle habits and body weight, as well as sociodemographic data of their family. The present study shows that during the lockdown, children's/adolescents' sleep duration and screen time increased, while their physical activity decreased. Their consumption of fruits and fresh fruit juices, vegetables, dairy products, pasta, sweets, total snacks, and breakfast increased, while fast-food consumption decreased. Body weight increased in 35% of children/adolescents. A multiple regression analysis showed that the body weight increase was associated with increased consumption of breakfast, salty snacks, and total snacks and with decreased physical activity. The COV-EAT study revealed changes in children's and adolescents' lifestyle behaviors during the first COVID-19 lockdown in Greece. Effective strategies are needed to prevent excessive body weight gain in future COVID-19 lockdowns.

Keywords: COVID-19; obesity; children; lifestyle; determinants; diet; physical activity; sedentary behavior; COV-EAT

Citation: Androutsos, O.; Perperidi, M.; Georgiou, C.; Chouliaras, G. Lifestyle Changes and Determinants of Children's and Adolescents' Body Weight Increase during the First COVID-19 Lockdown in Greece: The COV-EAT Study. *Nutrients* **2021**, *13*, 930. https://doi.org/10.3390/nu13030930

Academic Editor: Amelia Martí

Received: 7 January 2021
Accepted: 10 March 2021
Published: 13 March 2021

Publisher's Note: MDPI stays neutral with regard to jurisdictional claims in published maps and institutional affiliations.

Copyright: © 2021 by the authors. Licensee MDPI, Basel, Switzerland. This article is an open access article distributed under the terms and conditions of the Creative Commons Attribution (CC BY) license (https://creativecommons.org/licenses/by/4.0/).

1. Introduction

Since December 2019, the world is facing a new disease (coronavirus disease 2019 (COVID-19)), caused by the severe acute respiratory syndrome coronavirus 2 (SARS-CoV-2). The WHO declared COVID-19 a pandemic in March 2020. In Greece, a number of regulatory measures have been implemented, including the closing of schools on 11 March and finally a lockdown, imposed on 23 March as a "last-resort" preventive measure to halt the spreading of the disease until COVID-19 vaccines would be available. This unprecedented situation led to significant changes in children's daily routine, who no longer attended school and out-of-school activities (e.g., participation in sports, free play at playgrounds, etc.), but were isolated at home with their families.

Studies conducted during the COVID-19 pandemic in adults have shown that self-isolation at home due to the lockdown was associated with lower level of physical activity, longer sedentary time, modifications in eating behavior, and sleeping disturbances [1–3]. Furthermore, an increase of food purchased before the pandemic was reported in some countries, which increased the availability of foods during the lockdown [4]. Self-isolation has been also linked to boredom and stress, which in turn may lead to higher energy intake, consumption of energy-dense "comfort foods", and emotional eating [5]. To date, there is a lack of studies focusing on changes of children's lifestyle behaviors during the COVID-19 lockdown. However, there are studies which have examined the impact of school closing in the summer period, which is a condition similar to the COVID-19 lockdown, on children's eating behavior and weight status [3,6–9]. The majority of these studies concluded that children's body mass index (BMI) increased more rapidly during summer vacation compared to school period [7]. Moreover, it was revealed that children tend to consume less vegetables and more sugar, spend more time on TV-watching, and be more active during summer breaks compared to school time [8]. Interestingly, the study of Von Hippel et al. showed that the prevalence of childhood obesity increased only during summer vacations and not during any other time period of the year [6].

Factors that may influence children's eating behavior have been previously reported and include certain lifestyle behaviors, such as sedentary behavior [10–15], insufficient sleep duration [10,12–14], and inactivity [10–13,15–17], as well as determinants from children's social and physical environment, such as parental modeling [10,11,16,17] and availability of foods at home [11,16]. It is also known that retaining higher energy intake compared to energy expenditure for long periods of time increases the risk of overweight/obesity [18].

The scientific community raises concerns about the health implications that may be caused by the COVID-19 lockdown [1,2,19–22]. The present study aims to report changes in children's and adolescents' lifestyle behaviors during the first lockdown that was implemented in Greece due to COVID-19 and explore potential associations with changes of their body weight.

2. Materials and Methods

2.1. Study Design and Participants

The COV-EAT study was a cross-sectional study, which was conducted across 63 municipalities in Greece. Parents having children aged 2–18 years were invited to participate. The following inclusion criteria were applied: living in Greece, being able to complete the study questionnaire in Greek language, having children aged 2–18 years, and providing a consent form. The COV-EAT study adhered to the Declaration of Helsinki and the conventions of the Council of Europe on human rights and Biomedicine. The study protocol was approved by the Ethical Committee of the Department of Physical Education and Sport Science in the School of Physical Education, Sport Science, and Dietetics, University of Thessaly, and registered at clinicaltrials.org (NCT04437121). All parents electronically signed an informed consent form prior to their participation in the study. Only one child per family was included in this study.

2.2. Instruments and Variables

An online survey was conducted in a sample of families, who were invited to electronically fill in a questionnaire which included 70 questions divided in 3 sections. The first section focused on participants' sociodemographic data and included 15 questions about child's gender, parents' and child's age, number of children in the family, city of residence, and socioeconomic status. The second section contained 20 questions about parents' dietary and lifestyle habits before and during the lockdown. Specifically, parents had to answer questions about the frequency of cooking at home and their fast-food consumption, the number of meals and snacks consumed per day, the reasons of snacking, and their body weight and height. The third section contained 35 questions about their child's eating habits and its sedentary behavior. Parents were asked to report their child's body weight and height, the number of meals and snacks during the day, the frequency of breakfast, fast-food, fruits, juices, vegetables, dairy, red meat, poultry, fish, pasta, legumes, sweets, salty snacks, and beverages consumption, the servings of fruits, juices, vegetables, and dairy consumed per day, vitamin supplementation, as well as screen time, sleep duration, and changes in physical activity. All answers were given about the period before and during the lockdown. According to the difference between the values of each lifestyle behavior before and during the lockdown, each parameter was categorized as "decrease" (i.e., before-lockdown value of lifestyle behavior higher than during-lockdown value), "stable" (i.e., same values of lifestyle behavior before and during the lockdown), or "increase" (i.e., before-lockdown value of lifestyle behavior lower than during-lockdown value).

The questionnaire is available as a Supplementary Materials.

2.3. Procedure

All data were collected between 30 April and 24 May 2020. The questionnaire was created using the Google Forms tool and was distributed electronically via networks of dietitians/nutritionists in Greece, personal networks, and social media.

2.4. Statistical Analyses

Continuous data are presented as mean $\pm$ standard deviation (SD). Categorical variables are presented as absolute (n) and relative (%) frequencies. Mean values of consumption of food groups before and during the quarantine were compared using the Student's test for paired data. Associations between categorical data were evaluated with Fisher's exact test. For paired pre- vs. post-comparisons of sleeping time, the extended McNemar's test (allowing for 3×3 contingency tables in matched observations) was used. For paired pre- vs. post-comparisons of screen time, the Wilcoxon matched-pairs signed-rank test was applied. A stepwise, backwards, regression approach was utilized to assess the effect of dietary data on the probability of body weight increase versus no change or decrease (logistic regression). Participants that answered "don't know" were treated as missing values. The initial, full model included dietary data, gender, age, area of residency, change in sleep and screen time, and change in physical activity. For logistic regression analysis, results are reported as odds ratios, along with 95% confidence intervals (CI) and p-values. The level of statistical significance was set to 0.05 for analyses, and in cases of multiple comparisons, the Bonferroni correction was applied. All analyses were run in Stata 11 MP statistical software (StataCorp., College Station, TX, USA).

3. Results

In total, 397 dyads of children/adolescents (51.4% boys) with an average age of 7.8 (4.1) years were recruited. Families' characteristics are presented in Table 1, and detailed demographic and socioeconomic data are presented in Table 2.

Tables 3 and 4 present children's/adolescents' changes of lifestyle behaviors before vs. during the lockdown. Specifically, during the lockdown, more children/adolescents tended to sleep longer than 10 h/night, and fewer slept less than 8 h/night than before the lockdown. Similarly, the children/adolescents who spent more than 3 h/day in front of a screen were more during home isolation, whereas those who did not spent time on a screen were less during the confinement than before the confinement. Moreover, 66.9% of the parents reported that their child's physical activity level was decreased during the lockdown, and 35% that their child's body weight increased. Regarding children's eating behavior, the consumption of fruits and fresh fruit juices, vegetables, dairy products, pasta, sweets, total snacks, and breakfast significantly increased ($p < 0.05$). In contrast, fast-food consumption was significantly decreased ($p < 0.001$). No significant changes were observed in core foods used for lunch and dinner, such as red meat, poultry, fish, and legumes. Similarly, no significant changes were observed in the consumption of prepacked juices and sodas and salty snacks.

Table 1. Families' age and anthropometric characteristics. The COV-EAT study.

Characteristics	Mean $\pm$ SD ($n = 397$)
Children's/adolescents' age (years)	7.8 $\pm$ 4.1
Children's/adolescents' body weight (Kg)	32.3 $\pm$ 16.9
Fathers' age (years)	43.2 $\pm$ 6.4
Fathers' body weight (Kg)	88.7 $\pm$ 12.9
Fathers' body height (cm)	179.2 $\pm$ 6.3
Mothers' age (years)	39.8 $\pm$ 5.3
Mothers' body weight (Kg)	70.1 $\pm$ 14.1
Mothers' body height (cm)	165.5 $\pm$ 5.9

Table 2. Family socio-demographic status. The COV-EAT study.

Variables		N (%)
	Urban	331 (83.4%)
Area of residence	Semi-urban	35 (8.8%)
	Rural	31 (7.8%)
Parental marital status	Core families—married parents	370 (93.2%)
	Single-parent families	27 (6.8%)
Fathers' occupation before lockdown	Employee	378 (95.2%)
	Unemployed	11 (2.8%)
	Retired	8 (2.0%)
Fathers who lost their job during lockdown		11 (2.9%)
Fathers who increased their working hours during the lockdown		12 (3.2%)
Mothers' occupation before lockdown	Employee	311 (78.3%)
	Unemployed	84 (21.2%)
	Retired	2 (0.5%)
Mothers who lost their job during lockdown		16 (5.1%)
Mothers who increased their working hours during the lockdown		13 (4.2%)

Data are shown as absolute (n) and relative (%) frequencies. Missing values were not included in the statistical analyses.

Table 3. Changes of children's and adolescents' lifestyle habits * and body weight in the first coronavirus disease 2019 (COVID-19) lockdown in Greece. The COV-EAT study.

Lifestyle Habits		Before Lockdown		During Lockdown	
		Sample ($n = 397$)	Sample (%)	Sample ($n = 397$)	Sample (%)
Sleep duration before and during the first COVID-19 lockdown **	<8 h	61	15.4%	19	4.8%
	8–10 h	283	71.3%	282	71.0%
	>10 h	53	13.3%	96	24.2%
Screen time before and during the first COVID-19 lockdown ***	0 h	19	4.8%	4	1.0%
	1 h	135	34.0%	43	10.8%
	2 h	150	37.8%	79	19.9%
	3 h	66	16.6%	121	30.5%
	>3 h	27	6.8%	150	37.8%
Physical activity change during the COVID-19 lockdown ****	No Change			71	18.2%
	Increase			58	14.9%
	Decrease			261	66.9%
Body weight change during the COVID-19 lockdown *****	No Change			214	58.9%
	Increase			127	35%
	Decrease			22	6.1%

* Data are shown as absolute (n) and relative (%) frequencies. ** Extended McNemar's test: $p < 0.001$. *** Wilcoxon matched-pairs signed-rank test: $p < 0.001$. **** Seven missing values for the variable (1.8% "don't know" responses of the total). ***** Thirty-four missing values for the variable (8.6% "don't know" responses of the total).

Table 4. Changes of children's * and adolescents' eating habits in the first COVID-19 lockdown in Greece. The COV-EAT study.

Food Groups	Before Lockdown	During Lockdown	*p*-Value **
Salty snacks	0.18 (0.10)	0.19 (0.11)	0.12
Fruits and Fresh juices	1.80 (1.21)	2.08 (1.39)	<0.001
Vegetables	0.69 (0.73)	0.76 (0.77)	<0.001
Prepacked juices and sodas	0.26 (0.51)	0.28 (0.51)	0.33
Dairy	1.80 (0.93)	1.92 (0.97)	<0.001
Red meat	0.29 (0.16)	0.29 (0.16)	0.57
Poultry	0.23 (0.11)	0.23 (0.11)	0.64
Fish	0.15 (0.09)	0.15 (0.10)	0.26
Pasta	0.47 (0.27)	0.48 (0.27)	0.014
Legumes	0.20 (0.10)	0.20 (0.11)	0.57
Sweets	0.65 (0.24)	0.73 (0.24)	<0.001
Total snacks	1.95 (0.67)	2.41 (0.86)	<0.001
Fast-food	0.13 (0.13)	0.08 (1.43)	<0.001
Breakfast	6.13 (1.85)	6.56 (1.33)	<0.001

* Data presented as mean (SD) consumption (in servings/day) of each food. Breakfast consumption indicates the frequency of consumption on a weekly level. ** *t*-test for paired data/students test.

Table 5 presents the bivariate correlations between body weight increase and changes in lifestyle behaviors. More specifically, body weight increase was correlated with increase of consumption of salty snacks and red meat ($p < 0.05$). Similarly, increase of sleep duration ($p = 0.012$) and screen time ($p < 0.001$) and decrease of physical activity ($p < 0.001$) were associated with body weight increase. No significant associations were observed between body weight change and consumption of fresh fruits and fruit juices, vegetables, poultry, fish, pasta, and legumes.

Table 5. Associations between dietary or lifestyle changes and children's and adolescents' body weight (BW) changes during the first COVID-19 lockdown in Greece. The COV-EAT study.

BW Change	Lifestyle Determinants			*p*-Value
	Decrease **	Stable **	Increase **	
Salty snack consumption				
Non-increased BW * (*n* = 236)	27 (77.1%)	199 (70.1%)	10 (22.7%)	<0.001
Increased BW (*n* = 127)	8 (22.9%)	85 (29.9%)	34 (77.3%)	
Fruits and fresh juices				
Non-increased BW * (*n* = 236)	33 (60.0%)	124 (68.9%)	79 (61.7%)	0.3
Increased BW (*n* = 127)	22 (40.0%)	56 (31.1%)	49 (38.3%)	
Vegetables Consumption				
Non-increased BW * (*n* = 236)	10 (52.6%)	192 (66.4%)	34 (61.8%)	0.4
Increased BW (*n* = 127)	9 (47.4%)	97 (33.6%)	21 (38.2%)	
Prepacked juiced and sodas				
Non-increased BW * (*n* = 236)	30 (60.0%)	182 (70.3%)	24 (44.4%)	<0.001
Increased BW (*n* = 127)	20 (40.0%)	77 (29.7%)	30 (55.6%)	
Dairy Consumption				
Non-increased BW * (*n* = 236)	10 (55.6%)	199 (69.1%)	27 (47.4%)	0.005
Increased BW (*n* = 127)	8 (44.4%)	89 (30.9%)	30 (52.6%)	
Red meat Consumption				
Non-increased BW * (*n* = 236)	13 (72.2%)	215 (66.6%)	8 (36.4%)	0.016
Increased BW (*n* = 127)	5 (27.8%)	108 (33.4%)	14 (63.6%)	

Table 5. *Cont.*

BW Change	Lifestyle Determinants			*p*-Value
	Decrease **	Stable **	Increase **	
Poultry Consumption				
Non-increased BW * (*n* = 236)	8 (80.0%)	221 (64.8%)	7 (58.3%)	0.6
Increased BW (*n* = 127)	2 (20.0%)	120 (35.2%)	5 (41.7%)	
Fish Consumption				
Non-increased BW * (*n* = 236)	12 (80.0%)	214 (65.2%)	10 (50.0%)	0.2
Increased BW (*n* = 127)	3 (20.0%)	114 (34.8%)	10 (50.0%)	
Pasta Consumption				
Non-increased BW * (*n* = 236)	7 (58.3%)	216 (66.3%)	13 (52.0%)	0.3
Increased BW (*n* = 127)	5 (41.7%)	110 (33.7%)	12 (48.0%)	
Legumes Consumption				
Non-increased BW * (*n* = 236)	8 (61.5%)	218 (65.5%)	10 (58.8%)	0.8
Increased BW (n = 127)	5 (38.5%)	115 (34.5%)	7 (41.2%)	
Sweets Consumption				
Non-increased BW * (*n* = 236)	26 (65.0%)	158 (72.5%)	52 (49.5%)	<0.001
Increased BW (*n* = 127)	14 (35.0%)	60 (27.5%)	53 (50.5%)	
Total Snacks Consumption				
Non-increased BW * (*n* = 236)	12 (63.2%)	159 (80.7%)	65 (44.2%)	<0.001
Increased BW (*n* = 127)	7 (36.8%)	38 (19.3%)	82 (55.8%)	
Fast-food Frequency				
Non-increased BW * (*n* = 236)	100 (62.5%)	128 (69.6%)	8 (42.1%)	0.043
Increased BW (n = 127)	60 (37.5%)	56 (30.4%)	11 (57.9%)	
Breakfast Frequency				
Non-increased BW * (*n* = 236)	10 (47.6%)	200 (69.9%)	26 (46.4%)	0.001
Increased BW (*n* = 127)	11 (52.4%)	86 (30.1%)	30 (53.6%)	
Sleep Duration				
Stable BW	12 (60.0%)	176 (69.8%)	48 (52.7%)	0.012
Increased BW	8 (40.0%)	76 (30.2%)	43 (47.3%)	
Screen Time				
Stable BW	2 (40.0%)	83 (79.1%)	151 (59.7%)	<0.001
Increased BW	3 (60.0%)	22 (20.9%)	102 (40.3%)	
Physical Activity Changes				
Stable BW	132 (55.0%)	59 (89.4%)	43 (79.6%)	<0.001
Increased BW	108 (45.0%)	7 (10.6%)	11 (20.4%)	

Data are shown as absolute (n) and relative (%) frequencies. * Non-increased body weight means either stable or decreased. ** According to the difference between the values of each lifestyle behavior before and during lockdown, they were categorized as "decrease", "stable, or "increase".

The results of a multiple, stepwise, backwards, logistic regression analysis of the associations between children's and adolescents' body weight increase and changes of their lifestyle behaviors during the lockdown are shown in Table 6. Based on these findings, increase of consumption of breakfast, salty snacks, and total snacks along with decrease of physical activity were significantly associated with increase of children's and adolescents' body weight.

Table 6. Multiple regression analysis between the probability of children's and adolescent's body weight increase and dietary and lifestyle changes during the first COVID-19 lockdown in Greece. The COV-EAT study.

		OR	95% CI	*p*-Values
Breakfast frequency	Increase vs. No Change	2.3	1.8–4.4	0.015
	Increase vs. Decrease	1.7	0.5–1.5	0.359
Salty Snacks Consumption	Increase vs. No Change	4.2	1.9–9.3	0.001
	Increase vs. Decrease	6.7	2.1–20.9	0.001
Total Snack Consumption	Increase vs. No Change	3.2	1.9–5.4	<0.001
	Increase vs. Decrease	1.6	0.5–4.7	0.399
Physical Activity	No change vs. increase	2.4	0.8–7.1	0.116
	Decrease vs. Increase	5.1	2.1–12.2	<0.001

Data are shown as odds ratios (OR), along with 95% confidence intervals (95% CI) and *p*-values.

4. Discussion

The COV-EAT study is the first study in Greece and one of the few globally that examined changes of lifestyle behaviors in children and adolescents during the first lockdown that was implemented due to COVID-19 and explored their associations with children's/adolescents' body weight gain. The main findings of the present study showed that during the lockdown period, children and adolescents in Greece: (1) increased their consumption of certain foods, such as fruits and fresh juices, vegetables, dairy, pasta, sweets, total snacks, and decreased their fast-food consumption, (2) increased their screen time, (3) increased their sleep duration, (4) decreased their physical activity, and (5) 35% of them gained body weight. According to the results of a multiple regression analysis conducted in this study, increased consumption of breakfast, salty snacks, and total snacks along with decreased physical activity was significantly associated with increase of children's and adolescents' body weight.

The findings of the present study suggest that the COVID-19 lockdown, with the concomitant closure of schools, negatively affected children's lifestyle behaviors, which are some of the predominant risk factors for obesity [3]. In line with the findings of the current study, Pietrobelli et al. showed that during the lockdown, children and adolescents with obesity in Italy significantly increased their consumption of certain foods (chips, red meat, and sugary drinks), their sleep duration, and the time they devoted to screen activities, while they decreased the time they spent in sports [3]. Similarly, Ng et al. in a sample of 1214 Irish adolescents, showed that half of the participants tended to decrease their physical activity during the lockdown, especially those with overweight or obesity [23]. Furthermore, Jia et al. conducted a survey among 10,082 participants from high schools, colleges, and graduate schools (aged 19.8 ± 2.3 years) and showed that individuals' BMI, screen time, and sedentary and sleeping time on weekdays and weekends increased, while the frequency of engaging in active transport, moderate/vigorous-intensity housework, leisure-time moderate/vigorous-intensity physical activity, and leisure-time walking were decreased [24]. Also, the study by Ruiz-Roso et al. in a multinational sample of adolescents from Italy, Spain, Chile, Colombia, and Brazil indicated that families had more time to cook and improved eating habits by increasing legumes, vegetables and fruits intake and reducing fast-food consumption, but that was not enough to increase the overall diet quality, because of the higher sweet food and fried food consumption [25]. Similarly, in our study, fast-food consumption decreased ($p < 0.001$), which might have resulted from the fear of being affected by the coronavirus that could be transmitted from the person delivering the food. The COV-EAT study was conducted during the first quarantine, where ignorance of the protective measures against COVID-19 was excessive. Studies in adults are also in line with the findings of the COV-EAT study. According to the preliminary results of the ECLB-COVID19 international study in 1047 adults, the COVID-19 lockdown had a negative effect on physical activity and eating behavior and led to a significant increase in sitting time [26].

The alterations in children's and adolescent's lifestyle behaviors may be explained in different ways. The decrease of physical activity may be attributed to home confinement, which does not allow individuals to attend sport clubs and organized physical activity or visit schoolyards, parks, and recreational areas. Ng et al. reported that Irish adolescents with overweight were more likely to be less physically active during the COVID-19 lockdown [23]. In contrast, the increase of screen time may be due to the longer duration of distance learning replacing both school lessons and private lessons, in addition to more free time at home and to boredom. The increase of sleep duration may be linked to the fact that children did not have to go to school in the morning. Changes of eating behavior may be caused by several different factors. First, the insecurity caused by COVID-19 may have led families to change the home food environment and feeding practices. Indeed, Adams et al. reported that families experiencing food insecurity exerted greater pressure to their children to eat, while 30% of the families increased the amount of high-calorie snack foods, desserts/sweets, and fresh foods, and almost half of the study sample increased the availability of non-perishable processed foods in their homes [27]. In addition to the physical environment, the social environment at home may have changed because of COVID-19. In the present study, a number of parents (5.1% of mothers and 2.9% of fathers) lost their job, while others (4.2% of mothers and 3.2% of fathers) experienced an increase of working time during the COVID-19 lockdown. These changes might be associated with parental stress and disturbances of family interactions, parental modeling, and parenting feeding practices at home [28]. Furthermore, the psychological impact of self-isolation may have triggered boredom and stress, which are determinants of the consumption of energy-dense "comfort foods" and emotional eating [5]. Especially children and adolescents with obesity may be more susceptible to overeating, as observed in Polish adults with overweight and obesity [29]. It is also noted that cooking and preparation of new recipes for snacks might be used as a recreational activity by the family during the lockdown, which in turn increases the availability of home-made sweets, snacks, and foods. Additionally, a home does not always provide a steady environment for mealtimes, physical activity, and sleep schedule [3].

Changes of lifestyle behaviors may lead to an increase of energy intake over energy expenditure, a condition which results in body weight gain when lasting for long periods of time. As expected, increased consumption of energy-dense foods (i.e., total snacks, including sweets) and decreased physical activity were associated with an increase of children's and adolescents' body weight. Still, the present study also showed that the increases of breakfast consumption and total snacks were associated with an increase of participants' body weight. These observations may be attributed to the fact that children/adolescents increased the number of meals consumed per day and that, possibly, they consumed unhealthy foods/snacks in these extra meals. Future studies should shed more light on these associations. Moreover, increased body weight in 35% of children and adolescents could be a natural trend due to children's growth if the increase of body weight was about 0.5 kg. The mean body weight increase of 2 kg indicates an abnormal weight gain.

Since obesity and its complications (diabetes, heart disease, pulmonary disease, hypertension, etc.) can worsen the implications of COVID-19, it is critical to implement measures, during the lockdown, to promote healthy eating and physical activity and prevent obesity [3,9,19,30–32]. To achieve these goals, an umbrella of telehealth (e-health and m-health) obesity prevention and treatment actions should be implemented, in addition to the measures taken to tackle the expansion of COVID-19 [30,33]. Policy interventions to oversee food advertisements and behavioral strategies to promote nutrition education, appetite control, and family meal planning should be applied. Vulnerable groups, such as children and adolescents with overweight or obesity, lower socioeconomic groups, and families with food insecurity should be prioritized.

The findings of the current study should be interpreted under the light of its strengths and limitations. Regarding the strengths, the COV-EAT study was the first study in Greece to explore the potential effect of the first COVID-19 lockdown in Greece on children's and adolescents' lifestyle behaviors, using data from 397 families from urban, semi-urban, and rural areas. Regarding the limitations, firstly due to its cross-sectional design, no causal relationships could be established. Secondly, the study sample was not representative of all children and adolescents in Greece; therefore, the results cannot be generalized to the whole population of Greek children and adolescents. The sampling procedure, which was based on an online survey, may have also produced a selection bias regarding the recruited participants. Moreover, the questionnaire used in the COV-EAT study was not validated, while data were self-reported, and thus subject to recall bias and socially desirable answers, and only weight change was reported. It was also not feasible to conduct comparisons between maternal and paternal reports, which may have an effect on the results. Still, 90% of the reports were taken from mothers, which limits the possibility of such bias.

5. Conclusions

The COV-EAT study reported unfavorable changes in children's and adolescents' lifestyle behaviors during the first COVID-19 lockdown that was implemented in Greece in spring 2020. Certain lifestyle changes were associated with children's/adolescents' body weight gain. Considering that the COVID-19 pandemic may lead to further lockdowns, effective e-health and m-health strategies and programs to tackle the adoption of unhealthy lifestyle behaviors and prevent excessive body weight gain are urgently needed.

Supplementary Materials: The supplementary materials are available online at https://www.mdpi.com/2072-6643/13/3/930/s1.

Author Contributions: Conceptualization, O.A. and M.P.; methodology, O.A., statistical analysis, G.C.; data curation, O.A., M.P., and C.G.; writing—original draft preparation, O.A.; writing—review and editing, M.P., C.G., and G.C.; supervision, O.A. All authors have read and agreed to the published version of the manuscript.

Funding: This research received no external funding.

Institutional Review Board Statement: The study was conducted according to the guidelines of the Declaration of Helsinki and the conventions of the Council of Europe on human rights and Biomedicine. The study protocol was approved by the Ethical Committee of the Department of Physical Education and Sport Science in the School of Physical Education, Sport Science, and Dietetics, University of Thessaly (protocol code 1655 and date of approval: 6 June 2020), and registered at clinicaltrials.org (NCT04437121).

Informed Consent Statement: Informed consent was obtained from all subjects involved in the study.

Data Availability Statement: The data presented in this study are available on request from the corresponding author. The data are not publicly available due to ethical restrictions.

Acknowledgments: The authors would like to thank the study participants.

Conflicts of Interest: The authors declare no conflict of interest.

References

1. Naja, F.; Hamadeh, R. Nutrition amid the COVID-19 pandemic: A multi-level framework for action. *Eur. J. Clin. Nutr.* **2020**, *74*, 1117–1121. [CrossRef]
2. Butler, M.J.; Barrientos, R.M. The impact of nutrition on COVID-19 susceptibility and long-term consequences. *Brain Behav. Immun.* **2020**, *87*, 53–54. [CrossRef] [PubMed]

3. Pietrobelli, A.; Pecoraro, L.; Ferruzzi, A.; Heo, M.; Faith, M.; Zoller, T.; Antoniazzi, F.; Piacentini, G.; Fearnbach, S.N.; Heymsfield, S.B. Effects of COVID-19 Lockdown on Lifestyle Behaviors in Children with Obesity Living in Verona, Italy: A Longitudinal Study. *Obesity (Silver Spring)* **2020**, *28*, 1382–1385. [CrossRef]

4. Rodriguez-Perez, C.; Molina-Montes, E.; Verardo, V.; Artacho, R.; García-Villanova, B.; Guerra-Hernández, E.J.; Ruíz-López, M.D. Changes in Dietary Behaviours during the COVID-19 Outbreak Confinement in the Spanish COVIDiet Study. *Nutrients* **2020**, *12*, 1730. [CrossRef]

5. Di Renzo, L.; Gualtieri, P.; Pivari, F.; Soldati, L.; Attinà, A.; Cinelli, G.; Leggeri, C.; Caparello, G.; Barrea, L.; Scerbo, F.; et al. Eating habits and lifestyle changes during COVID-19 lockdown: An Italian survey. *J. Transl. Med.* **2020**, *18*, 229. [CrossRef]

6. Von Hippel, P.T.; Workman, J. From Kindergarten Through Second Grade, U.S. Children's Obesity Prevalence Grows Only During Summer Vacarions. *Obesity* **2016**, *24*, 2296–2300. [CrossRef] [PubMed]

7. Von Hippel, P.T.; Powell, B.; Downey, D.B.; Rowland, N.J. The effect of school on overweight in Childhood: Gain in body mass index during the school year and during summer vacation. *Am. J. Public Health* **2007**, *97*, 696–702. [CrossRef] [PubMed]

8. Wang, Y.C.; Hsiao, V.S.; Rundle, A.; Goldsmith, J. Weight-related behaviors when children are in school versus in summer breaks: Does income matter? *J. Sch. Health* **2015**, *85*, 458–466. [CrossRef] [PubMed]

9. Rundle, A.G.; Park, Y.; Herbstman, J.B.; Kinsey, E.W.; Wang, Y.C. COVID-19–Related School Closings and Risk of Weight Gain Among Children. *Obesity (Silver Spring)* **2020**, *28*, 1008–1009. [CrossRef]

10. Tenjin, K.; Sekine, M.; Yamada, M.; Tatsuse, T. Relationship Between Parental Lifestyle Dietary Habits of Children: A Cross-Sectional Study. *J. Epidemiol.* **2020**, *30*, 253–259. [CrossRef]

11. Koletzko, B.; Fishbein, M.; Lee, W.S.; Moreno, L.; Mouane, N.; Mouzaki, M.; Verduci, E. Prevention of Childhood Obesity: A Position Paper of the Global Federation of International Societies of Paediatric Gastroenterology, Hepatology and Nutrition (FISPGHAN). *J. Pediatr. Gastroenterol. Nutr.* **2020**, *70*, 702–710. [CrossRef] [PubMed]

12. Barnett, T.A.; Kelly, A.S.; Young, D.R.; Perry, C.K.; Pratt, C.A.; Edwards, N.M.; Rao, G.; Vos, M.B. Sedentary Behaviors in Today's Youth: Approaches to the Prevention and Management of Childhood Obesity: A Scientific Statement from the American Heart Association. *Circulation* **2018**, *138*, e142–e159. [CrossRef]

13. Robinson, T.N.; Banda, J.A.; Hale, L.; Robinson, T.N.; Banda, J.A.; Hale, L.; Lu, A.S.; Fleming-Milici, F.; Calvert, S.L.; Wartella, E. Screen Media Exposure and Obesity in Children and Adolescents. *Pediatrics* **2017**, *140* (Suppl. 2), S97–S101. [CrossRef] [PubMed]

14. Tambalis, K.D.; Panagiotakos, D.B.; Psarra, G.; Sidossis, L.S. Insufficient Sleep Duration Is Associated with Dietary Habits, Screen Time and Obesity in Children. *J. Clin. Sleep Med.* **2018**, *14*, 1689–1696. [CrossRef] [PubMed]

15. Avery, A.; Anderson, C.; McCullough, F. Associations between children's diet quality and watching television during meal or snack consumption: A systematic review. *Matern. Child Nutr.* **2017**, *13*, e12428. [CrossRef] [PubMed]

16. Scaglioni, S.; De Cosmi, V.; Ciappolino, V.; Parazzini, F.; Brambilla, P.; Agostoni, C. Factors Influencing Children's Eating Behaviours. *Nutrients* **2018**, *10*, 706. [CrossRef]

17. Gubbels, J.S. Environmental Influences on Dietary Intake of Children and Adolescents. *Nutrients* **2020**, *12*, 922. [CrossRef] [PubMed]

18. Van Stralen, M.M.; te Velde, S.J.; Singh, A.S.; De Bourdeaudhuij, I.; Martens, M.K.; van der Sluis, M.; Manios, Y.; Grammatikaki, E.; Chinapaw, M.J.; Maes, L.; et al. EuropeaN Energy balance Research to prevent excessive weight Gain among Youth (ENERGY) project: Design and methodology of the ENERGY cross-sectional survey. *BMC Public Health* **2011**, *11*, 65. [CrossRef]

19. Chen, P.; Mao, L.; Nassis, G.P.; Harmer, P.; Ainsworth, B.E.; Li, F. Coronavirus disease (COVID-19): The need to maintain regular physical activity while taking precautions. *J. Sport Health Sci.* **2020**, *9*, 103–104. [CrossRef]

20. Maffetone, P.B.; Laursen, P.B. The Perfect Storm: Coronavirus (Covid-19) Pandemic Meets Overfat Pandemic. *Front. Public Health* **2020**, *8*, 131. [CrossRef]

21. Bhutani, S.; Cooper, J.A. COVID-19 related home confinement in adults: Weight gain risks and opportunities. *Obesity (Silver Spring)* **2020**, *28*, 1576–1577. [CrossRef]

22. Frühbeck, G.; Baker, J.L.; Busetto, L.; Dicker, D.; Goossens, G.H.; Halford, J.C.G.; Handjieva-Darlenska, T.; Hassapidou, M.; Holm, J.C.; Lehtinen-Jacks, S.; et al. European Association for the Study of Obesity Position Statement on the Global COVID-19 Pandemic. *Obes. Facts* **2020**, *13*, 292–296. [CrossRef]

23. Ng, K.; Cooper, J.; McHale, F.; Clifford, J.; Woods, C. Barriers and facilitators to changes in adolescent physical activity during COVID-19. *BMJ Open Sport Exerc. Med.* **2020**, *6*, e000919. [CrossRef]

24. Jia, P.; Zhang, L.; Yu, W.; Yu, B.; Liu, M.; Zhang, D.; Yang, S. Impact of COVID-19 lockdown on activity patterns and weight status among youths in China: The COVID-19 Impact on Lifestyle Change Survey (COINLICS). *Int. J. Obes. (Lond.)* **2020**, *4*, 1–5. [CrossRef]

25. Ruiz-Roso, M.B.; de Carvalho Padilha, P.; Mantilla-Escalante, D.C.; Ulloa, N.; Brun, P.; Acevedo-Correa, D.; Arantes Ferreira Peres, W.; Martorell, M.; Aires, M.T.; de Oliveira Cardoso, L.; et al. Covid-19 Confinement and Changes of Adolescent's Dietary Trends in Italy, Spain, Chile, Colombia and Brazil. *Nutrients* **2020**, *12*, 1807. [CrossRef] [PubMed]

26. Ammar, A.; Brach, M.; Trabelsi, K.; Chtourou, H.; Boukhris, O.; Masmoudi, L.; Bouaziz, B.; Bentlage, E.; How, D.; Ahmed, M.; et al. Effects of COVID-19 Home Confinement on Eating Behaviour and Physical Activity: Results of the ECLB-COVID-19 International Online Survey. *Nutrients* **2020**, *12*, 1583. [CrossRef] [PubMed]

27. Adams, E.L.; Caccavale, L.J.; Smith, D.; Bean, M.K. Food insecurity, the home food environment, and parent feeding practices in the era of COVID-19. *Obesity (Silver Spring)* **2020**, *28*, 2056–2063. [CrossRef]

28. Browne, N.T.; Snethen, J.A.; Greenberg, C.S.; Frenn, M.; Kilanowski, J.F.; Gance-Cleveland, B.; Burke, P.J.; Lewandowski, L. When pandemics collide: The impact of COVID-19 on childhood obesity. *J. Pediatr. Nurs.* **2020**. [CrossRef]
29. Sidor, A.; Rzymski, P. Dietary Choices and Habits during COVID-19 Lockdown: Experience from Poland. *Nutrients* **2020**, *12*, 1657. [CrossRef]
30. Woo Baidal, J.A.; Chang, J.; Hulse, E.; Turetsky, R.; Parkinson, K.; Rausch, J.C. Zooming Towards a Telehealth Solution for Vulnerable Children with Obesity During Coronovirus Disease 2019. *Obesity (Silver Spring)* **2020**, *28*, 1184–1186. [CrossRef] [PubMed]
31. Ribeiro, K.D.D.S.; Garcia, L.R.S.; Dametto, J.F.D.S.; Assunção, D.G.F.; Maciel, B.L.L. COVID-19 and Nutrition: The Need for Initiatives to Promote Healthy Eating and Prevent Obesity in Childhood. *Child Obes.* **2020**, *16*, 235–237. [CrossRef] [PubMed]
32. Guan, H.; Okely, A.D.; Aguilar-Farias, N.; Del Pozo Cruz, B.; Draper, C.E.; El Hamdouchi, A.; Florindo, A.A.; Jáuregui, A.; Katzmarzyk, P.T.; Kontsevaya, A.; et al. Promoting healthy movement behaviours among children during the COVID-19 pandemic. *Lancet Child Adolesc. Health* **2020**, *4*, 416–418. [CrossRef]
33. Berg, E.A.; Picoraro, J.A.; Miller, S.D.; Srinath, A.; Franciosi, J.P.; Hayes, C.E.; Farrell, P.R.; Cole, C.R.; LeLeiko, N.S. COVID-19—A Guide to Rapid Implementation of Telehealth Services: A Playbook for the Pediatric Gastroenterologist. *J. Pediatr. Gastroenterol. Nutr.* **2020**, *70*, 734–740. [CrossRef] [PubMed]

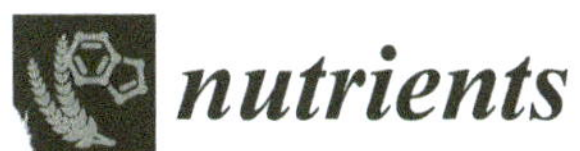

nutrients

Review

The Influence of Parental Dietary Behaviors and Practices on Children's Eating Habits

Lubna Mahmood [1], Paloma Flores-Barrantes [1], Luis A. Moreno [1,2,3,4,*], Yannis Manios [5,6] and Esther M. Gonzalez-Gil [1,4,7]

1   Growth, Exercise, Nutrition and Development (GENUD) Research Group, Instituto Agroalimentario de Aragón (IA2), University of Zaragoza, 50009 Zaragoza, Spain; lmahmood400@gmail.com (L.M.); pfloba@unizar.es (P.F.-B.); esthergg@ugr.es (E.M.G.-G.)
2   Instituto Agroalimentario de Aragón (IA2), 50009 Zaragoza, Spain
3   Instituto de Investigación Sanitaria de Aragón (IIS Aragón), 50009 Zaragoza, Spain
4   Centro de Investigación Biomédica en Red de Fisiopatología de la Obesidad y Nutrición (CIBERObn), Instituto de Salud Carlos III, 28040 Madrid, Spain
5   Department of Nutrition and Dietetics, School of Health Science & Education, Harokopio University, 17671 Athens, Greece; manios@hua.gr
6   Institute of Agri-food and Life Sciences, Hellenic Mediterranean University Research Centre, 71410 Heraklion, Greece
7   Department of Biochemistry and Molecular Biology II, Instituto de Nutrición y Tecnología de los Alimentos, Center of Biomedical Research (CIBM), Universidad de Granada, 18071 Granada, Spain
*   Correspondence: lmoreno@unizar.es; Tel.: +34-(97)-676-1000

Abstract: Poor dietary habits established during childhood might persist into adulthood, increasing the risk of developing obesity and obesity-related complications such as Type 2 Diabetes Mellitus. It has been found that early modifications in eating habits, especially during childhood, might promote health and decrease the risk of developing diseases during later life. Various studies found a great influence of parental dietary habits on dietary behaviors of their children regardless of demographic characteristics such as gender, age, socioeconomic status and country; however, the exact mechanism is still not clear. Therefore, in this review, we aimed to investigate both parents' and children's dietary behaviors, and to provide evidence for the potential influence of parents' dietary behaviors and practices on certain children's eating habits. Family meals were found to contribute the most in modeling children's dietary habits as they represent an important moment of control and interaction between parents and their children. The parental practices that influenced their children most were role modeling and moderate restriction, suggesting that the increase of parental encouragement and decrease of excessive pressure could have a positive impact in their children's dietary behaviors. This narrative review highlights that parental child-feeding behaviors should receive more attention in research studies as modifiable risk factors, which could help to design future dietary interventions and policies to prevent dietary-related diseases.

Keywords: parents; dietary intake; feeding practices; children; family meals; breakfast; snacking habits

Citation: Mahmood, L.; Flores-Barrantes, P.; Moreno, L.A.; Manios, Y.; Gonzalez-Gil, E.M. The Influence of Parental Dietary Behaviors and Practices on Children's Eating Habits. *Nutrients* **2021**, *13*, 1138. https://doi.org/10.3390/nu13041138

Academic Editor: Marilyn Cornelis

Received: 11 February 2021
Accepted: 26 March 2021
Published: 30 March 2021

Publisher's Note: MDPI stays neutral with regard to jurisdictional claims in published maps and institutional affiliations.

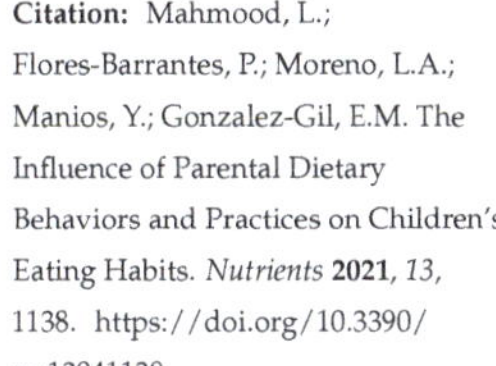

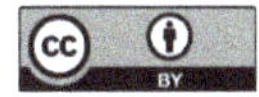

Copyright: © 2021 by the authors. Licensee MDPI, Basel, Switzerland. This article is an open access article distributed under the terms and conditions of the Creative Commons Attribution (CC BY) license (https://creativecommons.org/licenses/by/4.0/).

1. Introduction

Obesity is a complex condition influenced by both genetic and environmental factors [1]. Dietary intake has been linked with obesity in terms of volume, composition, meals' frequency, snacking habits and diet quality [2]. Additionally, there is indication that children are likely to maintain their dietary habits into adulthood [2]. Thus, understanding children's eating habits is very important in terms of children's health [3]. There are some factors that could influence children's eating habits such as the home food environment, as well as the social environment, contexts where perceptions, knowledge and eating habits are established [4]. However, parental dietary patterns seem to affect children most, as parents are the ones who shape the home food environment, influence how a child thinks about food, and, accordingly, start forming their own food preferences and eating behavior [4].

Out of the dietary habits, family mealtime becomes the main social context in which children can eat with their parents, who are considered as their main role-models [5]. Sharing meals with children, having breakfast together regularly and encouraging children to have healthy snacks with moderate restrictions have shown positive impacts on children's dietary behaviors [6]. Furthermore, one review study evaluated these practices and found that they were associated with higher consumption of dairy products, fruits and vegetables (FV), along with healthier breakfast patterns among children [7]. Also, the same review stated that encouragement practice gives children a chance of making decisions, whereas the moderate restriction practice help parents to imply clearer instructions to their children. Therefore, it was recommended to use a combination of the two practices, so that both parents and children would have the ability to contribute to determining food choices [8]. In this narrative review, we focus on the effect of parental dietary habits on children's eating behaviors, including family meals, breakfast routine and snacking habits.

2. Method for Literature Search

Serial literature searches for articles of interest were performed between August and December 2020. PubMed, Scopus, Education Resources Information Center (ERIC), Science Direct and Google scholar databases were searched using the following keywords: "parents", "dietary intake", "feeding practices", "children", "family meals", "breakfast", "snacking habits", "food choices", "food consumption", "role model", "diabetes", "parenting style", "behavior". We included both original researches and review articles published between 2000 and 2020. Studies were eligible if they were published in English and included preschoolers (ages 2–5 years), or school-age children (ages 6–13 years). A total of 2590 studies were identified, 508 duplicates were removed, 455 related titles were chosen, 92 articles met the inclusion criteria and 83 studies were included in this review.

3. Definitions

"Eating habits" can be defined as the conscious and repetitive way a person eats, and this includes what types of food are eaten, their quantities and timing of consumption, in response to cultural and social influences [9]. On the other hand, "eating behaviors" have been considered as a group of actions starting from a simple food chewing to food shopping, food preparation and food policy decision-making [10]. Food patterns or dietary patterns refer to the quantity, quality and variety of foods and beverages consumed as well as the frequency with which they are habitually consumed, and it refers to the diet as a whole [10]. A balanced diet is characterized by high intake of fresh FV, whole grains, legumes, nuts, fiber, polyunsaturated fatty acids and low in both refined grains as well as saturated fatty acids [11]. However, guidelines may differ in their recommendations regarding the consumption of processed meat and dairy products, probably relating to the national food culture, sustainable food choices and food safety [11].

4. Children's Eating Habits

Dietary habits from childhood track into adulthood, so understanding children's eating habits is very important in terms of children's health [12]. Nutrition is the main factor of interaction between parents and children, especially during the first year of life, starting by breastfeeding [12]. By the end of the first year of life, children start learning to feed themselves and make the transition to the family diet and meal patterns [12]. A review study that assessed both national and international research articles on child nutrition and eating behaviors concluded that as children switch to the family diet, recommendations from parents address not only food, but also the eating context, which refers to the immediate environment of each eating occasion [12]. Moreover, the same study suggested that a variety of healthy food items provided to children can promote their diet quality and food acceptance [12].

A study across 11 countries suggested that the nutritional status of children from birth to the age of 2 years was positively associated with dietary variety [13]. Furthermore, exposures to FV in early childhood have been associated with higher acceptance of these foods at later ages [13]. A longitudinal study of 120 2-year-old children and their parents followed for 9 years found that around 25% of children experienced some eating problems such as being hesitant to try new foods or insist on a limited number of food items (no variety), concluding that those problems may lead them to become picky eaters [14].

However, children with eating problems (i.e., picky eaters, meal skippers) may be at risk for behavioral problems, as well as impaired growth and development [14], whereas repeated exposure was found to be the main way for children to recognize the food. Thus, parents are advised to keep introducing food items more than once, and to avoid getting discouraged or giving up [12].

5. Home Food Environment

The home food environment includes the availability and accessibility of food, as well as other factors such as frequency of eating out, and parents' perception of food costs [15]. In addition, the home food environment was found to have remarkable effects on eating behaviors of parents and their children as most of the food consumed is stored and prepared at home [15]. Although children are likely to be influenced by their home food environment and the community, they may have limited control over it [16]. Results from the Quebec Longitudinal Study of Child Development, which included 1492 children, found that children who had a better family environment, i.e., less family pressure to eat, had low levels of soft-drinks consumption (unstandardized $\beta = -0.43$, $p < 0.001$, 95% confidence interval (CI), -0.62 to -0.23), and high level of fitness (unstandardized $\beta = 0.24$, $p < 0.001$, 95% CI, 0.12–0.36) [16]. In the same vein, the baseline survey of the Identification and prevention of Dietary- and lifestyle-induced health Effects in Children and infants (IDEFICS) study, which included 1435 families from eight European countries, found that home food environment plays a stronger role in shaping children's intake of healthy foods than unhealthy foods, especially for younger children [17].

As previously mentioned, the home food environment determines what kind of foods are available and accessible to children [15]. While availability and accessibility are often merged into a single construct, the content map presented in Vaughn's study [18] considered them separately because they may have differential effects on children's diet and eating behaviors. Accordingly, these diverse definitions could explain the differences found in the results of studies. Availability is related to the physical presence of food [18], whereas accessibility refers to parental actions to control how easy or difficult it is for children to access food by themselves or with limited assistance [18]. A review about the availability and accessibility of FV at home found that both availability and accessibility were associated with FV consumption among children and adolescents and inversely associated with children's total energy and fat intake [19].

Besides, low consumption of nutrient-poor, energy-dense food items, like sugar-sweetened beverages, cookies, packed snacks, food high in saturated/transfat, simple sugars and sodium, were noticed when these items were and were not available at home [19]. However, low-income families seem to have low access to healthy foods and possibly greater access to fast food due to dietary costs, which could explain some of the relationships between Socioeconomic Status (SES) and nutrient density of consumed foods [19].

Frequency of eating out is one of the dietary habits that are most influenced by the household environment [20]. Ready-to-eat and out-of-home (OH) foods include vending machines, take-away, cafes, restaurants, supermarkets and convenience stores [20]. Nowadays, families seem to prepare less food at home and spend more money on foods prepared away from home [20], and food prepared OH tends to be more energy-dense than food prepared at home, particularly in terms of fat and sugar content [20]. In addition, focus groups among the urban community in the US found that parents desire easy, convenient and tasteful meals that are culturally appropriate and low-cost, while some families may believe that food eaten out is lower in cost and tastier [21]. These beliefs would encourage parents to eat out and thus perpetuate the cycle of decreased home-prepared meals. Consequently, children may have less opportunities to learn culinary skills, have access to healthy diet, or reinforce healthy eating habits [21]. Cross-sectional data from the UK National Diet and Nutrition Survey Rolling Program of 4636 children and adolescents aged 1.5–18 years showed that consuming food prepared outside the home was associated with a greater intake of foods with high levels of fat and sugar in children [20]. Also, a systematic review documented the nutritional characteristics of eating away from home and its relations with the diet quality and energy intake. The results of this review concluded that eating outside the home is associated with lower diet quality and micronutrients intake, like vitamin C, Fe and Ca. However, the conclusion needed further confirmation as the review was based on studies from national surveys from Belgium and the United States only [22]. Similar results were obtained in a cross-sectional study conducted in Japan among 4258 caregivers, where children with obesity had a lower frequency of shared home-made meals, after adjusting for confounding factors.

However, validity and reliability of the questionnaire used to assess the frequency of cooking were not examined [23]. Unfortunately, these studies have only considered the effect of eating out without concerning the effect of ready-to-eat (unhealthy) meals prepared at home.

6. Parenting Styles and Feeding Practices

In the literature, parenting styles have been defined as psychological constructs representing the more general interactions between parents and children, whereas parental feeding practices includes specific rules or behaviors used by parents to control when, what and how much their children eat [24,25].

It has been previously stated by Horst and Sleddens [26] that according to Baumrind's taxonomy, parenting styles have been divided into three categories: authoritarian, permissive and authoritative. Whereas authoritarian styles are highly demanding but less responsive, permissive styles include less demanding but high responsiveness, and authoritative styles present both demanding and responsive [26].

Studies examining the direct role of parenting styles on children's eating behaviors are limited. However, a recent review of the evidence found that less parental monitoring was presented in the permissive style, whereas more restrictive food and high pressure on children to eat were linked to authoritarian parenting style. On the other hand, preferable parental monitoring of the child's food intake was associated with the authoritative parenting style [27]. Another two systematic reviews concluded that children tend to eat more healthily with a healthy body mass index (BMI) if they raised in authoritative households. However, the effects of these generic parenting styles were generally indirect and weak [28,29].

One review critically summarized previous research on parental feeding practices and found that role models can play a really important part in shaping children's eating habits. Therefore, role modeling behaviors were recommended for parents such as: providing healthy foods, modeling healthy eating and increasing encouragement to eat healthy foods [30]. Results from a study that used the Parental Feeding Style Questionnaire (PFSQ), which included 100 children (aged 2–5) in Hong Kong, showed that encouraging children to consume a variety of foods was associated with healthier eating behaviors, like meal frequency, better food choices and higher intake of fruits (Odd Ratio (OR) = 1.357; 95% confidence interval (CI) = 1.188 to 1.551) and vegetables (OR = 1.335; 95% CI = 1.128 to 1.579) [31]. Whereas, using foods as rewards could increase the child's preferences for these food items. Thus, using unhealthy foods as rewards may promote children's consumption of unhealthy energy-dense palatable foods [31]. Likewise, a cross-sectional study conducted in 17 primary schools in Dunedin city in New Zealand found that through a good parental role modeling, higher parental diet quality was associated with lower consumption of cakes, chocolate, biscuits and savory dishes in children [32]. A cross-sectional study included 13,305 children in nine European countries and found associations (OR between 1.40 and 2.42, $p < 0.02$) between parental role modeling of healthful foods with children's dietary habits, food intake and preferences for fruits and vegetables [33].

The results of these studies highlighted the importance of parental modeling in terms of their dietary behaviors and food choices on the diet of their children. However, parental role modeling studies have employed different methods, with varying validity, to measure children's dietary intake, such as 24 h dietary recalls, food frequency questionnaires, parent report of child dietary intake and child report of parental role modeling. This could explain why correlations between parent and child reports for these studies have also been mixed, whereas studies that have utilized both parent and child report are very limited.

A review study summarizing previous results on parental strategies and practices concluded that a "moderate restriction" could be beneficial as children of moderately restrictive parents were found to consume fewer calories, eat more fruits, and eat less fatty snacks and sweets [34]. Besides, the "prompting and encouragement" feeding practice made by parents could help their children to have healthier dietary habits [34]. The term "moderate restrictions" indicates a careful use of restrictions by parents in which unhealthy food items were gradually decreased and limited rather than being strictly forbidden, whereas the word 'encouragement' refers to the situation when parents offer more types of food with positive messages, but at the same time, children can still make decisions in combination with their parents [31].

On the other hand, restricted parental feeding practice seemed to be related to overeating, especially among preschool-age children [35]. One longitudinal study assessed the maternal influences on picky eating behaviors and diet of 173 9-year-old non-Hispanic white girls [36]. The results of this study suggested that with mothers who were less likely to pressure their children to eat, their children were less likely to be picky eaters or overweight [36]. While, when parents highly restrict energy-dense foods from their children's diet hoping children choose healthful alternatives, children usually increase their desire for it and start to eat when they are not hungry [34]. Therefore, various research studies discourage pressuring practice as it can create a negative family eating environment and make children pickier eaters [37,38].

Evidence suggests that high involvement and role-modeling practices are more favorable for supporting positive food-related behaviors, especially among young children. But unfortunately, these studies cannot be taken as proof of causality. Thus, long-term studies are needed to determine the causal link between parental feeding practices and children's eating habits.

Household food rules is another factor which is usually established by parents to guide youth behaviors and achieve goals for their growth [39]. To explain further, for example, both "limited fast food" and "limited portion sizes at meals" were significantly linked with improved food consumption and weight status [39]. Whereas a rule of "no fried snacks" was positively associated with percent body fat (PBF), however, the link between fat intake, snacking and excess weight was unclear as snack foods are often grouped as one item (e.g., chips, candies, ice cream and cookies) [39]. Besides, the "no snacking while watching television" rule was found to be an effective one as children tend to eat more when they are distracted and eating while watching TV also prolongs the eating period [39]. In a School of Public Health Project, Eating and Activity over Time (EAT) researchers found that children in families who watch TV while eating meals had a lower-quality diet than the children of families who turned the TV off during meals [40]. In the same study, children who watched TV while eating family meals seemed to consume fewer grains and vegetables, and more soft drinks, than those who did not watch TV. Similar results were also found among Australian children in which watching TV was associated with the consumption of energy-dense foods and drinks [41]. However, these studies do not definitively prove direct causal effects of household food rules on unhealthy food preferences and overall unhealthy diet.

7. Parental Dietary Behaviors Influence on Children's Eating Habits

Dietary preferences are formed by a combination of a complex interplay of genetic, familiar and environmental factors. However, parents seemed to have a high degree of control in modeling their children's eating behaviors [42]. During the first year of life, children's dietary patterns undergo a rapid evolution since parents are the ones who select the foods of the family and serve as models of eating. Thus, children tend to imitate their parents' behaviors as well as eating habits [42]. As illustrated in Figure 1, children's eating behaviors are affected by social, physical and intra-individual factors. In the family environment, parents establish more than 70% of their children's dietary behaviors by their own intake and the methods followed to socialize their children [42]. To systematically assess the effect of parental dietary patterns on children, several studies have been revised, which summarize how parental eating habits and feeding styles have been significantly associated with children's eating behaviors, food preferences, intake and consumption (Supplementary Table S1).

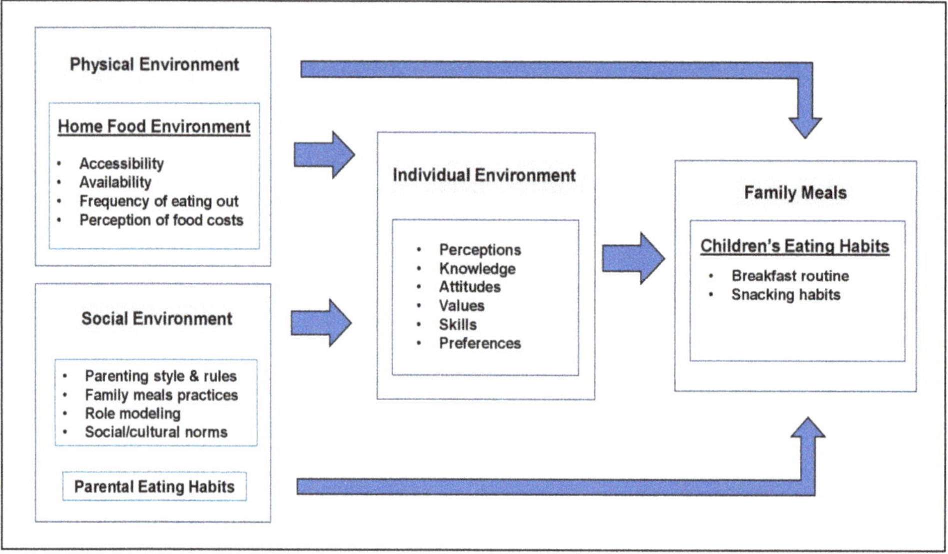

Figure 1. Summary of home/family-related determinants of children's eating habits.

Parental dietary behaviors refer to the passive processes that influence their children's dietary behaviors and food environment [43]. Various cross-sectional studies have indicated the close similarity between parents and children in the intakes of some healthy and unhealthy foods and beverages, as well as dietary composition, especially when more meals are eaten together [44–48]. Although this association has demonstrated that parents' dietary behavior might influence children's intake, these studies cannot be used to conclude causality. Therefore, the process by which parents affect their children's food intake remains largely unclear.

Four focus groups were conducted in Belgium among parents and caregivers showing that the influence of parental practices differs by age. The younger the child, especially at preschool age and first years of primary education, the stronger the role of parental practices [43]. The same study found that children may consider parents' norms and perceptions as a reference for what is appropriate to consume [43].

Various cross-sectional studies found showed a significant positive association and substantial correlation between children's and parent's intake of various foods [49–51]. Thus, parents' eating behaviors have proven to be a part of the whole process of establishing and promoting healthy or unhealthy dietary patterns among children and adolescents [42]. A Parent Mealtime Action Scale (PMAS) was developed among 439 fathers and 541 mothers in the USA to examine the dimensions of mealtime behaviors used by parents on children's diet and weight status. The results showed that parents could be influenced by their environment and culture, which may also affect their food choices, suggesting that their children's dietary patterns and nutritional status may also be altered accordingly [52]. Whereas the same study found that obliging a child to accept healthy food through giving advice only, without eating it themselves, is a dead end in nutrition education [52].

Previous studies concluded that parents' influence is thought to be strongest during childhood, especially in early ages, when parents act as role models, enforcers and providers. Therefore, intervention programs should consider what parents consume as well as the parental influence in terms of what parents feed their children and how they feed them.

7.1. Family Meals

Family meal has been defined as a meal being shared with family members or when one, or both, of the parents are present [53]. There are differences when analyzing the frequency of family meals: some considered it as having ≥ 3 and others ≥ 5 family meals taken weekly [53]. Thus, the lack of specificity and consistency in measuring, analyzing and defining family meals makes it difficult to come up with definite results and to compare results [53].

A systematic review [54] that focused on the effects of family meal frequency and psychosocial consequences in youth concluded that more frequent family meals were inversely associated with disordered eating, violent behaviors and depression in children. Additionally, in the same review, it was found that more frequent family meals were positively associated with an increased self-esteem among children [54]. It is agreed that family meals represent an important moment of both control and interaction in the family [55]. A study of family mealtime characteristics of Australian families with children aged 6 months to 6 years old showed that parents place high value on mealtime when they share meals with their children, which helps children to promote healthy eating behaviors. An important strength of this study was the reliable survey measures, but the used online, self-report surveys can be affected by respondent interpretation bias [55]. The presence of parents during mealtime has been linked to decreased meal skipping and increased consumption of dairy products and FV [43]. Correspondingly, results of the Next Generation Health Study in the US showed a higher FV consumption among children whose parents were eating the same food items and sharing their meals with them. This study included a large, nationally representative and generalizable sample; however, the self-estimation and self-report assessment were susceptible to recall bias [56].

In Scotland, a cohort of young children followed-up for 10 years suggested that determining the characteristics of family mealtime practices is needed to increase diet quality and improve children' eating behaviors, such as reduced access to TV viewing during meals, portion sizes, sitting at a table, besides social engagement between parents and children [57]. Similarly, the Quebec Longitudinal Study of Child Development investigated the effect of frequent family meals on children, and results showed that children who had a better family meal environment at the age of 6 years had lower levels of soft-drinks consumption and higher levels of fitness when they reached 10 years [16]. In the same vein, a Harvard cohort study found that children who eat together with their parents are twice as likely to eat their five servings of FV compared to families who do not share their meals. Moreover, in the same study, family meals seemed to help parents to perform as role models and be considered as an example of polite table manners and healthy eating habits [58]. In addition, results from the same study also showed that shared meals seem to help in childhood obesity prevention as children tend to eat less when they eat in the presence of their parents [58]. Participants in this study were children of nurses, hence, they all came from highly educated families compared to the general population [58].

One meta-analysis concluded that higher frequency of shared family meals in children and adolescents was significantly associated with a normal body weight and healthier dietary habits when they shared family meals 3 or more times per week [59]. Additionally, home cooking and shared family meals have been considered as a key strategy to promote healthy dietary habits and prevent obesity among children [60,61]. A family meals-focused randomized controlled trial in 160 families of 12-year-old children followed-up for about 5 years. Data were collected at baseline, post-intervention and follow-up, and results indicated that promoting healthy shared family meals could lead to a moderate reduction in excess body weight, especially among young children.

Despite the rigorous design, quality measurement and strong theoretical framework used in this study, the generalizability of study findings is limited [61], while engagement in family meals has been considered as the simplest and easiest independent intervention that could be applied to establish a healthy family environment [61]. Therefore, eating environment should be taken into account as it usually affects family communication, parents and children interactions, what kind of food is served, how much is eaten at meals and frequency and lengths of meals. However, it seems that the specific mechanisms of how family mealtimes influence children's nutritional outcomes are yet unclear and should be investigated.

7.2. Breakfast Routine

"Breakfast" refers to the first meal of the day, or a meal often eaten in the early morning [62]. The findings from the "Anthropometry, Intake and Energy Balance" (ANIBES) Study [62] reported that around 85% of the Spanish population (9–75 years) were regular breakfast consumers, although one in five adolescents were breakfast skippers. It has also been found in the same study that breakfast provides only 16–19% of the daily energy intake. Among the specific foods, the most commonly consumed breakfast foods among children and teenagers were chocolate, pastries and milk [62]. Additionally, a review studied the benefits of breakfast by involving national dietary survey data from various countries including Spain, the UK, Canada, the USA, Denmark and France. Its results found that a healthy regular breakfast has been associated with improved cognitive health, nutritional status and lower plasma cholesterol levels among children and adolescents [63]. These results were supported by a cross-sectional study conducted among 126 children in four elementary schools in Indonesia. Results from that study found that breakfast habits of children were significantly associated with the parent's breakfast habits [64]. Moreover, in the same study, 23% of fathers and 15.9% of mothers were not having breakfast daily, whereas, 17% of children reported that they are not taking their breakfast because no food was available at home in the morning [64].

One of the most wide-reaching reports is that of the European branch of the World Health Organization, who conducted a health behavior survey of over 200,000 male and female schoolchildren, 11–13 and 15 years of age in 39 European states in 2009/2010 [63]. Overall, 61% of 13-year-olds consumed a breakfast on each school day, while the figure fell to 55% among 15-year-olds. In general, breakfast consumption was most common among boys and declined with lower socio-economic status [63]. These data showed that about half to one third of children do not have breakfast every day, although the data does not reveal the actual frequency of breakfast intake [63]. The report also indicates that regular breakfast consumption is associated with higher intakes of micronutrients, a better diet that includes FV and less frequency of consumption of soft drinks [63]. According to the Health Sponsorship Council (HSC), there are more than 100,000 children worldwide aged 1–5 years missing breakfast at least once per week, while their parents are also skipping this meal. Besides, over 36,000 children worldwide never consume breakfast at home. It has been revealed that children of parents who skip breakfast are more likely to skip their breakfast, consume more energy-dense nutrient-poor food and are more likely to be overweight [65]. A cross-sectional study including 426 children aged 10–14 years from 4 local schools in Queensland found that skipping breakfast among children was associated with the lack of perceived parental emphasis on consuming breakfast (OR = 3.67, 95% CI: 1.75–7.68) [66].

Another cross-sectional survey conducted among preschoolers aged 2–5 years in Hong Kong showed that most children were having their breakfast daily but less than half of them consumed the recommended number of dairy products and FV [31]. Consequently, these studies suggested that parental breakfast-skipping habits are strongly associated with breakfast skipping among their children. Thus, findings underline the importance of addressing parental habits and their children's in the intervention plan.

7.3. Snacking Habits

"Snack" has been defined as a small portion of foods or drinks that is taken between regular meals [67]. Another study considered snacks as food items consumed at different times of the day [68]. A study conducted in Spain defined snacking as the process of consuming any food intake outside the three main meals, including mid-morning snack "between breakfast and lunch" and mid-afternoon snack "between lunch and dinner", and nibbling, "disorganized and without defined timing" [69]. The term "snack" seems not to have a static definition [67]. Thus, the impact of snacking is difficult to be assessed due to the variety of its definitions in the literature [67].

In Spain, it has been found that 84.4% of younger and 78.3% of older children were mid-afternoon snack consumers. Specifically, sandwich was the most common food item consumed [69]. Excessive consumption of soft drinks and high-fat-containing snacks and low intake of fruits and vegetables was reported among Mexican children in five Baja California counties [70]. Similar findings were found in a cross-sectional study which involved 109 students and their parents in Milan. Results showed that more than 35% of snacks consumed by school-age children were sweets, 23.8% sugary drinks, 9.4% savory snacks, whereas consumption of nuts, yogurt and fresh fruits was very low [71].

Despite limited data, a systematic review concluded that parents' eating behaviors, whether positive or negative, have an impact on the quality of snacks consumed by their children [72]. Whereas consumptions of lower-quality snacks were associated with increased prevalence of overweight among children [73–75]. Some research studies found that the influence of parents on children's snacking habits depends on the children's life stage and age. For instance, parental influence decreases in the transition from childhood to adolescence [76,77]. The nationally representative surveys of food intake in US children demonstrated a positive association between parents' and children's snack consumption, where children tend to consume more snacks if their parents prefer to have more snacks throughout the day [78]. A cross-sectional study which included 1632 elementary school children in Japan showed that their snacking habits were affected by paternal eating habits, for example, children did not consume vegetables as snacks as it was not offered by their parents. Nonetheless, since data were collected only from children in Takaoka city in Japan, the results may not be generalizable to a global population [79], whereas children's consumptions of FV as snacks were high in homes with greater FV intake among parents as well as FV availability [79]. These results were confirmed by another study which used a Web-based survey among 9842 students in Australia and found that when parents offered more snacks, children consumed more snacks [80]. Another cross-sectional study conducted among 667 students selected from schools in West-Flanders (Belgium) confirmed that parental monitoring and child's eating schedule or routine set by parents were associated with more FV intake among girls ($p \leq 0.001$, 95% CI: −1.8 to −0.5) and boys ($p \leq 0.001$, 95% CI: −1.7 to −0.5), and reduced negative eating behaviors such as less unhealthy snacking [81]. Results of comprehensive questionnaires, completed by parents of children aged 4–8 years ($n = 203$) in New Zealand, found that the lack of rules regarding the offering of foods to children was associated with a higher intake of fatty snacks [82].

Based on previous studies, it is suggested that during school age, parents play an important role in the control of children's food intake and food choices. Thus, the whole family is encouraged to be involved in the educational interventions to prevent imbalanced snacking behaviors in children.

8. Conclusions

Multiple parental factors influence a child's dietary habits and are reciprocally interacting, so they cannot be considered separately. The family environment that surrounds a child's domestic life has an active role in establishing and promoting behaviors that will persist throughout their life. Family meals seem to represent an important moment of both control and interaction, which contributes the most in modeling children's dietary habits. Parents should avoid excessive pressure or restriction as it can create a negative social and emotional experience that could affect children's acceptance of the food. Instead, parents should encourage their children on healthy snacking as well as not to skip their breakfast. This can be achieved through positive and active social modeling as well as moderate restriction. Given the considerable evidence for the strong effect of parents on their children's dietary habits, we believe that parents' child-feeding behaviors should receive more attention in childhood obesity prevention policies. We recommend that parents should be provided with information and guidance on how, as well as what, to feed their children, and these promotion strategies should be particularly aimed at parents' unhealthy eating too so they can improve their diet and so their children will imitate them.

Supplementary Materials: The following are available online at https://www.mdpi.com/article/10.3390/nu13041138/s1, Table S1: Studies assessing the influence of parental dietary behaviors on children's eating habits.

Author Contributions: L.M. completed the literature searches, review and drafted the manuscript. P.F.-B. revised the manuscript. E.M.G.-G., Y.M. and L.A.M. reviewed, edited and approved the manuscript. All authors have read and agreed to the published version of the manuscript.

Funding: This research received no external funding.

Institutional Review Board Statement: Not applicable.

Informed Consent Statement: Not applicable.

Data Availability Statement: No new data were created or analyzed in this study. Data sharing is not applicable to this article.

Conflicts of Interest: The authors declare no conflict of interest.

References

1. Albuquerque, D.; Nóbrega, C.; Manco, L.; Padez, C. The contribution of genetics and environment to obesity. *Br. Med. Bull.* **2017**, *123*, 159–173. [CrossRef]
2. ESPGHAN Committee on Nutrition; Agostoni, C.; Braegger, C.; Decsi, T.; Kolacek, S.; Koletzko, B.; Michaelsen, K.F.; Mihatsch, W.; Moreno, L.A.; Puntis, J.; et al. Breast-feeding: A commentary by the ESPGHAN Committee on Nutrition. *J. Pediatr. Gastroenterol. Nutr.* **2009**, *49*, 112–125. [CrossRef] [PubMed]
3. Moreno, L.A.; Rodríguez, G. Dietary risk factors for development of childhood obesity. *Curr. Opin. Clin. Nutr. Metab. Care* **2007**, *10*, 336–341. [CrossRef] [PubMed]
4. Scaglioni, S.; De Cosmi, V.; Ciappolino, V.; Parazzini, F.; Brambilla, P.; Agostoni, C. Factors Influencing Children's Eating Behaviours'. *Nutrients* **2018**, *10*, 706. [CrossRef]
5. Utter, J.; Scragg, R.; Mhurchu, C.N.; Schaaf, D. At-home breakfast consumption among New Zealand children: Associations with body mass index and related nutrition behaviors. *J. Am. Diet Assoc.* **2007**, *107*, 570–576. [CrossRef]
6. Keski-Rahkonen, A.; Kaprio, J.; Rissanen, A.; Virkkunen, M.; Rose, R.J. Breakfast skipping and health-compromising behaviors in adolescents and adults. *Eur. J. Clin. Nutr.* **2003**, *57*, 842–853. [CrossRef]
7. Blissett, J. Relationships between parenting style, feeding style and feeding practices and fruit and vegetable consumption in early childhood. *Appetite* **2011**, *57*, 826–831. [CrossRef]
8. Jansen, E.; Mulkens, S.; Jansen, A. Do not eat the red food prohibition of snacks leads to their relatively higher consumption in children. *Appetite* **2007**, *49*, 572–577. [CrossRef]

9. Rivera Medina, C.; Briones Urbano, M.; de Jesús Espinosa, A.; Toledo López, Á. Eating Habits Associated with Nutrition-Related Knowledge among University Students Enrolled in Academic Programs Related to Nutrition and Culinary Arts in Puerto Rico. *Nutrients* **2020**, *12*, 1408. [CrossRef]
10. Hu, F.B. Dietary pattern analysis: A new direction in nutritional epidemiology. *Curr. Opin. Lipidol.* **2002**, *13*, 3–9. [CrossRef]
11. Wirt, A.; Collins, E. Diet quality-what is it and does it matter. *Public Health Nutr.* **2009**, *12*, 2473–2492. [CrossRef]
12. Ramos, M.; Stein, L.M. Development Children's Eating Behavior. *J. Pediatr.* **2002**, *76*, 229–237. [CrossRef]
13. Arimond, M.; Ruel, M.T. Dietary diversity is associated with child nutritional status: Evidence from 11 demographic and health survey. *J. Nutr.* **2004**, *134*, 2579–2585. [CrossRef]
14. Mascola, A.J.; Bryson, S.W.; Agras, W.S. Picky eating during childhood: A longitudinal study to age 11 years. *Eat Behav.* **2010**, *11*, 253–257. [CrossRef] [PubMed]
15. Sallis, J.F.; Owen, N.; Fisher, E.B. Ecological Models of Health Behaviour. In *Health Behaviour and Health Education*, 4th ed.; Glanz, Z., Rimer, B.K., Viswanath, K., Eds.; Jossey-Bass: San Francisco, CA, USA, 2008; pp. 435–461.
16. Harbec, M.J.; Pagani, L.S. Associations between Early Family Meal Environment Quality and Later Well-Being in School-Age Children. *J. Dev. Behav. Pediatr.* **2018**, *39*, 136–143. [CrossRef] [PubMed]
17. Bogl, L.H.; Silventoinen, K.; Hebestreit, A.; Intemann, T.; Williams, G.; Michels, N.; Molnár, D.; Page, A.S.; Pala, V.; Papoutsou, S.; et al. Familial Resemblance in Dietary Intakes of Children, Adolescents, and Parents: Does Dietary Quality Play a Role? *Nutrients* **2017**, *9*, 892. [CrossRef]
18. Vaughn, A.E.; Ward, D.S.; Fisher, J.O.; Faith, M.S.; Hughes, S.O.; Kremers, S.P.; Musher-Eizenman, D.R.; O'Connor, T.M.; Patrick, H.; Power, T.G. Fundamental constructs in food parenting practices: A content map to guide future research. *Nutr. Rev.* **2016**, *74*, 98–117. [CrossRef]
19. Story, M.; Kaphingst, K.M.; Robinson-O'Brien, R.; Glanz, K. Creating healthy food and eating environments: Policy and environmental approaches. *Annu. Rev. Public Health* **2008**, *29*, 253–272. [CrossRef]
20. Ziauddeen, N.; Page, P.; Penney, T.L.; Nicholson, S.; Kirk, S.F. Almiron-Roig, E. Eating at food outlets and leisure places and "on the go" is associated with less-healthy food choices than eating at home and in school in children: Cross-sectional data from the UK National Diet and Nutrition Survey Rolling Program (2008–2014). *Am. J. Clin. Nutr.* **2018**, *107*, 992–1003. [PubMed]
21. Fulkerson, J.A.; Kubik, M.Y.; Rydell, S.; Boutelle, K.N.; Garwick, A.; Story, M.; Dudovitz, B. Focus groups with working parents of school-age children: What's needed to improve family meals. *J. Nutr. Educ. Behav.* **2011**, *43*, 189–193. [CrossRef]
22. Lachat, C.; Nago, E.; Verstraeten, R.; Roberfroid, D.; Van Camp, J.; Kolsteren, P. Eating out of home and its association with dietary intake: A systematic review of the evidence'. *Obes. Rev.* **2012**, *13*, 329–346. [CrossRef]
23. Tani, Y.; Fujiwara, T.; Doi, S.; Isumi, A. Home Cooking and Child Obesity in Japan: Results from the A-CHILD Study. *Nutrients* **2019**, *11*, 2859. [CrossRef]
24. Baranowski, T.; O'Connor, T.; Hughes, S.; Sleddens, E.; Beltran, A.; Frankel, L.; Mendoza, J.A.; Baranowski, J. Houston... We have a problem! Measurement of parenting. *Child Obes.* **2013**, *9*, S1–S4. [CrossRef]
25. Hughes, S.O.; Frankel, L.A.; Beltran, A.; Hodges, E.; Hoerr, S.; Lumeng, J.; Tovar, A.; Kremers, S. Food parenting measurement issues: Working group consensus report. *Child Obes.* **2013**, *9*, S95–S102. [CrossRef]
26. van der Horst, K.; Sleddens, E.F.C. Parenting styles, feeding styles and food-related parenting practices in relation to toddlers' eating styles: A cluster-analytic approach. *PLoS ONE* **2017**, *12*, e0178149. [CrossRef] [PubMed]
27. Collins, C.; Duncanson, K.; Burrows, T. A systematic review investigating associations between parenting style and child feeding behaviours. *J. Hum. Nutr. Diet. Off. J. Br. Diet. Assoc.* **2014**, *27*, 557–568. [CrossRef] [PubMed]
28. Sleddens, E.F.; Gerards, S.M.; Thijs, C.; de Vries, N.K.; Kremers, S.P. General parenting, childhood overweight and obesity-inducing behaviors: A review. *Int. J. Pediatr. Obes.* **2011**, *6*, e12–e27. [CrossRef]
29. Shloim, N.; Edelson, L.R.; Martin, N.; Hetherington, M.M. Parenting Styles, Feeding Styles, Feeding Practices, and Weight Status in 4–12-Year-Old Children: A Systematic Review of the Literature. *Front. Psychol* **2015**, *6*, 1849. [CrossRef] [PubMed]
30. Pearson, N.; Biddle, S.; Gorely, T. Family correlates of fruit and vegetable consumption in children and adolescents: A systematic review. *Public Health Nutr.* **2009**, *12*, 267–283. [CrossRef] [PubMed]
31. Lo, K.; Cheung, C.; Lee, A.; Tam, W.W.; Keung, V. Associations between Parental Feeding Styles and Childhood Eating Habits: A Survey of Hong Kong Pre-School Children. *PLoS ONE* **2015**, *10*, e0124753. [CrossRef] [PubMed]
32. Davison, B.; Saeedi, P.; Black, K.; Harrex, H.; Haszard, J.; Meredith-Jones, K.; Quigg, R.; Skeaff, S.; Stoner, L.; Wong, J.E.; et al. The Association between Parent Diet Quality and Child Dietary Patterns in Nine- to Eleven-Year-Old Children from Dunedin, New Zealand. *Nutrients* **2017**, *9*, 483. [CrossRef] [PubMed]
33. De Bourdeaudhuij, I.; te Velde, S.; Brug, J.; Due, P.; Wind, M.; Sandvik, C.; Maes, L.; Wolf, A.; Perez Rodrigo, C.; Yngve, A.; et al. Personal, social and environmental predictors of daily fruit and vegetable intake in 11-year-old children in nine European countries. *Eur. J. Clin. Nutr.* **2008**, *62*, 834–841. [CrossRef] [PubMed]
34. Gibson, E.L.; Kreichauf, S.; Wildgruber, A.; Vögele, C.; Summerbell, C.D.; Nixon, C.; Moore, H.; Douthwaite, W.; Manios, Y.; ToyBox-Study Group. A narrative review of psychological and educational strategies applied to young children's eating behaviours aimed at reducing obesity risk. *Obes. Rev.* **2012**, *13*, 85–95. [CrossRef] [PubMed]
35. Birch, L.L.; Fisher, J.O.; Davison, K.K. Learning to Overeat: Maternal Use of Restrictive Feeding Practices Promotes Girls' Eating in the Absence of Hunger. *Am. J. Clin. Nutr.* **2003**, *78*, 215–220. [CrossRef] [PubMed]

36. Galloway, A.T.; Fiorito, L.; Lee, Y.; Birch, L.L. Parental Pressure, Dietary Patterns, and Weight Status among Girls Who are 'Picky Eaters. *J. Am. Diet. Assoc.* **2005**, *105*, 541–548. [CrossRef]

37. Hennessy, E.; Hughes, S.O.; Goldberg, J.P.; Hyatt, R.R.; Economos, C.D. Permissive Parental Feeding Behavior Is Associated with an Increase in Intake of Low-Nutrient-Dense Foods among American Children Living in Rural Communities. *J. Acad. Nutr. Diet.* **2012**, *112*, 142–148. [CrossRef]

38. Fisher, J.O.; Birch, L.L. Parents' restrictive feeding practices are associated with young girls' negative self-evaluation of eating. *J. Am. Diet. Assoc.* **2000**, *100*, 1341–1346. [CrossRef]

39. Bailey-Davis, L.; Poulsen, M.N.; Hirsch, A.G.; Pollak, J.; Glass, T.A.; Schwartz, B.S. Home Food Rules in Relation to Youth Eating Behaviors, Body Mass Index, Waist Circumference, and Percent Body Fat. *J. Adolesc. Health* **2017**, *60*, 270–276. [CrossRef]

40. Feldman, S.; Eisenberg, M.E.; Neumark-Sztainer, D.; Story, M. Associations between watching TV during family meals and dietary intake among adolescents. *J. Nutr. Educ. Behav.* **2007**, *39*, 257–263. [CrossRef]

41. Norman, J.; Kelly, B.; McMahon, A.; Boyland, E.; Baur, A.; Chapman, A.; King, L.; Hughes, C.; Bauman, A. Sustained impact of energy-dense TV and online food advertising on children's dietary intake: A within-subject, randomized, crossover, counter-balanced trial. *Int. J. Behav. Nutr. Phys.* **2018**, *15*, 1–11. [CrossRef]

42. Scaglioni, S.; Arrizza, C.; Vecchi, F.; Tedeschi, S. Determinants of children's eating behavior. *Am. J. Clin. Nutr.* **2011**, *94*, 2006S–2011S. [CrossRef] [PubMed]

43. Vandeweghe, L.; Moens, E.; Braet, C.; Van Lippevelde, W.; Vervoort, L.; Verbeken, S. Perceived effective and feasible strategies to promote healthy eating in young children: Focus groups with parents, family child care providers and daycare assistants. *BMC Public Health* **2016**, *16*, 1–12. [CrossRef] [PubMed]

44. Fisk, M.; Crozier, R.; Inskip, M.; Godfrey, M.; Cooper, C.; Robinson, M. Influences on the quality of young children's diets. The importance of maternal food choices. *Br. J. Nutr.* **2011**, *105*, 287–296. [CrossRef]

45. McGowan, L.; Croker, H.; Wardle, J.; Cooke, J. Environmental and individual determinants of core and non-core food and drink intake in preschool-aged children in the United Kingdom. *Eur. J. Clin. Nutr.* **2012**, *66*, 322–328. [CrossRef]

46. Sonneville, R.; Rifas-Shiman, L.; Kleinman, P.; Gortmaker, L.; Gillman, W.; Taveras, M. Associations of obesogenic behaviors in mothers and obese children participating in a randomized trial. *Obesity* **2012**, *20*, 1449–1454. [CrossRef]

47. Wroten, C.; O'Neil, E.; Stuff, E.; Liu, Y.; Nicklas, A. Resemblance of dietary intakes of snacks, sweets, fruit, and vegetables among mother-child dyads from low-income families. *Appetite* **2012**, *59*, 316–323. [CrossRef]

48. Zuercher, L.; Wagstaff, A.; Kranz, S. Associations of food group and nutrient intake, diet quality, and meal sizes between adults and children in the same household. A cross-sectional analysis of U.S. households. *Nutr. J.* **2011**, *10*, 131. [CrossRef]

49. Hansson, L.M.; Heitmann, B.L.; Larsson, C.; Tynelius, P.; Willmer, M.; Rasmussen, F. Associations between Swedish Mothers' and 3- and 5-Year-Old Children's Food Intake. *J. Nutr. Educ. Behav.* **2016**, *48*, 520–529. [CrossRef]

50. Hall, L.; Collins, C.E.; Morgan, P.J.; Burrows, T.L.; Lubans, D.R.; Callister, R. Children's intake of fruit and selected energy-dense nutrient-poor foods is associated with fathers' intake. *J. Am. Diet. Assoc.* **2011**, *111*, 1039–1044. [CrossRef]

51. Miller, P.; Moore, R.H.; Kral, T.V. Children's daily fruit and vegetable intake: Associations with maternal intake and child weight status. *J. Nutr. Educ. Behav.* **2011**, *43*, 396–400. [CrossRef]

52. Hendy, H.M.; Williams, K.E.; Camise, T.S.; Eckman, N.; Hedemann, A. The Parent Mealtime Action Scale (PMAS). Development and association with children's diet and weight. *Appetite* **2009**, *52*, 328–339. [CrossRef]

53. Martin-Biggers, J.; Spaccarotella, K.; Berhaupt-Glickstein, A.; Hongu, N.; Worobey, J.; Byrd-Bredbenner, C. Come and get it! A discussion of family mealtime literature and factors affecting obesity risk. *Adv. Nutr.* **2014**, *5*, 235–247. [CrossRef]

54. Harrison, M.E.; Norris, M.L.; Obeid, N.; Fu, M.; Weinstangel, H.; Sampson, M. Systematic review of the effects of family meal frequency on psychosocial outcomes in youth. *Can. Fam. Physician Med. Fam. Can.* **2015**, *61*, e96–e106.

55. Litterbach, E.V.; Campbell, K.J.; Spence, A.C. Family meals with young children: An online study of family mealtime characteristics, among Australian families with children aged six months to six years. *BMC Public Health* **2017**, *17*, 1–9. [CrossRef]

56. Lipsky, L.M.; Haynie, D.L.; Liu, D.; Chaurasia, A.; Gee, B.; Li, K.; Iannotti, R.J.; Simons-Morton, B. Trajectories of eating behaviors in a nationally representative cohort of U.S. adolescents during the transition to young adulthood. *Int. J. Behav. Nutr. Phys. Act.* **2015**, *12*, 1–11. [CrossRef]

57. Skafida, V. The family meal panacea: Exploring how different aspects of family meal occurrence, meal habits and meal enjoyment relate to young children's diets. *Sociol. Health Illn.* **2013**, *35*, 906–923. [CrossRef]

58. Harte, S.; Theobald, M.; Trost, S.G. Culture and community: Observation of mealtime enactment in early childhood education and care settings. *Int. J. Behav. Nutr. Phys. Act.* **2019**, *16*, 69. [CrossRef]

59. Hammons, A.J.; Fiese, B.H. Is frequency of shared family meals related to the nutritional health of children and adolescents. *Pediatrics* **2011**, *127*, e1565–e1574. [CrossRef]

60. Sen, B. Frequency of family dinner and adolescent body weight status: Evidence from the national longitudinal survey of youth, 1997. *Obesity* **2006**, *14*, 2266–2276. [CrossRef]

61. Fulkerson, J.; Friend, S.; Flattum, C.; Horning, M.; Draxten, M.; Neumark-Sztainer, D.; Gurvich, O.; Story, M.; Garwick, A.; Kubik, M. Promoting healthful family meals to prevent obesity: HOME Plus, a randomized controlled trial. *Int. J. Behav. Nutr. Phys. Act.* **2015**, *12*, 1–12. [CrossRef]

62. Ruiz, E.; Ávila, J.M.; Valero, T.; Rodriguez, P.; Varela-Moreiras, G. Breakfast Consumption in Spain: Patterns, Nutrient Intake and Quality. Findings from the ANIBES Study, a Study from the International Breakfast Research Initiative. *Nutrients* **2018**, *10*, 1324. [CrossRef]

63. Gibney, M.J.; Barr, S.I.; Bellisle, F.; Drewnowski, A.; Fagt, S.; Livingstone, B.; Masset, G.; Varela Moreiras, G.; Moreno, L.A.; Smith, J. Breakfast in Human Nutrition: The International Breakfast Research Initiative. *Nutrients* **2018**, *10*, 559. [CrossRef]

64. Irwanti, W.; Paratmanitya, Y. Children's breakfast habit related to their perception towards parent's breakfast habits (study in Sedayu District, Bantul Regency. *J. Gizi Dan Diet. Indones.* **2016**, *4*, 63–70.

65. The Health Sponsorship Council's Breakfast-eaters Promotion. Encouraging Children to Eat Breakfast. Available online: https://www.google.com/url?sa=t&rct=j&q=&esrc=s&source=web&cd=&cad=rja&uact=8&ved=2ahUKEwin4 YTu3dXuAhXb6OAKHW_cAR0QFjAAegQIAxAC&url=http%3A%2F%2Fwww.hpa.org.nz%2Fsites%2Fdefault%2Ffiles% 2Fbreakfast-fact-pack-fnl-110204.pdf&usg=AOvVaw1fYwYu6NDcyLKHjTj6RLHT (accessed on 18 December 2020).

66. Cheng, T.S.; Tse, L.A.; Yu, I.; Griffiths, S. Children's perceptions of parental attitude affecting breakfast skipping in primary sixth-grade students. *J. Sch. Health* **2008**, *78*, 203–208. [CrossRef]

67. Johnson, G.H.; Anderson, G.H. Snacking definitions: Impact on interpretation of the literature and dietary recommendations. *Crit. Rev. Food Sci. Nutr.* **2010**, *50*, 848–871. [CrossRef] [PubMed]

68. Gregori, D.; Maffeis, C. Snacking and obesity: Urgency of a definition to exp lore such a relationship. *J. Am. Diet. Assoc.* **2007**, *107*, 562–563. [CrossRef] [PubMed]

69. Julian, C.; Santaliestra-Pasías, A.M.; Miguel-Berges, M.L.; Moreno, L.A. Frequency and quality of mid-afternoon snack among Spanish children. *Nutr. Hosp.* **2017**, *34*, 827–833. [CrossRef]

70. Jiménez-Cruz, A.; Bacardí-Gascón, M.; Jones, E.G. Consumption of fruits, vegetables, soft drinks, and high fat-containing snacks among Mexican children on the Mexico-US border. *Arch. Med. Res.* **2002**, *33*, 74–80. [CrossRef]

71. Spadafranca, A.; Bertoli, S.; Battezzati, A. Association between Snack Energy Intake in Children Aged 8–11 and Maternal Body Mass Index: Results from an Observational Study in an Elementary School of Milan. *SDRP J. Food Sci. Technol.* **2018**, *3*, 1–7.

72. Blaine, R.E.; Kachurak, A.; Davison, K.K.; Klabunde, R.; Fisher, J.O. Food parenting and child snacking: A systematic review. *Int. J. Behav. Nutr. Phys. Act.* **2017**, *14*, 146. [CrossRef]

73. Black, R.E.; Victora, C.G.; Walker, S.P.; Bhutta, Z.; Christian, P.; de Onis, M.; Ezzati, M.; Grantham-McGregor, S.; Katz, J.; Martorell, R.; et al. Maternal and child undernutrition and overweight in low-income and middle-income countries. *Lancet* **2013**, *382*, 427–451. [CrossRef]

74. Pries, A.M.; Huffman, S.L.; Mengkheang, K.; Kroeun, H.; Champeny, M.; Roberts, M.; Zehner, E. High use of commercial food products among infants and young children and promotions for these products in Cambodia. *Matern. Child Nutr.* **2016**, *12*, 52–63. [CrossRef]

75. Huffman, S.L.; Piwoz, E.G.; Vosti, S.A.; Dewey, K.G. Babies, soft drinks and snacks: A concern in low- and middle-income countries? *Matern. Child Nutr.* **2014**, *10*, 562–574. [CrossRef]

76. Salvy, S.J.; Elmo, A.; Nitecki, L.A.; Kluczynski, M.A.; Roemmich, J.N. Influence of parents and friends on children's and adolescents' food intake and food selection. *Am. J. Clin. Nutr.* **2011**, *93*, 87–92. [CrossRef]

77. Van Ansem, W.J.; Schrijvers, C.T.; Rodenburg, G.; van de Mheen, D. Children's snack consumption: Role of parents, peers and child snack-purchasing behaviour. Results from the INPACT study. *Eur. J. Public Health* **2015**, *25*, 1006–1011. [CrossRef]

78. Piernas, C.; Popkin, B.M. Trends in snacking among U.S. children. *Health Aff.* **2010**, *29*, 398–404. [CrossRef]

79. Tenjin, K.; Sekine, M.; Yamada, M.; Tatsuse, T. Relationship between Parental Lifestyle and Dietary Habits of Children: A Cross-Sectional Study. *J. Epidemiol.* **2020**, *30*, 253–259. [CrossRef]

80. Pearson, N.; Ball, K.; Crawford, D. Predictors of changes in adolescents' consumption of fruits, vegetables and energy-dense snacks. *Br. J. Nutr.* **2011**, *105*, 795–803. [CrossRef]

81. Haerens, L.; Craeynest, M.; Deforche, B.; Maes, L.; Cardon, C.; De Bourdeaudhuij, I. The contribution of psychosocial and home environmental factors in explaining eating behaviors in adolescents. *Eur. J. Clin. Nutr.* **2008**, *62*, 51–59. [CrossRef]

82. Haszard, J.J.; Skidmore, P.M.; Williams, S.M.; Taylor, R.W. Associations between parental feeding practices, problem food behaviors and dietary intake in New Zealand overweight children aged 4–8 years. *Public Health Nutr.* **2015**, *18*, 1036–1043. [CrossRef]

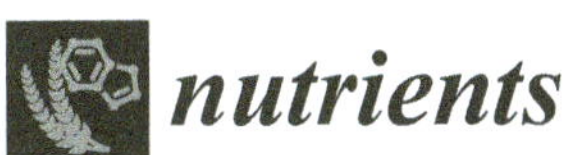

Article

Antenatal Determinants of Childhood Obesity in High-Risk Offspring: Protocol for the DiGest Follow-Up Study

Danielle Jones [1,2], Emanuella De Lucia Rolfe [3], Kirsten L. Rennie [3], Linda M. Oude Griep [3], Laura C. Kusinski [2], Deborah J. Hughes [2,5], Soren Brage [1,3], Ken K. Ong [1], Kathryn Beardsall [4,5] and Claire L. Meek [2,5,*]

[1] MRC Epidemiology Unit, University of Cambridge, Cambridge CB2 0QQ, UK;
    Danielle.Jones@mrc-epid.cam.ac.uk (D.J.); soren.brage@mrc-epid.cam.ac.uk (S.B.);
    Ken.Ong@mrc-epid.cam.ac.uk (K.K.O.)
[2] Institute of Metabolic Science, University of Cambridge, Cambridge CB2 0QQ, UK;
    lck34@medschl.cam.ac.uk (L.C.K.); deborah.hughes8@nhs.net (D.J.H.)
[3] NIHR Cambridge Biomedical Research Centre—Diet, Anthropometry and Physical Activity Group,
    MRC Epidemiology Unit, University of Cambridge, Cambridge CB2 0QQ, UK;
    Emanuella.De-Lucia-Rolfe@mrc-epid.cam.ac.uk (E.D.L.R.); Kirsten.Rennie@mrc-epid.cam.ac.uk (K.L.R.);
    Linda.OudeGriep@mrc-epid.cam.ac.uk (L.M.O.G.)
[4] Department of Paediatric Medicine, University of Cambridge, Cambridge CB2 0QQ, UK; kb274@cam.ac.uk
[5] Cambridge Universities NHS Foundation Trust, Cambridge Biomedical Campus, Cambridge CB2 0QQ, UK
*   Correspondence: clm70@cam.ac.uk

Citation: Jones, D.; De Lucia Rolfe, E.; Rennie, K.L.; Griep, L.M.O.; Kusinski, L.C.; Hughes, D.J.; Brage, S.; Ong, K.K.; Beardsall, K.; Meek, C.L. Antenatal Determinants of Childhood Obesity in High-Risk Offspring: Protocol for the DiGest Follow-Up Study. *Nutrients* **2021**, *13*, 1156. https://doi.org/10.3390/nu13041156

Academic Editor: Louise Brough

Received: 30 January 2021
Accepted: 29 March 2021
Published: 31 March 2021

Publisher's Note: MDPI stays neutral with regard to jurisdictional claims in published maps and institutional affiliations.

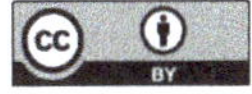

Copyright: © 2021 by the authors. Licensee MDPI, Basel, Switzerland. This article is an open access article distributed under the terms and conditions of the Creative Commons Attribution (CC BY) license (https://creativecommons.org/licenses/by/4.0/).

Abstract: Childhood obesity is an area of intense concern internationally and is influenced by events during antenatal and postnatal life. Although pregnancy complications, such as gestational diabetes and large-for-gestational-age birthweight have been associated with increased obesity risk in offspring, very few successful interventions in pregnancy have been identified. We describe a study protocol to identify if a reduced calorie diet in pregnancy can reduce adiposity in children to 3 years of age. The dietary intervention in gestational diabetes (DiGest) study is a randomised, controlled trial of a reduced calorie diet provided by a whole-diet replacement in pregnant women with gestational diabetes. Women receive a weekly dietbox intervention from enrolment until delivery and are blinded to calorie allocation. This follow-up study will assess associations between a reduced calorie diet in pregnancy with offspring adiposity and maternal weight and glycaemia. Anthropometry will be performed in infants and mothers at 3 months, 1, 2 and 3 years post-birth. Glycaemia will be assessed using bloodspot C-peptide in infants and continuous glucose monitoring with HbA1c in mothers. Data regarding maternal glycaemia in pregnancy, maternal nutrition, infant birthweight, offspring feeding behaviour and milk composition will also be collected. The DiGest follow-up study is expected to take 5 years, with recruitment finishing in 2026.

Keywords: gestational diabetes mellitus; pregnancy; study protocol; randomised controlled trial; large for gestational age; complex intervention; calorie restriction; maternal weight gain; childhood obesity; adiposity; type 2 diabetes; prevention

1. Introduction

Gestational diabetes, a common complication of pregnancy, is associated with short-term and long-term health implications for the baby [1,2]. Infants are commonly large-for-gestational-age at birth (LGA; >90th centile) and have a higher risk of obesity in childhood [2,3]. Unfortunately, very few interventions are available with proven efficacy to reduce the likelihood of childhood obesity in these high-risk children. The early development of obesity in children with existing environmental and genetic susceptibilities to type 2 diabetes is a major public health concern [4].

Events in pregnancy, perinatal and early postnatal periods may be important for future childhood obesity, but are relatively understudied, particularly in specific high-risk populations [5]. Babies born to mothers with gestational diabetes often have multiple risk factors for childhood obesity, which appear to have an additive effect upon risk. Maternal obesity in pregnancy [6,7], maternal excessive gestational weight gain [6], maternal postnatal weight retention [6], exposure to hyperglycaemia in utero [8–10], perinatal complications such as large-for-gestational age at birth [9,11,12], infant formula feeding [13] and increased growth trajectory in early life [14] are all established risk factors for childhood obesity or adiposity and are common features of a pregnancy affected by gestational diabetes.

It is therefore possible that an intervention which addresses maternal weight in pregnancy may reduce obesity rates in offspring. Family interventions (which target at least one parent to improve obesity rates in children) are already well-established in the prevention of childhood obesity [5]. However, many interventions to reduce the risk of childhood obesity target older children (2–10 years) and may miss the opportunity to intervene in early years [5,15]. The DiGest study, a currently ongoing dietary intervention in pregnant diagnosed with gestational diabetes, provides the opportunity to study the influence of a pregnancy weight intervention upon risk factors for childhood obesity in early life [16].

The DiGest Study is a randomised, double-blind controlled trial of a reduced calorie diet using a novel dietary intervention to assess the benefits of controlling maternal weight gain in late pregnancy in gestational diabetes. The trial is described in detail elsewhere [16]. Briefly, women are randomised to receive a weekly dietbox containing all meals and snacks and are blinded to the overall calorie content (1200 kcal/day for intervention group and 2000 kcal/day for control group; 40% carbohydrate, 25% protein, 35% fat). The dietbox commences at enrolment, typically 28–32 weeks' gestation, and continues until delivery of the infant. The clinical care team and research team are also blinded to calorie allocation. Dietboxes are nutritionally balanced and low in glycaemic index, low in saturated fat, high in vegetables and protein and suitable for use in pregnancy. Data will be collected to assess the impact upon maternal weight gain, infant birthweight and a range of obstetric and glycaemic outcomes during late pregnancy up to 3 months postnatally [16]. The design of the DiGest trial provides the opportunity for a controlled and blinded dietary study and reduces potential bias due to differences in maternal educational level, cooking ability, income and kitchen facilities.

In this manuscript we describe a follow up study to the DiGest trial which investigates the effect of the reduced calorie dietary intervention in pregnant women upon the development of obesity in a high-risk population of children from birth to 3 years of age. The hypothesis is that a reduced calorie diet in late pregnancy in women with gestational diabetes reduces offspring adiposity and improves maternal weight at 1, 2 and 3 years postpartum.

2. Materials and Methods

Study design and ethical approval: The DiGest Follow up study is an observational study on the effects of a multicentre, prospective, randomised double-blind controlled dietary intervention trial conducted in late pregnancy. In summary, participants of the follow up study will have been exposed to either the intervention diet of 1200 kcal/day, or the control diet of 2000 kcal/day as part of the DiGest study. Macronutrient ratios were identical for each diet; 40% carbohydrate, 25% protein, 35% fat. Meals were prepared from the same recipes, with a factor of 1.667 used to convert portion size to obtain meals of two different sizes. This diet it provided from enrolment (typically 28–32 weeks' gestation) to delivery of the infant. Participants will have attended 4 study visits in total to provide blood samples, blood pressure, body weight and anthropometry measurements, and to complete a series of questionnaires. Randomisation for the original DiGest study was stratified for centre. Throughout the DiGest intervention and Follow-up study, both mothers and children will receive standard NHS care, as described in the NICE guidelines [17]. The study is being conducted in accordance with the Declaration of Helsinki, and the protocol has been submitted to the Research Ethics Committee (UK Bloomsbury REC 21/PR/0213) and the NHS Health Research Authority (IRAS 281062).

Recruitment: The DiGest trial recruitment occurs at 5 hospital trusts in East Anglia, UK. The same study sites will be used for the follow-up study. At 3 months postpartum, DiGest trial participants will be given information about the follow-up study and invited to participate by the research midwives, nurses, clinical research staff or by their physician/obstetrician. For training purposes, students in healthcare disciplines (e.g., medicine, biomedical science, nursing, midwifery) may also occasionally recruit patients under appropriate supervision. Informed consent will be obtained at the final visit of the DiGest dietary intervention, with the mothers providing consent on their infant's behalf. Participants (or mother-infant dyad) can withdraw from the study at any time without reason without affecting their clinical care. There is no financial incentive for this study, but a small token of appreciation is provided for the child at each visit in line with guidelines of the Royal College of Paediatrics and Child Health [18].

Eligibility criteria: All women from the DiGest cohort (confirmed gestational diabetes and BMI 25 kg/m^2 or above at enrolment) are eligible to enrol in the follow-up study, however, they must be recruited within 12 months of the baby's birth. Mothers would be excluded if they are unwilling or unable to provide informed consent, if they experienced stillbirth, neonatal death or had an infant born with severe congenital anomaly.

Follow-up visit structure: The study timeline is outlined in Figure 1. Study visits will be carried out in the participants' home, local hospital or at another place convenient for the participant. The initial follow-up visit will coincide with the final DiGest visit at 3 months after the birth, where the consent form will be signed for both the mother and infant. Maternal and infant anthropometry will be measured at this visit as part of the DiGest study. Further Follow-up visits will take place at 1, 2 and 3 years postnatally and will take approximately 45 min.

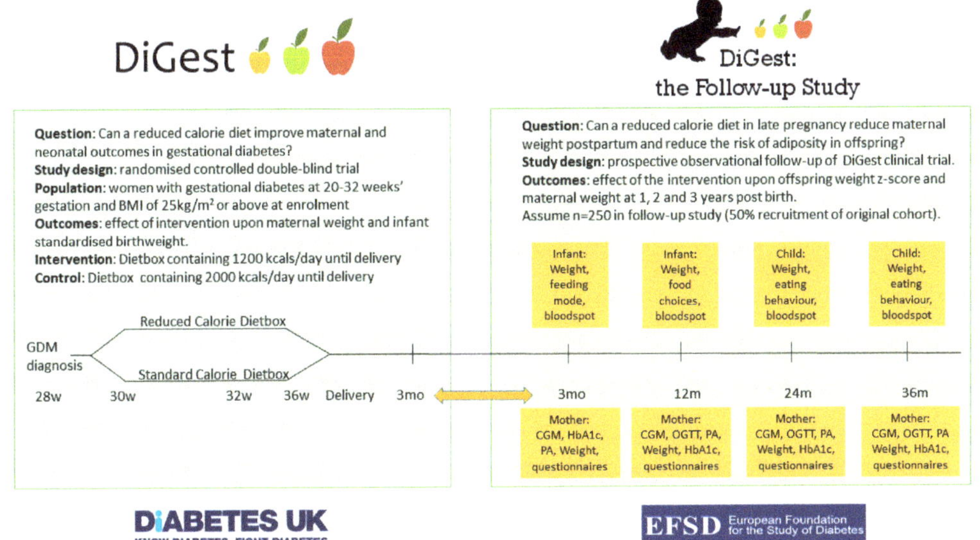

Figure 1. Summary of protocol and links between the DiGest trial and the follow up study.

Anthropometry Measurements: At all visits, maternal height and weight will be measured using a routinely calibrated stadiometer and weight scale (Seca Hammer Steindamm, Birmingham, U.K.). Waist and hip circumference will be measured to the nearest 0.1 cm with a fibreglass tape, in accordance with the World Health Organisation criteria [19]. Waist circumference is located at the midpoint between the lowest palpable rib and the iliac crest. Hip circumference is measured at the greater trochanters, or at the widest extension of the buttocks. Other maternal anthropometry that will be measured include mid upper arm circumference and skinfold thickness, using Harpenden calipers recorded to the nearest 0.2 mm. Infant length and weight will be taken in a supine position, measured to the nearest 0.1 cm using fibreglass tape, and 0.01 kg using scales (SECA 757 Infant digital scale, Seca, Birmingham, UK). Infant abdominal circumference, head circumference, skinfold thickness (Holtain calipers, Crosswell, Wales, U.K.), mid upper arm circumference will also be measured by trained research staff according to methods described elsewhere [16]. All equipment used to measure anthropometry are routinely calibrated.

Maternal Glucose Assessment: Due to the COVID-19 pandemic, a home-based OGTT using continuous glucose monitoring (CGM) will replace the gold standard OGTT for assessment of maternal glucose tolerance postnatally. An HbA1c will also be performed to replace mothers' annual diabetes check in primary care. We have previously assessed the feasibility and efficacy of the home-based OGTT with good results (Kusinski et al., submitted to press). In brief, a Dexcom G6 CGM sensor is sited during the study visit with a masked receiver so participants do not see their glucose results in real time. On day 3, participants are asked to eat normally, and fast overnight for at least 10 h. On the morning of day 4, at 09.00, participants are asked to drink a sachet of Rapilose (Galen, Craigavon, UK) containing 75 g of anhydrous glucose. Participants can have sips of water but are asked to consume no other foods or drinks for 3 h after the test. The timing of the home OGTT is chosen to coincide with peak sensor accuracy. Glucose readings are taken automatically every 5 min and transmit to the CGM receiver. Results from the OGTT at 0, 1 and 2 h are included in the analysis. Other CGM metrics will also be used to assess glycaemia as described in a recent CGM consensus statement. CGM metrics will be reported using both adult non-pregnant and pregnant ranges to allow comparison with pregnancy data gathered in the DiGest trial (also using a Dexcom G6 system).

Physical Activity Assessment

Participants will be asked to wear a wrist-worn accelerometer continuously for 7 days concurrently with the CGM. The triaxial accelerometer is waterproof and does not have a visual display, nor any auditory or vibrational cues, which means that participants will not be able to influence their activity level based on what is recorded by the device and nor will they be prompted to move about during periods of inactivity. These accelerometers have been used in in women during and after pregnancy to assess their daily physical activity with high compliance and produce reliable estimates of energy expenditure, overall physical activity and moderate-vigorous intensity activity [20–22]. Accelerometry data at 100 Hz will be collected and downloaded from the monitors for analysis. At the end of the recording period, mothers will be asked to complete the Recent Physical Activity Questionnaire (RPAQ), a self-completion questionnaire designed to assess an individual's physical activity over the previous four weeks. The questionnaire contains questions about physical activity in four domains: at home, at work, commuting and during leisure time. RPAQ has been validated against doubly labelled water and individually calibrated heart rate and movement sensing to assess physical activity energy expenditure (PAEE) in adults [23,24]. It has been used in diabetes prevention trials [25] and in longitudinal studies of pregnant women [26].

Other Biochemistry samples: A blood spot sample will be taken from mothers and frozen at −80 °C for future batch analysis of C-peptide and metabolomics. An optional heelprick blood spot will also be taken from infants, for future batch analysis of C-peptide and metabolomics. If a genetic sample has not been taken already as part of the DiGest trial, a cheek swab will be taken from both mothers and infants. Mothers will be asked to provide a sample of milk (formula or breast) which will be collected onto filter paper for assessment of infant nutrition including lipidomic profiling. To protect participant's privacy, this can be performed after the visit.

Questionnaires: Mothers will be asked to complete validated questionnaires about quality of life (EuroQuol EQ5D), eating behaviour (three factor eating questionnaire—

TFEQ-18) [27], physical activity (RPAQ) [24] and web-based multiple pass 24 h dietary recalls to assess habitual dietary intake (Intake24; [28,29]). These questionnaires have been used during the DiGest trial and participants will be familiar with them. In addition, mothers will be asked to complete questionnaires about parental feeding style (PFSQ) and their baby or child's eating behaviour (CEBQ) [30–33]. Information will be collected about infant feeding choice and if relevant, duration of breastfeeding.

3. Results

The aim of the study is to investigate the effects of a reduced calorie diet in late pregnancy in women diagnosed with gestational diabetes upon longer-term maternal and offspring metabolic outcomes. The primary outcome for child health is standardised weight at 1, 2 and 3 years of age. The primary outcome for the maternal population is maternal weight at 1, 2 and 3 years postpartum.

Offspring secondary outcomes at 1, 2 and 3 years of age: There are multiple secondary outcomes for children including weight, BMI, growth trajectory, and blood spot biomarkers such as C-peptide or metabolomics at 1, 2 and 3 years. Questionnaire data will be assessed to identify effects of the intervention in pregnancy upon child eating behaviour, with assessment for confounding factors including maternal BMI, maternal eating behaviour and parental feeding style.

Maternal secondary outcomes at 1, 2 and 3 years postpartum: Maternal outcomes to be studied include maternal weight and weight change, BMI, anthropometry measures of adiposity, glycaemia (CGM metrics, HbA1c, OGTT results, indices of insulin production and sensitivity, including HOMA-IR and HOMA-B, Matsuda score and Stumvoll index [34,35], cardiometabolic health (blood pressure, heart rate, lipids, fasting insulin, fasting glucose), maternal food intake, food nutritional content and quality, eating behaviour, quality of life, and incidence of type 2 diabetes or gestational diabetes in a future pregnancy.

Analysis Plan: An intention to treat analysis of the primary outcome for child health (standardised weight at 1, 2 and 3 years of age) will be based on linear regression with adjustment for the stratification variable of study centre through a fixed effects model. The potential role of other explanatory variables such as pre-pregnancy BMI, infant nutrition, infant postnatal growth trajectory or information from the questionnaires will be investigated. A per protocol analysis will also be performed in participants with >80% compliance and at least 4 weeks' exposure to the intervention. Secondary outcomes will also be examined through regression analyses (linear or logistic) appropriate for the type of outcome being considered.

Power calculation: All eligible women and their infants will be invited to join the follow-up study. However, calculations are based on assuming a 50% recruitment rate (n = 250 women and their infants) and a 20% withdrawal rate. For the maternal primary endpoint, data from earlier work suggest that typical values for maternal BMI outside of pregnancy in women with a history of gestational diabetes is mean 28.7 kg/m^2 (SD 7.1; n = 416) and maternal postpartum HbA1c 37.5 mmol/mol (SD 7.5; n = 157) [36]. Using these figures, recruitment of 250 women, will give 90% power to identify a 3 kg/m^2 difference in BMI (e.g., 29 vs. 32 kg/m^2) and a 3 mmol/mol difference in HbA1c postnatally while allowing for a 10–20% withdrawal rate. At 80% power, this sample size is sufficient to identify a 2 kg/m^2 difference in BMI (e.g., 30 vs. 32 kg/m^2) and a 2 mmol/mol difference in HbA1c postnatally.

For the offspring primary endpoint, assessment of infant weight will be based upon z-(SD) scores. At the sample size of 250 infants, there will be 90% power to identify a 0.45 SD increase in weight with 80% power to identify 0.4 SD increase in weight. At the age of 2 years old, a z-score of 0.4 is equivalent to 0.5 kg.

4. Discussion

This follow-up study of the DiGest randomised controlled trial provides a unique opportunity to assess the potential benefits of a dietary intervention in late pregnancy upon the development of obesity in children with multiple risk factors. The availability of data from mid pregnancy until the age of 3 years also allows detailed characterisation of the relative importance of pregnancy and postnatal risk factors in the development of adiposity in early childhood.

Rates of maternal obesity are increasing in the antenatal population throughout the world, and pre-pregnancy BMI is a strong predictor of both birthweight and future childhood obesity. A recent metanalysis identified that maternal obesity was significantly associated with overweight/obesity in early, mid and late childhood with odds ratios 2.43, 3.12 and 4.47, respectively [6]. Weight gain in pregnancy is also important and has repercussions for women's BMI for 15 years or more after the pregnancy [37]. Landon and colleagues found that gestational weight gain was strongly related to obesity in children aged 5–10 years old [10].

In addition to the effects of maternal obesity, exposure to intrauterine hyperglycaemia appears to further increase the risk of childhood obesity. There is evidence that maternal glycaemia in gestational diabetes is associated with childhood obesity at 10–14 years [2] and altered anthropometry at 5–10 years, favouring obesity [10]. Maternal hyperglycaemia can also indirectly increase childhood obesity rates, by increasing the risk of LGA in offspring. Data from the UK and Canada suggest that childhood obesity rates in LGA infants are at least twice that of children born appropriate for gestational age [11,38]. The exact mechanisms behind these intrauterine exposures and later life obesity are unclear. It is possible that altered placental secretary function, offspring hyperinsulinism and genetic susceptibilities all play a role.

The design of the DiGest and DiGest follow-up studies also allows longitudinal assessment of the effects of other pregnancy exposures upon longer-term offspring growth and health. For example, metformin use in pregnancy has been associated with lower birth weight but increased postnatal catch-up growth, but the consequences of this upon longer-term offspring cardiometabolic outcomes remain less clear [39,40]. The collection of anthropometric measures in offspring exposed to metformin in utero with paired blood samples, and a comparable unexposed control group, provides opportunity to explore this issue in greater depth.

Serum and cord blood stored for biomarkers such as leptin, adiponectin and placental hormones provides opportunities to identify infants at an earlier stage who are at risk of obesity in childhood. Previous work has demonstrated that cord blood leptin levels are associated with pregnancy diet, physical activity and neonatal body composition in a comparable population [41,42]. Cord blood adiponectin has also been associated with body composition effects which may be distinct in male and female neonates [43] and may additionally provide information about neonatal beta cell function [44]. Placental growth factors and metabolic function have also shown relevance for pregnancy outcomes [45,46]. Taken together, it is feasible that biomarkers in cord blood or maternal serum may facilitate early identification of offspring at risk of obesity and diabetes in later life, who could be prioritized for health interventions.

Although maternal physical activity levels in pregnancy and postpartum are likely to be vital for determining offspring habitual exercise levels, relatively few modifiable factors have been identified in children's physical activity levels in the very young [47,48]. Findings to date suggest that parents' physical activity levels are associated with children's activity levels in pre-school aged children and role-modelling by mothers appears to be one of the strongest associations [48]. However, relatively few studies have examined exercise after gestational diabetes in mothers and children. The DiGest Follow-Up study uses both questionnaires and accelerometers to assess physical activity, information which could inform future interventional studies.

Infant feeding and growth trajectory in the first year of life are also important. Although randomised studies of feeding modality in early life are not possible, observational analyses in unselected populations suggest consistent benefits of breastfeeding upon rates of childhood obesity [49,50]. There is also evidence that breastfeeding reduces childhood obesity risk in offspring of mothers with gestational diabetes and obesity [13,51]. Stettler and colleagues reported that similar benefits may persist until adulthood in a study of offspring to age 20 years [52]. The study also includes questionnaires about child eating behaviour, child food preferences and parental feeding style to examine behavioural associations with obesity and feeding behaviour in children aged up to 3 years.

The aetiology of childhood obesity is therefore complex and multifactorial. In infants of mothers with gestational diabetes, multiple risk factors are often evident at birth. Successful interventions are urgently needed to reduce the risk of obesity and future metabolic disease in these high-risk children.

5. Conclusions

The DiGest follow-up study provides the opportunity to assess pregnancy and postnatal risk factors for the development of childhood obesity, and to describe the potential impact of a dietary intervention in pregnancy. Early intervention in offspring with existing environmental and genetic susceptibilities to type 2 diabetes will be vital to break the intergenerational cycle of obesity.

6. Patents

No patents are relevant to the study described in this manuscript.

Author Contributions: C.L.M. designed the study, developed the methodology and wrote and revised the manuscript. C.L.M. acquired funding for the study and has overall responsibility for study conduct. D.J. contributed to writing the manuscript and read and revised the final manuscript. E.D.L.R., K.L.R., L.M.O.G., L.C.K., S.B., D.J.H., K.K.O. and K.B. contributed to aspects of study design, and read and revised the final manuscript. All authors have read and agreed to the published version of the manuscript.

Funding: This paper presents a study protocol for a follow-up study which was funded by the European Foundation for the Study of Diabetes and Novo Nordisk Foundation through the Future Leaders' Award (NNF19SA058974). The DiGest trial is funded by Diabetes UK (17/0005712).

Institutional Review Board Statement: The study will be conducted according to the guidelines of the Declaration of Helsinki, and is under review by the Bloomsbury Research Ethics Committee (protocol v.1; REC 21/PR/0213 and date 3/3/2021).

Informed Consent Statement: Informed consent will be obtained from all subjects involved in the study. Consent for infants was given by parents.

Data Availability Statement: No applicable.

Acknowledgments: We thank the National Institute of Health Research (NIHR) Clinical Research Network (CRN Eastern) for supporting research personnel at study sites who are involved in performing this research study. We are grateful to funding to E.D.L.R., K.R. and L.O.G., who are supported by the NIHR Cambridge Biomedical Research Centre (IS-BRC-1215-20014). Thank you also to Søren Brage for constructive comments and input to the physical activity aspects to the study.

Conflicts of Interest: The authors declare no conflict of interest.

References

1. Metzger, B.E.; Coustan, D.R. Summary and recommendations of the Fourth International Workshop-Conference on Gestational Diabetes Mellitus. The Organizing Committee. *Diabetes Care* **1998**, *21* (Suppl. 2), B161–167.
2. Lowe, W.L., Jr.; Lowe, L.P.; Kuang, A.; Catalano, P.M.; Nodzenski, M.; Talbot, O.; Tam, W.H.; Sacks, D.A.; McCance, D.; Linder, B.; et al. Maternal glucose levels during pregnancy and childhood adiposity in the Hyperglycemia and Adverse Pregnancy Outcome Follow-up Study. *Diabetologia* **2019**, *62*, 598–610. [CrossRef] [PubMed]
3. Metzger, B.E.; Lowe, L.P.; Dyer, A.R.; Trimble, E.R.; Chaovarindr, U.; Coustan, D.R.; Hadden, D.R.; McCance, D.R.; Hod, M.; McIntyre, H.D.; et al. Hyperglycemia and adverse pregnancy outcomes. *N. Engl. J. Med.* **2008**, *358*, 1991–2002. [CrossRef] [PubMed]
4. Blake-Lamb, T.L.; Locks, L.M.; Perkins, M.E.; Woo Baidal, J.A.; Cheng, E.R.; Taveras, E.M. Interventions for Childhood Obesity in the First 1000 Days A Systematic Review. *Am. J. Prev. Med.* **2016**, *50*, 780–789. [CrossRef]

5. Ash, T.; Agaronov, A.; Young, T.; Aftosmes-Tobio, A.; Davison, K.K. Family-based childhood obesity prevention interventions: A systematic review and quantitative content analysis. *Int. J. Behav. Nutr. Phys. Act.* **2017**, *14*, 113. [CrossRef]
6. Voerman, E.; Santos, S.; Patro Golab, B.; Amiano, P.; Ballester, F.; Barros, H.; Bergstrom, A.; Charles, M.A.; Chatzi, L.; Chevrier, C.; et al. Maternal body mass index, gestational weight gain, and the risk of overweight and obesity across childhood: An individual participant data meta-analysis. *PLoS Med.* **2019**, *16*, e1002744. [CrossRef]
7. Litwin, L.; Sundholm, J.K.M.; Rönö, K.; Koivusalo, S.B.; Eriksson, J.G.; Sarkola, T. Transgenerational effects of maternal obesity and gestational diabetes on offspring body composition and left ventricle mass: The Finnish Gestational Diabetes Prevention Study (RADIEL) 6-year follow-up. *Diabet Med.* **2020**, *37*, 147–156. [CrossRef] [PubMed]
8. Gu, Y.; Lu, J.; Li, W.; Liu, H.; Wang, L.; Leng, J.; Zhang, S.; Wang, S.; Tuomilehto, J.; Yu, Z.; et al. Joint Associations of Maternal Gestational Diabetes and Hypertensive Disorders of Pregnancy With Overweight in Offspring. *Front. Endocrinol.* **2019**, *10*, 645. [CrossRef]
9. Hammoud, N.M.; Visser, G.H.A.; van Rossem, L.; Biesma, D.H.; Wit, J.M.; de Valk, H.W. Long-term BMI and growth profiles in offspring of women with gestational diabetes. *Diabetologia* **2018**, *61*, 1037–1045. [CrossRef] [PubMed]
10. Landon, M.B.; Mele, L.; Varner, M.W.; Casey, B.M.; Reddy, U.M.; Wapner, R.J.; Rouse, D.J.; Tita, A.T.N.; Thorp, J.M.; Chien, E.K.; et al. The relationship of maternal glycemia to childhood obesity and metabolic dysfunction(double dagger). *J. Matern. Fetal Neonatal Med.* **2018**. [CrossRef]
11. Kaul, P.; Bowker, S.L.; Savu, A.; Yeung, R.O.; Donovan, L.E.; Ryan, E.A. Association between maternal diabetes, being large for gestational age and breast-feeding on being overweight or obese in childhood. *Diabetologia* **2019**, *62*, 249–258. [CrossRef]
12. Boney, C.M.; Verma, A.; Tucker, R.; Vohr, B.R. Metabolic syndrome in childhood: Association with birth weight, maternal obesity, and gestational diabetes mellitus. *Pediatrics* **2005**, *115*, e290–e296. [CrossRef] [PubMed]
13. Patel, N.; Dalrymple, K.V.; Briley, A.L.; Pasupathy, D.; Seed, P.T.; Flynn, A.C.; Poston, L. Mode of infant feeding, eating behaviour and anthropometry in infants at 6-months of age born to obese women—A secondary analysis of the UPBEAT trial. *BMC Pregnancy Childbirth* **2018**, *18*, 355. [CrossRef] [PubMed]
14. Wells, J.C.; Haroun, D.; Levene, D.; Darch, T.; Williams, J.E.; Fewtrell, M.S. Prenatal and postnatal programming of body composition in obese children and adolescents: Evidence from anthropometry, DXA and the 4-component model. *Int. J. Obes.* **2011**, *35*, 534–540. [CrossRef] [PubMed]
15. Lowe, W.L., Jr.; Scholtens, D.M.; Lowe, L.P.; Kuang, A.; Nodzenski, M.; Talbot, O.; Catalano, P.M.; Linder, B.; Brickman, W.J.; Clayton, P.; et al. Association of Gestational Diabetes With Maternal Disorders of Glucose Metabolism and Childhood Adiposity. *JAMA* **2018**, *320*, 1005–1016. [CrossRef]
16. Kusinski, L.C.; Murphy, H.R.; De Lucia Rolfe, E.; Rennie, K.L.; Oude Griep, L.M.; Hughes, D.; Taylor, R.; Meek, C.L. Dietary Intervention in Pregnant Women with Gestational Diabetes; Protocol for the DiGest Randomised Controlled Trial. *Nutrients* **2020**, *12*, 1165. [CrossRef]
17. Diabetes in pregnancy: Management of Diabetes and Its Complications from Preconception to the Postnatal Period. In *National Institute of Clinical Excellence (NICE) Guideline NG3*; 2015. Available online: https://www.nice.org.uk/guidance/ng3 (accessed on 30 March 2021).
18. Royal College of Paediatrics and Child Health Guidelines for the Ethical Conduct of Medical Research Involving Children. Available online: https://www.nihr.ac.uk/documents/children-payment-for-participation-report/12085 (accessed on 21 January 2021).
19. World Health Organisation. Noncommunicable Diseases and Their Risk Factors. The STEPS Manual. Available online: https://www.who.int/ncds/surveillance/steps/panammanual/en/ (accessed on 30 January 2017).
20. van Hees, V.T.; Renström, F.; Wright, A.; Gradmark, A.; Catt, M.; Chen, K.Y.; Löf, M.; Bluck, L.; Pomeroy, J.; Wareham, N.J.; et al. Estimation of daily energy expenditure in pregnant and non-pregnant women using a wrist-worn tri-axial accelerometer. *PLoS ONE* **2011**, *6*, e22922. [CrossRef]
21. Hesketh, K.R.; Evenson, K.R.; Stroo, M.; Clancy, S.M.; Østbye, T.; Benjamin-Neelon, S.E. Physical activity and sedentary behavior during pregnancy and postpartum, measured using hip and wrist-worn accelerometers. *Prev. Med. Rep.* **2018**, *10*, 337–345. [CrossRef]
22. da Silva, S.G.; Evenson, K.R.; Ekelund, U.; da Silva, I.C.M.; Domingues, M.R.; da Silva, B.G.C.; Mendes, M.A.; Cruz, G.I.N.; Hallal, P.C. How many days are needed to estimate wrist-worn accelerometry-assessed physical activity during the second trimester in pregnancy? *PLoS ONE* **2019**, *14*, e0211442. [CrossRef]
23. Besson, H.; Brage, S.; Jakes, R.W.; Ekelund, U.; Wareham, N.J. Estimating physical activity energy expenditure, sedentary time, and physical activity intensity by self-report in adults. *Am. J. Clin. Nutr.* **2010**, *91*, 106–114. [CrossRef]
24. Golubic, R.; May, A.M.; Benjaminsen Borch, K.; Overvad, K.; Charles, M.A.; Diaz, M.J.; Amiano, P.; Palli, D.; Valanou, E.; Vigl, M.; et al. Validity of electronically administered Recent Physical Activity Questionnaire (RPAQ) in ten European countries. *PLoS ONE* **2014**, *9*, e92829. [CrossRef]
25. Yates, T.; Griffin, S.; Bodicoat, D.H.; Brierly, G.; Dallosso, H.; Davies, M.J.; Eborall, H.; Edwardson, C.; Gillett, M.; Gray, L.; et al. PRomotion Of Physical activity through structured Education with differing Levels of ongoing Support for people at high risk of type 2 diabetes (PROPELS): Study protocol for a randomized controlled trial. *Trials* **2015**, *16*, 289. [CrossRef] [PubMed]
26. McParlin, C.; Robson, S.C.; Tennant, P.W.G.; Besson, H.; Rankin, J.; Adamson, A.J.; Pearce, M.S.; Bell, R. Objectively measured physical activity during pregnancy: A study in obese and overweight women. *BMC Pregnancy Childbirth* **2010**, *10*, 76. [CrossRef]

27. Bond, M.J.; McDowell, A.J.; Wilkinson, J.Y. The measurement of dietary restraint, disinhibition and hunger: An examination of the factor structure of the Three Factor Eating Questionnaire (TFEQ). *Int. J. Obes. Relat. Metab. Disord.* **2001**, *25*, 900–906. [CrossRef]

28. Bradley, J.; Simpson, E.; Poliakov, I.; Matthews, J.N.; Olivier, P.; Adamson, A.J.; Foster, E. Comparison of INTAKE24 (an Online 24-h Dietary Recall Tool) with Interviewer-Led 24-h Recall in 11-24 Year-Old. *Nutrients* **2016**, *8*, 358. [CrossRef] [PubMed]

29. Foster, E.; Lee, C.; Imamura, F.; Hollidge, S.E.; Westgate, K.L.; Venables, M.C.; Poliakov, I.; Rowland, M.K.; Osadchiy, T.; Bradley, J.C.; et al. Validity and reliability of an online self-report 24-h dietary recall method (Intake24): A doubly labelled water study and repeated-measures analysis. *J. Nutr. Sci.* **2019**, *8*, e29. [CrossRef] [PubMed]

30. Carnell, S.; Wardle, J. Measuring behavioural susceptibility to obesity: Validation of the child eating behaviour questionnaire. *Appetite* **2007**, *48*, 104–113. [CrossRef] [PubMed]

31. Llewellyn, C.H.; van Jaarsveld, C.H.; Johnson, L.; Carnell, S.; Wardle, J. Development and factor structure of the Baby Eating Behaviour Questionnaire in the Gemini birth cohort. *Appetite* **2011**, *57*, 388–396. [CrossRef]

32. Wardle, J.; Guthrie, C.A.; Sanderson, S.; Rapoport, L. Development of the Children's Eating Behaviour Questionnaire. *J. Child Psychol. Psychiatry* **2001**, *42*, 963–970. [CrossRef] [PubMed]

33. Wardle, J.; Sanderson, S.; Guthrie, C.A.; Rapoport, L.; Plomin, R. Parental feeding style and the inter-generational transmission of obesity risk. *Obes. Res.* **2002**, *10*, 453–462. [CrossRef] [PubMed]

34. Stumvoll, M.; Mitrakou, A.; Pimenta, W.; Jenssen, T.; Yki-Jarvinen, H.; Van Haeften, T.; Renn, W.; Gerich, J. Use of the oral glucose tolerance test to assess insulin release and insulin sensitivity. *Diabetes Care* **2000**, *23*, 295–301. [CrossRef]

35. Matsuda, M.; DeFronzo, R.A. Insulin sensitivity indices obtained from oral glucose tolerance testing: Comparison with the euglycemic insulin clamp. *Diabetes Care* **1999**, *22*, 1462–1470. [CrossRef]

36. Aiken, C.E.M.; Hone, L.; Murphy, H.R.; Meek, C.L. Improving outcomes in gestational diabetes: Does gestational weight gain matter? *Diabet Med.* **2019**, *36*, 167–176. [CrossRef]

37. Nehring, I.; Schmoll, S.; Beyerlein, A.; Hauner, H.; von Kries, R. Gestational weight gain and long-term postpartum weight retention: A meta-analysis. *Am. J. Clin. Nutr.* **2011**, *94*, 1225–1231. [CrossRef] [PubMed]

38. Asher, P. Fat babies and fat children. The prognosis of obesity in the very young. *Arch. Dis. Child.* **1966**, *41*, 672–673. [CrossRef] [PubMed]

39. Tarry-Adkins, J.L.; Aiken, C.E.; Ozanne, S.E. Neonatal, infant, and childhood growth following metformin versus insulin treatment for gestational diabetes: A systematic review and meta-analysis. *PLoS Med.* **2019**, *16*, e1002848. [CrossRef]

40. Tarry-Adkins, J.L.; Aiken, C.E.; Ozanne, S.E. Comparative impact of pharmacological treatments for gestational diabetes on neonatal anthropometry independent of maternal glycaemic control: A systematic review and meta-analysis. *PLoS Med.* **2020**, *17*, e1003126. [CrossRef] [PubMed]

41. van Poppel, M.N.M.; Simmons, D.; Devlieger, R.; van Assche, F.A.; Jans, G.; Galjaard, S.; Corcoy, R.; Adelantado, J.M.; Dunne, F.; Harreiter, J.; et al. A reduction in sedentary behaviour in obese women during pregnancy reduces neonatal adiposity: The DALI randomised controlled trial. *Diabetologia* **2019**. [CrossRef]

42. Okereke, N.C.; Uvena-Celebrezze, J.; Hutson-Presley, L.; Amini, S.B.; Catalano, P.M. The effect of gender and gestational diabetes mellitus on cord leptin concentration. *Am. J. Obs. Gynecol.* **2002**, *187*, 798–803. [CrossRef] [PubMed]

43. Basu, S.; Laffineuse, L.; Presley, L.; Minium, J.; Catalano, P.M.; Hauguel-de Mouzon, S. In utero gender dimorphism of adiponectin reflects insulin sensitivity and adiposity of the fetus. *Obesity* **2009**, *17*, 1144–1149. [CrossRef] [PubMed]

44. Zhang, D.L.; Du, Q.; Djemli, A.; Julien, P.; Fraser, W.D.; Luo, Z.C. Cord blood insulin, IGF-I, IGF-II, leptin, adiponectin and ghrelin, and their associations with insulin sensitivity, β-cell function and adiposity in infancy. *Diabet Med.* **2018**, *35*, 1412–1419. [CrossRef] [PubMed]

45. Musial, B.; Vaughan, O.R.; Fernandez-Twinn, D.S.; Voshol, P.; Ozanne, S.E.; Fowden, A.L.; Sferruzzi-Perri, A.N. A Western-style obesogenic diet alters maternal metabolic physiology with consequences for fetal nutrient acquisition in mice. *J. Physiol.* **2017**, *595*, 4875–4892. [CrossRef]

46. Sferruzzi-Perri, A.N.; Owens, J.A.; Pringle, K.G.; Robinson, J.S.; Roberts, C.T. Maternal insulin-like growth factors-I and -II act via different pathways to promote fetal growth. *Endocrinology* **2006**, *147*, 3344–3355. [CrossRef] [PubMed]

47. Hnatiuk, J.A.; Hesketh, K.R.; van Sluijs, E.M. Correlates of home and neighbourhood-based physical activity in UK 3-4-year-old children. *Eur. J. Public Health* **2016**, *26*, 947–953. [CrossRef] [PubMed]

48. Hesketh, K.R.; O'Malley, C.; Paes, V.M.; Moore, H.; Summerbell, C.; Ong, K.K.; Lakshman, R.; van Sluijs, E.M.F. Determinants of Change in Physical Activity in Children 0-6 years of Age: A Systematic Review of Quantitative Literature. *Sports Med.* **2017**, *47*, 1349–1374. [CrossRef]

49. Rito, A.I.; Buoncristiano, M.; Spinelli, A.; Salanave, B.; Kunešová, M.; Hejgaard, T.; García Solano, M.; Fijałkowska, A.; Sturua, L.; Hyska, J.; et al. Association between Characteristics at Birth, Breastfeeding and Obesity in 22 Countries: The WHO European Childhood Obesity Surveillance Initiative—COSI 2015/2017. *Obes. Facts* **2019**, *12*, 226–243. [CrossRef] [PubMed]

50. Wang, L.; Collins, C.; Ratliff, M.; Xie, B.; Wang, Y. Breastfeeding Reduces Childhood Obesity Risks. *Child. Obes.* **2017**, *13*, 197–204. [CrossRef]

51. Bider-Canfield, Z.; Martinez, M.P.; Wang, X.; Yu, W.; Bautista, M.P.; Brookey, J.; Page, K.A.; Buchanan, T.A.; Xiang, A.H. Maternal obesity, gestational diabetes, breastfeeding and childhood overweight at age 2 years. *Pediatr. Obes.* **2017**, *12*, 171–178. [CrossRef]
52. Stettler, N.; Kumanyika, S.K.; Katz, S.H.; Zemel, B.S.; Stallings, V.A. Rapid weight gain during infancy and obesity in young adulthood in a cohort of African Americans. *Am. J. Clin. Nutr.* **2003**, *77*, 1374–1378. [CrossRef]

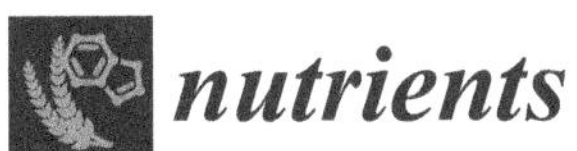

nutrients

Article

Complementary Feeding and Overweight in European Preschoolers: The ToyBox-Study

Natalya Usheva [1,*], Sonya Galcheva [2], Greet Cardon [3], Marieke De Craemer [4,5], Odysseas Androutsos [6], Aneta Kotowska [7], Piotr Socha [7], Berthold V. Koletzko [8], Luis A. Moreno [9], Violeta Iotova [2], Yannis Manios [10] and on behalf of the ToyBox-study Group [†]

[1] Department of Social Medicine and Health Care Organization, Medical University of Varna, 9002 Varna, Bulgaria
[2] Department of Pediatrics, Medical University of Varna, 9002 Varna, Bulgaria; sonya_galcheva@mail.bg (S.G.); iotova_v@yahoo.com (V.I.)
[3] Department of Movement and Sports Sciences, Ghent University, 9000 Ghent, Belgium; greet.cardon@ugent.be
[4] Department of Rehabilitation Sciences, Ghent University, 9000 Ghent, Belgium; marieke.decraemer@ugent.be
[5] Research Foundation Flanders, 1000 Brussels, Belgium
[6] Department of Nutrition and Dietetics, School of Physical Education, Sport Science and Dietetics, University of Thessaly, 382 21 Volos, Greece; oandrou@hua.gr
[7] Public Health Department, Children's Memorial Health Institute, 04-730 Warsaw, Poland; A.kotowska@ipczd.pl (A.K.); p.socha@ipczd.pl (P.S.)
[8] Division of Metabolic and Nutritional Medicine, Department Paediatrics, Dr. von Hauner Children's Hospital, LMU University Hospitals, 80337 Munich, Germany; berthold.koletzko@med.uni-muenchen.de
[9] GENUD (Growth, Exercise, Drinking Behaviour and Development) Research Group, University of Zaragoza, 50009 Zaragoza, Spain; lmoreno@unizar.es
[10] Department of Nutrition and Dietetics, Harokopio University, 176 76 Athens, Greece; manios@hua.gr
* Correspondence: nataly_usheva@mu-varna.bg; Tel.: +359-5267-7164
† Membership of the ToyBox-study Group is provided in the Acknowledgments.

Citation: Usheva, N.; Galcheva, S.; Cardon, G.; De Craemer, M.; Androutsos, O.; Kotowska, A.; Socha, P.; Koletzko, B.V.; Moreno, L.A.; Iotova, V.; et al. Complementary Feeding and Overweight in European Preschoolers: The ToyBox-Study. *Nutrients* **2021**, *13*, 1199. https://doi.org/10.3390/nu13041199

Academic Editors: Maria Luz Fernandez and Jennifer T. Smilowitz

Received: 31 January 2021
Accepted: 30 March 2021
Published: 5 April 2021

Publisher's Note: MDPI stays neutral with regard to jurisdictional claims in published maps and institutional affiliations.

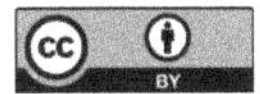

Copyright: © 2021 by the authors. Licensee MDPI, Basel, Switzerland. This article is an open access article distributed under the terms and conditions of the Creative Commons Attribution (CC BY) license (https://creativecommons.org/licenses/by/4.0/).

Abstract: Complementary feeding (CF) should start between 4–6 months of age to ensure infants' growth but is also linked to childhood obesity. This study aimed to investigate the association of the timing of CF, breastfeeding and overweight in preschool children. Infant-feeding practices were self-reported in 2012 via a validated questionnaire by >7500 parents from six European countries participating in the ToyBox-study. The proportion of children who received breast milk and CF at 4–6 months was 51.2%. There was a positive association between timing of solid food (SF) introduction and duration of breastfeeding, as well as socioeconomic status and a negative association with smoking throughout pregnancy ($p < 0.005$). No significant risk to become overweight was observed among preschoolers who were introduced to SF at 1–3 months of age compared to those introduced at 4–6 months regardless of the type of milk feeding. Similarly, no significant association was observed between the early introduction of SF and risk for overweight in preschoolers who were breastfed for ≥ 4 months or were formula-fed. The study did not identify any significant association between the timing of introducing SF and obesity in childhood. It is likely that other factors than timing of SF introduction may have impact on childhood obesity.

Keywords: complementary feeding; solid food; breastfeeding; overweight; obesity

1. Introduction

Obesity is an increasing worldwide problem with an estimate of 340 million overweight or obese children and adolescents aged 5–19 in 2016 and 38.2 million children under the age of 5 years being overweight or obese worldwide in 2019. Moreover, health expenditures for the adult population are constantly increasing, €70 billion per year in Europe (2017) and $342.2 billion in the US (2013). Direct medical costs related to childhood obesity alone were approximately $14 billion in 2013 and they are expected to rise significantly, especially because today's obese children are likely to become tomorrow's obese adults [1–5].

One of the risk factors for childhood obesity is inappropriate nutrition during infancy. The advantages of exclusive breastfeeding (EBF) compared to partial breastfeeding in the first months of life have been recognized. The World Health Organization's global public health recommendations promote "exclusive breastfeeding for 6 months" with continued breastfeeding up to the age of two years or beyond. Complementary feeding (CF) should occur when a baby is both developmentally ready and when breast milk is no longer able to fulfil the nutritional requirements of the child [6,7]. The recommended period for starting CF as stated by the European Society for Pediatric Gastroenterology, Hepatology and Nutrition is at week 17–26 (between the beginning of the fifth month and the beginning of the seventh month of life) [8].

The protective role of breastfeeding (BF) against overweight and obesity has been reported in many studies, showing a greater effect with longer duration of breastfeeding [9–11]. However, the association of timing of CF introduction and the quantity and quality of CF with childhood obesity is controversial [12–18]. Some studies reported an association of very early CF introduction before four months of age with later obesity in formula-fed infants whereas there was little effect in breastfed infants [19]; overweight and obesity at 2–12 years; obesity at three years [20,21]. An association between early CF introduction and overweight in children aged 1–17 has also been reported as being modified by the duration of breastfeeding in a birth cohort study in the Netherlands (Prevention and Incidence of Asthma and Mite Allergy—PIAMA) [22]. These findings are not consistent with the conclusions of the systematic review by Pearce et al. who found no consistent association between very early introduction of CF (prior to the age of four months) and childhood body mass index (BMI) [23].

Since there is no consensus yet on a possible relationship between introduction of solid foods (SF) and overweight in childhood, the aim of this study was to investigate the association between the timing of CF, breastfeeding status and overweight in a large pan-European sample of preschool children.

2. Materials and Methods

The ToyBox-study was conducted between May and June 2012 in six European countries (Belgium, Bulgaria, Germany, Greece, Poland and Spain) among parents/caregivers of preschoolers born between January 2007 and December 2008. The ToyBox-study (www.toybox-study.eu; accessed on 20 September 2020) adhered to the Declaration of Helsinki and the conventions of the Council of Europe on human rights and biomedicine. All the countries (Belgium, Bulgaria, Germany, Greece, Poland and Spain) obtained ethical clearance from the relevant ethics committees and local authorities and all parents/caregivers provided a signed consent form before being enrolled in the study. Detailed information about the ToyBox-study design has been previously reported [24].

Data about perinatal information of preschoolers (including anthropometric measurements at birth, breastfeeding and complementary feeding practices during the first year of life) were obtained through a standardized self-administered questionnaire for primary caregivers. They also aimed to include sociodemographic characteristics of the participants. The questions about children's nutrition during the first year of life were formulated with a focus on the presence/absence of breastfeeding at each month after birth and the age at which water, tea, juice, formula milk and solid/semi-solid foods were introduced. For the purpose of limiting the recall bias, parents/caregivers were advised to use the child's medical records for the questions in the perinatal section, resulting in an excellent value of ICC (intraclass correlation coefficient) in the test–retest reliability study—0.75, whereas the questions on parental weight and height had "moderate-to-excellent reliability" (i.e., ICC ranged from 0.489 to 0.911) [25]. Data on health-related behaviors (dietary habits, physical activity and sedentary behavior) of preschoolers and their parents were collected using validated questionnaires and the results regarding this topic are presented in other papers [26,27].

Family socioeconomic status (SES) was categorized according to maternal years of education as "low SES" ($\leq$12 years), "medium SES" (13–16 years) and "high SES" ($\geq$16 years of education). Preterm birth was defined as <37 gestational weeks, full-term birth—as $\geq$37 gestational weeks. Breastfeeding status was defined according to the WHO indicators [28]. Exclusive breastfeeding indicated breastfeeding with no other food or liquid given, except for medical drops and syrups (vitamins, minerals, medicines). Predominant breastfeeding applied if the infant received additional water or water-based liquids. The inclusion of other milks and foods (formula milk and/or semi-solids) was considered partial breastfeeding. The ever breastfed rate was the proportion of infants aged less than 12 months who were ever breastfed. Complementary feeding included liquids and SF (fruit juice, fruits, vegetables, meat, fish, eggs, milk products, creams and soup). Timely complementary feeding rate was defined as the proportion of infants 4–6 months of age who received breast milk and CF. Children without any information about feeding in the first two months (n = 454) and without information about the time of solid foods' introduction (n = 300) were excluded from the analyzed study sample (n = 7554). Both the analyzed and the excluded samples have similar distribution by country and participating status (intervention or control groups).

2.1. Anthropometric Data

Children's weight (to the nearest 0.1 kg) and height (to the nearest 0.1 cm) were measured using a standardized protocol and standardized equipment which was calibrated before and during the period of data collection [29]. All measurements were taken by research assistants who were thoroughly trained before the initiation of the study to achieve very good intra- and interobserver reliability agreement [30]. Overweight including obesity was defined on the basis of the WHO criteria as BMI z-score > 2 standard deviations (SD) and BMI z-score > 3 SDs, respectively, for children aged < 5 years. For children aged > 5 years, overweight was defined as BMI z-score > 1 SD and obesity as BMI z-score > 2 SDs. Calculation of the ponderal index (PI = weight/height^3) was used for assessment of the weight status of children at birth, with a PI range of 2.0–3.0 g/cm^3 considered normal. Children with a PI > 3.0 were considered overweight, and those with PI < 2.0 were classified as small for gestational age (SGA). Parental weight and height were self-reported by parents/caregivers and their BMI was calculated. Parents/caregivers were categorized according to their BMI as "under-/normal weight" ($\leq$24.9 kg/m^2), "overweight" ($\geq$25 and $\leq$29.9 kg/m^2) or "obese" ($\geq$30 kg/m^2) [31].

2.2. Statistical Analyses

Normal distribution of variables was tested with Shapiro–Wilk tests. Continuous variables are presented as the means $\pm$ standard deviation in case they were normally distributed (e.g., age of preschoolers, age of mothers, introduction of solid foods) and as the medians and IQR (interquartile range) for non-normally distributed variables (duration of breastfeeding, introduction of tea, introduction of fruit juices). Statistical analysis of parameters' distribution of the original samples by country was not applied as their number was small (n = 6). Post-sampling or bootstrapping were not considered.

Categorical variables were analyzed using the χ^2 test regarding country and children's BMI categories. An independent samples t-test was applied for comparison of the means and percentages from two samples while the one-way ANOVA (analysis of variance) for the means of more than two samples (birth weight; mother's age).

Comparison of the medians was performed using the median test. The association of feeding practices and children's BMI as well as mother's characteristics was determined by the correlation analysis. Logistic regression analysis with 95% confidence intervals (CIs) was used to estimate the odds of being overweight/obese (dependent variable) in relation to different infant-feeding practices. The results were adjusted for mother's age and BMI before pregnancy, SES, smoking habits during pregnancy and country. In order to quantify the probability of complying with current recommendations for the introduction of CF at 4–6 months of age, logistic regression analysis was performed and adjusted for mother's age and BMI before pregnancy, SES, smoking habits during pregnancy and country. Compliance to recommendations for introduction of CF at 4–6 months of age (yes/no) was considered as a dependent variable.

In the logistic regression models, the variables were selected based on their relevance for the research topic and being tested for absence of collinearity, hence the presented model coefficients correspond to variables with no significant impact as well. Thus, we can reach a conclusion about the existence of meaningful links. The regression analyses of the current data were targeted at identification of the relevant links between the study variables, but not at constituting a universal model which may be applied for analysis of other populations or for establishing new theories. The data were analyzed using the Statistical Package for Social Sciences (IBM SPSS v. 20, Chicago, IL, USA). The level of significance was set at $p < 0.05$.

3. Results

The total number of analyzed eligible questionnaires from the six countries was 6800 (mean age of the participants, 4.75 ± 0.43 years; 47.7% girls with no statistically significant difference in gender distribution between the participating countries). The sociodemographic characteristics of responders are presented in Table 1. Additional information regarding characteristics of the ToyBox-study sample were previously reported [24,31].

Table 1. Characteristics of participants by country (* χ^2 test; ** ANOVA).

	Belgium	Bulgaria	Germany	Greece	Poland	Spain	Total	p
				Country, n (%)				
				Gender				
Male	600 (53.2)	438 (50.1)	577 (52.3)	841 (51.1)	707 (53.0)	392 (55.0)	3555 (52.3)	0.37 *
Female	528 (46.8)	436 (49.9)	527 (47.7)	806 (48.9)	627 (47.0)	321 (45.0)	3245 (47.7)	
	1128 (100)	874 (100)	1104 (100)	1647 (100)	1334 (100)	713 (100)	6800 (100)	
				Mean birth weight ($\pm$SD)				
	3.34 (0.51)	3.26 (0.53)	3.32 (0.54)	3.14 (0.53)	3.44 (0.55)	3.32 (0.50)	3.29 (0.54)	<0.001 **
				Ponderal index at birth				
Low	121 (10.7)	142 (16.2)	28 (2.6)	339 (20.7)	754 (59.6)	95 (13.2)	1633 (24.3)	
Normal	914 (81.0)	690 (78.9)	883 (80.8)	1267 (77.2)	499 (39.5)	554 (77.7)	4806 (71.6)	<0.001 *
High	93 (8.3)	42 (4.9)	28 (2.6)	34 (2.1)	12 (0.9)	66 (9.1)	274 (4.1)	
				BMI at month 6				
Under-/normal	788 (94.9)	445 (90.6)	917 (91.7)	1334 (92.8)	818 (89.1)	545 (92.1)	4897 (92.0)	
Overweight	35 (4.2)	21 (4.3)	65 (6.5)	85 (5.9)	75 (8.2)	41 (6.9)	322 (6.1)	<0.001 *
Obese	7 (0.9)	25 (5.1)	18 (1.8)	17 (1.3)	25 (2.7)	6 (1.0)	98 (1.9)	
				BMI at month 12				
Under-/normal	607 (94.4)	400 (82.1)	902 (91.0)	1231 (88.2)	749 (82.6)	515 (88.9)	4404 (88.0)	
Overweight	27 (4.2)	60 (12.4)	62 (6.3)	130 (9.3)	131 (14.4)	55 (9.5)	465 (9.3)	<0.001 *
Obese	9 (1.4)	27 (5.5)	27 (2.7)	35 (2.5)	27 (3.0)	9 (1.6)	134 (2.7)	
				BMI categories of preschoolers, n (%)				
Underweight	8 (0.7)	5 (0.6)	4 (0.4)	11 (0.7)	7 (0.5)	2 (0.3)	37 (0.5)	
Normal weight	1059 (93.9)	764 (87.4)	1024 (92.8)	1356 (82.3)	1214 (91.0)	613 (86.0)	6030 (87.8)	
Overweight	47 (4.2)	76 (8.7)	61 (5.5)	200 (12.1)	83 (6.2)	75 (10.5)	542 (8.0)	<0.001 *
Obese	14 (1.2)	29 (3.3)	14 (1.3)	80 (4.9)	30 (2.2)	23 (3.2)	190 (2.8)	
				SES, n (%)				
Low SES	453 (40.2)	124 (14.2)	243 (22.0)	790 (48.0)	445 (33.4)	290 (40.7)	2345 (34.5)	
Medium SES	341 (30.2)	300 (34.3)	388 (35.1)	448 (27.2)	395 (29.6)	256 (35.9)	2128 (31.3)	
High SES	334 (29.6)	450 (51.5)	473 (42.8)	409 (24.8)	494 (37.0)	167 (23.4)	2327 (34.2)	<0.001 *
	1128 (100)	874 (100)	1104 (100)	1647 (100)	1334 (100)	713 (100)	6800 (100)	
				Mother's age—mean ($\pm$SD)				
	33.7 (4.7)	33.9 (4.4)	35.7 (5.1)	37.1 (4.4)	34.5 (4.3)	37.7 (4.6)	35.4 (4.7)	<0.001 **
				BMI categories, n (%)				
Under-/normal	755 (70.4)	667 (78.9)	727 (70.9)	1101 (70.1)	1011 (78.6)	503 (74.2)	4764 (73.5)	
Overweight	217 (20.2)	133 (15.7)	213 (20.8)	328 (20.9)	204 (15.9)	134 (19.8)	1229 (19.0)	<0.001 *
Obese	100 (9.3)	45 (5.3)	86 (8.4)	142 (9.0)	72 (5.6)	41 (6.0)	486 (7.5)	

Table 1. *Cont.*

	Country, *n* (%)							
	Belgium	Bulgaria	Germany	Greece	Poland	Spain	Total	*p*
Tobacco use during pregnancy								
No smoking	1011 (90.7)	687 (79.8)	956 (89.2)	1340 (82.7)	1220 (93.2)	574 (81.0)	5788 (86.6)	
Smoking, 2nd trimester	2 (0.2)	12 (1.4)	4 (0.4)	40 (2.5)	1 (0.1)	2 (0.3)	61 (0.9)	<0.0001 *
Smoking, 1st and 3rd trimester	6 (0.5)	46 (5.3)	29 (2.7)	54 (3.3)	29 (2.2)	25 (3.5)	189 (2.8)	
Smoking throughout pregnancy	96 (8.6)	116 (13.5)	83 (7.7)	187 (11.5)	59 (4.5)	108 (15.2)	649 (9.7)	

Tea (chamomile and other types of tea, especially for baby colics) was the first CF for most of the children in our study, introduced at a median age of three months (IQR, 2–5 months), resulting in a low proportion of exclusively breastfed children at four months of age (Table 2).

Table 2. Infant feeding practices among pre-school children from the six countries, participating in the ToyBox-study.

Infant-Feeding Practice	Country, *n* (%)							*p*
	Belgium	Bulgaria	Germany	Greece	Poland	Spain	Total	
Exclusive breastfeeding at 4–6 months of age, *n* (%)	32 (2.8)	47 (5.4)	163 (14.8)	44 (2.7)	105 (7.9)	37 (5.2)	428 (6.3)	<0.001
Ever breastfed rate, *n* (%)	751 (66.7)	811 (92.8)	928 (84.1)	1418 (86.1)	1263 (94.7)	606 (85.0)	5777 (85.0)	<0.001
Duration of BF (median; months; IQR)	4 (2–6)	5 (3–9)	7 (4–11)	3 (2–6)	9 (4–13)	5 (2–9)	5 (2–9)	<0.001
Continued BF rate (>12 months)	31 (3.9)	87 (10.3)	134 (12.1)	84 (5.9)	347 (26.3)	95 (15.7)	778 (12.8)	<0.001
Introduction of tea (median; months; IQR)	3 (2–4)	2 (2–4)	3 (1–6)	3 (1–6)	3 (2–5)	3 (2–6)	3 (2–5)	<0.001
Introduction of fruit juices (Median; months; IQR)	6 (4–12)	4 (3–6)	8 (6–13)	8 (6–13)	6 (5–7)	6 (5–8)	6 (5–8)	<0.001
Introduction of SF, months (mean ± SD)	4.6 ± 1.8	6.6 ± 2.0	6.3 ± 1.8	5.8 ± 1.2	5.8 ± 1.6	5.6 ± 1.5	5.8 ± 1.7	<0.001 *
Introduction of SF at 1–3 months of age, *n* (%)	197 (17.5)	19 (2.2)	18 (1.6)	15 (0.8)	15 (1.1)	16 (2.2)	279 (4.1)	
Introduction of SF at 4–6 months of age, *n* (%)	839 (74.4)	485 (55.5)	694 (63.9)	1385 (84.1)	995 (74.6)	596 (83.6)	4994 (73.4)	<0.001 †
Introduction of SF at 7–12 months of age, *n* (%)	92 (8.1)	370 (42.3)	392 (35.5)	248 (15.1)	324 (24.3)	101 (14.2)	1527 (22.5)	
Exclusive BF at 4–6 months of age + introduction of SF and BF < 12 months	32 (2.84)	47 (5.38)	163 (14.76)	44 (2.67)	105 (7.87)	37 (5.19)	428 (6.29)	<0.001
Exclusive BF at 4–6 months of age + introduction of SF and BF ≥ 12 months	15 (1.15)	24 (2.90)	74 (7.86)	18 (1.09)	142 (10.64)	18 (2.52)	225 (3.31)	<0.001

* Introduction of solid foods is significantly different with exception of the following comparisons: Greece and Spain (*p* = 0.13); Greece and Poland (*p* = 0.9); Poland and Spain (*p* = 0.18) (ANOVA); † *p*-value of the χ^2 test; EBF—exclusive breastfeeding; SF—solid foods; IQR—interquartile range.

In the study sample, the median introduction to fruit juices was at six months of age (IQR, 5–8 months), with the earliest introduction being among Bulgarian children (median, four months of age; IQR, 3–6 months). In the total sample, the proportion of 4–6-month-old infants who received breast milk and CF (timely complementary feeding rate) was 51.2% (35.4%, Belgians; 50.4%, Spanish; 53.7%, Polish; 67.8%, Bulgarians; 72.3%, Germans (*p* < 0.01)). The median age of SF introduction was six months (IQR, 5–6 months), with the earliest introduction in Belgium (median, four months of age, IQR, 4–5 months). Some 26.6% (*n* = 1806) introduced CF outside of the recommended age range, with 4.1% (*n* = 279) before the 16th postnatal week and 22.5% (*n* = 1527) after the 25th week. The time of CF introduction was correlated with breastfeeding duration (Spearman's $\rho = 0.2$; $p < 0.001$). There was a weak positive relationship between the introduction of CF and SES (Spearman's $\rho = 0.08$; $p < 0.001$) and a negative relationship with smoking during pregnancy (Pearson's r $= -0.04$; $p = 0.003$). Stratifying by country, a negative relationship with smoking during pregnancy was identified only in the Bulgarian sample (Spearman's $\rho = 0.12$; $p < 0.001$).

The prevalence of overweight and obesity according to the WHO I criteria was 8.0% ($n = 542$) and 2.8% ($n = 190$), respectively (Table 1). Infant-feeding practices showed a different relationship to the prevalence of overweight and obesity at different stages of childhood. Timely introduction of CF at 4–6 months of age had a negative association with the prevalence of overweight and obesity at six and 12 months of age, with no differences between breastfed and non-breastfed children ($p < 0.05$) (Table 3).

Table 3. Breastfeeding practices and weight status of children (χ^2 and independent samples *t*-test).

	Weight at Month 6			Weight at Month 12			Weight, Preschoolers		
	Under-/Normal	Overweight	Obese	Under-/Normal	Overweight	Obese	Under-/Normal	Overweight	Obese
EBF at 0–3 months of age; *n* (%)	1672 (91.7)	116 (6.4)	35 (1.9)	1557 (88.6)	163 (9.3)	37 (2.1)	2104 (90.8)	170 (7.3)	43 (1.9)
EBF at 4–6 months of age; *n* (%)	304 (90.2)	23 (6.8)	10 (3.0)	299 (88.7)	29 (8.6)	9 (2.7)	392 (91.6)	29 (6.8)	7 (1.6)
Introduction of CF at 0–3 months of age; *n* (%)	187 (93.5)	7 (3.5)	6 (3.0)	147 (92.5)	7 **(4.4) ***	5 (3.1)	262 (93.9)	12 **(4.3) ***	5 **(1.8) ***
Introduction of CF at 4–6 months of age; *n* (%)	3655 (92.5)	241 **(6.1) ***	54 **(1.4) ***	3310 (88.4)	349 **(9.3) ***	86 (2.3)	4447 (89.1)	401 **(8.0) ***	145 **(2.9) ***
Introduction of CF at 7–12 months of age; *n* (%)	1005 (90.0)	74 **(6.6) ***	38 **(3.4) ***	947 (86.2)	109 (9.9)	43 (3.9)	1358 (88.9)	129 (8.4)	40 (2.6)

EBF—exclusive breastfeeding; significant comparisons of the prevalence of overweight and obesity (independent samples *t*-test) at 6 months of age: * introduction of CF (complementary foods) at 4–6 and ≥ 7 months of age—t $= 2.71$; $p < 0.01$; at 12 months of age: * introduction of CF at 4–6 and 0–3 months of age—t $= 4.32$; $p < 0.001$; pre-school age: * introduction of CF at 4–6 and 0–3 months of age—t $= 2.98$; $p < 0.01$.

On the country level, the significant difference in the prevalence of overweight and obesity at preschool age was observed only in two countries—late CF introduction (after seven months) compared to earlier introduction is related to higher prevalence of obesity in Belgium ($p < 0.001$) and to higher prevalence of overweight in Poland ($p < 0.05$) (Table 4).

Table 4. Breastfeeding practices and weight status of preschool children by country (χ^2).

Country		Weight, Preschoolers, *n* (%)		
		Under-/Normal Weight	Overweight	Obese
Belgium	EBF at 0–3 months of age	304 (93.3)	17 (5.2)	5 (1.5)
	EBF at 4–6 months of age	29 (90.6)	1 (3.1)	2 (6.3)
	Introduction of CF at 0–3 months of age	187 (94.9)	8 (4.1)	2 (1.0) *
	Introduction of CF at 4–6 months of age	801 (95.5)	32 (3.8)	6 (0.7) **
	Introduction of CF at 7–12 months of age	79 (85.9)	7 (7.6)	6 (6.5) *
Bulgaria	EBF at 0–3 months of age	190 (91.8)	16 (7.7)	1 (0.5)
	EBF at 4–6 months of age	43 (91.5)	4 (8.5)	0
	Introduction of CF at 0–3 months of age	19 (100)	0	0
	Introduction of CF at 4–6 months of age	416 (85.8)	49 (10.1)	20 (4.1)
	Introduction of CF at 7–12 months of age	334 (90.3)	27 (7.3)	9 (2.4)

Table 4. Cont.

Country		Weight, Preschoolers, n (%)		
		Under-/Normal Weight	Overweight	Obese
Germany	EBF at 0–3 months of age	458 (94.0)	23 (4.7)	6 (1.2)
	EBF at 4–6 months of age	158 (96.9)	4 (2.5)	1 (0.6)
	Introduction of CF at 0–3 months of age	16 (88.9)	1 (5.6)	1 (5.6)
	Introduction of CF at 4–6 months of age	643 (92.8)	43 (6.2)	7 (1.0)
	Introduction of CF at 7–12 months of age	369 (94.1)	17 (4.3)	6 (1.5)
Greece	EBF at 0–3 months of age	305 (84.7)	44 (12.2)	11 (3.1)
	EBF at 4–6 months of age	36 (81.8)	6 (13.6)	2 (4.5)
	Introduction of CF at 0–3 months of age	12 (85.7)	0	2 (14.3)
	Introduction of CF at 4–6 months of age	1156 (83.5)	164 (11.8)	65 (4.7)
	Introduction of CF at 7–12 months of age	199 (80.2)	36 (14.5)	13 (5.2)
Poland	EBF at 0–3 months of age	575 (92.3)	37 (5.9)	11 (1.8)
	EBF at 4–6 months of age	95 (90.5)	9 (8.6)	1 (1.0)
	Introduction of CF at 0–3 months of age	14 (93.3)	1 (6.7)	0
	Introduction of CF at 4–6 months of age	916 (92.1)	53 (5.3) *	26 (2.6)
	Introduction of CF at 7–12 months of age	291 (89.8)	29 (9.0) *	4 (1.2)
Spain	EBF at 0–3 months of age	272 (86.6)	33 (10.5)	9 (2.9)
	EBF at 4–6 months of age	31 (83.8)	5 (13.5)	1 (2.7)
	Introduction of CF at 0–3 months of age	14 (87.5)	2 (12.5)	0
	Introduction of CF at 4–6 months of age	515 (86.4)	60 (10.1)	21 (3.5)
	Introduction of CF at 7–12 months of age	86 (85.1)	13 (12.9)	2 (2.0)

Significant comparisons of the prevalence of overweight and obesity in preschool age (independent samples *t*-test): Belguim: obesity; * introduction of CF (complementary foods) at 0–3 and 7–12 months of age (t = 2.06; $p < 0.02$); ** introduction of CF at 4–6 and 7–12 months of age (t = 2.27; $p < 0.001$); Poland: overweight; * introduction of CF at 4–6 and $\geq$ 7 months of age (t = 2.12; $p = 0.03$).

Table 5 presents results of the logistic regression analysis identifying one single risk factor connected to inappropriate timing of CF introduction (<4 months of age or >6 months of age)—lower SES (OR = 1.25; 95% CI, 1.08–1.45).

Table 5. Maternal characteristics associated with non-compliance to the recommendation for introduction of complementary foods (CF) at 4–6 months of age.

	Introduction of SF at 4–6 Months of Age (n = 4266) OR (95% CI), p	
Smoking habits throughout pregnancy [1]		
No smoking	1 (reference)	
Smoking, 2nd trimester	1.50 (0.75–3.01)	0.25
Smoking, 1st and 3rd trimesters	1.07 (0.75–1.53)	0.71
Smoking throughout pregnancy	1.22 (0.98–1.52)	0.08
BMI before pregnancy [2]		
Underweight	1.04 (0.85–1.29)	0.68
Normal weight	1 (reference)	
Overweight	1.16 (0.97–1.39)	0.11
Obese	1.20 (0.89–1.62)	0.24
SES [3]		
Low	1.25 (1.08–1.45)	0.002
Medium	1.11 (0.96–1.28)	0.17
High	1 (reference)	

[1] Adjusted for age and BMI before pregnancy, country and SES. [2] Adjusted for age before pregnancy, smoking habits during pregnancy, country and SES. [3] Adjusted for age and BMI before pregnancy, smoking habits during pregnancy, country.

The logistic regression analysis showed that the odds of becoming overweight at preschool age among children who had early introduction of SF (1–3 months of age) compared to those with CF introduction at 4–6 months of age was 0.69 (OR = 0.69; 95% CI,

0.41–1.16; $p = 0.16$). The children introduced to SF before four months of age had a trend for a different overweight risk at preschool age according to their BF status which was not significant when adjusted for the mother's characteristics (SES, education, pre-pregnancy weight and smoking habits during pregnancy). For the children breastfed for ≥ 4 months, early introduction of CF was associated with a trend for higher later overweight (OR = 1.23; 95% CI, 0.29–5.14; $p = 0.78$), while among the exclusively formula-fed breastfed children, this risk tended to be lower (OR = 0.39; 95% CI, 0.052–3.12; $p = 0.38$). Late CF introduction at 7–12 months of age was not related to a difference in later overweight and obesity risk when adjusted for country, age and gender (OR = 0.98; 95% CI, 0.83–1.21; $p = 0.99$).

4. Discussion

Our study investigated the association between the timing of CF, breastfeeding status and overweight among European preschool children. Breastfed children (any type of breastfeeding) throughout the first 4–6 months of life and after the 12th month had a lower prevalence of overweight/obesity in childhood compared to formula-fed children. This finding is consistent with the European studies reporting similar results in previous cohorts [9,14,32,33]. The main findings point at a lower prevalence of overweight/obesity at six months of age ($p < 0.001$) in children with introduction of solid foods between 4–6 months of age compared to late introduction (7–12 months of age). However, there were no significant findings for the prevalence at one year and at preschool age ($p > 0.05$). A late SF introduction is related to a higher prevalence of overweight and obesity at six months of age, 12 months of age and at preschool age. Our results are consistent with the previously reported findings [15,18].

Pluymen et al. and Huh et al. reported that the duration of breastfeeding modifies the association between CF introduction and overweight: BF for less than four months and CF introduction before four months of age increased the risk for overweight by 37% compared to those with CF introduction ≥ 4 months of age [21,22]. We found a non-significant trend for an association of early introduction of SF and preschool overweight in breastfed children but not in formula-fed children.

Different previous studies aimed at identification of predictors of children's dietary intake such as SES and geographic region [34,35]. SES is one of the most commonly identified factors associated with childhood overweight and obesity and reflects a child's living conditions. However, there is uncertainty as to the mechanisms through which SES influences the child's weight. Breastfeeding practices and timing of CF introduction are related to SES and other maternal characteristics such as BMI, age at birth, tobacco use during pregnancy, gestational weight gain, depression and use of day care [36–39]. Results from the ToyBox-study show that mothers with low SES are more likely to have overweight/obese children compared to those with medium/high SES (OR = 1.41; 95% CI, 1.17–1.71 [31].

The current analysis supports the findings of other studies that significant risk factors associated with non-compliance to the recommendation for introduction of CF at 4–6 months of age are low SES and smoking throughout pregnancy ($p < 0.05$) [14,40–42]. Maternal educational level did not modify the association of CF < 4 months of age and overweight in the PIAMA cohort as well [19]. Rose et al., based on the data of the Infant Feeding Practices Study II and Year 6 Follow-Up Studies, suggested that the mother's decisions about milk-feeding and the types and quality of solid foods introduced in infancy can shape dietary patterns and obesity risk later in childhood. Infants who were offered foods high in energy density at nine months of age had a higher intake of these foods at six years of age and a higher prevalence of overweight compared to other classes of dietary patterns [43].

Our results, which hopefully will be useful for improving effectiveness of childhood obesity prevention programs in Europe, can also be utilized in low developed and developing countries. Although malnutrition is still a major challenge across the African continent, the largest growth of obesity among 5- to 19-year-olds in the world between 1975 and 2016 was observed in southern Africa (about 400% per decade) [44].

A methodological limitation of the report is the cross-sectional study design of our study which does not enable identifying cause–effect associations. Another limitation is the parental self-reporting of weight, height, gestational weight gain, infant's birth weight, as well as BF practices and timing of CF introduction by mothers' some 3–4 years later. The use of the mean educational level as a single indicator for SES is another limitation of the study. Furthermore, the mother's alcohol consumption during pregnancy which was not investigated as a risk factor for child health may be added to the list of the study limitations. The strengths of our study are the large number of study participants, the inclusion of children from several European countries adding external validity and the standardization of measurement approaches [25,31].

5. Conclusions

We conclude that other variables have a greater impact on the risk for childhood obesity than the timing of CF introduction. Therefore, intervention programs for childhood obesity should be conducted, including educating mothers about healthy eating practices and other possible risk factors for overweight.

Author Contributions: Conceptualization, V.I. and N.U.; methodology, G.C., N.U. and V.I.; formal analysis, S.G., N.U.; investigation, S.G. and M.D.C.; writing—original draft preparation, N.U., V.I. and M.D.C.; writing—review and editing, B.V.K., M.D.C., O.A., V.I., G.C., A.K., S.G., Y.M., L.A.M. and P.S.; supervision, V.I., Y.M. and the Toy-Box-study group. All authors have read and agreed to the published version of the manuscript.

Funding: The ToyBox-study was funded by the Seventh Framework Program (The Community Research and Development Information Service (CORDIS; FP7)) of the European Commission under grant agreement No. 245200. B.V.K. is the Else Kröner Seniorprofessor of Paediatrics at LMU— University of Munich, financially supported by the Else Kröner-Fresenius-Foundation, the LMU Medical Faculty and the LMU University Hospitals. The content of this article reflects only the authors' views and the European Community is not liable for any use that may be made of the information contained therein.

Institutional Review Board Statement: The ToyBox-study (www.toybox-study.eu; accessed on 20 September 2020) adhered to the Declaration of Helsinki and the conventions of the Council of Europe on human rights and biomedicine. All the countries (Belgium, Bulgaria, Germany, Greece, Poland and Spain) obtained ethical clearance from the relevant ethics committees and local authorities: 1. Ethics Committee of Ghent University Hospital (Belgium)—EC/2010/037; 2. Committee for the Ethics of Scientific Studies (KENI) at the Medical University of Varna (Bulgaria)— 15/21.07.2011; 3. Ethics Committee of the Medical Faculty at LMU Munich (Ethikkommission der Ludwig-Maximilians-Universität München) (Germany)—400-11 (2012); 4. Bioethics Committee of the Harokopio University of Athens (Greece) (28/02-12-2010) and the Ministry of Education of Greece (approval code 29447/Γ7 (05-05-2011)); 5. Ethics Committee of the Children's Memorial Health Institute (Poland)— 1/KBE/2012; 6. CEICA (Comité Ético de Investigación Clínica de Aragón (Spain))—PI11/056 30.08.2011. The ToyBox-study is registered with the clinical trials registry: clinicaltrials.gov, ID: NCT02116296.

Informed Consent Statement: All parents/caregivers provided a signed consent form before being enrolled in the study.

Data Availability Statement: The data presented in this study are available on request from the corresponding author. The data are not publicly available due to restrictions of informed consent and the requirement of IRB review and approval.

Acknowledgments: We gratefully acknowledge all the members of the ToyBox-study Group. Coordinator: Yannis Manios; project manager: Odysseas Androutsos; steering committee: Yannis Manios, Berthold Koletzko, Ilse de Bourdeaudhuij, Mai Chin A Paw, Luis Moreno, Carolyn Summerbell, Tim Lobstein, Lieven Annemans and Goof Buijs; external advisors: John Reilly, Boyd Swinburn and Dianne Ward; Harokopio University (Greece): Yannis Manios, Odysseas Androutsos, Eva Grammatikaki, Christina Katsarou, Eftychia Apostolidou, Anastasia Livaniou, Eirini Efstathopoulou, Paraskevi–Eirini Siatitsa, Angeliki Giannopoulou, Effie Argyri, Konstantina Maragkopoulou, Athanasios Douligeris and Roula Koutsi; Ludwig-Maximilians-Universität München (Germany): Berthold Koletzko, Kristin Duvinage, Sabine Ibrügger, Angelika Strauß, Birgit Herbert, Julia Birnbaum, Annette Payr and Christine Geyer; Ghent University (Belgium): Department of Movement and Sports Sciences: Ilse de Bourdeaudhuij, Greet Cardon, Marieke de Craemer and Ellen de Decker; Department of Public Health: Lieven Annemans, Stefaan de Henauw, Lea Maes, Carine Vereecken, Jo van Assche and Lore Pil; Vrije Universiteit Amsterdam (VU University) Medical Center, The Institute for Research in Extramural Medicine (EMGO) Institute for Health and Care Research (The Netherlands): Mai Chin A Paw and Saskia te Velde; University of Zaragoza (Spain): Luis Moreno, Theodora Mouratidou, Juan Fernandez, Maribel Mesana, Pilar de Miguel–Etayo, Esther M. González-Gil, Luis Gracia–Marco and Beatriz Oves; Oslo and Akershus University College of Applied Sciences (Norway): Agneta Yngve, Susanna Kugelberg, Christel Lynch, Annhild Mosdøl and Bente B. Nilsen; University of Durham (UK): Carolyn Summerbell, Helen Moore, Wayne Douthwaite and Catherine Nixon; State Institute of Early Childhood Research (Germany): Susanne Kreichauf and Andreas Wildgruber; Children's Memorial Health Institute (Poland): Piotr Socha, Zbigniew Kulaga, Kamila Zych, Magdalena Góźdź, Beata Gurzkowska and Katarzyna Szott; Medical University of Varna (Bulgaria): Violeta Iotova, Mina Lateva, Natalya Usheva, Sonya Galcheva, Vanya Marinova, Zhaneta Radkova and Nevyana Feschieva; International Association for the Study of Obesity (UK): Tim Lobstein and Andrea Aikenhead; CBO B.V. (the Netherlands): Goof Buijs, Annemiek Dorgelo, Aviva Nethe and Jan Jansen; AOK-Verlag (Germany): Otto Gmeiner, Jutta Retterath, Julia Wildeis and Axel Günthersberger; Roehampton University (UK): Leigh Gibson; University of Luxembourg (Luxembourg): Claus Voegele.

Conflicts of Interest: The authors declare no conflict of interest.

References

1. WHO. *Interim Report of the Commission on Ending Childhood Obesity*; 2015; pp. 5–9.
2. Biener, A.; Cawley, J.; Meyerhoefer, C. The High and Rising Costs of Obesity to the US Health Care System. *J. Gen. Intern. Med.* **2017**, *32*, 6–8. [CrossRef]
3. Erixon, F. Europe's Obesity Challenge. *ECIPE Policy Brief* **2016**, *7*, 1–3.
4. Singh, A.S.; Mulder, C.; Twisk, J.W.; van Mechelen, W.; Chinapaw, M.J. Tracking of childhood overweight into adulthood: A systematic review of the literature. *Obes Rev.* **2008**, *9*, 474–488. [CrossRef]
5. WHO. *Obesity and Overweight*. 2020. Available online: https://www.who.int/news-room/fact-sheets/detail/obesity-and-overweight (accessed on 20 September 2020).
6. WHO. The Optimal Duration of Exclusive Breastfeeding: Report of an Expert Consultation. 28–30 March 2001. Available online: www.who.int/nutrition/publications/optimal_duration_of_exc_bfeeding_report_eng.pdf (accessed on 20 September 2020).
7. WHO. *Complementary Feeding: Report of the Global Consultation*; WHO: Switzerland, Geneva, 2002.
8. Fewtrell, M.; Bronsky, J.; Campoy, C.; Domellöf, M.; Embleton, N.; Mis, N.F.; Hojsak, I.; Hulst, J.M.; Indrio, F.; Lapillonne, A.; et al. Complementary feeding: A position paper by the European Society for Paediatric Gastroenterology, Hepatology and Nutrition (ESPGHAN) Committee on nutrition. *J. Pediatr. Gastroenterol. Nutr.* **2017**, *64*, 119–132. [CrossRef]
9. Arenz, S.; Rückerl, R.; Koletzko, B.; von Kries, R. Breast-feeding and childhood obesity—A systematic review. *Int. J. Obes. Relat. Metab. Disord.* **2004**, *28*, 1247–1256. [CrossRef] [PubMed]
10. Programme, E.C.O. *EU Childhood Obesity Programme Press Pack—20 April 2007*; Budapest, Hungary, 2007.
11. Owen, C.G.; Martin, R.M.; Whincup, P.H.; Smith, G.D.; Cook, D.G. Effect of infant feeding on the risk of obesity across the life course: A quantitative review of published evidence. *Pediatrics* **2005**, *115*, 1367–1377. [CrossRef] [PubMed]
12. Grote, V.; Theurich, M.; Koletzko, B. Do complementary feeding practices predict the later risk of obesity? *Curr. Opin. Clin. Nutr. Metab. Care* **2012**, *15*, 293–297. [CrossRef] [PubMed]
13. Grote, V.; Theurich, M.; Luque, V.; Gruszfeld, D.; Verduci, E.; Xhonneux, A.; Koletzko, B. Complementary Feeding, Infant Growth, and Obesity Risk: Timing, Composition, and Mode of Feeding. *Nestle Nutr. Inst. Workshop Ser.* **2018**, *89*, 93–103. [PubMed]
14. Papoutsou, S.; Savva, S.C.; Hunsberger, M.; Jilani, H.; Michels, N.; Ahrens, W.; Tornaritis, M.; Veidebaum, T.; Molnár, D.; Siani, A.; et al. Timing of solid food introduction and association with later childhood overweight and obesity: The IDEFICS study. *Matern. Child Nutr.* **2017**, *1*, e12471. [CrossRef]
15. Moorcroft, K.E.; Marshall, J.L.; McCormick, F.M. Association between timing of introducing solid foods and obesity in infancy and childhood: A systematic review. *Matern. Child Nutr.* **2010**, *7*, 3–26. [CrossRef]
16. Barrera, C.M.; Perrine, C.G.; Li, R.; Scanlon, K.S. Age at Introduction to Solid Foods and Child Obesity at 6 Years. *Child Obes.* **2016**, *12*, 188–192. [CrossRef] [PubMed]
17. Koletzko, B.; Hirsch, N.L.; Jewell, J.M.; Caroli, M.; Breda, J.R.D.S.; Weber, M. Pureed Fruit Pouches for Babies: Child Health under Squeeze. *J. Pediatr. Gastroenterol. Nutr.* **2018**, *67*, 561–563. [CrossRef] [PubMed]

18. A Theurich, M.; Grote, V.; Koletzko, B. Complementary feeding and long-term health implications. *Nutr. Rev.* **2020**, *78*, 6–12. [CrossRef] [PubMed]
19. Moss, B.G.; Yeaton, W.H. Early Childhood Healthy and Obese Weight Status: Potentially Protective Benefits of Breastfeeding and Delaying Solid Foods. *Matern. Child Heal. J.* **2013**, *18*, 1224–1232. [CrossRef]
20. Wang, J.; Wu, Y.; Xiong, G.; Chao, T.; Jin, Q.; Liu, R.; Hao, L.; Wei, S.; Yang, N.; Yang, X. Introduction of complementary feeding before 4 months of age increases the risk of childhood overweight or obesity: A metaanalysis of prospective cohort studies. *Nutr. Res.* **2016**, *36*, 759–770. [CrossRef]
21. Huh, S.Y.; Rifas-Shiman, S.L.; Taveras, E.M.; Oken, E.; Gillman, M.W. Timing of solid food introduction and risk of obesity in preschool-aged children. *Pediatrics* **2011**, *127*, e544–e551. [CrossRef]
22. Pluymen, L.P.; Wijga, A.H.; Gehring, U.; Koppelman, G.H.; Smit, H.A.; Van Rossem, L. Early introduction of complementary foods and childhood overweight in breastfed and formula-fed infants in the Netherlands: The PIAMA birth cohort study. *Eur. J. Nutr.* **2018**, *57*, 1985–1993. [CrossRef]
23. Pearce, J.; Taylor, M.A.; Langley-Evans, S.C. Timing of the introduction of complementary feeding and risk of childhood obesity: A systematic review. *Int. J. Obes.* **2013**, *37*, 1295–1306. [CrossRef]
24. Manios, Y.; Androutsos, O.; Katsarou, C.; Iotova, V.; Socha, P.; Geyer, C.; Moreno, L.; Koletzko, B.; De Bourdeaudhuij, I.; ToyBox-Study Group. Designing and implementing a kindergarten-based, family-involved intervention to prevent obesity in early childhood. The ToyBox-study. *Obes. Rev.* **2014**, *15*, 5–13. [CrossRef]
25. González-Gil, E.M.; Mouratidou, T.; Cardon, G.; Androutsos, O.; De Bourdeaudhuij, I.; Góźdź, M.; Usheva, N.; Birnbaum, J.; Manios, Y.; Moreno, L.A.; et al. Reliability of primary caregivers reports on lifestyle behaviours of European pre-school children: The ToyBox-study. *Obes. Rev.* **2014**, *15*, 61–66. [CrossRef]
26. Cardon, G.; De Bourdeaudhuij, I.; Iotova, V.; Latomme, J.; Socha, P.; Koletzko, B.; Moreno, L.; Manios, Y.; Androutsos, O.; De Craemer, M.; et al. Health Related Behaviours in Normal Weight and Overweight Preschoolers of a Large Pan-European Sample: The ToyBox-Study. *PLoS ONE* **2016**, *11*, e0150580. [CrossRef] [PubMed]
27. Pinket, A.S.; De Craemer, M.; Maes, L.; De Bourdeaudhuij, I.; Cardon, G.; Androutsos, O.; Koletzko, B.; Moreno, L.; Socha, P.; Iotova, V.; et al. Water intake and beverage consumption of pre-schoolers from six European countries and associations with socio-economic status: The ToyBox-study. *Public Health Nutr.* **2016**, *19*, 2315–2325. [CrossRef] [PubMed]
28. WHO/UNICEF/IFPRI/UCDavis/FANTA/AED/USAID. *Indicators for Assessing Infant and Young Child Feeding Practicies*; World Health Organization: Geneva, Switazerland, 2008.
29. Mouratidou, T.; Miguel, M.L.; Androutsos, O.; Manios, Y.; De Bourdeaudhuij, I.; Cardon, G.; Kulaga, Z.; Socha, P.; Galcheva, S.; Iotova, V.; et al. Tools, harmonization and standardization procedures of the impact and outcome evaluation indices obtained during a kindergarten-based, family-involved intervention to prevent obesity in early childhood: The ToyBox-study. *Obes. Rev.* **2014**, *15*, 53–60. [CrossRef] [PubMed]
30. De Miguel-Etayo, P.; Mesana, M.I.; Cardon, G.; De Bourdeaudhuij, I.; Góźdź, M.; Socha, P.; Lateva, M.; Iotova, V.; Koletzko, B.V.; Duvinage, K.; et al. Reliability of anthropometric measurements in European preschool children: The ToyBox-study. *Obes. Rev.* **2014**, *15*, 67–73. [CrossRef] [PubMed]
31. Manios, Y.; Androutsos, O.; Katsarou, C.; Vampouli, E.A.; Kulaga, Z.; Gurzkowska, B.; Iotova, V.; Usheva, N.; Cardon, G.; Koletzko, B.; et al. Prevalence and sociodemographic correlates of overweight and obesity in a large Pan-European cohort of preschool children and their families. The ToyBox-study. *Nutrition* **2018**, *55*, 55–56. [CrossRef] [PubMed]
32. Rito, A.I.; Buoncristiano, M.; Spinelli, A.; Salanave, B.; Kunešová, M.; Hejgaard, T.; García Solano, M.; Fijałkowska, A.; Sturua, L.; Breda, J.; et al. Association between Characteristics at Birth, Breastfeeding and Obesity in 22 Countries: The WHO European Childhood Obesity Surveillance Initiative—COSI 2015/2017. *Obes. Facts* **2019**, *12*, 226–243. [CrossRef] [PubMed]
33. Von Kries, R.; Koletzko, B.; Sauerwald, T.; Von Mutius, E.; Barnert, D.; Grunert, V.; Von Voss, H. Breast feeding and obesity: Cross sectional study. *BMJ* **1999**, *319*, 147–150. [CrossRef]
34. Bammann, K.; Gwozdz, W.; Lanfer, A.; Barba, G.; De Henauw, S.; Eiben, G.; Fernandez-Alvira, J.; Kovács, E.; Lissner, L.; Moreno, L.; et al. Socioeconomic factors and childhood overweight in Europe: Results from the multi-centre IDEFICS study. *Pediatr. Obes.* **2012**, *8*, 1–12. [CrossRef]
35. Olaya, B.; Moneta, M.V.; Pez, O.; Bitfoi, A.; Carta, M.G.; Eke, C.; Goelitz, D.; Keyes, K.M.; Kuijpers, R.; Lesinskiene, S.; et al. Country-level and individual correlates of overweight and obesity among primary school children: A cross-sectional study in seven European countries. *BMC Public Health* **2015**, *15*, 475. [CrossRef]
36. Shrewsbury, V.; Wardle, J. Socioeconomic Status and Adiposity in Childhood: A Systematic Review of Cross-sectional Studies 1990–2005. *Obesity* **2008**, *16*, 275–284. [CrossRef]
37. Mech, P.; Hooley, M.; Skouteris, H.; Williams, J. Parent-related mechanisms underlying the social gradient of childhood overweight and obesity: A systematic review. *Child Care Heal. Dev.* **2016**, *42*, 603–624. [CrossRef]
38. Gross, R.S.; Mendelsohn, A.L.; Fierman, A.H.; Racine, A.D.; Messito, M.J. Food Insecurity and Obesogenic Maternal Infant Feeding Styles and Practices in Low-Income Families. *Pediatrics* **2012**, *130*, 254–261. [CrossRef]
39. Androutsos, O.; Moschonis, G.; Ierodiakonou, D.; Karatzi, K.; De Bourdeaudhuij, I.; Iotova, V.; Zych, K.; Moreno, L.A.; Koletzko, B.; Manios, Y.; et al. Perinatal and lifestyle factors mediate the association between maternal education and preschool children's weight status: The ToyBox study. *Nutrition* **2018**, *48*, 6–12. [CrossRef] [PubMed]

40. van Rossem, L.; Oenema, A.; Steegers, E.A.; Moll, H.A.; Jaddoe, V.W.; Hofman, A.; Mackenbach, J.P.; Raat, H. Are starting and continuing breastfeeding related to educationalbackground? The Generation R study. *Pediatrics* **2009**, *123*, e1017–e1027. [PubMed]
41. Gibbs, B.G.; Forste, R. Socioeconomic status, infant feeding practices and early childhood obesity†. *Pediatr. Obes.* **2014**, *9*, 135–146. [CrossRef] [PubMed]
42. Grummer-Strawn, L.M.; Scanlon, K.S.; Fein, S.B. Infant Feeding and Feeding Transitions During the First Year of Life. *Pediatrics* **2008**, *122*, S36–S42. [CrossRef] [PubMed]
43. Rose, C.M.; Birch, L.; Savage, J.S. Dietary patterns in infancy are associated with child diet and weight outcomes at 6 years. *Int. J. Obes.* **2017**, *41*, 783–788. [CrossRef] [PubMed]
44. UNICEF-WHO-The World Bank Group. *Joint Child Malnutrition Estimates-Levels and Trends*; World Health Organization: Geneva, Switzerland, 2018. Available online: https://www.who.int/nutgrowthdb/estimates2017/en/ (accessed on 20 September 2020).

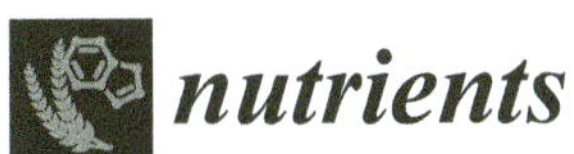

Review

Management of Childhood Obesity—Time to Shift from Generalized to Personalized Intervention Strategies

Mohamad Motevalli [1,*]**, Clemens Drenowatz** [2]**, Derrick R. Tanous** [1]**, Naim Akhtar Khan** [3]
and Katharina Wirnitzer [1,4,5,6]

[1]   Department of Sport Science, Leopold-Franzens University of Innsbruck, A-6020 Innsbruck, Austria;
     derrick.tanous@student.uibk.ac.at (D.R.T.); katharina.wirnitzer@ph-tirol.ac.at (K.W.)
[2]   Division of Sport, Physical Activity and Health, University College of Teacher Education Upper Austria,
     A-4020 Linz, Austria; clemens.drenowatz@ph-ooe.at
[3]   Nutritional Physiology & Toxicology Division, INSERM UMR 1231, Université de Bourgogne,
     F-21000 Dijon, France; naim.khan@u-bourgogne.fr
[4]   Department of Subject Didactics and Educational Research & Development, University College of Teacher
     Education Tyrol, A-6020 Innsbruck, Austria
[5]   Life and Health Science Cluster Tirol, Subcluster Health/Medicine/Psychology, A-6020 Innsbruck, Austria
[6]   Research Center Medical Humanities, Leopold-Franzens University of Innsbruck, A-6020 Innsbruck, Austria
*   Correspondence: mohamad_motevali@yahoo.com

Citation: Motevalli, M.; Drenowatz, C.; Tanous, D.R.; Khan, N.A.; Wirnitzer, K. Management of Childhood Obesity—Time to Shift from Generalized to Personalized Intervention Strategies. *Nutrients* **2021**, *13*, 1200. https://doi.org/10.3390/nu13041200

Academic Editors: Odysseas Androutsos and Evangelia Charmandari

Received: 30 January 2021
Accepted: 2 April 2021
Published: 6 April 2021

Publisher's Note: MDPI stays neutral with regard to jurisdictional claims in published maps and institutional affiliations.

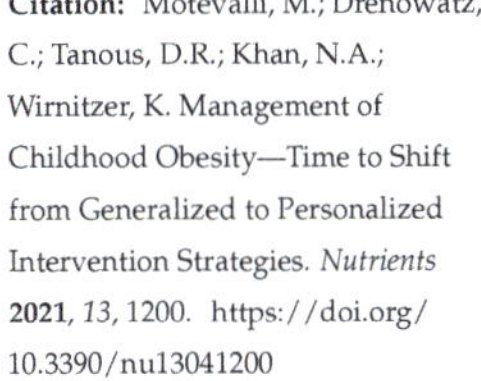

Copyright: © 2021 by the authors. Licensee MDPI, Basel, Switzerland. This article is an open access article distributed under the terms and conditions of the Creative Commons Attribution (CC BY) license (https://creativecommons.org/licenses/by/4.0/).

Abstract: As a major public health concern, childhood obesity is a multifaceted and multilevel metabolic disorder influenced by genetic and behavioral aspects. While genetic risk factors contribute to and interact with the onset and development of excess body weight, available evidence indicates that several modifiable obesogenic behaviors play a crucial role in the etiology of childhood obesity. Although a variety of systematic reviews and meta-analyses have reported the effectiveness of several interventions in community-based, school-based, and home-based programs regarding childhood obesity, the prevalence of children with excess body weight remains high. Additionally, researchers and pediatric clinicians are often encountering several challenges and the characteristics of an optimal weight management strategy remain controversial. Strategies involving a combination of physical activity, nutritional, and educational interventions are likely to yield better outcomes compared to single-component strategies but various prohibitory limitations have been reported in practice. This review seeks to (i) provide a brief overview of the current preventative and therapeutic approaches towards childhood obesity, (ii) discuss the complexity and limitations of research in the childhood obesity area, and (iii) suggest an Etiology-Based Personalized Intervention Strategy Targeting Childhood Obesity (EPISTCO). This purposeful approach includes prioritized nutritional, educational, behavioral, and physical activity intervention strategies directly based on the etiology of obesity and interpretation of individual characteristics.

Keywords: children; adolescents; overweight; obesity; weight management; lifestyle; body composition

1. Introduction

The examination of the etiology of childhood obesity is a growing area of research aiming to yield important insights for public health [1,2]. During the last three decades, the annual growth rate of publications on childhood obesity (average of 11.6% per year) has been generally higher than other sub-areas in the pediatric field and biomedical research [3]. Given the rising prevalence of childhood obesity in most developed and developing countries, it is now considered a global pandemic [4]. Worldwide, an estimated 170 million children are considered overweight or obese currently [5], and approximately more than half of them are predicted to become obese adults [6].

These trends in excess body weight may also contribute to an increase in chronic cardio-metabolic disorders, typically observed only in adults (e.g., hypertension, hyperglycemia, and dyslipidemia), but are becoming increasingly common in children and adolescents with obesity [7]. Additionally, pediatric populations with obesity are known to have several psychosocial problems including discrimination, social isolation, and low self-esteem, which affect their health, education, and quality of life [6,8]. Furthermore, the crosstalk between obesity and many viral pandemics, such as the 2009 swine flu [9] or the current COVID-19 pandemic [10,11], has provided new insights into mortal characteristics of this chronic syndrome.

The etiology of obesity is complicated and multifactorial, which indicates that excess body weight results from a complex interaction of a broad range of factors [12]. In addition to genetic vulnerability as a well-recognized internal factor contributing to excess body weight, a wide range of physiological disorders, as well as modifiable environmental factors and obesogenic behaviors, play key roles in the development of obesity [11,13,14]. Amongst children, the most common obesogenic behavior includes high consumption of unhealthy foods, low levels of physical activity (PA), high levels of mental stress, high levels of screen time, and poor sleep patterns [1,2,15]. These behaviors are influenced by several factors and interactions involving genetics, interpersonal relationships, and the environment [16,17]. Additionally, some evidence indicates that obesity-related behaviors are highly context-dependent and are influenced by several biopsychosocial factors [18]. When discussing the gene–environment interplay in the etiology of obesity, it is believed that the contribution to an obese phenotype is not "nature or nurture", but rather "nature via nurture" [12]. Recently, Jackson et al. emphasized in their review that biology plays a fundamental role in determining the amount of body fat in addition to environmental factors [12]. Moreover, genetically predetermined obesogenic behavior seems to have a significant relationship with environmental influence on body weight [12], which could add to the complexity of obesity. This complex interaction is exemplified further by the role of energy flux (the rate of energy expenditure and energy intake) in the regulation of energy balance [19]. The complicated nature of childhood obesity which leads to a wide range of inter-individual differences highlights the importance of child-centered specific approaches, particularly personalized interventions, for managing childhood obesity.

Current scientific insights are limited in successfully decelerating the rise of the childhood obesity pandemic; the present review's primary goal is to establish a novel translational link between the literature and practice by introducing applied strategies targeting childhood obesity. Therefore, the purpose of this narrative review is to provide a brief overview of the current preventative and therapeutic approaches towards the management of childhood obesity (focusing on their limitations and complexity), and accordingly, to suggest an Etiology-Based Personalized Intervention Strategy Targeting Childhood Obesity (EPISTCO) as a purposeful approach to prioritize and implement nutritional, PA, and lifestyle intervention strategies based on the etiology of obesity and interpretation of individual characteristics. These objectives are based on the limited success of previous efforts targeting childhood obesity.

2. Weight-Related Behaviors in Children

Comprehensive clinical guidelines and recommendations to diagnose, prevent, and treat childhood obesity have been well documented for pediatric specialists to implement at different stages in obesity prevention and treatment programs [20,21].

Nutrition and dietary pattern not only affect anthropometry and body composition in children and adolescents, but they also influence neurocognitive and psychomotor development [22,23]. Evidence indicates that when compared to adults, children and adolescents are at a higher risk of insufficient intake of certain food groups (e.g., whole grains and/or unprocessed foods) [7,24], which may contribute to the increased risk of obesity [7]. Calorically restricted diets are widely used to target childhood obesity [22], but potentially contribute to nutrient deficiencies, which may impair growth and development [22,25]. The importance of adequate nutrient consumption for growth and development also emphasizes the need for targeting energy expenditure by ensuring sufficient PA. Even though detrimental effects of insufficient PA on various health and weight outcomes are well-documented, results from a comprehensive analysis including 1.6 million adolescents from a pooled number of 298 school-based studies from 146 countries show that 80% of adolescents do not meet PA recommendations of at least 60 min of PA with moderate to vigorous intensity over 5 d/w, which puts their current and future health at risk [26].

In addition to poor nutrition and low PA, results from different studies show that most children and adolescents do not meet obesity-associated lifestyle guidelines, such as recommendations for sleep and screen time [27,28]. According to the Centers for Disease Control and Prevention (CDC), 60% to 70% of the American pediatric population does not meet the American Academy of Pediatrics (AAP) sleep recommendations [1,27] of 10–13 h for 3- to 5-year-olds, 9–12 h for 6- to 12-year-olds, and 8–10 h for 13- to 18-year-olds [29]. Short duration and late sleep timing can contribute to the onset and development of childhood obesity [30], particularly by altering appetite-regulating hormones and con-sequential eating disorders [31]. Parents can play an important role in fostering healthy sleep patterns by arranging sleep time, providing a calm atmosphere, and keeping screens away before bedtime [32]. Higher amounts of daily screen time contribute to obesity due to their association with a reduced feeling of satiety, increased consumption of unhealthy and energy-dense snacks [33], and poor sleep patterns [34]. The AAP recommends that daily nonacademic screen time (TV, video games, and mobile phone) should not exceed one hour for 2- to 5-year-olds, and two hours for ≥6-year-old children, and there should be parental supervision of content watched [1]. Available data, however, indicates that the majority of children has an extraordinarily high daily screen time [28,35], up to an average of 6 h/day among 13- to 18-year-olds [36] and 7 h/day among 8- to 18-year-olds [37] when TV, computer, mobile devices, and web-based sources are combined. Sedentary behaviors, screen time, and sleep abnormalities can be even higher during annual vacation due to the absence of a regular schedule [38].

3. Strategies for the Prevention and Treatment of Childhood Obesity

To date, the safety and efficacy of various approaches on the management of childhood obesity have been reported by numerous experimental and cross-sectional studies as well as reviews and meta-analyses [2,6,15,39,40]. Nevertheless, pediatric clinicians and researchers are often encountering several challenges when applying preventative and therapeutic programs and the characteristics of an optimal and comprehensive weight management strategy remain controversial [1,41]. Evidence suggests that the management of childhood obesity requires consideration of genetic, biological, behavioral, psychological, interpersonal, and environmental factors to induce sustainable lifestyle changes along with an in-depth understanding of these interactions to identify opportunities for intervention strategies [39].

3.1. Intervention Components

The most common preventative and therapeutic interventions applied and suggested by investigations are nutritional, PA, lifestyle, and educational methods. In adolescents with a high degree of obesity or advanced metabolic disease, clinical treatments including pharmacological and surgical strategies have also been suggested [20]. Due to the potential side effects of medical interventions, a careful evaluation and comparison of risks and benefits are necessary before implementing such interventions for pediatric patients with obesity [42]. It has been emphasized that pharmacotherapy and bariatric surgery should never be implemented in adolescents with obesity (and those with other vital untreated disorders) who have not engaged in healthy dietary and PA practices [20].

3.1.1. Diet

It should be considered that nutritional approaches targeting childhood obesity are not limited to restricted energy intake but rather, the most appropriate nutrition strat-egy for long-term weight reduction and the promotion of metabolic and mental health is shifting to healthy food choices [43] that include predominantly whole food plant-based sources [44,45]. This dietary pattern restricts added sugars, refined grains, sweetened beverages, fast foods, calorie-dense snacks, and high-fat processed foods and includes fruits, vegetables, nuts, and whole-grains along with well-structured meal frequencies [6,44,46]. The weight-related benefits rising from plant-based diets are attributable to a reduced caloric intake and an increase in postprandial energy expenditure by a higher thermogenic response [47,48]. Additionally, whole food plant-based diets lead to favorable changes in cardio-metabolic and digestive health, which are both associated with further weight-related advantages as well [49,50]. Increasing nutritional literacy of children and their parents (regarding agriculture, food industries, food safety, cooking, and theoretical knowledge of energy balance, nutrition, and diets) could further promote sustainable changes that contribute to healthier dietary patterns [51]. While these are general principles and recommendations, no single diet should be prescribed or recommended as the best for all children with obesity [43]. Researchers believe that the optimal macronutrient composition depends on factors such as appetite, thermogenesis, energy homeostasis, and gut microbiota [52]. Furthermore, the ideal diet for treating overweight and obesity should be safe, efficacious, nutritionally adequate, culturally acceptable, and economically affordable [43]. To date, however, the majority of nutritional strategies targeting childhood obesity are still based on a "one-size-fits-all" model, which does not take into account the inter-individual variability [53], which often results in a reduced adherence rate to dietary changes [54].

3.1.2. Physical Activity

On the other side of the energy balance equation, PA has been emphasized as a critical component for healthy body weight. Promoting PA is considered an effective intervention strategy in pediatric weight management [55,56], which attributes to the concept of energy flux [19]. Energy flux represents the rate of energy expenditure and energy intake [19,57], and a higher energy flux (obtained by increased PA) results in better regulation of energy balance during weight loss [57] and/or the prevention of weight gain [58]. PA could also result in favorable improvements in mental and physiological health, and both are indirectly associated with further weight-related advantages [59]. In children and adolescents with obesity, the most common barriers to engage in regular PA programs are lack of self-discipline, lack of someone to engage in PA with, self-consciousness about appearance [60], and decreased level of motivation due to the limited motor abilities and/or being out of shape [61]. Daily physical activities of children are not limited to regular physical education classes or sport/exercise engagements. Active travel to school, unstructured active play during school recess, and activities at home or playgrounds can be additional viable PA sources [32]. Currently, however, due to the COVID-19 pandemic and social lockdowns, the movement opportunities have been significantly diminished [62], and home exercises have been highly recommended [63].

3.1.3. Lifestyle and Education

In addition to diet and PA, other lifestyle parameters (e.g., psychological behaviors, modifying sleep patterns) are considered effective interventions in weight management programs. Independently or along with educational interventions, additional lifestyle behaviors could further increase the efficiency of PA and dietary interventions [1]. A controlled experimental study showed that a two-year, multi-component obesity intervention focusing on a lifestyle educational curriculum resulted in beneficial changes in Body Mass Index (BMI) percentiles in the intervention groups [64]. There is also evidence suggesting that mindfulness interventions [65,66] and forethoughtfulness (defined as being oriented more towards the future than the present) [67] might be advantageous for improving obesity-related eating and behavioral patterns. Mindfulness, defined as the awareness that arises from purposefully paying attention in the present moment with non-judgment [68], is suggested as an effective intervention strategy targeting childhood obesity [69]. Evidence also indicates that sleep is an important modifiable risk factor for managing childhood obesity, as eating and PA behaviors can be affected by the quality and duration of sleep [70]. Modifying sleep patterns in school-age children resulted in healthy dietary patterns via decreased food consumption, in particular, thus promoting favorable weight outcomes [71].

In general, it has been well-established that multi-component interventions including PA, nutritional, lifestyle, and educational strategies have been shown to yield better outcomes than single-component strategies [1,41,72]. In a systematic review of the effectiveness of lifestyle interventions targeting children's weight and cardio-metabolic health, beneficial outcomes were observed only following the multi-component interventions [73]. However, due to the complex interaction in these approaches, identifying the degree of effectiveness for each component remains controversial.

3.2. Intervention Settings

Almost all studies in the childhood obesity sector have critically investigated or discussed the environment where interventions are applied and the people who support and/or supervise weight management programs. It has been well-established that home, school, and community can all play important roles independently in shaping and stabilizing children's lifelong health- and weight-related behaviors [74,75].

3.2.1. Home

Parental beliefs, attitudes, behaviors, and social support are vital for a child's health and body composition [76]. Available evidence indicates that parents are involved in about half of the interventions targeting childhood obesity, and successful improvements on children's BMI are in 75% of studies with parental involvement [74]. Results show, from a meta-analysis of 22 randomized control trials examining home-based interventions to control childhood obesity, that parents can play a crucial role in managing children's weight by facilitating, motivating, and coaching the healthy behaviors of their children [77]. Due to the close familiarity of parents and their child, parents may better understand and consider the lifestyle parameters contributing to the development of obesity in their child [78]. Although parent-only interventions may be more cost-effective compared to school- and community-based programs [79], evidence suggests to combine home-based programs with other settings to deliver more favorable effects on anthropometry and BMI in children [80]. The effectiveness of grandparental supervision, on the other hand, has been reported to be close to zero with no association between children's BMI z-scores and grandparental child care (whether as the primary caregiver or co-residence) [81].

3.2.2. School

School is an important setting for improving child health behaviors, as children spend a significant part of their daily life in schools [82,83]. Moreover, the following conditions of the school environment also benefit the setting for implementing overweight/obesity-related interventions: schools offer a structured environment for applying interventions with ease; schools may provide one or two meals per day and, therefore, potentially dictate healthy food choices in their cafeteria; schools usually provide opportunities for PA and active games during recess and daytime; schools produce and expand extracurricular educational resources and wellness policies for both children and parents; schools could run an indirect competitive and encouraging atmosphere to promote children's motivation and adherence towards interventions; schools could introduce their physical education instructors and/or athletic trainers as role-models; schools benefit from the contribution of staff and teachers to facilitate, deliver, and supervise the interventions [74,84,85]. Interestingly, successful school-based interventions are also highly effective in improving children's anti-obesogenic behaviors at home [83]. However, because of time and budget constraints, many schools are not able to implement health and weight management programs [72].

3.2.3. Community and Clinics

In addition to home- and school-based strategies, the community environment and clinical settings are also common areas for managing childhood obesity and prevention [20,75]. Community interventions targeting obesity incorporate policies and strategies and aim to reduce the population risk of obesity [75]. These interventions involve but are not limited to the availability and use of health and fitness facilities, media-based activities, and health-oriented businesses by local and central administrations [1,86]. The EPODE program (Ensemble Prévenons l'Obésité Des Enfants: together, let us prevent childhood obesity) could be considered a successful example of a community-based intervention, which emphasizes a multifactorial approach targeting childhood obesity at different community levels [87]. Interventions using a community-based approach could achieve the long-term goals of reducing the prevalence of childhood obesity [88], especially for children who live in low-income societies [75]. Clinical or primary-care interventions, on the other hand, include any medical or non-medical strategies implemented by healthcare and pediatric specialists [89]. Clinical and community-level interventions can significantly improve lifestyle patterns when applied simultaneously [90]. Significant improvements in body weight have been achieved in pre-school children aged 2–5 years following multi-component clinical interventions (e.g., PA, nutrition, education) with parental involvement [91]. However, reports from different meta-analytic studies indicate poor effectiveness of primary-care programs on childhood obesity [89,92,93], which might be attributed to a dose-response relationship, where the frequency and duration of treatment contact highly affect the outcomes [1]. Additionally, the "sustainability" of intervention effects could be another limitation in clinical approaches, as the time of engagement is limited compared to other settings [94,95].

In general, it seems that due to the multi-factorial nature of childhood obesity, a maximally efficient strategy to manage childhood obesity requires integrating multiple settings for delivering multi-component interventions. Evidence shows that school-based interventions with family inclusion have the largest effect on weight outcomes when multi-component programs are implemented, including PA and diet [84,96]. Results from a study comparing the effectiveness of home versus school settings on nutritional habits, PA behaviors, and BMI changes showed that the home environment had a stronger association with health in general compared to the school setting [97]. It should be mentioned, however, that parental involvement in many preventive studies can be more effective in pre-school and early-school children, whereas school- and community-based intervention strategies lead to more favorable outcomes in older children and adolescents [1], particularly for those who are above twelve [98]. Nevertheless, to enhance the effectiveness of strategies, it appears important that parents permanently engage in supporting and reinforcing their children's health behaviors [99].

Some limitations can affect the progress of weight management programs, similar to any preventative and therapeutic strategy. Time and financial resources are major limitations for the implementation of multi-component weight management strategies [100]. In addition, poor awareness and lack of self-discipline have been reported as personal barriers when adhering to a healthy lifestyle [60]. Furthermore, difficult-to-reach goals set by parents and clinicians are considered a vital but hidden limitation, as it is well-established that strict targets may often lead to failure in weight control programs in children [101]. Age also appears to be an important moderator for weight control outcomes as older children displayed larger and more beneficial effects than younger children following weight-management interventions [92,93]. Beyond these limitations, the obesity prevention strategies seem to follow a dose-effective manner, as more intensive and longer-lasting interventions are associated with better outcomes in children [93]. Further, it appears that purposeless and/or unsupervised strategies not based on the individual needs and personal characteristics of the targeted child could minimize intervention effects [54].

4. Personalized Strategies

Despite a wealth of scientific information on a wide range of interventions and strategies targeting childhood obesity, the translation and transfer of this knowledge into a practical approach seem highly challenging. According to a comprehensive study by the Institute of Medicine (IOM), which analyzed more than 800 scientific reports, the progress of obesity prevention was not favorable in the national trend data, and data was not translatable into clearly scalable strategies [102,103]. It has been reported that meta-analytic approaches for identifying solutions to obesity, which is a complex health problem, could not deliver favorable practical information [102]. As a result of obesity's complexity, the condition seems not only limited to its etiology, but also to intervention strategies targeting childhood obesity. Given the interaction between various components of preventative/treatment approaches, the management of childhood obesity remains highly complex. Figure 1 shows a conceptual model that describes the complexity of interactions between key aspects of four research-derived categories ("What", "When", "Who", and "Where"), which are critical in the management of childhood obesity. "What" refers to the components including diet, PA, other lifestyle interventions, education, medication, and surgery. "When" stands for different age groups that are targeted (including pre-school, school-age, and puberty). "Who" represents the involved population such as the child, parents, teachers, and specialists. Finally, "Where" appoints different settings including home, school, community, and clinic (Figure 1).

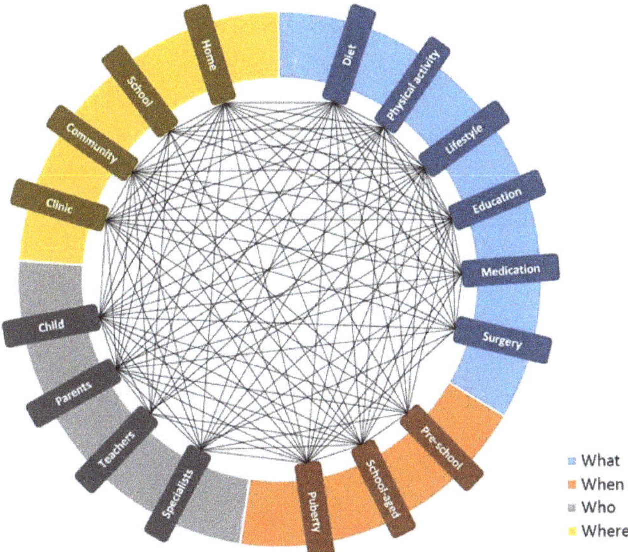

Figure 1. Conceptual 4W model describing the complexity of interactions between research-based modules contributing to the management of childhood obesity.

Recently, the implementation of personalized dietary approaches to managing complicated health problems (e.g., cardiovascular and metabolic disorders) has been increasing [104,105]. Personalized interventions could be defined as advanced and detailed models of clinical/primary care interventions. Given the available data, current clinical interventions seem to have some limitations. Clinical strategies focus primarily on treatment rather than prevention and thus are often conducted in close coordination with the primary healthcare system with high accessibility and frequency of visits mostly in the clinical setting [106]. Clinical approaches mainly focus on nutritional and medical interventions with lower attention on lifestyle, educational, and movement strategies [20]. Lifestyle counseling, including suggestions for PA by health specialists, remains below an acceptable level [107–109] even though the importance of lifestyle interventions by physicians and/or health care providers has been well-documented in patients' health- and weight-related behaviors [107,108]. This may be attributed to inadequate knowledge and training, office time constraints, and poor personal habits of specialists/physicians [107,109]. Rather than providing general information, a personalized strategy uses a broad range of info on individual characteristics to develop targeted nutritional and non-nutritional advice, products, or services assisting people to reach their goals via a purposeful approach based on their current behaviors, preferences, barriers, and objectives.

Personalized dietary approaches have been reported previously as a promising topic of research in the treatment of obesity [110]. To date, evidence supporting personalized strategies to manage obesity has come from clinical and observational studies mostly in the area of nutrition. The Academy of Nutrition and Dietetics developed the personalized nutritional approach NCP (Nutrition Care Process) based on nutritional assessment, diagnosis, planning, and monitoring. This multi-step model was designed to structure individualized nutritional care targeting childhood obesity and was effective in different investigations [22,111,112]. In a review study assessing the effects of NCP-based educational programs (including education on meal planning, portion control, healthy snack selection, and cooking with plant-based sources), favorable outcomes were reported regarding childhood obesity [113].

In addition to nutritional interventions, the limited available data supports the effectiveness of other personalized interventions on weight and/or health outcomes in children and adolescents. A 3-month personalized PA intervention using an internet-based program showed significant effects on psychosocial health and PA level in adolescents [114]. Evidence consistently indicates that when compared to generalized programs, personalized technology-based PA interventions are more effective at modifying health behaviors [115]. Results from a study on adolescents with obesity or diabetes show that 16 weeks of personalized exercise (based upon baseline fitness level of participants)—with parental support and ongoing motivation—can improve PA level and result in a sense of personal health [116]. Additionally, a controlled experimental study showed beneficial effects of personalized lifestyle coaching on childhood obesity [117], in which a health coach called child-parent pairs separately by telephone for a total of 21 sessions. There is also evidence indicating children's health behaviors, particularly sleep patterns, could be improved following personalized educational interventions for mothers with 3- to 5-year-old children [118].

In general, personalized recommendations on the personal needs of a child and his/her family could be a promising approach for the prevention and treatment of obesity. A comprehensive personalized approach targeting childhood obesity may include, among others, nutritional, educational, and PA-based intervention strategies at various settings to alter lifestyle patterns and attitudes. The overall consensus is that implementing a well-proposed personalized program not only maximizes desirable outcomes but also contributes to the sustainable adherence of a healthy lifestyle pattern [54]. In addition, due to the purposeful nature of personalized interventions, time and budget could be partially saved following this approach. Similar to other successful programs, a personalized program should further combine education and motivation to obtain slow but sustainable weight and health benefits [43].

5. EPISTCO Model

Considering the complicated facts in the etiology and management of childhood obesity and in order to establish a novel translational link between the literature and practice, this narrative review presents a basis for an Etiology-Based Personalized Intervention Strategy Targeting Childhood Obesity (EPISTCO) (Figure 2), to provide a framework for the purposeful prevention and treatment of childhood obesity.

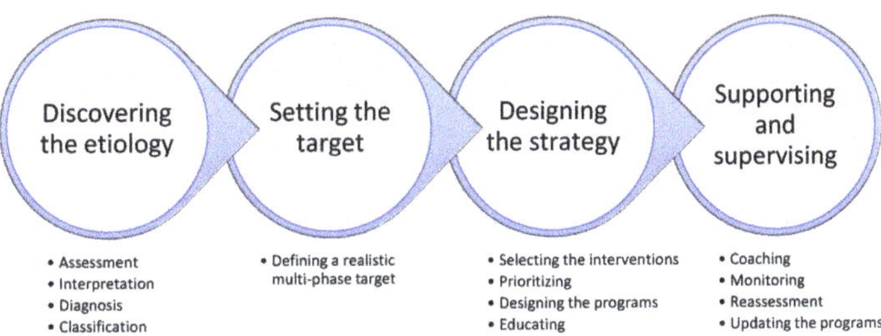

Figure 2. Schematic design of EPISTCO (Etiology-Based Personalized Intervention Strategy Targeting Childhood Obesity) model, which is based on four multi-stage steps.

The EPISTCO model highlights that the design of a personalized program targeting childhood obesity requires an understanding of the complex etiology of excess weight gain by assessing a series of biological, nutritional, behavioral, and environmental factors. Unlike previously described models, the EPISTCO model implements a multi-component intervention program within multiple settings and considers personalized priorities for the components and settings. In this structured multi-disciplinary and etiology-based approach, the programs are highly adaptable based on individual and environmental barriers and potentials.

The EPISTCO model includes four multi-stage steps (Figure 2). The first and probably the most important step is "discovering the etiology of obesity", which most likely requires a clinical setting. This step consists of four stages including (a) assessments, (b) interpretation of data, (c) diagnosis of the relevant causes, and (d) classification of the causes. Assessments (e.g., physical characteristics, eating habits and disorders, sleep patterns, etc.) can be made via questionnaires, field tests, and laboratory measurements and are depending on the availability of time, equipment, and specialists. Table 1 represents the most important assessment items summarized in nine general categories that provide viable information to design an EPISTCO.

Table 1. Essential prerequisite information to design and conduct an etiology-based personalized intervention strategy targeting childhood obesity.

	Questionnaire	Laboratory Tests	Field Tests
1. Individual and parental information	*		
2. Self-reported targets	*		
3. Facilities/limitations in personal environment	*		
4. Energy balance status with a short history	*	*	
5. Lifestyle behaviors with a short history	*		
6. Body composition status with a short history	*	*	
7. Clinical status with a short history	*	*	
8. Biochemistry status with a short history		*	
9. Physical fitness status with a short history		*	*

Step 2 is "setting the target", in which a multi-phase goal is defined according to the information obtained from Step 1. The emphasis is to set a realistic target, as difficult-to-reach targets often lead to failure. Step 3, "designing the strategy", consists of the following stages: (a) selecting the most appropriate interventions, (b) prioritizing interventions according to stage "d" from Step 1, (c) designing program schedules along with extra general recommendations, and (d) educating both the child and parents about the next step in conjugation with motivational incentives. At the end of Step 3, the next visit(s) must be set according to a time-based, target-based, or problem-based style. Accordingly, this step will also determine the role of different settings including home, schools and communities. Finally, Step 4, "supervising and supporting", consists of three stages: (a) individualized direct or indirect coaching and psychological supporting, (b) monitoring, (c) reassessment, analysis of the progress as well as evaluating problems, and (d) revising and updating the program. This step returns most likely to the clinical setting to connect Step 4 and Step 1. Rather than circling back, the intention is to continue the procedure to stabilize health behaviors.

To further enhance the understanding of the characteristics of this personalized approach, the following examples can be considered. For a child with obesity who has a proper quantity and quality of nutrition, interventions should prioritize PA and other lifestyle patterns. A more active child with excess body weight, on the other hand, with other causes (e.g., unhealthy food choices, sleep patterns, lifestyle, biochemistry) may require a different approach that should be scrutinized during initial assessments in order to design and suggest a purposeful etiology-based program. To reach favorable results, it is, nevertheless, highly recommended that all steps and stages of the EPISTCO approach are conducted and supervised by well-experienced pediatric specialists in different sub-disciplines of health. Moreover, every stage throughout the process should be well documented. The gathered data will also provide viable information that enhances the understanding of the etiology of obesity, which is critical for the improvement of the effectiveness of such personalized approaches.

6. Conclusions

The high prevalence of childhood obesity is a major threat to future public health and available literature indicates that weight-related nutritional, PA, and lifestyle recommendations are not met by the majority of children. Given the complex and multi-factorial nature of obesity in both etiology and management, it appears that there is a fundamental need to develop and apply personalized approaches to prevent and treat childhood obesity. As a practical, purposeful, and promising suggestion, the EPISTCO model emphasizes incorporating various approaches, including nutritional, lifestyle, and PA, that are prioritized, prescribed, and supervised based on the individual needs and personal characteristics within multiple settings.

In general, the EPISTCO model offers a purposeful framework for pediatric researchers and specialists that contributes to a better understanding of the interplay between various factors associated with childhood obesity, which can increase the efficacy of interventions. While it includes a comprehensive approach towards minimizing childhood obesity, not all aspects need to be implemented in every situation.

Author Contributions: Conceptualization, M.M., C.D. and K.W.; writing original draft and preparation, M.M.; reviewing and editing, C.D., K.W., D.R.T., N.A.K. and M.M.; supervision and general support, K.W. and N.A.K. All authors have read and agreed to the published version of the manuscript.

Funding: This research received no external funding.

Institutional Review Board Statement: Not applicable.

Informed Consent Statement: Not applicable.

Data Availability Statement: No new data were created or analyzed in this study. Data sharing is not applicable to this article.

Acknowledgments: There are no professional relationships with companies or manufacturers who will benefit from the results of the present study.

Conflicts of Interest: The authors declare no conflict of interest.

References

1. Smith, J.D.; Fu, E.; Kobayashi, M.A. Prevention and management of childhood obesity and its psychological and health comorbidities. *Annu. Rev. Clin. Psychol.* **2020**, *16*, 351–378. [CrossRef] [PubMed]
2. Baranowski, T.; Motil, K.J.; Moreno, J.P. Multi-etiological perspective on child obesity prevention. *Curr. Nutr. Rep.* **2019**, *8*, 1–10. [CrossRef]

3. Gehanno, J.-F.; Gehanno, B.; Schuers, M.; Grosjean, J.; Rollin, L. Analysis of publication trends in childhood obesity research in PubMed since 1945. *Child. Obes.* **2019**, *15*, 227–236. [CrossRef]
4. NCD Risk Factor Collaboration (NCD-RisC). Worldwide trends in body-mass index, underweight, overweight, and obesity from 1975 to 2016: A pooled analysis of 2416 population-based measurement studies in 128·9 million children, adolescents, and adults. *Lancet* **2017**, *390*, 2627–2642. [CrossRef]
5. Lobstein, T.; Baur, L.; Uauy, R. IASO International Obesity TaskForce. Obesity in children and young people: A crisis in public health. *Obes. Rev.* **2004**, *5*, 4–104. [CrossRef] [PubMed]
6. Liberali, R.; Kupek, E.; Assis, M.A.A. Dietary patterns and childhood obesity risk: A systematic review. *Child. Obes.* **2020**, *16*, 70–85. [CrossRef] [PubMed]
7. Ruiz, L.D.; Zuelch, M.L.; Dimitratos, S.M.; Scherr, R.E. Adolescent obesity: Diet quality, psychosocial health, and cardiometabolic risk factors. *Nutrients* **2019**, *12*, 43. [CrossRef] [PubMed]
8. Goñi, I.L.; Arenaza, L.; Medrano, M.; García, N.; Cadenas-Sanchez, C.; Ortega, F.B. Associations between the adherence to the Mediterranean diet and cardiorespiratory fitness with total and central obesity in preschool children: The PREFIT project. *Eur. J. Nutr.* **2018**, *57*, 2975–2983. [CrossRef] [PubMed]
9. Vaillant, L.; La Ruche, G.; Tarantola, A.; Barboza, P.; Epidemic Intelligence Team at InVS. Epidemiology of fatal cases associated with pandemic H1N1 influenza 2009. *Eurosurveillance* **2009**, *14*, 19309. [CrossRef]
10. Khan, A.S.; Hichami, A.; Khan, N.A. Obesity and COVID-19: Oro-naso-sensory perception. *J. Clin. Med.* **2020**, *9*, 2158. [CrossRef]
11. Ritter, A.; Kreis, N.-N.; Louwen, F.; Yuan, J. Obesity and COVID-19: Molecular mechanisms linking both pandemics. *Int. J. Mol. Sci.* **2020**, *21*, 5793. [CrossRef] [PubMed]
12. Jackson, S.E.; Llewellyn, C.H.; Smith, L. The obesity epidemic—Nature via nurture: A narrative review of high-income countries. *SAGE Open Med.* **2020**, *8*. [CrossRef] [PubMed]
13. Xu, S.; Xue, Y. Pediatric obesity: Causes, symptoms, prevention and treatment. *Exp. Ther. Med.* **2016**, *11*, 15–20. [CrossRef] [PubMed]
14. Ryder, J.R.; Fox, C.K.; Kelly, A.S. Treatment options for severe obesity in the pediatric population: Current limitations and future opportunities. *Obesity* **2018**, *26*, 951–960. [CrossRef]
15. Sisson, S.B.; Krampe, M.; Anundson, K.; Castle, S. Obesity prevention and obesogenic behavior interventions in child care: A systematic review. *Prev. Med.* **2016**, *87*, 57–69. [CrossRef]
16. Russell, C.G.; Russell, A. A biopsychosocial approach to processes and pathways in the development of overweight and obesity in childhood: Insights from developmental theory and research. *Obes. Rev.* **2019**, *20*, 725–749. [CrossRef] [PubMed]
17. Smith, J.D.; Egan, K.N.; Montaño, Z.; Dawson-McClure, S.; Jake-Schoffman, D.E.; Larson, M.; St. George, S.M. A developmental cascade perspective of paediatric obesity: A conceptual model and scoping review. *Health Psychol. Rev.* **2018**, *12*, 271–293. [CrossRef]
18. Rosenbaum, D.L.; White, K.S. Understanding the complexity of biopsychosocial factors in the public health epidemic of overweight and obesity. *Health Psychol. Open* **2016**, *3*. [CrossRef]
19. Drenowatz, C.; Greier, K. The role of energy flux in weight management. *Exerc. Med.* **2017**, *1*, 4. [CrossRef]
20. Styne, D.M.; Arslanian, S.A.; Connor, E.L.; Farooqi, I.S.; Murad, M.H.; Silverstein, J.H.; Yanovski, J.A. Pediatric obesity—Assessment, treatment, and prevention: An endocrine society clinical practice guideline. *J. Clin. Endocrinol. Metab.* **2017**, *102*, 709–757. [CrossRef]
21. Weihrauch-Blüher, S.; Kromeyer-Hauschild, K.; Graf, C.; Widhalm, K.; Korsten-Reck, U.; Jödicke, B.; Markert, J.; Müller, M.J.; Moss, A.; Wabitsch, M.; et al. Current guidelines for obesity prevention in childhood and adolescence. *Obes. Facts* **2018**, *11*, 263–276. [CrossRef]
22. Kim, J.; Lim, H. Nutritional management in childhood obesity. *J. Obes. Metab. Syndr.* **2019**, *28*, 225–235. [CrossRef] [PubMed]
23. Santacruz, A.; Marcos, A.; Wärnberg, J.; Martí, A.; Martin-Matillas, M.; Campoy, C.; Moreno, L.A.; Veiga, O.; Redondo-Figuero, C.; Garagorri, J.M.; et al. Interplay between weight loss and gut microbiota composition in overweight adolescents. *Obesity* **2009**, *17*, 1906–1915. [CrossRef] [PubMed]
24. Gu, X.; Tucker, K.L. Dietary quality of the US child and adolescent population: Trends from 1999 to 2012 and associations with the use of federal nutrition assistance programs. *Am. J. Clin. Nutr.* **2017**, *105*, 194–202. [CrossRef]
25. Suskind, D.L. Nutritional deficiencies during normal growth. *Pediatr. Clin. N. Am.* **2009**, *56*, 1035–1053. [CrossRef]
26. Guthold, R.; Stevens, G.A.; Riley, L.M.; Bull, F.C. Global trends in insufficient physical activity among adolescents: A pooled analysis of 298 population-based surveys with 1·6 million participants. *Lancet Child. Adolesc. Health* **2020**, *4*, 23–35. [CrossRef]
27. Centers for Disease Control and Prevention (CDC). Available online: https://www.cdc.gov/sleep/data_statistics.html (accessed on 18 December 2020).
28. Barnett, T.A.; Kelly, A.S.; Young, D.R.; Perry, C.K.; Pratt, C.A. Edwards, N.M.; Rao, G.; Vos, M.B. Sedentary behaviors in today's youth: Approaches to the prevention and management of childhood obesity: A scientific statement from the American Heart Association. *Circulation* **2018**, *138*, e142–e159. [CrossRef] [PubMed]
29. Paruthi, S.; Brooks, L.J.; D'Ambrosio, C.; Hall, W.A.; Kotagal, S.; Lloyd, R.M.; Malow, B.A.; Maski, K.; Nichols, C.; Quan, S.F.; et al. Recommended amount of sleep for pediatric populations: A consensus statement of the American Academy of Sleep Medicine. *J. Clin. Sleep Med.* **2016**, *12*, 785–786. [CrossRef] [PubMed]

30. Taveras, E.M.; Gillman, M.W.; Peña, M.M.; Redline, S.; Rifas-Shiman, S.L. Chronic sleep curtailment and adiposity. *Pediatrics* **2014**, *133*, 1013–1022. [CrossRef]
31. Miller, A.L.; Lumeng, J.C.; LeBourgeois, M.K. Sleep patterns and obesity in childhood. *Curr. Opin. Endocrinol. Diabetes Obes.* **2015**, *22*, 41–47. [CrossRef]
32. Guan, H.; Okely, A.D.; Aguilar-Farias, N.; Del Pozo Cruz, B.; Draper, C.E.; El Hamdouchi, A.; Florindo, A.A.; Jáuregui, A.; Katzmarzyk, P.T.; Kontsevaya, A.; et al. Promoting healthy movement behaviours among children during the COVID-19 pandemic. *Lancet Child Adolesc. Health* **2020**, *4*, 416–418. [CrossRef]
33. Robinson, T.N.; Banda, J.A.; Hale, L.; Lu, A.S.; Fleming-Milici, F.; Calvert, S.L.; Wartella, E. Screen media exposure and obesity in children and adolescents. *Pediatrics* **2017**, *140*, S97–S101. [CrossRef] [PubMed]
34. Hale, L.; Guan, S. Screen time and sleep among school-aged children and adolescents: A systematic literature review. *Sleep Med. Rev.* **2015**, *21*, 50–58. [CrossRef] [PubMed]
35. Atkin, A.J.; Sharp, S.J.; Corder, K.; van Sluijs, E.M.; ICAD Collaborators. Prevalence and correlates of screen time in youth: An international perspective. *Am. J. Prev. Med.* **2014**, *47*, 803–807. [CrossRef] [PubMed]
36. Jensen, M.; George, M.; Russell, M.; Odgers, C. Young adolescents' digital technology use and mental health symptoms: Little evidence of longitudinal or daily linkages. *Clin. Psychol. Sci.* **2019**, *7*, 1416–1433. [CrossRef] [PubMed]
37. Rideout, V. Measuring time spent with media: The common sense census of media use by US 8- to 18-year-olds. *J. Child. Media* **2016**, *10*, 138–144. [CrossRef]
38. Weaver, R.G.; Armstrong, B.; Hunt, E.; Beets, M.W.; Brazendale, K.; Dugger, R.; Turner-McGrievy, G.; Pate, R.R.; Maydeu-Olivares, A.; Saelens, B.; et al. The impact of summer vacation on children's obesogenic behaviors and body mass index: A natural experiment. *Int. J. Behav. Nutr. Phys. Act.* **2020**, *17*, 153. [CrossRef]
39. Kumar, S.; Kelly, A.S. Review of childhood obesity: From epidemiology, etiology, and comorbidities to clinical assessment and treatment. *Mayo Clin. Proc.* **2017**, *92*, 251–265. [CrossRef]
40. Brown, T.; Moore, T.H.; Hooper, L.; Gao, Y.; Zayegh, A.; Ijaz, S.; Elwenspoek, M.; Foxen, S.C.; Magee, L.; O'Malley, C.; et al. Interventions for preventing obesity in children. *Cochrane Database Syst. Rev.* **2019**, *7*, CD001871. [CrossRef]
41. Wang, Y.; Cai, L.; Wu, Y.; Wilson, R.F.; Weston, C.; Fawole, O.; Bleich, S.N.; Cheskin, L.J.; Showell, N.N.; Lau, B.D.; et al. What childhood obesity prevention programmes work? A systematic review and meta-analysis. *Obes. Rev.* **2015**, *16*, 547–565. [CrossRef]
42. Chao, A.M.; Wadden, T.A.; Berkowitz, R.I. The safety of pharmacologic treatment for pediatric obesity. *Expert Opin. Drug Saf.* **2018**, *17*, 379–385. [CrossRef] [PubMed]
43. Koliaki, C.; Spinos, T.; Spinou, M.; Brinia, M.E.; Mitsopoulou, D.; Katsilambros, N. Defining the optimal dietary approach for safe, effective and sustainable weight loss in overweight and obese adults. *Healthcare.* **2018**, *6*, 73. [CrossRef] [PubMed]
44. Baroni, L.; Goggi, S.; Battaglino, R.; Berveglieri, M.; Fasan, I.; Filippin, D.; Griffith, P.; Rizzo, G.; Tomasini, C.; Tosatti, M.A.; et al. Vegan nutrition for mothers and children: Practical tools for healthcare providers. *Nutrients* **2018**, *11*, 5. [CrossRef]
45. Wirnitzer, K.C. Vegan diet in sports and exercise—health benefits and advantages to athletes and physically active people: A narrative review. *Int. J. Sports Exerc. Med.* **2020**, *6*, 165. [CrossRef]
46. Kaisari, P.; Yannakoulia, M.; Panagiotakos, D.B. Eating frequency and overweight and obesity in children and adolescents: A meta-analysis. *Pediatrics* **2013**, *131*, 958–967. [CrossRef]
47. Barnard, N.; Kahleova, H.; Levin, S. The Use of Plant-Based Diets for Obesity Treatment. *Int. J. Dis. Reversal Prev.* **2019**, *1*, 12.
48. Greger, M. A whole food plant-based diet is effective for weight loss: The evidence. *Am. J. Lifestyle Med.* **2020**, *14*, 500–510. [CrossRef]
49. Tran, E.; Dale, H.F.; Jensen, C.; Lied, G.A. Effects of plant-based diets on weight status: A systematic review. *Diabetes Metab. Syndr. Obes.* **2020**, *13*, 3433–3448. [CrossRef]
50. Sabaté, J.; Wien, M. Vegetarian diets and childhood obesity prevention. *Am. J. Clin. Nutr.* **2010**, *91*, 1525S–1529S. [CrossRef]
51. Bailey, C.J.; Drummond, M.J.; Ward, P.R. Food literacy programmes in secondary schools: A systematic literature review and narrative synthesis of quantitative and qualitative evidence. *Public Health Nutr.* **2019**, *22*, 2891–2913. [CrossRef]
52. Dey, M.; Kashyap, P.C. A diet for healthy weight: Why reaching a consensus seems difficult. *Nutrients* **2020**, *12*, 2997. [CrossRef]
53. Franzago, M.; Santurbano, D.; Vitacolonna, E.; Stuppia, L. Genes and diet in the prevention of chronic diseases in future generations. *Int. J. Mol. Sci.* **2020**, *21*, 2633. [CrossRef] [PubMed]
54. Gibson, A.A.; Sainsbury, A. Strategies to improve adherence to dietary weight loss interventions in research and real-World settings. *Behav. Sci.* **2017**, *7*, 44. [CrossRef]
55. Hill, J.O.; Wyatt, H.R.; Peters, J.C. Energy balance and obesity. *Circulation* **2012**, *126*, 126–132. [CrossRef] [PubMed]
56. Chaput, J.P.; Lambert. M.; Mathieu. M.E.; Tremblay, M.S.; O' Loughlin, J.; Tremblay, A. Physical activity vs. sedentary time: Independent associations with adiposity in children. *Pediatr. Obes.* **2012**, *7*, 251–258. [CrossRef] [PubMed]
57. Melby, C.L.; Paris, H.L.; Sayer, R.D.; Bell, C.; Hill, J.O. Increasing energy flux to maintain diet-induced weight loss. *Nutrients* **2019**, *11*, 2533. [CrossRef]
58. Hand, G.A.; Shook, R.P.; Hill, J.O.; Giacobbi, P.R.; Blair, S.N. Energy flux: Staying in energy balance at a high level is necessary to prevent weight gain for most people. *Expert Rev. Endocrinol. Metab.* **2015**, *10*, 599–605. [CrossRef]
59. Warburton, D.E.R.; Bredin, S.S.D. Health benefits of physical activity: A systematic review of current systematic reviews. *Curr. Opin. Cardiol.* **2017**, *32*, 541–556. [CrossRef]

60. Thang, C.; Whitley, M.; Izadpanah, N.; DeUgarte, D.; Slusser, W. Barriers and comorbidities from a pediatric multidisciplinary tertiary care obesity program. *J. Child. Obes.* **2017**, *2*, 2. [CrossRef]
61. Teixeira, P.J.; Carraça, E.V.; Markland, D.; Silva, M.N.; Ryan, R.M. Exercise, physical activity, and self-determination theory: A systematic review. *Int. J. Behav. Nutr. Phys. Act.* **2012**, *9*, 78. [CrossRef]
62. Woods, J.A.; Hutchinson, N.T.; Powers, S.K.; Robertsd, W.O.; Gomez-Cabrera, M.C.; Radak, Z.; Berkes, I.; Boros, A.; Boldogh, I.; Leeuwenburgh, C.; et al. The COVID-19 pandemic and physical activity. *Sports Med. Health Sci.* **2020**, *2*, 55–64. [CrossRef]
63. Chen, P.; Mao, L.; Nassis, G.P.; Harmer, P.; Ainsworth, B.E.; Li, F. Coronavirus disease (COVID-19): The need to maintain regular physical activity while taking precautions. *J. Sport Health Sci.* **2020**, *9*, 103–104. [CrossRef]
64. Natale, R.A.; Messiah, S.E.; Asfour, L.S.; Uhlhorn, S.B.; Englebert, N.E.; Arheart, K.L. Obesity prevention program in childcare centers: Two-year follow-up. *Am. J. Health Promot.* **2017**, *31*, 502–510. [CrossRef] [PubMed]
65. O'Reilly, G.A.; Cook, L.; Spruijt-Metz, D.; Black, D.S. Mindfulness-based interventions for obesity-related eating behaviours: A literature review. *Obes. Rev.* **2014**, *15*, 453–461. [CrossRef] [PubMed]
66. Dunn, C.; Haubenreiser, M.; Johnson, M.; Nordby, K.; Aggarwal, S.; Myer, S.; Thomas, C. Mindfulness approaches and weight loss, weight maintenance, and weight regain. *Curr. Obes. Rep.* **2018**, *7*, 37–49. [CrossRef] [PubMed]
67. Chang, B.P.I.; Claassen, M.A.; Klein, O. The time is ripe: Thinking about the future reduces unhealthy eating in those with a higher BMI. *Foods* **2020**, *9*, 1391. [CrossRef]
68. Paulson, S.; Davidson, R.; Jha, A.; Kabat-Zinn, J. Becoming conscious: The science of mindfulness. *Ann. N. Y. Acad. Sci.* **2013**, *1303*, 87–104. [CrossRef]
69. Black, D.S.; Fernando, R. Mindfulness Training and classroom behavior among lower-income and ethnic minority elementary school children. *J. Child Fam. Stud.* **2014**, *23*, 1242–1246. [CrossRef] [PubMed]
70. Hart, C.N.; Hawley, N.L.; Wing, R.R. Development of a behavioral sleep intervention as a novel approach for pediatric obesity in school-aged children. *Pediatr. Clin. N. Am.* **2016**, *63*, 511–523. [CrossRef]
71. Hart, C.N.; Carskadon, M.A.; Considine, R.V.; Fava, J.L.; Lawton, J.; Raynor, H.A.; Jelalian, E.; Owens, J.; Wing, R. Changes in children's sleep duration on food intake, weight, and leptin. *Pediatrics* **2013**, *132*, e1473–e1480. [CrossRef]
72. Shirley, K.; Rutfield, R.; Hall, N.; Fedor, N.; McCaughey, V.K.; Zajac, K. Combinations of obesity prevention strategies in US elementary schools: A critical review. *J. Prim. Prev.* **2015**, *36*, 1–20. [CrossRef] [PubMed]
73. Ho, M.; Garnett, S.P.; Baur, L.; Burrows, T.; Stewart, L.; Neve, M.; Collins, C. Effectiveness of lifestyle interventions in child obesity: Systematic review with meta-analysis. *Pediatrics* **2012**, *130*, e1647–e1671. [CrossRef] [PubMed]
74. Ickes, M.J.; McMullen, J.; Haider, T.; Sharma, M. Global school-based childhood obesity interventions: A review. *Int. J. Environ. Res. Public Health* **2014**, *11*, 8940–8961. [CrossRef]
75. Bleich, S.N.; Segal, J.; Wu, Y.; Wilson, R.; Wang, Y. Systematic review of community-based childhood obesity prevention studies. *Pediatrics* **2013**, *132*, e201–e210. [CrossRef]
76. Ayine, P.; Selvaraju, V.; Venkatapoorna, C.M.K.; Geetha, T. Parental feeding practices in relation to maternal education and childhood obesity. *Nutrients* **2020**, *12*, 1033. [CrossRef]
77. Pamungkas, R.A.; Chamroonsawasdi, K. Home-based interventions to treat and prevent childhood obesity: A systematic review and meta-analysis. *Behav. Sci.* **2019**, *9*, 38. [CrossRef] [PubMed]
78. Mazzeschi, C.; Pazzagli, C.; Laghezza, L.; Battistini, D.; Reginato, E.; Perrone, C.; Ranucci, C.; Fatone, C.; Pippi, R.; Giaimo, M.D.; et al. Description of the EUROBIS program: A combination of an Epode community-based and a clinical care intervention to improve the lifestyles of children and adolescents with overweight or obesity. *Biomed. Res. Int.* **2014**, *2014*, 546262. [CrossRef] [PubMed]
79. Janicke, D.M.; Sallinen, B.J.; Perri, M.G.; Lutes, L.D.; Silverstein, J.H.; Brumback, B. Comparison of program costs for parent-only and family-based interventions for pediatric obesity in medically underserved rural settings. *J. Rural Health* **2009**, *25*, 326–330. [CrossRef]
80. Mehdizadeh, A.; Nematy, M.; Vatanparast, H.; Khadem-Rezaiyan, M.; Emadzadeh, M. Impact of parent engagement in childhood obesity prevention interventions on anthropometric indices among preschool children: A systematic review. *Child. Obes.* **2020**, *16*, 3–19. [CrossRef]
81. An, R.; Xiang, X.; Xu, N.; Shen, J. Influence of grandparental child care on childhood obesity: A systematic review and meta-analysis. *Child. Obes.* **2020**, *16*, 141–153. [CrossRef] [PubMed]
82. Benjamins, M.R.; Whitman, S. A culturally appropriate school wellness initiative: Results of a 2-year pilot intervention in 2 Jewish schools. *J. Sch. Health* **2010**, *80*, 378–386. [CrossRef]
83. Bogart, L.M.; Elliott, M.N.; Cowgill, B.O.; Klein, D.J.; Hawes-Dawson, J.; Uyeda, K.; Schuster, M.A. Two-year BMI outcomes from a school-based intervention for nutrition and exercise: A randomized trial. *Pediatrics* **2016**, *137*, e20152493. [CrossRef]
84. Khambalia, A.Z.; Dickinson, S.; Hardy, L.L.; Gill, T.; Baur, L.A. A synthesis of existing systematic reviews and meta-analyses of school-based behavioural interventions for controlling and preventing obesity. *Obes. Rev.* **2012**, *13*, 214–233. [CrossRef] [PubMed]
85. Pyle, S.A.; Sharkey, J.; Yetter, G.; Felix, E.; Furlong, M.J.; Poston, W.S.C. Fighting an epidemic: The role of schools in reducing childhood obesity. *Psychol. Sch.* **2006**, *43*, 361–376. [CrossRef]
86. Karacabeyli, D.; Allender, S.; Pinkney, S.; Amed, S. Evaluation of complex community-based childhood obesity prevention interventions. *Obes. Rev.* **2018**, *19*, 1080–1092. [CrossRef] [PubMed]

87. Borys, J.M.; Le Bodo, Y.; Jebb, S.A.; Seidell, J.C.; Summerbell, C.; Richard, D.; De Henauw, S.; Moreno, L.A.; Romon, M.; Visscher, T.L.; et al. EPODE approach for childhood obesity prevention: Methods, progress and international development. *Obes. Rev.* **2012**, *13*, 299–315. [CrossRef] [PubMed]

88. Economos, C.D.; Hammond, R.A. Designing effective and sustainable multifaceted interventions for obesity prevention and healthy communities. *Obesity* **2017**, *25*, 1155–1156. [CrossRef]

89. Mitchell, T.B.; Amaro, C.M.; Steele, R.G. Pediatric weight management interventions in primary care settings: A meta-analysis. *Health Psychol.* **2016**, *37*, 704–713. [CrossRef]

90. Hoffman, J.; Frerichs, L.; Story, M.; Jones, J.; Gaskin, K.; Apple, A.; Skinner, A.; Armstrong, S. An integrated clinic-community partnership for child obesity treatment: A randomized pilot trial. *Pediatrics* **2018**, *141*, e20171444. [CrossRef] [PubMed]

91. Ling, J.; Robbins, L.B.; Wen, F. Interventions to prevent and manage overweight or obesity in preschool children: A systematic review. *Int. J. Nurs. Stud.* **2016**, *53*, 270–289. [CrossRef] [PubMed]

92. Janicke, D.M.; Steele, R.G.; Gayes, L.A.; Lim, C.S.; Clifford, L.M.; Schneider, E.M.; Carmody, J.K.; Westen, S. Systematic review and meta-analysis of comprehensive behavioral family lifestyle interventions addressing pediatric obesity. *J. Pediatr. Psychol.* **2014**, *39*, 809–825. [CrossRef] [PubMed]

93. Whitlock, E.P.; O'Connor, E.A.; Williams, S.B.; Beil, T.L.; Lutz, K.W. Effectiveness of weight management interventions in children: A targeted systematic review for the USPSTF. *Pediatrics* **2010**, *125*, e396–e418. [CrossRef] [PubMed]

94. McGowan, B.M. A practical guide to engaging individuals with obesity. *Obes. Facts* **2016**, *9*, 182–192. [CrossRef] [PubMed]

95. Hampl, S.; Paves, H.; Laubscher, K.; Eneli, I. Patient engagement and attrition in pediatric obesity clinics and programs: Results and recommendations. *Pediatrics* **2011**, *128*, S59–S64. [CrossRef] [PubMed]

96. Bleich, S.N.; Vercammen, K.A.; Zatz, L.Y.; Frelier, J.M.; Ebbeling, C.B.; Peeters, A. Interventions to prevent global childhood overweight and obesity: A systematic review. *Lancet Diabetes Endocrinol.* **2018**, *6*, 332–346. [CrossRef]

97. Haddad, J.; Ullah, S.; Bell, L.; Leslie, E.; Magarey, A. the influence of home and school environments on children's diet and physical activity, and body mass index: A structural equation modelling approach. *Matern. Child. Health J.* **2018**, *22*, 364–375. [CrossRef]

98. Kothandan, S.K. School based interventions versus family based interventions in the treatment of childhood obesity-a systematic review. *Arch. Public Health* **2014**, *72*, 3. [CrossRef]

99. Ward, D.S.; Welker, E.; Choate, A.; Henderson, K.E.; Lott, M.; Tovar, A.; Wilson, A.; Sallis, J.F. Strength of obesity prevention interventions in early care and education settings: A systematic review. *Prev. Med.* **2017**, *95*, S37–S52. [CrossRef]

100. Mauro, M.; Taylor, V.; Wharton, S.; Sharma, A.M. Barriers to obesity treatment. *Eur. J. Intern. Med.* **2008**, *19*, 173–180. [CrossRef]

101. Byrne, S.; Cooper, Z.; Fairburn, C. Weight maintenance and relapse in obesity: A qualitative study. *Int. J. Obes. Relat. Metab. Disord.* **2003**, *27*, 955–962. [CrossRef]

102. Institute of Medicine (IOM). *Bridging the Evidence Gap in Obesity Prevention: A Framework to Inform Decision Making*; The National Academies Press: Washington, DC, USA, 2010; pp. 227–267. [CrossRef]

103. Accelerating Progress in Obesity Prevention. Available online: https://www.ncbi.nlm.nih.gov/books/NBK201141/ (accessed on 18 December 2020).

104. Barrea, L.; Annunziata, G.; Bordoni, L.; Muscogiuri, G.; Colao, A.; Savastano, S.; OPERA Group. Nutrigenetics-personalized nutrition in obesity and cardiovascular diseases. *Int. J. Obes. Suppl.* **2020**, *10*, 1–13. [CrossRef] [PubMed]

105. Drabsch, T.; Holzapfel, C. A scientific perspective of personalised gene-based dietary recommendations for weight management. *Nutrients* **2019**, *11*, 617. [CrossRef] [PubMed]

106. Davis, M.M.; Gance-Cleveland, B.; Hassink, S.; Johnson, R.; Paradis, G.; Resnicow, K. Recommendations for prevention of childhood obesity. *Pediatrics* **2007**, *120*, S229–S253. [CrossRef]

107. Belfrage, A.S.V.; Grotmol, K.S.; Tyssen, R.; Moum, T.; Finset, A.; Isaksson Rø, K.; Lien, L. Factors influencing doctors' counselling on patients' lifestyle habits: A cohort study. *BJGP Open* **2018**, *2*, bjgpopen18X101607. [CrossRef]

108. Smith, A.W.; Borowski, L.A.; Liu, B.; Galuska, D.A.; Signore, C.; Klabunde, C.; Huang, T.T.; Krebs-Smith, S.M.; Frank, E.; Pronk, N.; et al. primary care physicians' diet-, physical activity-, and weight-related care of adult patients. *Am. J. Prev. Med.* **2011**, *41*, 33–42. [CrossRef]

109. Lobelo, F.; de Quevedo, I.G. The evidence in support of physicians and health care providers as physical activity role models. *Am. J. Lifestyle Med.* **2016**, *10*, 36–52. [CrossRef]

110. Bray, M.S.; Loos, R.J.; McCaffery, J.M.; Ling, C.; Franks, P.W.; Weinstock, G.M.; Snyder, M.P.; Vassy, J.L.; Agurs-Collins, T.; Conference Working Group. NIH working group report-using genomic information to guide weight management: From universal to precision treatment. *Obesity* **2016**, *24*, 14–22. [CrossRef] [PubMed]

111. Swan, W.I.; Vivanti, A.; Hakel-Smith, N.A.; Hotson, B.; Orrevall, Y.; Trostler, N.; Beck Howarter, K.; Papoutsakis, C. Nutrition care process and model update: Toward realizing people-centered care and outcomes management. *J. Acad. Nutr. Diet.* **2017**, *117*, 2003–2014. [CrossRef]

112. Thompson, K.L.; Davidson, P.; Swan, W.I.; Hand, R.K.; Rising, C.; Dunn, A.V.; Lewis, N.; Murphy, W.J. Nutrition care process chains: The "missing link" between research and evidence-based practice. *J. Acad. Nutr. Diet.* **2015**, *115*, 1491–1498. [CrossRef]

113. Kim, J.; Kim, Y.M.; Jang, H.B.; Lee, H.J.; Park, S.I.; Park, K.H.; Lim, H. Evidence-based nutritional intervention protocol for korean moderate-severe obese children and adolescents. *Clin. Nutr. Res.* **2019**, *8*, 184–195. [CrossRef] [PubMed]

114. Cook, T.L.; De Bourdeaudhuij, I.; Maes, L.; Haerens, L.; Grammatikaki, E.; Widhalm, K.; Kwak, L.; Plada, M.; Moreno, L.A.; Zampelas, A.; et al. Moderators of the effectiveness of a web-based tailored intervention promoting physical activity in adolescents: The HELENA Activ-O-Meter. *J. Sch. Health* **2014**, *84*, 256–266. [CrossRef] [PubMed]
115. Ghanvatkar, S.; Kankanhalli, A.; Rajan, V. User models for personalized physical activity interventions: Scoping review. *JMIR mHealth uHealth* **2019**, *7*, e11098. [CrossRef]
116. Faulkner, M.S.; Michaliszyn, S.F.; Hepworth, J.T.; Wheeler, M.D. Personalized exercise for adolescents with diabetes or obesity. *Biol. Res. Nurs.* **2014**, *16*, 46–54. [CrossRef] [PubMed]
117. Heerman, W.J.; Teeters, L.; Sommer, E.C.; Burgess, L.E.; Escarfuller, J.; Van Wyk, C.; Barkin, S.L.; Duhon, A.A.; Cole, J.; Samuels, L.R.; et al. Competency-based approaches to community health: A randomized controlled trial to reduce childhood obesity among latino preschool-aged children. *Child. Obes.* **2019**, *15*, 519–531. [CrossRef] [PubMed]
118. Koulouglioti, C.; Cole, R.; McQuillan, B.; Moskow, M.; Kueppers, J.; Pigeon, W. Feasibility of an individualized, home-based obesity prevention program for preschool-age children. *Child. Health Care* **2013**, *42*, 134–152. [CrossRef]

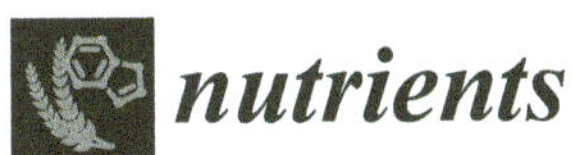 *nutrients*

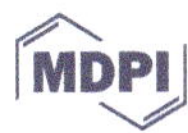

Article

Resting Energy Expenditure Is Not Altered in Children and Adolescents with Obesity. Effect of Age and Gender and Association with Serum Leptin Levels

J. Karina Zapata [1], Victoria Catalán [2,3,4], Amaia Rodríguez [2,3,4], Beatriz Ramírez [2,3,4], Camilo Silva [1,3,4], Javier Escalada [1,3,4], Javier Salvador [1,3,4], Giuseppe Calamita [5], M. Cristina Azcona-Sanjulian [4,6], Gema Frühbeck [1,2,3,4,*] and Javier Gómez-Ambrosi [2,3,4,*]

[1] Department of Endocrinology and Nutrition, Clínica Universidad de Navarra, 31008 Pamplona, Spain; jzapatac@unav.es (J.K.Z.); csilvafr@unav.es (C.S.); fescalada@unav.es (J.E.); jsalvador@unav.es (J.S.)
[2] Metabolic Research Laboratory, Clínica Universidad de Navarra, 31008 Pamplona, Spain; vcatalan@unav.es (V.C.); arodmur@unav.es (A.R.); bearamirez@unav.es (B.R.)
[3] Centro de Investigación Biomédica en Red-Fisiopatología de la Obesidad y Nutrición (CIBERobn), Instituto de Salud Carlos III, 31008 Pamplona, Spain
[4] Instituto de Investigación Sanitaria de Navarra (IdiSNA), 31008 Pamplona, Spain; cazcona@unav.es
[5] Department of Biosciences, Biotechnologies and Biopharmaceutics, University of Bari "Aldo Moro", 70125 Bari, Italy; giuseppe.calamita@uniba.it
[6] Paediatric Endocrinology Unit, Department of Paediatrics, Clínica Universidad de Navarra, 31008 Pamplona, Spain
[*] Correspondence: gfruhbeck@unav.es (G.F.); jagomez@unav.es (J.G.-A.); Tel.: +34-948-255400 (ext. 4484) (G.F.); +34-948-425600 (ext. 806567) (J.G.-A.)

Citation: Zapata, J.K.; Catalán, V.; Rodríguez, A.; Ramírez, B.; Silva, C.; Escalada, J.; Salvador, J.; Calamita, G.; Azcona-Sanjulian, M.C.; Frühbeck, G.; et al. Resting Energy Expenditure Is Not Altered in Children and Adolescents with Obesity. Effect of Age and Gender and Association with Serum Leptin Levels. *Nutrients* **2021**, *13*, 1216. https://doi.org/10.3390/nu13041216

Academic Editor: Odysseas Androutsos and Evangelia Charmandari

Received: 11 February 2021
Accepted: 5 April 2021
Published: 7 April 2021

Publisher's Note: MDPI stays neutral with regard to jurisdictional claims in published maps and institutional affiliations.

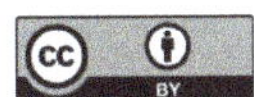

Copyright: © 2021 by the authors. Licensee MDPI, Basel, Switzerland. This article is an open access article distributed under the terms and conditions of the Creative Commons Attribution (CC BY) license (https://creativecommons.org/licenses/by/4.0/).

Abstract: In children and adolescents, obesity does not seem to depend on a reduction of resting energy expenditure (REE). Moreover, in this young population, the interactions between either age and obesity or between age and gender, or the role of leptin on REE are not clearly understood. To compare the levels of REE in children and adolescents we studied 181 Caucasian individuals (62% girls) classified on the basis of age- and sex-specific body mass index (BMI) percentile as healthy weight (n = 50), with overweight (n = 34), or with obesity (n = 97) and in different age groups: 8–10 (n = 38), 11–13 (n = 50), and 14–17 years (n = 93). REE was measured by indirect calorimetry and body composition by air displacement plethysmography. Statistically significant differences in REE/fat-free mass (FFM) regarding obesity or gender were not observed. Absolute REE increases with age (p < 0.001), but REE/FFM decreases (p < 0.001) and there is an interaction between gender and age (p < 0.001) on absolute REE showing that the age-related increase is more marked in boys than in girls, in line with a higher FFM. Interestingly, the effect of obesity on absolute REE is not observed in the 8–10 year-old group, in which serum leptin concentrations correlate with the REE/FFM (r = 0.48; p = 0.011). In conclusion, REE/FFM is not affected by obesity or gender, while the effect of age on absolute REE is gender-dependent and leptin may influence the REE/FFM in 8–10 year-olds.

Keywords: children; adolescents; resting energy expenditure; obesity; age; leptin

1. Introduction

The prevalence of obesity among children and adolescents has increased dramatically in the last decades [1–4]. Overweight and obesity in children and adolescents are independent risk factors for cardiovascular diseases (CVD), type 2 diabetes, hypertension, dyslipidemia, certain types of cancer, and sleep-disorders [5–8]. Moreover, the presence of overweight and obesity during childhood and adolescence is associated with increased risk of adult comorbidities [9,10].

Obesity has a multifactorial nature resulting from an imbalance between energy intake and expenditure during an extended time period [11]. Daily total energy expenditure (TEE)

is composed of resting energy expenditure (REE), which represents 55–75% of TEE, thermic effect of food (TEF), which accounts for 7–15% of TEE, and the energy expended during physical activities, representing between 15–30% of TEE [12–14]. TEE is difficult to measure and can be assessed by direct calorimetry [15] or by doubly labelled water [16], complex techniques that are usually performed for research only. Indirect calorimetry measures the oxygen consumed and carbon dioxide produced as an estimator of energy expended and has been recognized as the gold standard for assessing REE in clinical practice [17].

Overweight and obesity are consequences of excess of calories intake and/or low levels of energy expenditure [18]. However, whether energy expenditure is actually different in patients with obesity is controversial being dependent on how it is expressed. Most studies have found that REE, the main component of TEE, is higher in individuals with obesity as compared with normal weight subjects. However, when body size and composition are taken into account the effect of obesity is unclear or disappears [19]. The fat-free mass (FFM) compartment, including skeletal muscle, bone and other highly active metabolic organs, is the major determinant of REE. About 80% of the interindividual variability in REE can be accounted for by FFM, fat mass, age, and gender [20,21]. In addition, other factors such as the levels of catecholamines or the concentrations of thyroid hormones or leptin may contribute to the variability in REE [22,23]. A portion of the remaining variability can be ascribed to still unidentified genetic factors. When REE is related to FFM, the increased REE observed in subjects with obesity disappears in most studies [20,24–27]. However, some studies still find increased REE in individuals with obesity when REE is expressed as REE/FFM [20,28].

Leptin is an adipokine mainly produced by adipose tissue in proportion to the amount of fat mass, being involved in the regulation of food intake, glucose and lipid homeostasis, reproduction, angiogenesis, and blood pressure, among others [29,30]. Circulating leptin concentrations are closely correlated with the total amount of fat mass being, therefore, elevated in individuals with obesity [31]. However, individuals with obesity exhibit an impaired response to leptin despite their hyperleptinemia, suggesting a state of leptin resistance [32]. Some studies have shown a positive association of serum leptin concentrations and energy expenditure in adults [33,34], while others did not find such a relation [35,36]. Studies in mice have suggested that leptin has direct thermogenic effects on skeletal muscle [37] and that it increases energy expenditure through actions on the sympathetic nervous system modulating the activity of brown, white, and beige adipose tissues via the hypothalamus [38,39]. However, this thermogenic effect has been recently questioned stating that leptin is not a thermogenic hormone, but has effects on body temperature regulation, by opposing torpor bouts and by shifting thermoregulatory thresholds [40].

Previous studies have shown that, similar to what happens in adults, REE expressed in absolute terms is increased in children and adolescents with obesity, but in most of them there are no statistically significant differences when REE is adjusted by FFM [41–44]. REE in children and adolescents is also determined by age and gender, being increased with age and reduced in females when it is expressed in absolute values, but when expressed adjusted by FFM the differences are not so clear [45]. Moreover, the interactions between age and obesity or between age and gender and the potential influence of leptin on REE are not completely understood. Therefore, we hypothesized that in children and adolescents age and gender may interact with the degree of obesity in the regulation of REE and that REE may be influenced by leptin. The aim of the present study was to establish whether obesity in children and adolescents is associated or not with reduced REE and whether there are interactions regarding gender and age. In addition, we also analyzed the potential association of serum leptin concentrations and other cardiometabolic factors with REE.

2. Materials and Methods

2.1. Patient Selection and Study Design

To compare the levels of REE in children and adolescents with overweight and obesity we studied 181 Caucasian individuals (62% girls) from an age range of 8–17 years (mean ±

SEM, 13.3 ± 0.2). Volunteers were recruited from children and adolescents attending the Department of Paediatrics at the Clínica Universidad de Navarra, Spain for conventional check-up. Each child and adolescent was classified on the basis of age- and sex-specific body mass index (BMI) percentile as with normal weight (BMI < 85th percentile), with overweight (BMI $\geq$ 85th and < 95th percentile), or with obesity (BMI $\geq$ 95th percentile) [46] based on the Centers for Disease Control (CDC) 2000 growth charts. With these criteria, the study included 50 subjects with healthy weight, 34 with overweight, and 97 with obesity. The children and adolescents were also classified in different age groups: 8–10 ($n = 38$), 11–13 ($n = 50$), and 14–17 years ($n = 93$). The experimental design was approved by the Hospital's Ethical Committee responsible for research (protocol 2020.236). Informed consent was obtained from all parents or guardians and from all participants over 12 years old. Children under 12 years willingly agreed to participate in the study.

2.2. Anthropometric Measurements and Resting Energy Expenditure

Body weight was measured with a digital scale to the nearest 0.1 kg, and height was measured to the nearest 0.1 cm with a Harpenden stadiometer (Holtain Ltd., Crymych, UK). BMI was calculated as weight in kg divided by the square of height in meters. Waist circumference was measured with a non-elastic tape at the midpoint between the iliac crest and the rib cage. Body fat and FFM were estimated by air displacement plethysmography (Bod-Pod®, Life Measurements, Concord, CA, USA) and converted to a body composition estimate using the Lohman equation. Data for estimation of body fat by this plethysmographic method has been reported to agree closely with the traditional gold standard hydrodensitometry (underwater weighing) [47]. Blood pressure was measured after a 5-min rest in the semi-sitting position with a sphygmomanometer. Blood pressure was determined at least 3 times at the right upper arm and the mean was used in the analyses. REE was measured after a period of 12-h fasting. Following a 30-min rest and after achieving steady state, REE was measured through indirect calorimetry (Vmax29, SensorMedics Corporation, Yorba Linda, CA, USA) in a thermostable (21–23 °C) environment [48].

2.3. Blood Analyses

Blood samples were collected after an overnight fast in the morning in order to avoid potential confounding influences due to hormonal rhythmicity. Plasma glucose was analyzed by an automated analyzer (Roche/Hitachi Modular P800) as previously described [49], with quantification being based on enzymatic colorimetric reactions. Insulin was measured by means of an enzyme-amplified chemiluminescence assay (Immulite®, Diagnostic Products Corp., Los Angeles, CA, USA). An indirect measure of insulin resistance was calculated using the homeostatic model assessment (HOMA). Total cholesterol and triglyceride concentrations were determined by enzymatic spectrophotometric methods (Roche, Basel, Switzerland). High-density lipoprotein (HDL-cholesterol) was quantified by a colorimetric method in a Beckman Synchron® CX analyzer (Beckman Instruments, Ltd., Bucks, UK). Low-density lipoprotein (LDL-cholesterol) was calculated by the Friedewald formula. High-sensitivity C-reactive protein (CRP) was measured using the Tina-quant® CRP (Latex) ultrasensitive assay (Roche, Basel, Switzerland). Thyroid-stimulating hormone (TSH) concentrations were measured by an electro-chemiluminescence immunoassay (ECLIA) using Roche Elecsys® E170 immunoassay analyzer (Roche). Leptin was quantified in a subsample of 113 children and adolescents by a double-antibody radioimmunoassay method (Linco Research, Inc., St. Charles, MO, USA); intra-and inter-assay coefficients of variation were 5.0% and 4.5%, respectively.

2.4. Statistical Analysis

Data are presented as mean $\pm$ standard error of the mean (SEM). Differences between groups were analyzed by ANOVA followed by Fisher's LSD (Least Significant Difference). Two-way ANOVA was used in order to analyze the interaction between age and gender or age and the degree of obesity. CRP concentrations did not fulfill the normality criteria and were therefore logarithmically transformed. We used crude Pearson's correlation coefficients to test the statistical relation between REE and REE/FFM with any other variable. The calculations were performed using SPSS 23 (SPSS, Chicago, IL, USA) and GraphPad Prism 8 (GraphPad Software, Inc., La Jolla, CA, USA). A *p* value lower than 0.05 was considered statistically significant.

3. Results

3.1. Clinical Characteristics of the Cohort

Clinical characteristics of the children and adolescents enrolled in the study are summarized in Table 1. There were statistically significant differences regarding age, with the overweight and obese groups being slightly younger than the healthy weight group. As expected, body fat percentage was significantly elevated in the subjects with overweight and still further increased in the individuals with obesity ($p < 0.001$). Waist circumference was significantly higher in the subjects with either overweight or obesity ($p < 0.001$). Blood pressure was within the normal range in all groups, exhibiting a small though significant increase in the overweight group, being further increased in the obese group compared to the healthy weight group ($p < 0.001$). Children and adolescents with obesity exhibited normoglycemia, but showed insulin resistance as evidenced by the increased insulin concentrations ($p = 0.006$) and HOMA values ($p = 0.004$). Circulating concentrations of triglycerides were increased ($p < 0.001$), while HDL-cholesterol was decreased ($p = 0.019$) in the group with obesity. Patients with obesity exhibited increased circulating concentrations of CRP as compared to both groups with either normal weight or overweight ($p < 0.001$). Leptin levels were increased in the overweight and obese groups ($p < 0.001$).

Table 1. Demographic, biochemical and metabolic characteristics of the children and adolescents classified according to ponderal status.

	Healthy Weight	Overweight	Obesity	*p*
n	50	34	97	
Sex, M/F	15/35	8/26	46/51	0.018
Age, years	14.5 ± 0.3	13.2 ± 0.5 *	13.3 ± 0.3 *	0.002
Height, cm	161 ± 2	156 ± 2	156 ± 2	0.120
Weight, kg	53.5 ± 1.5	60.1 ± 2.5	75.2 ± 2.4 *,†	<0.001
BMI, kg/m^2	20.5 ± 0.3	24.2 ± 0.4 *	29.9 ± 0.5 *,†	<0.001
Body fat, %	24.0 ± 1.3	33.3 ± 1.3 *	40.4 ± 0.7 *,†	<0.001
FFM, kg	40.4 ± 1.2	40.1 ± 2.1	44.2 ± 1.3	0.083
Waist circumference, cm	74 ± 1	80 ± 1 *	92 ± 1 *,†	<0.001
SBP, mm Hg	99 ± 2	105 ± 2 *	110 ± 1 *,†	<0.001
DBP, mm Hg	60 ± 1	62 ± 1	67 ± 1 *,†	<0.001
REE, kcal/d	1439 ± 24	1523 ± 39	1756 ± 35 *,†	<0.001
REE/FFM, kcal/d/kg	36.6 ± 0.8	39.6 ± 1.1 *	41.2 ± 0.6 *	<0.001
Glucose, mg/dL	86 ± 1	87 ± 1	89 ± 1	0.104
Insulin, μU/mL	11.7 ± 2.1	10.2 ± 1.1	19.8 ± 1.9 *,†	0.006
HOMA	2.6 ± 0.5	2.2 ± 0.3	4.4 ± 0.4 *,†	0.004
Triglycerides, mg/dL	65 ± 3	75 ± 6	89 ± 4 *	<0.001
Total cholesterol, mg/dL	159 ± 4	160 ± 5	165 ± 3	0.502
LDL-cholesterol, mg/dL	89 ± 4	91 ± 4	96 ± 3	0.347
HDL-cholesterol, mg/dL	57 ± 2	54 ± 2	51 ± 1 *	0.019
CRP, mg/L	0.8 ± 0.2	1.3 ± 0.3	3.9 ± 1.1 *,†	<0.001
TSH, μU/mL	2.16 ± 0.20	2.55 ± 0.31	2.62 ± 0.15	0.273
Leptin, ng/mL	10.0 ± 1.2	26.0 ± 2.9 *	35.2 ± 2.8 *	<0.001

Data presented as mean ± SEM. BMI, body mass index; FFM, fat-free mass; SBP, systolic blood pressure; DBP, diastolic blood pressure; REE, resting energy expenditure; HOMA, homeostatic model of assessment; CRP, C-reactive protein; TSH, thyroid-stimulating hormone. Differences between groups were analyzed by ANOVA followed by LSD tests. * $p < 0.05$ vs normal BMI. † $p < 0.05$ vs. Overweight. Differences in gender distribution were analyzed by χ^2 analysis. CRP concentrations were logarithmically transformed for statistical analysis.

3.2. Obesity Is Associated with Increased REE, but Not REE/FFM

Total REE was significantly increased ($p < 0.001$) in children and adolescents with obesity as compared to the overweight and healthy weight groups (Figure 1A). When REE is normalized by FFM, the primary determinant of REE variation [50–53] (Supplementary Figure S1A), we found that REE/FFM was significantly increased in overweight ($p < 0.05$) and obese ($p < 0.001$) children and adolescents as compared to the healthy weight group (Figure 1B). Given their lower mass, REE was significantly ($p < 0.001$) decreased in females as compared to males (Figure 2A), however after normalization by FFM, no differences were observed (Figure 2B). Total REE were significantly increased with age in children and adolescents (Figure 2C). Interestingly, REE/FFM was markedly decreased in the 11–13 years ($p < 0.001$) and 14–17 years ($p < 0.001$) children and adolescents as compared to the 8–10 years group (Figure 2D). We observed a moderate positive correlation of age with REE ($r = 0.46$; $p < 0.001$) and a strong negative correlation with REE/FFM ($r = -0.74$; $p < 0.001$) in the global cohort (Table 2 and Supplementary Figure S1B). In this sense, after adjusting for age by ANCOVA the differences in REE between the healthy weight, overweight and obese groups were maintained ($p < 0.001$), but the differences in REE/FFM were lost ($p = 0.070$). Similarly, we reanalyzed the data matching by age ($n = 153$: 36 healthy weight, 34 overweight, 83 obese) finding statistically significant differences in REE ($p < 0.001$) (Supplementary Figure S2A) but not in REE/FFM ($p = 0.111$) (Supplementary Figure S2B). REE was significantly correlated with height ($r = 0.67$; $p < 0.001$), weight ($r = 0.88$; $p < 0.001$), BMI ($r = 0.73$; $p < 0.001$), fat mass ($r = 0.33$; $p < 0.001$), FFM ($r = 0.83$; $p < 0.001$), waist circumference ($r = 0.78$; $p < 0.001$), HOMA ($r = 0.37$; $p < 0.001$) and HDL-cholesterol ($r = -0.31$; $p < 0.001$), among others. REE/FFM was significantly correlated with height ($r = -0.76$; $p < 0.001$), weight ($r = -0.44$; $p < 0.001$), and fat mass ($r = 0.38$; $p < 0.001$), among others (Table 2).

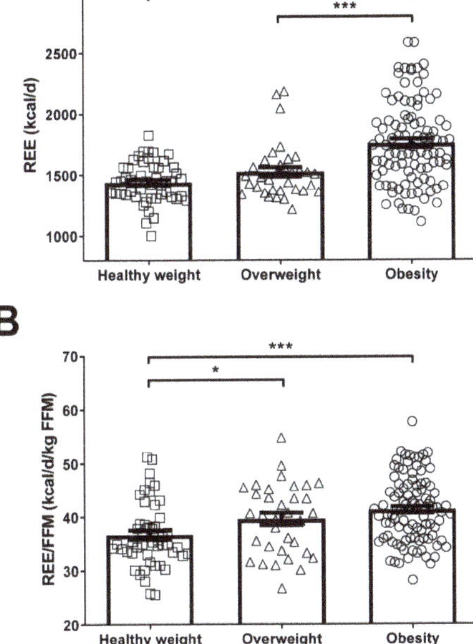

Figure 1. Comparison of absolute REE (**A**) and normalized by FFM (**B**) in children and adolescents with healthy weight, overweight or obesity. Values are means ± SEM. Statistical differences between groups were analyzed by ANOVA followed by LSD tests. * $p < 0.05$ and *** $p < 0.001$ between groups. REE, resting energy expenditure; FFM, fat-free mass.

Table 2. Simple correlation analysis between REE and REE/FFM with other variables.

	All (*n* = 181)		8–10 y (*n* = 38)		11–13 y (*n* = 50)		14–17 y (*n* = 93)	
	REE	**REE/FFM**	**REE**	**REE/FFM**	**REE**	**REE/FFM**	**REE**	**REE/FFM**
Age	**0.46**	**−0.74**	**0.33**	**−0.44**	0.19	**−0.45**	0.11	−0.07
	<0.001	**<0.001**	**0.042**	**0.005**	0.194	**<0.001**	0.285	0.507
Height	**0.67**	**−0.76**	**0.70**	**−0.57**	**0.67**	**−0.50**	**0.56**	**−0.36**
	<0.001	**<0.001**	**<0.001**	**<0.001**	**<0.001**	**<0.001**	**<0.001**	**<0.001**
Weight	**0.88**	**−0.44**	**0.86**	**−0.37**	**0.82**	−0.26	**0.88**	0.15
	<0.001	**<0.001**	**<0.001**	**<0.001**	**<0.001**	0.064	**<0.001**	0.145
BMI	**0.73**	−0.10	**0.63**	−0.08	**0.64**	−0.06	**0.74**	**0.31**
	<0.001	0.187	**<0.001**	0.652	**<0.001**	0.676	**<0.001**	**0.002**
Body fat%	**0.33**	**0.38**	0.29	**0.40**	**0.37**	**0.34**	**0.42**	**0.60**
	<0.001	**<0.001**	0.075	**0.014**	**0.009**	**0.015**	**<0.001**	**<0.001**
FFM	**0.83**	**−0.72**	**0.82**	**−0.73**	**0.83**	**−0.60**	**0.80**	**−0.34**
	<0.001	**<0.001**	**<0.001**	**<0.001**	**<0.001**	**<0.001**	**<0.001**	**0.001**
WC	**0.78**	**−0.18**	**0.62**	**−0.41**	**0.69**	0.01	**0.77**	**0.28**
	<0.001	**0.017**	**<0.001**	**0.010**	**<0.001**	0.942	**<0.001**	**0.007**
SBP	**0.49**	0.05	0.32	−0.13	**0.45**	0.03	**0.58**	**0.26**
	<0.001	0.515	0.059	0.462	**0.001**	0.859	**<0.001**	**0.015**
DBP	**0.50**	0.01	0.11	0.05	**0.44**	0.14	**0.54**	**0.27**
	<0.001	0.944	0.542	0.771	**0.002**	0.350	**<0.001**	**0.011**
Glucose	**0.22**	0.06	0.23	0.15	0.11	−0.08	**0.30**	0.20
	0.007	0.470	0.221	0.426	0.467	0.584	**0.008**	0.085
Insulin	**0.36**	**−0.20**	**0.53**	−0.01	**0.49**	−0.16	0.21	−0.04
	<0.001	**0.019**	**0.003**	0.972	**<0.001**	0.282	0.102	0.742
HOMA	**0.37**	**−0.20**	**0.54**	0.01	**0.49**	−0.17	0.23	−0.04
	<0.001	**0.019**	**0.002**	0.986	**<0.001**	0.277	0.079	0.759
Triglycerides	**0.25**	0.07	0.19	−0.30	0.23	0.17	**0.37**	0.18
	0.002	0.396	0.312	0.103	0.135	0.291	**<0.001**	0.125
T. cholest.	−0.04	**0.17**	0.15	−0.18	−0.26	**0.36**	0.08	0.13
	0.613	**0.037**	0.436	0.330	0.093	**0.018**	0.485	0.249
LDL-cholest.	0.01	**0.18**	0.13	−0.11	−0.23	**0.34**	0.17	0.13
	0.882	**0.028**	0.481	0.552	0.144	**0.027**	0.153	0.277
HDL-cholest.	**−0.31**	0.02	0.01	−0.03	**−0.34**	0.12	**−0.39**	−0.08
	<0.001	0.859	0.972	0.895	**0.027**	0.441	**<0.001**	0.502
CRP	**0.27**	**0.35**	0.29	0.18	0.29	**0.43**	**0.64**	**0.49**
	0.038	**0.006**	0.266	0.485	0.145	**0.027**	**0.005**	**0.046**
TSH	0.04	0.10	0.32	−0.27	0.17	0.03	0.03	0.15
	0.628	0.265	0.124	0.197	0.316	0.855	0.792	0.210
Leptin	**0.28**	−0.06	0.02	**0.48**	0.29	−0.01	0.20	0.15
	0.003	0.559	0.923	**0.011**	0.063	0.972	0.193	0.321

Values are Pearson's correlation coefficients and associated *p* values. CRP concentrations were logarithmically transformed for statistical analysis. BMI, body mass index; FFM, fat-free mass; WC, waist circumference; SBP, systolic blood pressure; DBP, diastolic blood pressure; HOMA, homeostatic model assessment; LDL, low-density lipoproteins; HDL, high-density lipoproteins; CRP, C-reactive protein; TSH, thyroid-stimulating hormone. Bold denotes statistically significant correlation.

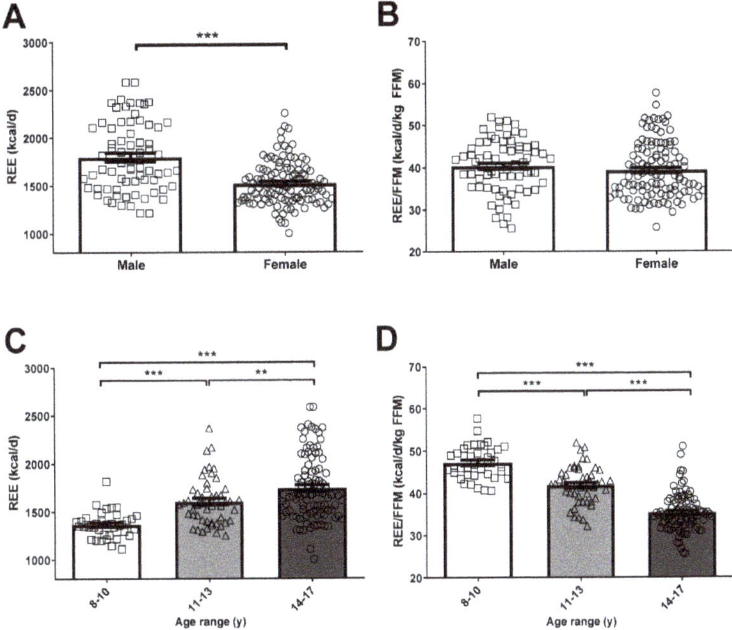

Figure 2. Comparison of absolute REE (**A,C**) and normalized by FFM (**B,D**) between male and female children and adolescents (**A,B**) or between different age groups (8–10, 11–13 and 14–17 years) (**C,D**). Values are means ± SEM. Statistical differences between groups were analyzed by ANOVA followed by LSD tests. ** $p < 0.01$ and *** $p < 0.001$ between groups. REE, resting energy expenditure; FFM, fat-free mass.

3.3. Age, but Not Gender, Influences REE/FFM in Children and Adolescents

When the global sample of children and adolescents was segregated by gender, the age-induced increase in total REE was more evident in males than in females ($p < 0.001$, for interaction between age and gender) as can be observed in Figure 3A, in line with the amount of FFM (Supplementary Figure S3A). However, the progressive decrease with age in REE adjusted by FFM was similar in males and females (Figure 3B). When the data were segregated by age and obesity degree, we found an effect on total REE of age ($p < 0.001$) and obesity ($p < 0.001$), with the latter being absent in the 8–10 years group (Figure 4A), again in line with the amount of FFM (Supplementary Figure S3B). On the contrary, we found a decrease due to age in REE/FFM but not due to obesity consistent across the three age groups (Figure 4B).

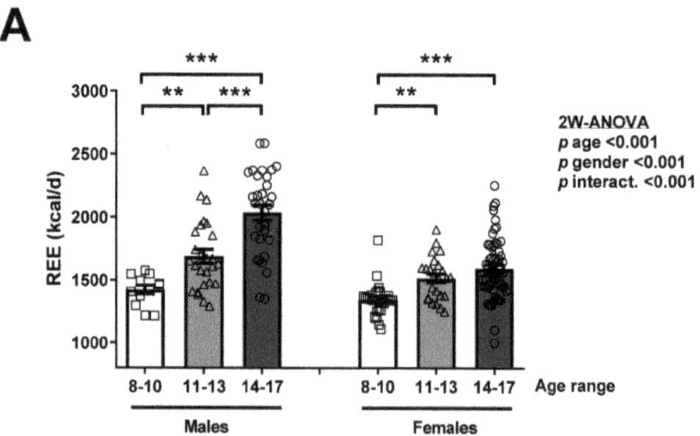

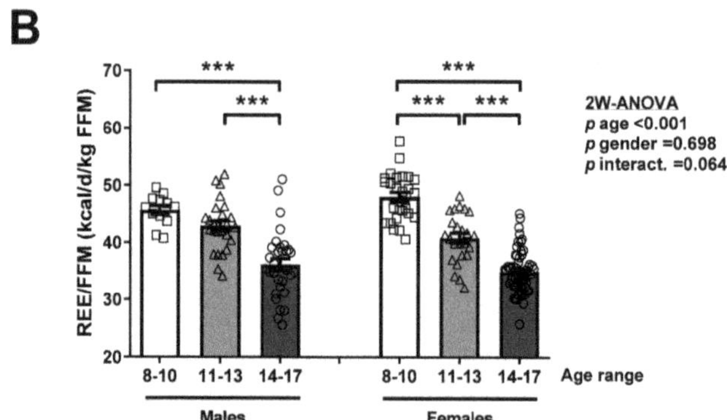

Figure 3. Comparison of absolute REE (**A**) and normalized by FFM (**B**) in the whole sample of children and adolescents (n = 181) segregated by gender and age groups (8–10, 11–13 and 14–17 years). Values are means ± SEM. Differences between groups were analyzed by two-way ANOVA (age x gender). Differences between age groups within each gender were analyzed by ANOVA followed by LSD tests. ** p < 0.01 and *** p < 0.001 between groups. REE, resting energy expenditure; FFM, fat-free mass.

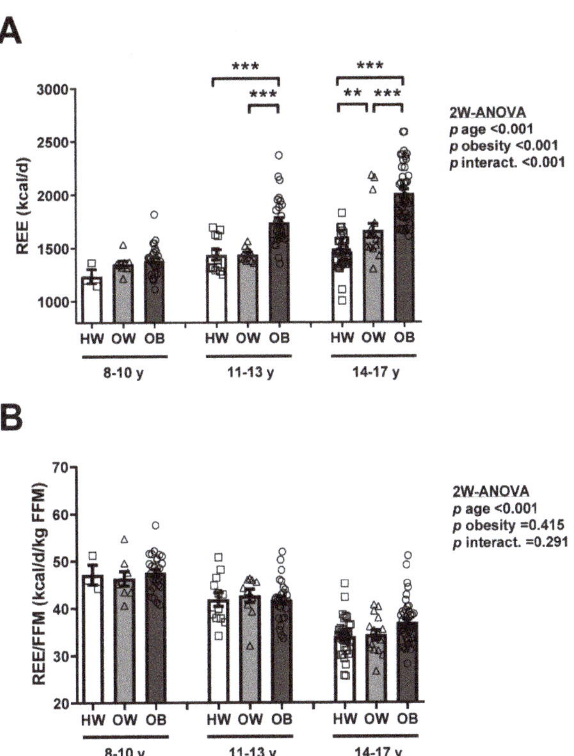

Figure 4. Comparison of absolute REE (**A**) and normalized by FFM (**B**) in the whole sample of children and adolescents (*n* = 181) segregated by age and weight groups (healthy weight, overweight and obesity). Values are means ± SEM. Differences between groups were analyzed by two-way ANOVA (age x obesity). Differences between groups of healthy weight, overweight and obesity within each age group were analyzed by ANOVA followed by LSD tests. ** *p* < 0.01 and *** *p* < 0.001 between groups. REE, resting energy expenditure; FFM, fat-free mass. HW, healthy weight; OW, overweight; OB, obesity.

3.4. Association between Serum Leptin Concentrations and REE/FFM in Children and Adolescents

Serum leptin concentrations were available in 113 children and adolescents. Leptin levels were significantly higher in females (*p* = 0.003) and, although a slight trend was observed, we found no effect due to age (*p* = 0.182) (Figure 5A). Serum leptin concentrations were significantly correlated with fat mass (*r* = 0.66; *p* < 0.001) in both boys (*r* = 0.72; *p* < 0.001) and girls (*r* = 0.64; *p* < 0.001). In the global sample, we found a statistically significant positive correlation of serum leptin concentrations with REE (*r* = 0.28; *p* = 0.003), but not with REE/FFM (*r* = −0.06; *p* = 0.559) as can be observed in Table 2 and Figure 5B. However, when segregated by age groups we observed no global correlation of leptin levels with REE but, interestingly, a significant positive correlation of serum leptin with REE/FFM (*r* = 0.48; *p* = 0.011) was found in the 8–10 years age group (Figure 5B).

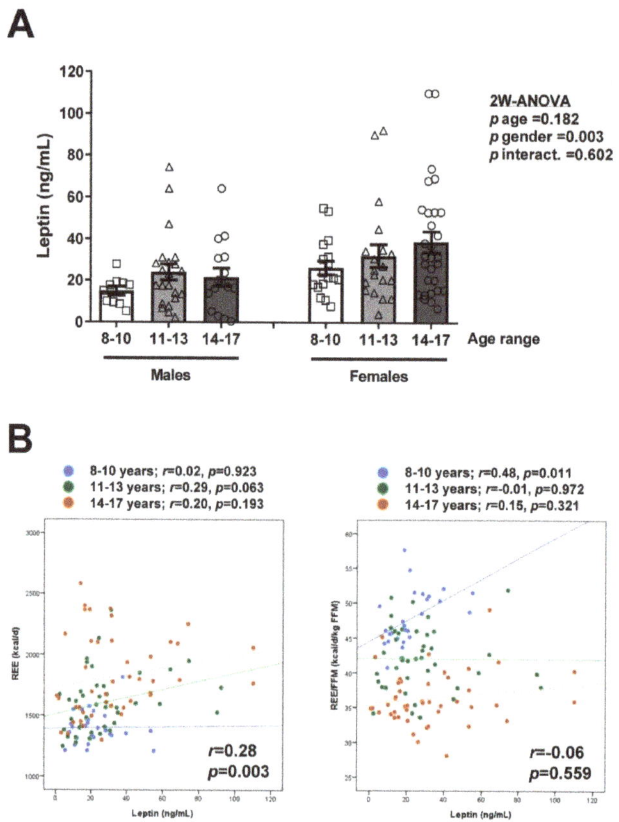

Figure 5. (**A**) Comparison of serum leptin concentrations in the subsample of children and adolescents (*n* = 113) segregated by gender and age groups (8–10, 11–13, and 14–17 years). Values are means ± SEM. Differences between groups were analyzed by two-way ANOVA (age × gender). (**B**) Scatter diagrams showing the correlations of serum leptin levels with REE (left) and REE/FFM (right) segregated by age groups (8–10, 11–13 and 14–17 years). Pearson's correlation coefficient (*r*) and *p* values are indicated.

4. Discussion

The major findings of the present study are that (i) obesity is associated with an increased REE in children and adolescents that is not observed after adjusting REE to FFM; (ii) REE is higher in males but similar to females after adjustment by FFM; (iii) absolute REE increases with age but decreases when referred to FFM; (iv) there is an interaction on absolute REE showing that the age-related increment is more marked in males than in females, which is not observed for REE/FFM; (v) the effect of obesity on REE is not observed in the 8–10 years age range; and that (vi) serum leptin levels correlate with REE/FFM in the 8–10 years age group only.

Previous studies in adults have shown that the increased REE observed in obesity is not observed when REE is adjusted by FFM, the major determinant of REE [24–27]. However, a reduced number of studies reported decreased REE in individuals with obesity when REE is expressed as REE/FFM [28], which would agree with the initial theory of a reduced energy expenditure in people with obesity as a cause of their obesity or as an obstacle to lose weight [19]. In the present study, we used air displacement plethysmography to determine FFM, a method shown to be useful for measuring body composition in children and adolescents with good accuracy [54,55]. Similar to adults, children and adolescents with obesity have increased REE in absolute terms, but in most cases, when adjusting REE by FFM, there are no statistically significant differences [41–44,56]. The work by Bandini et al showed increased REE in adolescents with obesity even after adjustment by FFM [20,57], while Molnár and Schutz in another study with one of the largest sample of adolescents found no differences in REE after adjusting for both FFM and fat mass [58]. Our data show that obesity in children and adolescents is associated with an increase in REE that is not observed after adjusting by FFM, which suggests that reduced energy expenditure is not the cause of obesity in children and adolescents.

Gender is another factor that may be contributing to REE variability in children and adolescents. In our hands, absolute values of REE are higher in males than in females, but the differences are lost after adjustment by FFM. Some studies have found a significant influence of gender on REE when FFM is accounted for [52,59,60] or after adjustment for FFM and fat mass [61]. The contribution of gender to REE variability has been established at 1.1% [59]. However, other studies have observed a lack of effect of gender on REE/FFM [43,62] and even on absolute REE values [63,64]. It is possible that the effect of gender on REE/FFM is age-dependent in children and adolescents. In this sense, age has been considered a clear determinant of REE being negatively correlated in adults [65] mostly due to the changes in body composition [66], and positively in children and adolescents due to the age-related increase in body size [67,68]. In the present study, REE showed a moderate positive correlation with age, while REE/FFM was negatively correlated with age, in agreement with previous studies [68]. Accordingly, REE/FFM was decreased in the group of children and adolescents of 11–13 years of age as compared to the 8–10 years group, and even reduced in the 14–17 years group, with a similar trend for boys and girls being found. The decrease in age-associated REE/FFM is probably more related to a decrease in REE relative to size with increasing body size than to an increase in FFM, since although total FFM increases with age, the FFM% was very similar between the different age groups. Interestingly, we found an interaction between age and gender in absolute REE values, showing that the age-related increase is more marked in males than in females. This finding is likely due to the higher amount of FFM in males associated with growth. In the same line, the interaction observed between age and the degree of obesity in REE, with a lack of effect of obesity in the 8–10 years group is, again, probably due to the amount of FFM. There was no interaction between age and the degree of obesity in REE/FFM supporting the notion that obesity is not associated with altered REE when REE is referred to FFM.

Data from the present study show that leptin exhibits a positive correlation with REE in children and adolescents in the whole sample, while the association is lost when REE is adjusted by FFM. Interestingly, when the analysis is performed by age groups we observe a significant positive correlation of leptin with REE/FFM in the youngest cohort (8–10 years of age). Several studies have shown that leptin is correlated with TEE in children and adolescents [22,69,70], something that can be expected since circulating leptin increases with body size as does TEE. Other studies have found a correlation of leptin with REE, but the correlation is lost after adjustment by FFM or FFM and fat mass [22,69,71]. In some studies leptin was significantly and positively correlated with REE after FFM adjustment [69], while other authors reported that TEE is independently influenced by leptin in overweight children [23]. The fact that we found association of leptin with REE/FFM only in the youngest group suggests that leptin may exert a thermogenic role at early ages or that its putative thermogenic effect is lost as FFM and fat mass increase with age. Interestingly, in this age group we did not observe an effect of obesity on absolute REE values. In this sense, a study performed in adolescent females reported a correlation between leptin and REE adjusted by FFM finding that those girls with the lowest amount of FFM and fat mass exhibited the closest association [72]. In agreement with this, leptin has been associated with energy expenditure during exercise in lean but not obese children aged 8–10 years [73]. Leptin therapy in leptin-deficient patients and in lean people does not affect energy expenditure, but in some cases leptin prevents the reductions in TEE in human cohorts after weight loss achieved by dietary restriction [40]. A recent study has shown that leptin treatment does not affect energy expenditure in humans, but its systemic effects may be more marked in individuals with low leptin levels [74]. Given that children aged 8–10 years was the group with the lower leptin levels without having less amount of fat mass than the other groups, we propose that a threshold of leptin concentration or leptin/fat mass may exist with leptin levels below that threshold paradoxically exerting effects on REE. Whether or not leptin is playing a role in energy expenditure is still controversial and deserves further research. Moreover, the adiponectin–leptin ratio has been established as a promising index to estimate adipose tissue dysfunction in adults [75] and might be useful also in children to assess functionality beyond the mere amount of fat mass.

Some potential limitations of our study should be pointed out. First, our study was conducted in Caucasian subjects and it would need to be determined whether our findings extend to other ethnicities. Second, the sample size of the group of lower age with healthy weight was not particularly big. However, the sample was of enough size in comparison to previous studies and the statistical analyses performed allowed us to detect statistically significant differences among groups. Third, some authors consider that although the normalization of REE to FFM (REE/FFM) is a commonly used method, this approach may be inappropriate when a comparison between lean and obese individuals is made. The logic behind this argument is that skeletal muscle increases with obesity proportionally more than other more metabolically active organs, which also form part of the FFM. Therefore, individuals with obesity tend to have lower REE/FFM than lean individuals because REE does not increase in the same proportion, because their FFM is proportionally less metabolically active than in lean individuals [19,76,77]. However, in our sample, although being slightly higher in the group with obesity, there were no statistically significant differences regarding FFM between groups. In this sense, it has been stated that a simple and practical ratio-based way of universally adjusting REE for differences in body size and composition does not exist [78]. The comparison of FFM metabolic activity and in particular the one from the skeletal muscle mass between healthy weight and obesity raises interesting questions for future studies.

5. Conclusions

In conclusion, our results indicate that obesity is not related to changes in REE when REE is adjusted for FFM. REE/FFM is similar in both genders. Absolute REE increases with age, but decreases when referred to FFM and there is an interaction between gender and age on absolute REE showing that age-related increment is more marked in boys than in girls, in relation to a higher FFM. Interestingly, the effect of obesity on REE is not observed in children aged 8–10 years, which is the only age group in which serum leptin levels are positively correlated with REE/FFM.

Supplementary Materials: The following are available online at https://www.mdpi.com/article/10.3390/nu13041216/s1, Figure S1: Correlations of FFM with REE and of age with REE and REE/FFM, Figure S2: REE and REE/FFM by ponderal status, Figure S3: FFM segregated by gender and age, or by age and ponderal status.

Author Contributions: G.F. and J.G.-A. designed the study and obtained the funds. J.K.Z., G.F., and J.G.-A. analyzed and interpreted the data. G.F. and J.G.-A. drafted the manuscript. J.K.Z., V.C., A.R., B.R., C.S., J.E., J.S., G.C., M.C.A.-S., G.F., and J.G.-A. provided study materials or performed experiments. J.K.Z., V.C., A.R., B.R., C.S., J.E., J.S., G.C., M.C.A.-S., G.F., and J.G.-A. critically revised the article for important intellectual content. All authors have read and agreed to the published version of the manuscript.

Funding: This work was supported by Plan Estatal I+D+I 2017–20 from the Spanish Instituto de Salud Carlos III–Subdirección General de Evaluación y Fomento de la investigación–FEDER (grants number PI17/02183, PI17/02188 and PI19/00785), and by CIBEROBN, ISCIII, Spain.

Institutional Review Board Statement: The study was conducted according to the guidelines of the Declaration of Helsinki, and approved by the Research Ethics Committee of the University of Navarra (protocol code 2020.236).

Informed Consent Statement: Informed consent was obtained from all subjects involved in the study.

Data Availability Statement: The data presented in this study are available on request from the corresponding author. The data are not publicly available due to privacy restrictions.

Acknowledgments: The authors gratefully acknowledge the valuable collaboration of all the members of the Nutrition Unit for their technical support. The authors also wish to thank all subjects who participated in this study.

Conflicts of Interest: The authors declare no conflict of interest.

References

1. The GBD 2015 Obesity Collaborators. Health effects of overweight and obesity in 195 countries over 25 years. *N. Engl. J. Med.* **2017**, *377*, 13–27. [CrossRef] [PubMed]
2. Skinner, A.C.; Ravanbakht, S.N.; Skelton, J.A.; Perrin, E.M.; Armstrong, S.C. Prevalence of Obesity and Severe Obesity in US Children, 1999–2016. *Pediatrics* **2018**, *141*, e20173459. [CrossRef] [PubMed]
3. Ogden, C.L.; Fryar, C.D.; Hales, C.M.; Carroll, M.D.; Aoki, Y.; Freedman, D.S. Differences in Obesity Prevalence by Demographics and Urbanization in US Children and Adolescents, 2013–2016. *JAMA* **2018**, *319*, 2410–2418. [CrossRef] [PubMed]
4. Garrido-Miguel, M.; Cavero-Redondo, I.; Alvarez-Bueno, C.; Rodriguez-Artalejo, F.; Moreno, L.A.; Ruiz, J.R.; Ahrens, W.; Martinez-Vizcaino, V. Prevalence and trends of overweight and obesity in european children from 1999 to 2016: A systematic review and meta-analysis. *JAMA Pediatr.* **2019**, *173*, e192430. [CrossRef]
5. Weiss, R.; Dziura, J.; Burgert, T.S.; Tamborlane, W.V.; Taksali, S.E.; Yeckel, C.W.; Allen, K.; Lopes, M.; Savoye, M.; Morrison, J.; et al. Obesity and the Metabolic Syndrome in Children and Adolescents. *N. Engl. J. Med.* **2004**, *350*, 2362–2374. [CrossRef]
6. Koren, D.; Chirinos, J.A.; Katz, L.E.L.; Mohler, E.R.; Gallagher, P.R.; Mitchell, G.F.; Marcus, C.L. Interrelationships between obesity, obstructive sleep apnea syndrome and cardiovascular risk in obese adolescents. *Int. J. Obes.* **2015**, *39*, 1086–1093. [CrossRef]
7. Furer, A.; Afek, A.; Sommer, A.; Keinan-Boker, L.; Derazne, E.; Levi, Z.; Tzur, D.; Tiosano, S.; Shina, A.; Glick, Y.; et al. Adolescent obesity and midlife cancer risk: A population-based cohort study of 2.3 million adolescents in Israel. *Lancet Diabetes Endocrinol.* **2020**, *8*, 216–225. [CrossRef]
8. Caprio, M.; Santoro, N.; Weiss, R. Childhood obesity and the associated rise in cardiometabolic complications. *Nat. Metab.* **2020**, *2*, 223–232. [CrossRef]
9. Bjerregaard, L.G.; Jensen, B.W.; Angquist, L.; Osler, M.; Sørensen, T.I.; Baker, J.L. Change in Overweight from Childhood to Early Adulthood and Risk of Type 2 Diabetes. *N. Engl. J. Med.* **2018**, *378*, 1302–1312. [CrossRef]
10. Bjerregaard, L.G.; Adelborg, K.; Baker, J.L. Change in body mass index from childhood onwards and risk of adult cardiovascular disease. *Trends Cardiovasc. Med.* **2020**, *30*, 39–45. [CrossRef]
11. Bray, G.A.; Frühbeck, G.; Ryan, D.H.; Wilding, J.P.H. Management of obesity. *Lancet* **2016**, *387*, 1947–1956. [CrossRef]
12. Soares, M.J.; Müller, M.J. Resting energy expenditure and body composition: Critical aspects for clinical nutrition. *Eur. J. Clin. Nutr.* **2018**, *72*, 1208–1214. [CrossRef] [PubMed]
13. Hall, K.D.; Heymsfield, S.B.; Kemnitz, J.W.; Klein, S.; Schoeller, D.A.; Speakman, J.R. Energy balance and its components: Implications for body weight regulation. *Am. J. Clin. Nutr.* **2012**, *95*, 989–994. [CrossRef] [PubMed]
14. Frühbeck, G. Does a NEAT difference in energy expenditure lead to obesity? *Lancet* **2005**, *366*, 615–616. [CrossRef]
15. Kenny, G.P.; Notley, S.R.; Gagnon, D. Direct calorimetry: A brief historical review of its use in the study of human metabolism and thermoregulation. *Eur. J. Appl. Physiol.* **2017**, *117*, 1765–1785. [CrossRef]
16. Westerterp, K.R. Doubly labelled water assessment of energy expenditure: Principle, practice, and promise. *Eur. J. Appl. Physiol.* **2017**, *117*, 1277–1285. [CrossRef]
17. Delsoglio, M.; Achamrah, N.; Berger, M.M.; Pichard, C. Indirect Calorimetry in Clinical Practice. *J. Clin. Med.* **2019**, *8*, 1387. [CrossRef] [PubMed]
18. Hopkins, M.; Blundell, J.E. Energy balance, body composition, sedentariness and appetite regulation: Pathways to obesity. *Clin. Sci.* **2016**, *130*, 1615–1628. [CrossRef]
19. Carneiro, I.P.; Elliott, S.A.; Siervo, M.; Padwal, R.; Bertoli, S.; Battezzati, A.; Prado, C.M. Is Obesity Associated with Altered Energy Expenditure? *Adv. Nutr.* **2016**, *7*, 476–487. [CrossRef]
20. Bandini, L.G.; Schoeller, D.A.; Dietz, W.H. Energy Expenditure in Obese and Nonobese Adolescents. *Pediatr. Res.* **1990**, *27*, 198–202. [CrossRef]
21. Goran, M.I.; Treuth, M.S. Energy expenditure, physical activity, and obesity in children. *Pediatr. Clin. N. Am.* **2001**, *48*, 931–953. [CrossRef]
22. Salbe, A.D.; Nicolson, M.; Ravussin, E. Total energy expenditure and the level of physical activity correlate with plasma leptin concentrations in five-year-old children. *J. Clin. Investig.* **1997**, *99*, 592–595. [CrossRef] [PubMed]
23. Butte, N.F.; Puyau, M.R.; Vohra, F.A.; Adolph, A.L.; Mehta, N.R.; Zakeri, I. Body Size, Body Composition, and Metabolic Profile Explain Higher Energy Expenditure in Overweight Children. *J. Nutr.* **2007**, *137*, 2660–2667. [CrossRef] [PubMed]
24. Ravussin, E.; Burnand, B.; Schutz, Y.; Jéquier, E. Twenty-four-hour energy expenditure and resting metabolic rate in obese, moderately obese, and control subjects. *Am. J. Clin. Nutr.* **1982**, *35*, 566–573. [CrossRef] [PubMed]

25. Prentice, A.M.; Black, A.E.; Coward, W.A.; Davies, H.L.; Goldberg, G.R.; Murgatroyd, P.R.; Ashford, J.; Sawyer, M.; Whitehead, R.G. High levels of energy expenditure in obese women. *BMJ* **1986**, *292*, 983–987. [CrossRef] [PubMed]
26. Verga, S.; Buscemi, S.; Caimi, G. Resting energy expenditure and body composition in morbidly obese, obese and control subjects. *Acta Diabetol.* **1994**, *31*, 47–51. [CrossRef] [PubMed]
27. Dal, U.; Erdoğan, A.T.; Cureoglu, A.; Beydağı, H.; Beydagi, H. Resting Energy Expenditure in Normal-Weight and Overweight/Obese Subjects Was Similar Despite Elevated Sympathovagal Balance. *Obes. Facts* **2012**, *5*, 776–783. [CrossRef]
28. Weijs, P.J.; VanSant, G.A. Validity of predictive equations for resting energy expenditure in Belgian normal weight to morbid obese women. *Clin. Nutr.* **2010**, *29*, 347–351. [CrossRef]
29. Frühbeck, G. Intracellular signalling pathways activated by leptin. *Biochem. J.* **2005**, *393*, 7–20. [CrossRef]
30. Blüher, M.; Mantzoros, C.S. From leptin to other adipokines in health and disease: Facts and expectations at the beginning of the 21st century. *Metabolism* **2015**, *64*, 131–145. [CrossRef]
31. Gómez-Ambrosi, J.; Salvador, J.; Silva, C.; Pastor, C.; Rotellar, F.; Gil, M.J.; Cienfuegos, J.A.; Frühbeck, G. Increased cardiovascular risk markers in obesity are associated with body adiposity: Role of leptin. *Thromb. Haemost.* **2006**, *95*, 991–996. [CrossRef] [PubMed]
32. Könner, A.C.; Brüning, J.C. Selective Insulin and Leptin Resistance in Metabolic Disorders. *Cell Metab.* **2012**, *16*, 144–152. [CrossRef]
33. Jørgensen, J.O.; Vahl, N.; Dall, R.; Christiansen, J.S. Resting metabolic rate in healthy adults: Relation to growth hormone status and leptin levels. *Metabolism* **1998**, *47*, 1134–1139. [CrossRef]
34. Bi, X.; Loo, Y.T.; Henry, C.J. Does circulating leptin play a role in energy expenditure? *Nutrition* **2019**, *60*, 6–10. [CrossRef]
35. Kennedy, A.; Gettys, T.W.; Watson, P.; Wallace, P.; Ganaway, E.; Pan, Q.; Garvey, W.T. The Metabolic Significance of Leptin in Humans: Gender-Based Differences in Relationship to Adiposity, Insulin Sensitivity, and Energy Expenditure. *J. Clin. Endocrinol. Metab.* **1997**, *82*, 1293–1300. [CrossRef]
36. Johnstone, A.M.; Murison, S.D.; Duncan, J.S.; Rance, K.A.; Speakman, J.R. Factors influencing variation in basal metabolic rate include fat-free mass, fat mass, age, and circulating thyroxine but not sex, circulating leptin, or triiodothyronine. *Am. J. Clin. Nutr.* **2005**, *82*, 941–948. [CrossRef]
37. Dulloo, A.G.; Stock, M.J.; Solinas, G.; Boss, O.; Montani, J.P.; Seydoux, J. Leptin directly stimulates thermogenesis in skeletal muscle. *FEBS Lett.* **2002**, *515*, 109–113. [CrossRef]
38. Pandit, R.; Beerens, S.; Adan, R.A.H. Role of leptin in energy expenditure: The hypothalamic perspective. *Am. J. Physiol. Regul. Integr. Comp. Physiol.* **2017**, *312*, R938–R947. [CrossRef]
39. Caron, A.; Lee, S.; Elmquist, J.K.; Gautron, L. Leptin and brain-adipose crosstalks. *Nat. Rev. Neurosci.* **2018**, *19*, 153–165. [CrossRef]
40. Fischer, A.W.; Cannon, B.; Nedergaard, J. Leptin: Is it thermogenic? *Endocr. Rev.* **2020**, *41*, 232–260. [CrossRef] [PubMed]
41. Laessle, R.G.; Wurmser, H.; Pirke, K.M. A Comparison of Resting Metabolic Rate, Self-Rated Food Intake, Growth Hormone, and Insulin Levels in Obese and Nonobese Preadolescents. *Physiol. Behav.* **1997**, *61*, 725–729. [CrossRef]
42. Treuth, M.; Figueroa-Colon, R.; Hunter, G.; Weinsier, R.; Butte, N.; Goran, M. Energy expenditure and physical fitness in overweight vs non-overweight prepubertal girls. *Int. J. Obes.* **1998**, *22*, 440–447. [CrossRef] [PubMed]
43. Ekelund, U.; Aman, J.; Yngve, A.; Renman, C.; Westerterp, K.; Sjöström, M. Physical activity but not energy expenditure is reduced in obese adolescents: A case-control study. *Am. J. Clin. Nutr.* **2002**, *76*, 935–941. [CrossRef] [PubMed]
44. Ekelund, U.; Franks, P.W.; Wareham, N.J.; Åman, J. Oxygen Uptakes Adjusted for Body Composition in Normal-Weight and Obese Adolescents. *Obes. Res.* **2004**, *12*, 513–520. [CrossRef] [PubMed]
45. Bitar, A.; Fellmann, N.; Vernet, J.; Coudert, J.; Vermorel, M. Variations and determinants of energy expenditure as measured by whole-body indirect calorimetry during puberty and adolescence. *Am. J. Clin. Nutr.* **1999**, *69*, 1209–1216. [CrossRef]
46. Barlow, S.E.; Expert, C. Expert committee recommendations regarding the prevention, assessment, and treatment of child and adolescent overweight and obesity: Summary report. *Pediatrics* **2007**, *120* (Suppl. S4), S164–S192. [CrossRef]
47. Fields, D.A.; Higgins, P.B.; Radley, D. Air-displacement plethysmography: Here to stay. *Curr. Opin. Clin. Nutr. Metab. Care* **2005**, *8*, 624–629. [CrossRef]
48. Añón-Hidalgo, J.; Catalán, V.; Rodríguez, A.; Ramírez, B.; Idoate-Bayón, A.; Silva, C.; Mugueta, C.; Galofré, J.C.; Salvador, J.; Frühbeck, G.; et al. Circulating Concentrations of GDF11 are Positively Associated with TSH Levels in Humans. *J. Clin. Med.* **2019**, *8*, 878. [CrossRef] [PubMed]
49. Gómez-Ambrosi, J.; Rodríguez, A.; Catalán, V.; Ramírez, B.; Silva, C.; Rotellar, F.; Gil, M.J.; Salvador, J.; Frühbeck, G. Serum retinol-binding protein 4 is not increased in obesity or obesity-associated type 2 diabetes mellitus, but is reduced after relevant reductions in body fat following gastric bypass. *Clin. Endocrinol.* **2008**, *69*, 208–215. [CrossRef]
50. Bogardus, C.; Lillioja, S.; Ravussin, E.; Abbott, W.; Zawadzki, J.K.; Young, A.; Knowler, W.C.; Jacobowitz, R.; Moll, P.P. Familial Dependence of the Resting Metabolic Rate. *N. Engl. J. Med.* **1986**, *315*, 96–100. [CrossRef]
51. Weinsier, R.L.; Schutz, Y.; Bracco, D. Reexamination of the relationship of resting metabolic rate to fat-free mass and to the metabolically active components of fat-free mass in humans. *Am. J. Clin. Nutr.* **1992**, *55*, 790–794. [CrossRef]
52. Goran, M.I.; Kaskoun, M.; Johnson, R. Determinants of resting energy expenditure in young children. *J. Pediatr.* **1994**, *125*, 362–367. [CrossRef]
53. Müller, M.J.; Geisler, C.; Hübers, M.; Pourhassan, M.; Braun, W.; Bosy-Westphal, A. Normalizing resting energy expenditure across the life course in humans: Challenges and hopes. *Eur. J. Clin. Nutr.* **2018**, *72*, 628–637. [CrossRef] [PubMed]

54. Elberg, J.; McDuffie, J.R.; Sebring, N.G.; Salaita, C.; Keil, M.; Robotham, D.; Reynolds, J.C.; Yanovski, J.A. Comparison of methods to assess change in children's body composition123. *Am. J. Clin. Nutr.* **2004**, *80*, 64–69. [CrossRef] [PubMed]
55. Wells, J.; Fuller, N. Precision of measurement and body size in whole-body air-displacement plethysmography. *Int. J. Obes.* **2001**, *25*, 1161–1167. [CrossRef] [PubMed]
56. Vermorel, M.; Lazzer, S.; Bitar, A.; Ribeyre, J.; Montaurier, C.; Fellmann, N.; Coudert, J.; Meyer, M.; Boirie, Y. Contributing factors and variability of energy expenditure in non-obese, obese, and post-obese adolescents. *Reprod. Nutr. Dev.* **2005**, *45*, 129–142. [CrossRef]
57. Oria, H.E.; Carrasquilla, C.; Cunningham, P.; Hess, D.S.; Johnell, P.; Kligman, M.D.; Moorehead, M.K.; Papadia, F.S.; Renquist, K.E.; American Society for Bariatric Surgery Standards Committee; et al. Guidelines for weight calculations and follow-up in bariatric surgery. *Surg. Obes. Relat. Dis.* **2005**, *1*, 67–68. [CrossRef]
58. Molnár, D.; Schutz, Y. Fat oxidation in nonobese and obese adolescents: Effect of body composition and pubertal development. *J. Pediatr.* **1998**, *132*, 98–104. [CrossRef]
59. Rodríguez, G.; Moreno, L.A.; Sarría, A.; Pineda, I.; Fleta, J.; Pérez-González, J.M.; Bueno, M. Determinants of resting energy expenditure in obese and non-obese children and adolescents. *J. Physiol. Biochem.* **2002**, *58*, 9–15. [CrossRef]
60. Henry, C.; Dyer, S.; Ghusain-Choueiri, A. New equations to estimate basal metabolic rate in children aged 10–15 years. *Eur. J. Clin. Nutr.* **1999**, *53*, 134–142. [CrossRef]
61. Lazzer, S.; Patrizi, A.; De Col, A.; Saezza, A.; Sartorio, A. Prediction of basal metabolic rate in obese children and adolescents considering pubertal stages and anthropometric characteristics or body composition. *Eur. J. Clin. Nutr.* **2014**, *68*, 695–699. [CrossRef] [PubMed]
62. Ribeyre, J.; Fellmann, N.; Montaurier, C.; Delaître, M.; Vernet, J.; Coudert, J.; Vermorel, M. Daily energy expenditure and its main components as measured by whole-body indirect calorimetry in athletic and non-athletic adolescents. *Br. J. Nutr.* **2000**, *83*, 355–362.
63. Gazzaniga, J.M.; Burns, T.L. Relationship between diet composition and body fatness, with adjustment for resting energy expenditure and physical activity, in preadolescent children. *Am. J. Clin. Nutr.* **1993**, *58*, 21–28. [CrossRef]
64. Grund, A.; Vollbrecht, H.; Frandsen, W.; Krause, H.; Siewers, M.; Rieckert, H.; Müller, M. No effect of gender on different components of daily energy expenditure in free living prepubertal children. *Int. J. Obes.* **2000**, *24*, 299–305. [CrossRef]
65. Cheng, Y.; Yang, X.; Na, L.-X.; Li, Y.; Sun, C.-H. Gender- and Age-Specific REE and REE/FFM Distributions in Healthy Chinese Adults. *Nutrients* **2016**, *8*, 536. [CrossRef] [PubMed]
66. Roberts, S.B.; Rosenberg, I. Nutrition and Aging: Changes in the Regulation of Energy Metabolism with Aging. *Physiol. Rev.* **2006**, *86*, 651–667. [CrossRef] [PubMed]
67. Maffeis, C.; Schutz, Y.; Micciolo, R.; Zoccante, L.; Pinelli, L. Resting metabolic rate in six- to ten-year-old obese and nonobese children. *J. Pediatr.* **1993**, *122*, 556–562. [CrossRef]
68. Molnár, D.; Schutz, Y. The effect of obesity, age, puberty and gender on resting metabolic rate in children and adolescents. *Eur. J. Nucl. Med. Mol. Imaging* **1997**, *156*, 376–381. [CrossRef] [PubMed]
69. Nagy, T.R.; Gower, B.A.; Trowbridge, C.A.; Dezenberg, C.; Shewchuk, R.M.; Goran, M.I. Effects of Gender, Ethnicity, Body Composition, and Fat Distribution on Serum Leptin Concentrations in Children. *J. Clin. Endocrinol. Metab.* **1997**, *82*, 2148–2152. [CrossRef]
70. Ten, S.; Bhangoo, A.; Ramchandani, N.; Mueller, C.; Vogiatzi, M.; New, M.; Lesser, M.; MacLaren, N. Resting Energy Expenditure in Insulin Resistance Falls with Decompensation of Insulin Secretion in Obese Children. *J. Pediatr. Endocrinol. Metab.* **2008**, *21*, 359–368. [CrossRef] [PubMed]
71. Arslanian, S.; Suprasongsin, C.; Kalhan, S.C.; Drash, A.L.; Brna, R.; Janosky, J.E. Plasma leptin in children: Relationship to puberty, gender, body composition, insulin sensitivity, and energy expenditure. *Metabolism* **1998**, *47*, 309–312. [CrossRef]
72. Haas, V.K.; Gaskin, K.J.; Kohn, M.R.; Clarke, S.D.; Müller, M.J. Different thermic effects of leptin in adolescent females with varying body fat content. *Clin. Nutr.* **2010**, *29*, 639–645. [CrossRef]
73. Souza, M.S.; Cardoso, A.L.; Yasbek, P., Jr.; Faintuch, J. Aerobic endurance, energy expenditure, and serum leptin response in obese, sedentary, prepubertal children and adolescents participating in a short-term treadmill protocol. *Nutrition* **2004**, *20*, 900–904. [CrossRef]
74. Chrysafi, P.; Perakakis, N.; Farr, O.M.; Stefanakis, K.; Peradze, N.; Sala-Vila, A.; Mantzoros, C.S. Leptin alters energy intake and fat mass but not energy expenditure in lean subjects. *Nat. Commun.* **2020**, *11*, 1–15. [CrossRef]
75. Frühbeck, G.; Catalán, V.; Rodríguez, A.; Gómez-Ambrosi, J. Adiponectin-leptin ratio: A promising index to estimate adipose tissue dysfunction. Relation with obesity-associated cardiometabolic risk. *Adipocyte* **2018**, *7*, 57–62. [CrossRef] [PubMed]
76. Hall, K.D. Modeling Metabolic Adaptations and Energy Regulation in Humans. *Annu. Rev. Nutr.* **2012**, *32*, 35–54. [CrossRef]
77. Browning, M.G.; Evans, R.K. The contribution of fat-free mass to resting energy expenditure: Implications for weight loss strategies in the treatment of adolescent obesity. *Int. J. Adolesc. Med. Health* **2015**, *27*, 241–246. [CrossRef] [PubMed]
78. Heymsfield, S.B.; Thomas, D.; Bosy-Westphal, A.; Shen, W.; Peterson, C.M.; Müller, M.J. Evolving concepts on adjusting human resting energy expenditure measurements for body size. *Obes. Rev.* **2012**, *13*, 1001–1014. [CrossRef] [PubMed]

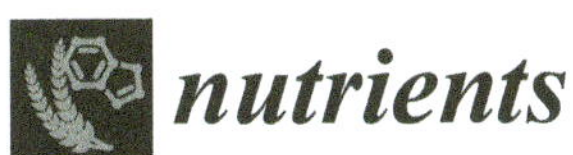 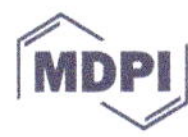

Article

Physical Activity, Sedentariness, Eating Behaviour and Well-Being during a COVID-19 Lockdown Period in Greek Adolescents

Ioannis D. Morres [1], Evangelos Galanis [1], Antonis Hatzigeorgiadis [1,*], Odysseas Androutsos [2] and Yannis Theodorakis [1]

[1] Department of Physical Education and Sport Science, University of Thessaly, 42100 Trikala, Greece; iomorres@pe.uth.gr (I.D.M.); v.galanis@hotmail.com (E.G.); theodorakis@pe.uth.gr (Y.T.)
[2] Department of Nutrition and Dietetics, University of Thessaly, 42132 Trikala, Greece; oandroutsos@uth.gr
[*] Correspondence: ahatzi@pe.uth.gr; Tel.: +30-243-104-7009

Abstract: Adolescents' daily life has dramatically changed during the COVID-19 era due to the social restrictions that have been imposed, including closures of schools, leisure centers and sport facilities. The purpose of this study was to examine levels of well-being and mood and their relations with physical (in)activity and eating behaviors in adolescents during a lockdown period in Greece. A total of 950 adolescents (Mean Age = 14.41 years $\pm$ 1.63) participated in a web-based survey while education was conducted online and organized sport activities were interrupted. Participants showed poor well-being, insufficient physical activity levels and moderate scores of healthy eating behavior. Hierarchical regression analysis showed that, after controlling for the effect of gender and body mass index, increased physical activity and healthier eating behavior predicted better well-being (b = 0.24, $p < 0.01$ and b = 0.19, $p < 0.01$, respectively), whereas sedentariness predicted worse well-being (b = -0.16, $p < 0.01$). Furthermore, it was revealed that days of physical activity per week was a stronger predictor of well-being than minutes of physical activity per week, and that both in-house and out-of-house physical activity were beneficial. Considering that well-being in our study was below the threshold recommended by the World Health Organization as indicative of possible depressive symptoms, measures to increase physical activity, decrease sedentariness and improve eating behavior should become a priority for communities and policy makers.

Keywords: pandemic; COVID-19; lockdown; exercise; sport; diet; mood; quality of life

Citation: Morres, I.D.; Galanis, E.; Hatzigeorgiadis, A.; Androutsos, O.; Theodorakis, Y. Physical Activity, Sedentariness, Eating Behaviour and Well-Being during a COVID-19 Lockdown Period in Greek Adolescents. *Nutrients* **2021**, *13*, 1449. https://doi.org/10.3390/nu13051449

Academic Editor: Sebastian Schmid

Received: 18 March 2021
Accepted: 21 April 2021
Published: 24 April 2021

Publisher's Note: MDPI stays neutral with regard to jurisdictional claims in published maps and institutional affiliations.

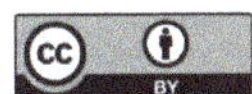

Copyright: © 2021 by the authors. Licensee MDPI, Basel, Switzerland. This article is an open access article distributed under the terms and conditions of the Creative Commons Attribution (CC BY) license (https://creativecommons.org/licenses/by/4.0/).

1. Introduction

Physical activity is defined as "any bodily movement produced by skeletal muscles that results in energy expenditure" [1] and includes various subsets such as walking, cycling or sport. A subset of physical activity that is planned, structured, repetitive and purposive to fitness gains is typically called "exercise" [1]. Physical activity is a preventive/therapeutic factor towards psychological well-being components or proxies while sedentariness an adverse factor. Particularly, large-scale cross sectional studies in adults have linked physical activity to lower risk of depression [2] and sedentariness to higher risk of depression [3]. Furthermore, systematic reviews or cross sectional studies found that exercise is related with lower depression [4,5] or anxiety [6] in adult samples. Various systematic reviews of cross sectional and empirical studies in young people (<18 years) have also demonstrated the positive and negative role, respectively, of physical activity and sedentariness in well-being [7,8]. Similarly, meta-analyses showed that physical activity in young people improves well-being components such as depression [9,10] or anxiety [11,12]. The World Health Organization (WHO) [13] guidelines for better mental health recommend physical activity of ≥420 min/week for adolescents, a larger amount of time than for adults (150–300 min/week). This highlights the importance of increased physical activity for better well-being in adolescents.

However, physical activity and well-being are decreasing worldwide after the COVID-19 pandemic declaration by the WHO in March 2020. Particularly, lockdown measures via social distance restrictions including closures of schools, leisure facilities and sport clubs have been repeatedly introduced to contain the spread of the SARS-CoV-2 virus but led adolescents to lower physical activity and well-being [14–19]. In spite of this rather somber reality, some encouraging findings were provided by a study conducted in China [16], which reported that even limited weekly physical activity (>60 min of weekly) was linked to lower risk of deteriorated well-being in young people during the COVID-19 pandemic. In line, the WHO [13] recommends >60 min/day of moderate-vigorous physical activity for better mental health in adolescents. The importance of physical activity for adolescents is highlighted further by a series of research findings in the era of COVID-19. Particularly, it has been found that physical activity lowers sedentariness and sleep disturbance [19], which are, in turn, linked to an improvement of the widely deteriorated dietary behavior [20,21]. The importance of addressing healthy dietary behavioral patterns should represent a constant concern. State-of-the-art outlines have reported an update for healthy eating across five continents and for Mediterranean diet, with physical activity being an inherent component [22,23].

In the imposed COVID-19 lockdown period in Greece (spring 2020), adults showed decreased physical activity [24] increased depressive symptoms [25], disturbed eating behavioral patterns [26] and the lowest well-being across the 27 European Union member states [27]. In the same period, 25.9% of Greek young adults (University students) have shown increased depressive symptoms corresponding to a threshold for clinical depression [28]. Despite these dramatic changes, the prevalence of well-being, the level of physical (in) activity, the status of eating behaviors and the predictive well-being effects of physical (in) activity and eating behaviors have not been explored in Greek adolescents during a COVID-19 lockdown period. This exploration is essential, as many Greek adolescents in the pre-COVID-19 era showed poor eating behavior [29] and of the lowest well-being levels across 31 countries [30]. This exploration should thus be prioritised to update decision-makers on effective policies for adolescents during a lockdown period, especially since 35% of the Greek families reported well-being decreases for their kids (<18 years) in the first lockdown during spring 2020 [31].

Therefore, this study aimed to explore the prevalence of poor well-being, and the levels and predictive effects of physical activity and eating behavior on well-being in adolescents during the second total lockdown period (November 2020–January 2021) in Greece.

2. Materials and Methods

The study was conducted in accordance with the Declaration of Helsinki and received ethical approval from the University of Thessaly ethics committee (Re: 1723;/09-12-2020). An online survey was prepared using Google Forms, which allowed gathering information during the COVID-19 pandemic lockdown period. Inclusion criteria for participating in this study were age, 12–17 years, and educational level, attending the secondary Greek education (Gymnasium or Lyceum). First, a social media search was conducted with the aim to allocate groups of interest for parents (schools, institutions, parent/guardian groups or associations). The survey was subsequently communicated to such lists. In this communication parents were informed regarding the aim of the survey, the procedures, and the expected benefits. They were also reassured that participation was voluntary and they, or their children, could withdraw from the completion of the survey if they wished. Parents were subsequently asked to provide their consent for their children's participation, and finally asked to forward the survey to their children. The completion of the survey took approximately 15 min and was based on self-reports. Data were collected between mid-January and the beginning of February 2021. Hence, the data captures the reactions of participants in the period of the second lockdown period, when school classes were conducted online and the vast majority of sport activities for our target group were interrupted.

2.1. Sample

Participants were 950 adolescents (518 boys) aged 12 to 17 years (Mage = 14.41, SD = 1.63), who attended secondary education in Greece (46% junior high school (Gymnasium), 54% high school (Lyceum)). Based on self-reports on weight and high, the mean Body Mass Index (BMI) of participants was 21.06 (SD = 2.30). Among them, 698 (73%) were members of sport clubs with mean sport experience 7.17 (SD = 2.89) years, mean competitive experience 4.70 (SD = 2.26) years; they were training between 3 and 6 days per week (M = 4.57, SD = 1.43 days) for an average of 6.94 (SD = 4.28) hours.

2.2. Measures

2.2.1. Physical Activity and Sedentary Behavior

The International Physical Activity Questionnaire Short Form (IPAQ-SF) [32], in particular, the Greek version previously implemented to adolescents [33], was used to assess participants' physical activity and sedentary behavior. The questionnaire assesses frequency (days/week) and duration (minutes/day) of light, moderate, and vigorous intensity physical activity, and in addition sedentary time per day. The amount of physical activity per week, per category of intensity, is calculated by multiplying the number of days/week reported by the minutes/day reported. Sedentary time is calculated by multiplying the average sedentary time per day by seven. The total physical activity per week was calculated by adding the minutes of the different intensities. Two items similar to the ones of the IPAQ-SF were added in this survey to better capture physical activity during the lockdown period; these asked participants to indicate frequency and duration of physical activity in the house and out of the house (e.g., street, park, sport venues). The scores for these additional items were calculated accordingly.

2.2.2. Mood

The Greek version of the 4-Dimensional Mood Scale (4DMS) [34] was used to assess participants' mood. The scale consists of 20 adjectives assessing positive energy (positive affectivity and high activation—four items), relaxation (positive affectivity and low activation—five items), negative arousal (negative affectivity and high activation—six items), and tiredness (negative affectivity and low activation—five items). Participants rated each adjective on the extent to which it generally described their mood during the previous seven days using a 5-point Likert format (1 = not at all, 5 = very much).

2.2.3. Psychological Well-Being

The World Health Organization Well-Being Index-5 [33] was used to assess participants' psychological well-being. This scale consists of five questions focusing on subjective quality of life based on positive mood (good spirits, relaxation), vitality (being active and waking up fresh and rested) and general interest (being interested in things). Participants were asked to indicate their levels of well-being during the previous seven days. Responses were given on a 6-point Likert scale (0 = at no time, 5 = all the time), with lower scores indicating worse well-being. According to the WHO, the Well-Being Index-5 has been translated in more than 30 languages including the Greek language and can be employed for children aged 9 years old and above [33].

2.2.4. Eating Behavior

A slightly modified version of the Short Diet Behaviour Questionnaire for Lockdowns (SDBQ-L) [35,36] was used to address eating behavior for the study population. Following a short description of what consists healthy eating, participants asked to indicate whether (a) they were following a healthy diet, (b) they were eating more than usual, (c) they were eating on a consistent schedule, and (d) they were eating out of control. Responses were provided on a 7-point Likert scale (1 = definitely no, 7 = definitely yes), with higher scores indicating better eating behavior after reversing scores for items 'b' and 'd'. The SDBQ-L has been previously administrated in Greek populations [35].

2.2.5. Data Analysis

Descriptive statistics, Cronbach's alpha coefficients for the scales, and correlations between all variables are presented in Table 1. The reliability of all scales was satisfactory, ranging from 0.80 to 0.87. Notably, first and foremost, participants' mean score on well-being index was close to the median point of the scale, below the WHO threshold (<13), indicating a poor well-being [33]. Scores for positive moods were moderate and for negative moods moderate to low. Moderate and vigorous physical activity combined were below the 50% of the recommended by WHO physical activity. Finally, scores on healthy eating habits were moderate. Well-being was strongly, positively related to positive moods and negatively to negative moods. Physical activity and healthy eating habits showed moderate positive correlations with well-being and positive moods, and negative low correlations with negative moods. Finally, sedentary behavior showed negative correlations with well-being and positive moods and positive correlations with negative moods.

Table 1. Descriptive statistics, Cronbach's alpha, and correlations.

	Descriptives		Alpha	Correlations									
	M	SD		1	2	3	4	5	6	7	8	9	10
1. Well-being	12.63	5.92	0.84	-									
2. Positive energy	3.00	0.98	0.87	0.67 **	-								
3. Relaxation	2.75	0.81	0.80	53 **	0.46 **	-							
4. Negative activation	2.07	0.89	0.87	−0.45 **	−0.25 **	−0.35 **	-						
5. Tiredness	2.03	0.80	0.85	−0.33 **	−0.17 **	−0.19 **	0.51 **	-					
6. Eating behaviour	4.45	1.21	0.75	0.24 **	0.29 **	0.13 **	−0.09 **	−0.09 **	-				
7. Light PA	247.78	209.30	-	0.28 **	0.30 **	0.11 **	−0.07 *	0.00	0.11 **	-			
8. Moderate PA	97.28	119.55	-	0.24 **	0.22 **	0.08 **	−0.07 *	−0.04	0.13 **	0.39 **	-		
9. Vigorous PA	70.23	104.06	-	0.27 **	0.29 **	0.06	−0.07 *	0.01	0.14 **	0.35 **	0.31 **	-	
10. Total PA	415.28	334.29	-	0.35 **	0.36 **	0.12 **	−0.10 **	−0.01	0.16 **	0.87 **	0.70 **	0.64 **	-
11. Sedentary time	439.11	216.57	-	−0.24 **	−0.27 **	−0.10 **	0.19 **	0.14 **	−0.10 **	−0.15 **	−0.03	−0.11 **	−0.14 **

$* p < 0.5$, $** p < 0.01$; M: Mean; SD: Standard Deviation.

3. Results

3.1. Preliminary Analyses

Descriptive statistics, Cronbach's alpha coefficients for the scales and correlations between all variables are presented in Table 1. The reliability of all scales was satisfactory, ranging from 0.80 to 0.87. Notably, first and foremost, participants' mean score on well-being index was close to the median point of the scale, below the WHO threshold, indicating a poor well-being. Scores for positive moods were moderate and for negative moods moderate to low. Moderate and vigorous physical activity combined were below the 50% of the recommended by WHO physical activity for adolescents. Finally, scores on healthy eating habits were moderate. Well-being was strongly, positively related to positive moods and negatively to negative moods. Physical activity and healthy eating habits showed moderate positive correlations with well-being and positive moods, and negative low correlations with negative moods. Finally, sedentary behavior showed negative correlations with well-being and positive moods and positive correlations with negative moods.

3.2. Group Differences

Two, two-way (2 × 2) multivariate analyses of variance, one for the psychometric variables (well-being and mood) and one for the behavioral variables (total physical activity, sedentary time, and healthy eating habits), were conducted to test for differences as a function of sex and sport participation. Mean scores for all subgroups are presented in Table 2.

Table 2. Mean scores for all subgroups.

	Boys		Girls		Athletes		Non-Athletes	
	M	SD	M	SD	M	SD	M	SD
1. Well-being	14.41	5.55	10.47	5.63	13.22	5.90	10.96	5.65
2. Positive energy	3.22	0.95	2.73	0.96	3.07	1.00	2.86	0.91
3. Relaxation	2.95	0.76	2.50	0.79	2.77	0.83	2.70	0.75
4. Negative activation	1.83	0.72	2.36	0.97	2.03	0.84	2.18	0.99
5. Tiredness	1.93	0.71	2.16	0.89	2.01	0.77	2.11	0.89
6. Eating behaviour	4.38	1.18	4.53	1.24	4.49	1.23	4.34	1.14
7. Light PA	281,96	221,42	205,71	184,62	267,57	209,79	190,99	196,03
8 Moderate PA	106,74	123,19	85,80	114,24	112,57	128,05	54,58	77,79
9. Vigorous PA	85,42	118,82	51,74	79,26	80,40	108,28	41,51	85,16
10. Total PA	474.12	359.28	343.25	288.00	460.55	339.34	287.09	281.84
11. Sedentary time	413.73	210.68	469.55	219.82	429.29	211.53	466.37	228.19

M: Mean; SD: Standard Deviation; PA: Physical Activity.

Regarding the psychometric variables, the analyses showed significant multivariate effects for sex, $F(5, 941) = 22.21$, $p < 0.01$, partial $\eta2 = 0.11$, and sport participation, $F(5, 941) = 4.87$, $p < 0.01$, partial $\eta2 = 0.03$, and a non-significant interaction effect, $F(5, 941) = 1.45$, $p = 0.20$. Examination of the univariate effects for sex revealed significant differences in well-being, $F(1, 949) = 74.99$, $p < 0.01$, partial $\eta2 = 0.07$, positive energy, $F(1, 949) = 29.68$, $p < 0.01$, partial $\eta2 = 0.03$, relaxation, $F(1, 949) = 55.76$, $p < 0.01$, partial $\eta2 = 0.06$, negative activation, $F(1, 949) = 66.87$, $p < 0.01$, partial $\eta2 = 0.07$, and tiredness, $F(1, 949) = 18.52$, $p < 0.01$, partial $\eta2 = 0.02$, with boys scoring higher than girls on well-being and positive moods, and lower on negative moods. Examination of the univariate effects for sport participation revealed significant differences in well-being, $F(1, 949) = 18.17$, $p < 0.01$, partial $\eta2 = 0.02$, and positive energy, $F(1, 949) = 11.40$, $p < 0.01$, partial $\eta2 = 0.01$, with athletes scoring higher than non-athletes, and non-significant effects for relaxation, $F(1, 949) = 0.03$, $p = 0.86$, negative activation, $F(1, 949) = 1.72$, $p = 0.19$, and tiredness, $F(1, 949) = 1.21$, $p = 0.27$.

Regarding the behavioral variables, the analyses showed significant multivariate effects for sex, $F(3, 942) = 11.23$, $p < 0.01$, partial $\eta2 = 0.04$, and sport participation, $F(3, 942) = 15.26$, $p < 0.01$, partial $\eta2 = 0.05$, and a non-significant interaction effect, $F(3, 942) = 0.78$, $p = 0.51$. Examination of the univariate effects for sex revealed significant differences in total physical activity, $F_{(1, 948)} = 21.56$, $p < 0.01$, partial $\eta2 = 0.02$, and sedentary time, $F_{(3, 942)} = 9.46$, $p < 0.01$, partial $\eta2 = 0.01$, with boys scoring higher in physical activity and lower on sedentary time, and a non-significant effect on healthy eating habits, $F_{(1, 948)} = 1.66$, $p = 0.20$. Examination of the univariate effects for sport participation revealed significant differences in physical activity, $F_{(1, 948)} = 43.95$, $p < 0.01$, partial $\eta2 = 0.04$, and healthy eating habits, $F_{(1, 948)} = 3.89$, $p < 0.01$, partial $\eta2 = 0.01$, with athletes scoring higher than non-athletes, and a non-significant effect on sedentary time, $F_{(1, 948)} = 3.54$, $p = 0.06$.

3.3. Prediction of Well-Being

Three sets of hierarchical regressions analyses were performed to examine the predictive strength of the behavioral variables for well-being, and the specifics of physical activity in predicting well-being. In all analyses, sex and BMI were entered in the first step to account for sex differences and the effect of BMI on well-being, which were identified in the preliminary analyses.

In the first hierarchical analysis, total physical activity, sedentary time and healthy eating habits were entered in the second step of the analysis. In the first step of the analysis, sex and BMI predicted 13% of the well-being variance, with both predictors being significant ($b = -0.34$, $p < 0.01$ and $b = -0.15$, $p < 0.01$, respectively). In the second step, the introduction of the behavioral variables raised the prediction to 27.5% of the variance. All predictors were significant; among the behavior variables, total physical activity was the stronger ($b = 0.24$, $p < 0.01$), followed by eating habits ($b = 0.19$, $p < 0.01$) and sedentary time ($b = -0.15$, $p < 0.01$). The results of this regression analysis are presented in Table 3.

Table 3. Prediction of well-being from behavioral variables.

	Beta	**t**	**R^2**	**F**
step 1			13	$(2, 914) = 68.40$ **
Sex	−0.33	−10.95 **		
BMI	−0.15	−4.89 **		
step 2			27.5	$(5, 914) = 68.96$ **
Sex	−0.27	−9.54 **		
BMI	−0.09	−3.28 **		
Total PA	0.24	8.03 **		
Sedentary time	−0.16	−5.49 **		
Eating behavior	0.19	6.57 **		

** $p < 0.01$; BMI: Body Mass Index; PA: Physical Activity.

The purpose of the second regression was to identify (a) the role of physical activity intensity and (b) whether frequency (i.e., number of days/week) or duration (total number of minutes/week) of physical activity were stronger predictors of well-being. Thus, in this hierarchical analysis, days and total time of light, moderate and vigorous physical activity were entered in the second step of the analysis. In the second step of the model, the introduction of the physical activity raised the prediction from 13.1% to 23.4% of the variance. Interestingly, the frequency of light, moderate and vigorous physical activity were all significant predictors of well-being, while the duration was not significant for any of them. Similar coefficients were revealed for all types of activity; for vigorous, $b = 0.12$, $p < 0.01$, for moderate, ($b = 0.10$, $p < 0.01$), and for light, ($b = 0.14$, $p < 0.01$). The results of this regression analysis are presented in Table 4.

Table 4. Prediction of well-being from physical activity intensity, frequency and duration.

	Beta	t	R^2	F
step 1			13.1	(2, 915) = 68.88 **
Sex	−0.33	−10.95 **		
BMI	−0.15	−4.89 **		
step 2			23.4	(8, 914) = 34.55 **
Sex	−0.26	−8.80 **		
BMI	−0.10	−3.57 **		
Light PA-days	0.13	4.01 **		
Light PA-time	0.03	0.92		
Moderate PA-days	0.10	2.55 *		
Moderate PA-time	0.04	1.25		
Vigorous PA-days	0.12	2.87 **		
Vigorous PA-time	0.01	0.36		

* $p < 05$; ** $p < 0.01$; BMI: Body Mass Index; PA: Physical Activity.

The purpose of the third regression analysis was to identify the role of physical activity location. Thus, in this hierarchical analysis, days of in-house physical activity and days of out-of-house physical activity were entered in the second step of the analysis. In the second step, the introduction of the physical activity raised the prediction from 13.1% to 22.6% of the variance. Both variables were significant predictors of well-being, with out-of-house physical activity (b = 0.23, $p < 0.01$) being stronger than in-house physical activity (b = 0.17, $p < 0.01$). The results of this regression analysis are presented in Table 5.

Table 5. Prediction of well-being from physical activity location.

	Beta	t	R^2	F
step 1			13.1	(2, 913) = 68.89
Sex	−0.34	10.99 **		
BMI	−0.15	4.92 **		
step 2			22.6	(4, 911) = 66.43
Sex	−0.27	9.10 **		
BMI	−0.11	3.79 **		
Home PA	0.17	5.59 **		
Out-of-home PA	0.23	7.41 **		

** $p < 0.01$; BMI: Body Mass Index; PA: Physical Activity.

4. Discussion

The present study aimed primarily at identifying relationships between physical activity, sedentariness, eating behavior and well-being among adolescents during a lockdown period, while school classes were delivered on-line and organized sport activities were interrupted. The most striking result was the worryingly low levels of well-being reported by participants. The average score on well-being, and accordingly the score of 49.5% of the participants, was below the threshold (total score < 13) identified by the WHO as requiring inspection for depressive symptoms [33]. Similarly, 48.3% of Australian adolescents in a COVID-19 lockdown showed mental distress corresponding to a probable mental illness [37]. Poor well-being components have also been recorded in Philippines where 27% to 40% of young people aged 12 to 21 years old showed increased levels of anxiety and/or depressive symptoms [38].

The signaling effects of the COVID-19 on Greek adolescents have been identified during the previous lockdown period, in spring 2020. In a study with parents, it was reported that the psychological health of children (<18 years) was considerably affected in 35% of the Greek families [31]. These findings are similar to the findings from Canada where 35.7% of parents were found to be experiencing high levels of anxiety due to COVID-19 [39]. Similarly discouraging findings were found for young people and/or parents in the previous lockdown period in Italy [40,41] or in Greece; for example, University students in

Greece showed considerable reduction of mental health, including increased anxiety and depressive symptoms corresponding to a threshold for clinical depression [28].

Encouragingly, physical activity and healthy patterns of eating behavior were positively related with participants' positive mood dimensions and well-being. Furthermore, adolescents who used to participate in organized sport reported higher levels of physical activity and better well-being compared to those not participating in organized sport, above the threshold suggested by the WHO for better well-being but still low. Despite the interruption of sport due to the restrictions, which should have had a more dramatic impact on athletes' physical activity and subsequently well-being, athletes managed to maintain a more active lifestyle and better well-being. Various studies have repeatedly related physical activity with better well-being components including lower depression and anxiety symptoms in adolescents [11,12] and adults [4,6]. In light of this repeated positive evidence, the WHO [13] guidelines recommend adolescents perform physical activity of 60 min/day ($\geq$420 min/week) for better mental health. Physical activity of participants in the present study was below the recommended by the WHO levels, nevertheless, was the stronger predictor of well-being, even after controlling for the effects of sex and BMI that were also found to influence well-being. The beneficial effects of physical activity for mental health during the COVID-19 pandemic have been also evidenced in young Chinese persons by the authors of [16], who reported that physical activity for >60 min/week was linked to lower risk of deteriorated well-being.

Healthy eating emerged as a secondary significant predictor of better well-being. Indeed, healthy eating in the COVID-19 pandemic is linked to improved well-being components such as lower depressive and anxious symptoms [42]. However, eating behavioral patterns have deteriorated in the COVID-19 pandemic (e.g., number of main meals or snacks between meals, eating out of control or type of food) [36]. Furthermore, data from Cyprus for the pre- and post-lockdown period due to COVID-19 reported a significant increase of young people (5–14 years old) consuming food items containing sugar [18]. Initiatives towards healthier eating behavior at home are thus essential, and relevant updates have been recently published for further action. In particular, the importance of addressing healthy dietary behavioral patterns represents a constant concern. State-of-the-art outlines have reported an update for healthy eating across five continents and for Mediterranean diet, with physical activity being an inherent component [22,23]. Such initiatives, however, seem to be potentially challenging due to adolescents' poor well-being. Despite this somber reality, the multiple benefits of physical activity reveal promising perspectives towards healthier eating. In particular, physical activity lowers sedentariness and sleep disturbance [19], which are, in turn, linked to less deteriorated dietary behavior [20,21]. This beneficial sequence seems to be supported, although not examined, in our study by the correlations amongst house-based physical activity, better eating behavior and improved well-being.

In contrast to physical activity and healthy eating behavior, sedentary time predicted well-being deterioration in our study. This is an unsurprising finding because sedentary time has been repeatedly associated with deteriorated well-being components (e.g., depression) in large-scale epidemiological studies across adolescents [7,8] and adult populations [3]. Moreover, adolescents living in COVID-19 lockdowns have demonstrated increased sedentariness and low well-being [14–19]; sitting time in particular has dramatically increased [36] and clearly related with deteriorated well-being components including sleeping patterns and depressive and anxiety symptoms [43]. Tackling sedentary time in Greek adolescents during the COVID-19 pandemic and involved lockdowns should thus be prioritized to decrease sitting time modalities such as the widespread screen time. Towards this direction, it would be interesting to consider the potentially detrimental effects of online schooling on physical activity, and address to school directors and policy makers the importance of physically active breaks between classes in the daily schedule.

A final issue deserving consideration is the relevant contribution of physical activity modalities towards the prediction of well-being. The first notable point is that frequency of physical activity (days/week) was a stronger predictor of duration (total minutes/week), for all physical activity intensity modes. The emerged importance of frequency in physical activity participation has significant implications for how the recommendations for physical activity that should be prioritized, at least during the pandemic times. Small bouts of physical activity may increase overall frequency (days/week) without increasing risks of injuries, which are typically linked to accumulated physical activity volume. In line with this, a recent study has reported the contribution of small bouts to increased frequency of physical activity among children [44]. The second issue is that out-of-house physical activity was a stronger predictor of well-being; yet, after accounting for that effect, in-house physical activity was still a significant predictor. Even though the superiority of the out-of-house activity is a reasonable finding, that in-house physical activity during a lockdown time, where the chances of going out of the house are limited, highlights the unique impact that physical activity per se, not combined with going out, can have on well-being. Therefore, the promotion of ideas and innovative ways to exercise in the house should be particularly emphasized during lockdown periods.

5. Limitations

The findings of the current study should be considered under the light of certain limitations. First, the cross-sectional design of the study does not allow causal conclusions with regard to the statistical prediction of well-being from physical activity, sedentariness and eating habits; second, the reliance on self-reported behavioral measures, including physical activity, sedentary behavior and eating habits, which are dependent on memory and, in cases, liable to social desirability; third, the consideration of additional, to gender and BMI, control variables that may have influenced the results; and finally the recruitment of the sample through the social media, which does not allow calculation of response rates and limits the participation of people without access to the internet or non-users of social media, thus limiting the generalizability of the findings. These limitations, despite being typical in large scale surveys, and in particular web-based surveys, suggest that our findings should be interpreted with caution.

6. Conclusions

Action needs to be taken by both researchers and policy makers to enhance well-being in Greek adolescents by providing guidance and opportunities for increased physical activity, decreased sedentary time and healthier eating behaviors. Such action is of high priority as 50% of our sample showed levels of well-being below the general population norms. These levels signify according to the WHO the need to subsequently investigate for potential depression; thus, prompt research is warranted to address this important health risk that emerged during the pandemic. Considering evidence suggesting that Greek adolescents' physical activity and well-being are among the lowest in Europe even before the emergence of the pandemic [30], initiatives targeting the improvement of healthy habits should be supported hereafter with consistency.

Author Contributions: Conceptualization, Y.T. and I.D.M.; methodology, A.H. and O.A.; formal analysis, E.G. and A.H.; writing—original draft preparation, I.D.M. and E.G.; writing—review and editing, A.H., O.A. and Y.T. All authors have read and agreed to the published version of the manuscript.

Funding: This research received no external funding.

Institutional Review Board Statement: The study was conducted according to the guidelines of the Declaration of Helsinki, and approved by the Ethics Committee of the Department of Physical Education & Sport Science, of the University of Thessaly (Re: 1723/09-12-2020).

Informed Consent Statement: Informed consent was obtained from parents of all subjects involved in the study.

Data Availability Statement: Data are available upon request from the first author.

Conflicts of Interest: The authors declare no conflict of interest.

References

1. Caspersen, C.J.; Powell, K.E.; Christenson, G. Physical activity, exercise and physical fitness: Definitions and distinctions for health-related research. *Public Health Rep.* **1985**, *100*, 126–131.
2. Harris, A.H.; Cronkite, R.; Moos, R. Physical activity, exercise coping, and depression in a 10-year cohort study of depressed patients. *J. Affect. Disord.* **2006**, *93*, 79–85. [CrossRef]
3. Zhai, L.; Zhang, Y.; Zhang, D. Sedentary behaviour and the risk of depression: A meta-analysis. *Br. J. Sports Med.* **2015**, *49*, 705–709. [CrossRef]
4. Morres, I.D.; Hatzigeorgiadis, A.; Stathi, A.; Comoutos, N.; Arpin-Cribbie, C.; Krommidas, C.; Theodorakis, Y. Aerobic exercise for adult patients with major depressive disorder in mental health services: A systematic review and meta-analysis. *Depress. Anxiety* **2019**, *36*, 39–53. [CrossRef]
5. Morres, I.D.; Hatzigeorgiadis, A.; Krommidas, C.; Comoutos, N.; Sideri, E.; Ploumpidis, D.; Economou, M.; Papaioannou, A.; Theodorakis, Y. Objectively measured physical activity and depressive symptoms in adult outpatients diagnosed with major depression. Clinical perspectives. *Psychiatry Res.* **2019**, *280*, 112489. [CrossRef] [PubMed]
6. Wipfli, B.M.; Rethorst, C.D.; Landers, D.M. The anxiolytic effects of exercise: A meta-analysis of randomized trials and dose–response analysis. *J. Sport Exerc. Psychol.* **2008**, *30*, 392–410. [CrossRef] [PubMed]
7. Burkhardt, J.; Brennan, C. The effects of recreational dance interventions on the health and well-being of children and young people: A systematic review. *Arts Health* **2012**, *4*, 148–161. [CrossRef]
8. Biddle, S.J.H.; Asare, M. Physical activity and mental health in children and adolescents: A review of reviews. *Br. J. Sports Med.* **2011**, *45*, 886–895. [CrossRef] [PubMed]
9. Carter, T.; Morres, I.D.; Meade, O.; Callaghan, P. The Effect of Exercise on Depressive Symptoms in Adolescents: A Systematic Review and Meta-Analysis. *J. Am. Acad. Child Adolesc. Psychiatry* **2016**, *55*, 580–590. [CrossRef]
10. Wegner, M.; Amatriain-Fernández, S.; Kaulitzky, A.; Murillo-Rodriguez, E.; Machado, S.; Budde, H. Systematic Review of Meta-Analyses: Exercise Effects on Depression in Children and Adolescents. *Front. Psychiatry* **2020**, *11*, 81. [CrossRef]
11. Philippot, A.; Meerschaut, A.; Danneaux, L.; Smal, G.; Bleyenheuft, Y.; De Volder, A.G. Impact of Physical Exercise on Symptoms of Depression and Anxiety in Pre-adolescents: A Pilot Randomized Trial. *Front. Psychol.* **2019**, *10*, 1820. [CrossRef] [PubMed]
12. Carter, T.; Pascoe, M.; Bastounis, A.; Morres, I.D.; Callaghan, P.; Parker, A.G. The effect of physical activity on anxiety in children and young people: A systematic review and meta-analysis. *J. Affect. Disord.* **2021**, *285*, 10–21. [CrossRef] [PubMed]
13. World Health Organization. *WHO Guidelines on Physical Activity and Sedentary Behaviour*; WHO: Geneva, Switzerland, 2020.
14. Vanderloo, L.M.; Carsley, S.; Aglipay, M.; Cost, K.T.; Maguire, J.; Birken, C.S. Applying Harm Reduction Principles to Address Screen Time in Young Children Amidst the COVID-19 Pandemic. *J. Dev. Behav. Pediatrics* **2020**, *41*, 335–336. [CrossRef]
15. Margaritis, I.; Houdart, S.; El Ouadrhiri, Y.; Bigard, X.; Vuillemin, A.; Duché, P. How to deal with COVID-19 epidemic-related lockdown physical inactivity and sedentary increase in youth? Adaptation of Anses' benchmarks. *Arch. Public Health* **2020**, *78*, 52. [CrossRef] [PubMed]
16. Qin, Z.; Shi, L.; Xue, Y.; Lin, H.; Zhang, J.; Liang, P.; Lu, Z.; Wu, M.; Chen, Y.; Zheng, X.; et al. Prevalence and Risk Factors Associated with Self-reported Psychological Distress among Children and Adolescents During the COVID-19 Pandemic in China. *JAMA Netw. Open* **2021**, *4*, e2035487. [CrossRef] [PubMed]
17. Stavridou, A.; Stergiopoulou, A.-A.; Panagouli, E.; Mesiris, G.; Thirios, A.; Mougiakos, T.; Troupis, T.; Psaltopoulou, T.; Tsolia, M.; Sergentanis, T.N.; et al. Psychosocial consequences of COVID-19 in children, adolescents and young adults: A systematic review. *Psychiatry Clin. Neurosci.* **2020**, *74*, 615–616. [CrossRef]
18. Konstantinou, C.; Andrianou, X.D.; Constantinou, A.; Perikkou, A.; Markidou, E.; Christophi, C.A.; Makris, K.C. Exposome changes in primary school children following the wide population non-pharmacological interventions implemented due to COVID-19 in Cyprus: A national survey. *EClinicalMedicine* **2021**, *32*, 100721. [CrossRef] [PubMed]
19. Bates, L.C.; Zieff, G.; Stanford, K.; Moore, J.B.; Kerr, Z.Y.; Hanson, E.D.; Barone Gibbs, B.; Kline, C.E.; and Stoner, L. COVID-19 Impact on Behaviors across the 24-Hour Day in Children and Adolescents: Physical Activity, Sedentary Behavior, and Sleep. *Children* **2020**, *7*, 138. [CrossRef]
20. Du, C.; Zan, M.C.H.; Cho, M.J.; Fenton, J.I.; Hsiao, P.Y.; Hsiao, R.; Keaver, L.; Lai, C.-C.; Lee, H.; Ludy, M.-J.; et al. Health Behaviors of Higher Education Students from 7 Countries: Poorer Sleep Quality during the COVID-19 Pandemic Predicts Higher Dietary Risk. *Clocks Sleep* **2021**, *3*, 12–30. [CrossRef]
21. Ruiz-Roso, M.B.; de Carvalho Padilha, P.; Mantilla-Escalante, D.C.; Ulloa, N.; Brun, P.; Acevedo-Correa, D.; Arantes Ferreira Peres, W.; Martorell, M.; Aires, M.T.; de Oliveira Cardoso, L.; et al. Covid-19 Confinement and Changes of Adolescent's Dietary Trends in Italy, Spain, Chile, Colombia and Brazil. *Nutrients* **2020**, *12*, 1807. [CrossRef]
22. Fernandez, M.L.; Raheem, D.; Ramos, F.; Carrascosa, C.; Saraiva, A.; Raposo, A. Highlights of Current Dietary Guidelines in Five Continents. *Int. J. Environ. Res. Public Health* **2021**, *18*, 2814. [CrossRef]
23. Serra-Majem, L.; Tomaino, L.; Dernini, S.; Berry, E.M.; Lairon, D.; Ngo de la Cruz, J.; Bach-Faig, A.; Donini, L.M.; Me-dina, F.-X.; Belahsen, R.; et al. Updating the Mediterranean Diet Pyramid towards Sustainability: Focus on Environmental Concerns. *Int. J. Environ. Res. Public Health* **2020**, *17*, 8758. [CrossRef] [PubMed]
24. Bourdas, D.I.; Zacharakis, E.D. Impact of COVID-19 Lockdown on Physical Activity in a Sample of Greek Adults. *Sports* **2020**, *8*, 139. [CrossRef] [PubMed]

25. Parlapani, E.; Holeva, V.; Voitsidis, P.; Blekas, A.; Gliatas, I.; Porfyri, G.N.; Golemis, A.; Papadopoulou, K.; Dimitriadou, A.; Chatzigeorgiou, A.F.; et al. Psychological and Behavioral Responses to the COVID-19 Pandemic in Greece. *Front. Psychiatry* **2020**, *11*, 821. [CrossRef] [PubMed]
26. Papandreou, C.; Arija, V.; Aretouli, E.; Tsilidis, K.K.; Bulló, M. Comparing eating behaviours, and symptoms of depression and anxiety between Spain and Greece during the COVID-19 outbreak: Cross-sectional analysis of two different confinement strategies. *Eur. Eat. Disord. Rev. J. Eat. Disord. Assoc.* **2020**, *28*, 836–846. [CrossRef] [PubMed]
27. European Foundation for the Improvement of Living Working Conditions. *Living, Working and COVID-19: First Findings, April 2020*; Publications Office of the European Union: Luxembourg, 2020. Available online: https://www.eurofound.europa.eu/publications/report/2020/living-working-and-covid-19-first-findings-april-2020 (accessed on 24 April 2020).
28. Kaparounaki, C.K.; Patsali, M.E.; Mousa, D.-P.V.; Papadopoulou, E.V.K.; Papadopoulou, K.K.K.; Fountoulakis, K.N. University students' mental health amidst the COVID-19 quarantine in Greece. *Psychiatry Res.* **2020**, *290*, 113111. [CrossRef]
29. World Health Organization. *Spotlight on Adolescent Health and Well-Being*; Findings from the 2017/2018 Health Behaviour in School-Aged Children (HBSC) Survey in Europe and Canada; WHO Regional Office for Europe: Copenhagen, Denmark, 2020.
30. Bruckauf, Z. *Adolescents' Mental Health*; United Nations: New York, NY, USA, 2017.
31. Magklara, K.; Lazaratou, H.; Barbouni, A.; Poulas, K.; Farsalinos, K. Impact of COVID-19 pandemic and lockdown measures on mental health of children and adolescents in Greece. *medRxiv* **2020**. [CrossRef]
32. Craig, C.L.; Marshall, A.L.; Sjöström, M.; Bauman, A.E.; Booth, M.L.; Ainsworth, B.E.; Pratt, M.; Ekelund, U.; Yngve, A.; Sallis, J.F. International physical activity questionnaire: 12-country reliability and validity. *Med. Sci. Sports Exerc.* **2003**, *35*, 1381–1395. [CrossRef]
33. World Health Organization. *Wellbeing Measures in Primary Health Care/the DEPCARE Project: Report on a WHO Meeting, Stockholm, Sweden, 12–13 February 1998*; World Health Organization: Geneva, Switzerland, 1998.
34. Huelsman, T.J.; Nemanick, R.C.; Munz, D.C. Scales to Measure Four Dimensions of Dispositional Mood: Positive Energy, Tiredness, Negative Activation, and Relaxation. *Educ. Psychol. Meas.* **1998**, *58*, 804–819. [CrossRef]
35. Ammar, A.; Trabelsi, K.; Brach, M.; Chtourou, H.; Boukhris, O.; Masmoudi, L.; Bouaziz, B.; Bentlage, E.; How, D.; Ahmed, M.; et al. Effects of home confinement on mental health and lifestyle behaviours during the COVID-19 outbreak: Insight from the "ECLB-COVID19" multi countries survey. *medRxiv* **2020**. [CrossRef]
36. Ammar, A.; Brach, M.; Trabelsi, K.; Chtourou, H.; Boukhris, O.; Masmoudi, L.; Bouaziz, B.; Bentlage, E. Effects of COVID-19 Home Confinement on Eating Behaviour and Physical Activity: Results of the ECLB-COVID19 International Online Survey. *Nutrients* **2020**, *12*, 1583. [CrossRef]
37. Li, S.H.; Beames, J.R.; Newby, J.M.; Maston, K.; Christensen, H.; Werner-Seidler, A. The impact of COVID-19 on the lives and mental health of Australian adolescents. *medRxiv* **2020**. [CrossRef]
38. Tee, M.L.; Tee, C.A.; Anlacan, J.P.; Aligam, K.J.G.; Reyes, P.W.C.; Kuruchittham, V.; Ho, R.C. Psychological impact of COVID-19 pandemic in the Philippines. *J. Affect. Disord.* **2020**, *277*, 379–391. [CrossRef] [PubMed]
39. McCormack, G.R.; Doyle-Baker, P.K.; Petersen, J.A.; Ghoneim, D. Parent anxiety and perceptions of their child's physical activity and sedentary behaviour during the COVID-19 pandemic in Canada. *Prev. Med. Rep.* **2020**, *20*, 101275. [CrossRef] [PubMed]
40. Cusinato, M.; Iannattone, S.; Spoto, A.; Poli, M.; Moretti, C.; Gatta, M.; Miscioscia, M. Stress, Resilience, and Well-Being in Italian Children and Their Parents during the COVID-19 Pandemic. *Int. J. Environ. Res. Public Health* **2020**, *17*, 8297. [CrossRef] [PubMed]
41. Maugeri, G.; Castrogiovanni, P.; Battaglia, G.; Pippi, R.; D'Agata, V.; Palma, A.; Di Rosa, M.; Musumeci, G. The impact of physical activity on psychological health during Covid-19 pandemic in Italy. *Heliyon* **2020**, *6*, e04315. [CrossRef] [PubMed]
42. Chi, X.; Liang, K.; Chen, S.-T.; Huang, Q.; Huang, L.; Yu, Q.; Jiao, C.; Guo, T.; Stubbs, B.; Hossain, M.M.; et al. Mental health problems among Chinese adolescents during the COVID-19: The importance of nutrition and physical activity. *Int. J. Clin. Health Psychol. IJCHP* **2020**, 100218. [CrossRef]
43. Lu, C.; Chi, X.; Liang, K.; Chen, S.-T.; Huang, L.; Guo, T.; Jiao, C.; Yu, Q.; Veronese, N.; Soares, F.C.; et al. Moving More and Sitting Less as Healthy Lifestyle Behaviors are Protective Factors for Insomnia, Depression, and Anxiety Among Adolescents During the COVID-19 Pandemic. *Psychol. Res. Behav. Manag.* **2020**, *13*, 1223–1233. [CrossRef]
44. Brooke, H.L.; Atkin, A.J.; Corder, K.; Brage, S.; van Sluijs, E.M.F. Frequency and duration of physical activity bouts in school-aged children: A comparison within and between days. *Prev. Med. Rep.* **2016**, *4*, 585–590. [CrossRef]

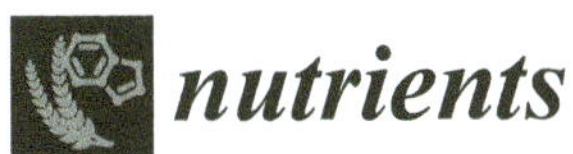
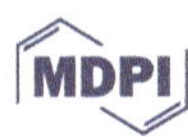

Article

Associations between Children's Genetic Susceptibility to Obesity, Infant's Appetite and Parental Feeding Practices in Toddlerhood

Claire Guivarch [1,*], Marie-Aline Charles [1,2], Anne Forhan [1], Ken K. Ong [3], Barbara Heude [1] and Blandine de Lauzon-Guillain [1]

[1] Université de Paris, CRESS, INSERM, INRAE, F-75004 Paris, France; marie-aline.charles@inserm.fr (M.-A.C.); anne.forhan@inserm.fr (A.F.); barbara.heude@inserm.fr (B.H.); blandine.delauzon@inserm.fr (B.d.L.-G.)
[2] Unité Mixte Inserm-Ined-EFS ELFE, Ined, F-75020 Paris, France
[3] MRC Epidemiology Unit and Department of Paediatrics, Institute of Metabolic Science, University of Cambridge, Cambridge CB2 0QQ, UK; Ken.Ong@mrc-epid.cam.ac.uk
* Correspondence: claire.guivarch@inserm.fr; Tel.: +33-145-595-019

Citation: Guivarch, C.; Charles, M.-A.; Forhan, A.; Ong, K.K.; Heude, B.; de Lauzon-Guillain, B. Associations between Children's Genetic Susceptibility to Obesity, Infant's Appetite and Parental Feeding Practices in Toddlerhood. *Nutrients* **2021**, *13*, 1468. https://doi.org/10.3390/nu13051468

Academic Editor: Odysseas Androutsos and Evangelia Charmandari

Received: 8 March 2021
Accepted: 23 April 2021
Published: 26 April 2021

Publisher's Note: MDPI stays neutral with regard to jurisdictional claims in published maps and institutional affiliations.

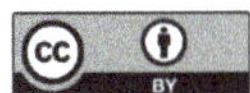

Copyright: © 2021 by the authors. Licensee MDPI, Basel, Switzerland. This article is an open access article distributed under the terms and conditions of the Creative Commons Attribution (CC BY) license (https://creativecommons.org/licenses/by/4.0/).

Abstract: Previous findings suggest that parental feeding practices may adapt to children's eating behavior and sex, but few studies assessed these associations in toddlerhood. We aimed to study the associations between infant's appetite or children's genetic susceptibility to obesity and parental feeding practices. We assessed infant's appetite (three-category indicator: low, normal or high appetite, labelled 4-to-24-month appetite) and calculated a combined obesity risk-allele score (genetic risk score of body mass index (BMI-GRS)) in a longitudinal study of respectively 1358 and 932 children from the EDEN cohort. Parental feeding practices were assessed at 2-year-follow-up by the CFPQ. Three of the five tested scores were used as continuous variables; others were considered as binary variables, according to the median. Associations between infant's appetite or child's BMI-GRS and parental feeding practices were assessed by linear and logistic regression models, stratified on child's sex if interactions were significant. 4-to-24-month appetite was positively associated with restrictive feeding practices among boys and girls. Among boys, high compared to normal 4-to-24-month appetite was associated with higher use of food to regulate child's emotions (OR [95% CI] = 2.24 [1.36; 3.68]). Child's BMI-GRS was not related to parental feeding practices. Parental feeding practices may adapt to parental perception of infant's appetite and child's sex.

Keywords: parental feeding practices; genetic susceptibility to obesity; eating behavior; birth cohort

1. Introduction

Childhood overweight and obesity are a major public health challenge of this century, affecting an estimated 38.2 million children under 5 years old worldwide in 2019 [1]. Childhood obesity is associated with short- and long-term adverse outcomes, such as adulthood obesity and cardio-metabolic disorders [2]. Obesity is mostly caused by interactions between genetic susceptibility and obesogenic environment [3,4]. A great number of the genes identified by genome-wide association study of obesity and also those from studies of monogenic forms of severe childhood obesity appear to be involved in the central regulation of food intake [5]. Moreover, several studies have shown that genetic susceptibility to obesity affects infant [6] and child's appetite [4,7] and that early appetite is related to the child's weight status later in childhood [8–10].

According to the Developmental Origins of Health and Disease concept, early childhood is a vulnerability window: the first years of life are characterized by a rapid change in infant feeding from milk to solid foods that will lay the foundation for future eating habits and behaviors [11,12]. Parents play a key role in the development of healthy eating habits and eating behavior in childhood in that they decide which foods the child is offered as well as the portion size, feeding time and meal environment [12,13]. Moreover, parents play a model role [14,15]. The influence of parents on their child's eating behavior development starts in the first weeks of life with breastfeeding. Indeed, previous studies suggest that breastfeeding is positively associated with infant's self-regulation capacities [12] and is also related to child's eating behavior [16] and parental feeding practices [17]. Other studies suggest that parental feeding practices may differ according to child's sex and that, for the same parental feeding practice, child's response may depend on their sex [18,19]. Moreover, several cross-sectional studies have found that coercive parental feeding practices, such as restriction or pressure to eat, are related to child's weight status (e.g., parental restrictive feeding practices are associated to higher child's BMI, whereas parental pressure to eat is associated to lower child's BMI) [20–22], child's intake (e.g., parental restrictive practices are associated with increased child's energy intake) [23–25] or eating behavior (e.g., parental pressure to eat may enhance food dislikes) [26,27]. Some longitudinal studies found that coercive feeding practices led to lower childhood BMI [28,29]. Recent longitudinal studies have highlighted that associations between child's weight status and eating behavior and parental feeding practices could be more complex, non-linear and bidirectional [13,30–32]. They have especially suggested that parents may adapt their feeding practices to the appetite of their child (i.e., using restriction if the infant's appetite is considered high) [31] and to the child's weight status [33–36]. The child's genetic susceptibility to obesity appeared positively related to infant's appetite [6] and to appetitive traits in childhood [7,37], but a recent review stated that it remains unclear how genetic and parental feeding practices interact to influence child's appetite [38].

In this context, we aimed to study the associations between infant's appetite or child's genetic susceptibility to obesity and parental feeding practices in toddlerhood with a longitudinal design. We hypothesized that (1) infants perceived as always asking for food during first years of life may lead to higher parental restrictive feeding practices and higher parental use of food for non-nutritional purposes (i.e., using food to manage infant's emotions or as a reward); (2) infants perceived as having low appetite during the first years of life may lead to greater parental pressure to eat, and (3) a higher child's genetic risk score of body mass index (BMI-GRS) may lead to higher use of restrictive parental feeding practices and lower use of pressure to eat.

2. Materials and Methods

2.1. Study Population

The EDEN mother-child study is a prospective cohort aiming at assessing prenatal and postnatal determinants of childhood growth, development and health [39]. Briefly, 2002 pregnant women under 24 weeks' amenorrhea were recruited from 2003 to 2006 in two French university hospitals, in Poitiers and Nancy. Exclusion criteria were multiple pregnancies, known diabetes before pregnancy, illiteracy and planning to move outside the region in the next 3 years. This study was approved by the ethics research committee of Bicêtre hospital (ID 0270 of 12 December 2002) and by the National Commission on Informatics and Liberty (CNIL, ID 902267 of 12 December 2002). Written consent was obtained from both parents.

Data collected during pregnancy and at birth included sociodemographic variables, maternal smoking and newborn characteristics (sex, gestational age, birthweight). At 4, 8, 12 and 24 months after birth, mothers completed mailed questionnaires that provided detailed information on their feeding practices.

2.2. Infant's Appetite

At ages 4, 8, 12 and 24 months, maternal perception of infant's appetite was assessed with a single item, translated as "Usually, would you say that your baby: (1) is always hungry or demanding to feed? (2) demands to feed the same as other babies of the same age? (3) needs to be stimulated to eat (at 4, 8 and 12 months) or is not often hungry (at 24 months)?" High appetite was defined by the category "is always hungry or demanding to feed", normal appetite by the second category "demands to feed the same as other babies of the same age" and low appetite by the third category "needs to be stimulated to eat/not often hungry". Using the four age-specific variables, infants were classified in the "low appetite" category when parents reported a low appetite at least once up to 24 months and never reported a high appetite during this period. Infants were classified in the "high appetite" category when parents reported a high appetite at least once up to 24 months and never reported a low appetite during this period. All other infants were classified in the "normal appetite" category.

2.3. Children's Genetic Susceptibility to Obesity

DNA was extracted from cord-blood samples collected at birth [39]. As previously described, genotyping candidate single nucleotide polymorphisms (SNPs) was conducted at the Medical Research Council Epidemiology Unit, Cambridge (iPLEX platform; Sequenom) [40]. Among the 32 loci identified by Speliotes et al. as having genome-wide significant associations with BMI in adults [41], in the present study, we considered the 16 SNPs also showing associations with childhood BMI in that original report [41] or in subsequent data [42], as in previous studies [6]. Briefly, a combined obesity risk-allele score, indicating genetic susceptibility to obesity (BMI-GRS), was calculated for each included infant as the sum of risk alleles (0, 1 or 2) associated with higher BMI across the 16 SNPs. In the present study, the score ranged from 5 to 22 from a possible range of 0 to 32.

2.4. Parental Feeding Practices

At the 2-year follow-up, parental feeding practices were evaluated by using the Comprehensive Feeding Practices Questionnaire (CFPQ) [43] translated in French and validated in French children [44]. In the present analysis, five scales of the questionnaire were used: restriction for health (4 items, e.g., if I did not guide or regulate my child's eating, s/he would eat too much of his/her favourite foods, Cronbach's $\alpha = 0.79$), restriction for weight (4 items, e.g., I encourage my child to eat less so he/she won't get fat, Cronbach's $\alpha = 0.67$), pressure to eat (3 items, e.g., my child should always eat all of the food on his/her plate, Cronbach's $\alpha = 0.59$), using food as a reward (3 items, e.g., I offer my child his/her favourite foods in exchange for good behaviour, Cronbach's $\alpha = 0.45$) and using food to regulate the child's emotions (3 items, e.g., do you give this child something to eat or drink if s/he is upset even if you think s/he is not hungry?, Cronbach's $\alpha = 0.66$). Each item is associated with a score between 1 (never or disagree) and 5 (always or agree). Scores of coercive parental feeding practices (restriction for health, restriction for weight and pressure to eat) were considered as continuous variables. Because scores were not normally distributed and transformations tested did not help to reach normality, parental feeding practices of using food as a reward or to regulate the child's emotions were considered as binary variables, according to the median in our sample. "Normal use" of a specific parental feeding practice was defined by a score below the median and "high use" by a score equal to or above the median.

2.5. Potential Confounders

The maternal characteristics were collected at the maternity ward and included maternal age at delivery (years), primiparity (yes/no), maternal education level (<high school diploma, high school diploma, 2-year university degree and 5-year university degree), household income (≤€1500, €1501 to €2300, €2301 to €3000 and >€3000) and smoking status during pregnancy (no smoker/ smoker). The child's characteristics were collected at birth and during the first year: sex, birth weight (kg), any breastfeeding duration (<1 month, 1 to <4 months and at least 4 months) and age at complementary food introduction (months). At each clinical examination (birth, 1, 3 and 5 years), the child's weight and length were measured. At each follow-up (4, 8 and 12 months, 2, 3, 4 and 5 years), weight and length data were collected from self-administered questionnaires and clinical visits when reported by health professionals in the child's health booklet. Individual growth curves for weight and length were predicted by using the Jenss growth curve model as previously described [45]. This method allows for calculating parameters for individual growth patterns, such as weight, length and body mass index (BMI). In the present study, we used the WHO weight-for-length z-score at 2 years as a covariate in sensitivity models.

2.6. Sample Selection

Of the 2002 women recruited, 76 were excluded because they left the study before or at the time of delivery; 24 because of miscarriages, intrauterine death or discontinuation of pregnancy for medical reasons; and nine because they delivered outside the study hospitals. Data on birthweight were available for 1899 newborns. Infants with missing data on at least one parental feeding practice or less than 2 time points for infant's appetite assessment (n = 499) and on potential confounders (n = 42) were then excluded (Figure 1). These exclusions lead to a sample of 1358 infants for complete-case analysis of the association between infant's appetite and parental feeding practices.

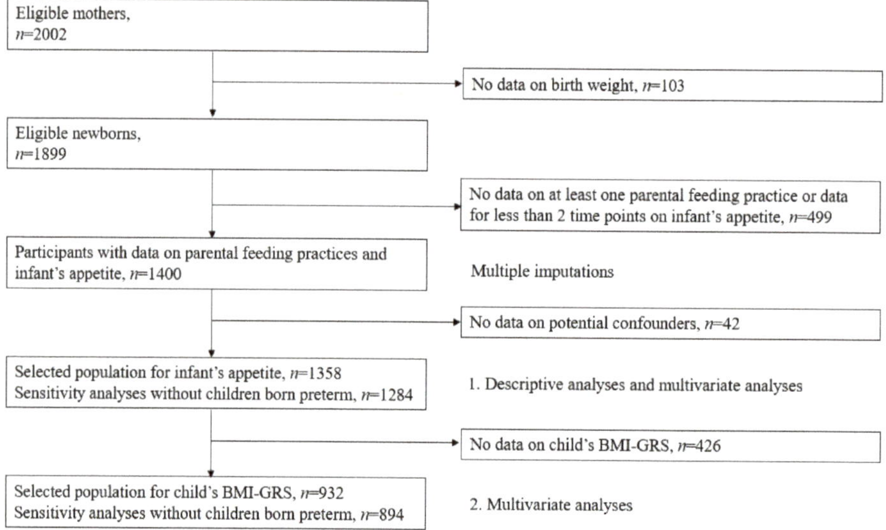

Figure 1. Flow of participants in the study.

Children with missing data on child's BMI-GRS were excluded for analyses involving BMI-GRS, leading to a sample of 932 infants.

2.7. Statistical Analyses
2.7.1. Main Analyses

Comparisons between included and excluded populations were assessed by chi-square and Student t-tests. Bivariate analyses between infant's appetite or child's BMI-GRS and parental feeding practices involved unadjusted linear and logistic regression models. Associations between infant's appetite or child's BMI-GRS and parental feeding practices were tested with linear regression models for coercive parental feeding practices and with logistic regression models for parental use of food for non-nutritional purposes. Analyses were run separately for each outcome. We tested the interaction between child's sex and infant's appetite for each parental feeding practice. Significant interactions were observed for the following feeding practices: restriction for health (p = 0.003), restriction for weight (p = 0.0004), emotional feeding (p = 0.02) and the interaction was almost significant for food as a reward (p = 0.08). Thus, analyses were performed separately among girls and boys for these feeding practices. As no significant interaction was found between child's BMI-GRS and child's sex (all $p > 0.2$), the associations between child's BMI-GRS and parental feeding practices were conducted on the whole sample.

For multivariable analyses, potential confounding factors included in the models were identified from the literature and selected by using the Directed Acyclic Graphs method. Then, models used to test the association between child's BMI-GRS and parental feeding practices were adjusted only for study center, whereas models used to test the associations between infant's appetite and parental feeding practices were adjusted for study center as well as for maternal characteristics (age at delivery, primiparity, education level, household income, smoking status during pregnancy) and child's characteristics (birth weight, any breastfeeding duration and age at complementary food introduction). Analyses conducted on the whole sample were also adjusted for child's sex.

2.7.2. Sensitivity Analyses

In the first sensitivity analysis, we excluded infants born before 37 gestational weeks because parental feeding practices may differ for pre-term infants [46], which led to samples of 1284 ($n = 667$ boys and $n = 617$ girls) for infant's appetite analyses and 894 infants for BMI-GRS analyses. For infant's appetite analyses, a second sensitivity analysis was performed by further adjusting on child's WHO weight-for-length z-score at 2 years. In the third sensitivity analysis, we considered 4-to-12-month appetite instead of the 4-to-24-month summary variable, to test the potential influence of children's current appetite. In another sensitivity analysis, we considered 1-year appetite instead of the 4-to-24-month summary variable, to test the stability of the main findings using a raw variable [6]. Another sensitivity analysis involved a weighted BMI-GRS (in which risk alleles were weighted by their reported effects size on adult BMI) [41,42] instead of the crude BMI-GRS.

We first conducted analyses on complete cases. Then, we used multiple imputations to deal with missing data on exposure variables and potential confounders. Missing data for child's BMI-GRS were only imputed if maternal BMI-GRS was available. The number of missing data ranged from 0% to 31.1% per variable (Supplementary Table S1). We assumed that data were missing at random and generated five independent datasets with the fully conditional specification method (MI procedure, FCS statement, NIMPUTE option), and then calculated pooled effect estimates (SAS MIANALYSE procedure). Continuous variables were imputed with predictive mean matching, and logistic regressions were used for categorical variables. To generate significance testing of categorical variables, the median of the p-values from the imputed data analyses in each dataset was used, as proposed by Eekhout et al. [47].

Analyses were conducted with SAS v9.4 (SAS Institute, Cary, NC, USA). $p < 0.05$ was considered statistically significant.

3. Results

Infants included in and excluded from the present study were similar concerning child's sex, birth weight and gestational age. However, infants included were breastfed longer and were born to older mothers, with lower BMI, higher education level, higher household income, higher rate of primiparity and lower rate of smoking during pregnancy than those excluded. The maternal and child's characteristics of the study population, parental feeding practices and infant's appetite are summarized in Tables 1 and 2.

Table 1. Characteristics of the study population (*n* = 1358).

	% (n), Mean (SD) or Median (Q1–Q3)
Maternal Characteristics	
Center	
Poitiers	46.8% (636)
Nancy	53.2% (722)
Age at delivery (years)	29.9 (4.7)
Primiparous	47.2% (641)
Education level	
<High school diploma	23.1% (314)
High school diploma	17.7% (240)
2 years university degree	23.2% (315)
5 years university degree	36.0% (489)
Household income (€/month)	
$\leq$1500	12.6% (171)
1501–2300	29.2% (397)
2301–3000	28.1% (382)
>3000	30.0% (408)
Smoker status during pregnancy	22.0% (299)
BMI before pregnancy (kg/m^2)	23.1 (4.4)
Parental Feeding Practices [a]	
Restriction for health	3.4 (1.0)
Restriction for weight	1.7 (0.6)
Pressure to eat	2.3 (0.8)
Food as a reward	1.33 (1.00–1.66)
Emotional feeding	1.33 (1.00–1.66)
Child Characteristics	
Boys	52.1% (707)
Birth weight (kg)	3.3 (0.5)
Gestational age (weeks)	39.2 (1.7)
Pre-term birth (<37 weeks)	5.4% (74)
Any breastfeeding duration, months	
<1	33.3% (452)
1 to <4	31.0% (421)
$\geq$4	35.7% (485)
BMI genetic risk score (0–32 score)	13.7 (2.5)
WHO weight for length z-score at 2 years	0.2 (1.7)

BMI, body mass index. [a] Parental feeding practices were assessed using the Comprehensive Feeding Practices Questionnaire [43] at the 2-year follow-up. Each studied parental feeding practice is associated to a score between 1 and 5. Scores of coercive parental feeding practices (restriction for health, restriction for weight and pressure to eat) were studied as continuous variables. Because scores of parental feeding practices of using food for non-nutritional purposes (as a reward or to regulate child's emotions) were not normally distributed and those transformations did not help to reach normality, these scores were studied as binary variables, according to the median.

Table 2. Description of infant's appetite from 4 to 24 months.

	4 Months	8 Months	12 Months	24 Months
Infant appetite				
Needs to be stimulated	2.7% (36)	2.7% (36)	4.8% (62)	6.6% (90)
Normal appetite	93.4% (1239)	95.2% (1252)	92.0% (1188)	88% (1194)
Always hungry	3.9% (52)	2.1% (27)	3.3% (42)	5.4% (73)
4-to-24-month appetite				
Low appetite	11.1% (151)			
Normal appetite	77.7% (1055)			
High appetite	11.2% (152)			

Data are % (n). 4-to-24-month appetite is an indicator of infant's appetite. Infants were classified in the low appetite category when parents reported a low appetite at least once up to 24 months and never reported a high appetite during this period. Infants were classified in the high appetite category when parents reported a high appetite at least once up to 24 months and never reported a low appetite during this period. All other infants were classified in the normal-appetite category.

3.1. Infant's Appetite and Parental Feeding Practices at 2 Years

In the main adjusted analyses, 4-to-24-month appetite was positively associated to parental restriction for weight among girls (linear trend $p < 0.001$) and boys (linear trend $p = 0.03$) at 2 years (Table 3). Among girls only, 4-to-24-month appetite was positively associated to parental restriction for health (linear trend $p < 0.001$) (Table 3) and to parental use of food as a reward (linear trend $p = 0.002$) at 2 years (Supplementary Table S2). Moreover, low compared to normal 4-to-24-month infant's appetite was related to higher parental pressure to eat (β [95% CI] = 0.15 [0.01; 0.28]) and high 4-to-24-month infant's appetite was related to higher parental pressure to eat (β [95% CI] = 0.14 [0.00; 0.28]) at 2 years (Table 3). Among boys only, low compared to normal 4-to-24-month appetite was related to higher use of food as a reward (OR [95% CI] = 2.69 [1.50; 4.81]) and high 4-to-24-month appetite was related to higher use of food as a reward (OR [95% CI] = 1.58 [1.01; 2.49]) (Supplementary Table S2) and to regulate the child's emotions (OR [95% CI] = 2.24 [1.36; 3.68]) at 2 years (Table 4).

Sensitivity analyses (Tables 3 and 4, Supplementary Table S2) revealed similar results after excluding infants born before 37 gestational weeks. Findings were similar after further adjustment on child's 2-year WHO weight-for-length z-score. When considering 4-to-12-month appetite instead of 4-to-24-month appetite, the main finding remained unchanged, but the associations between infant's appetite and parental pressure to eat were no longer significant. Moreover, among boys, for parental use of food as a reward, the association with low appetite was weakened and became non-significant, but the same tendency was observed. After multiple imputations, similar results were found, except concerning use of food as a reward: among boys, the association with high 4-to-24-month appetite was weakened and no more significant. When we assessed the association between appetite at 1 year and parental feeding practices at 2 years, low 1-year appetite was related to lower parental restriction for health among girls, and lower parental restriction for weight among boys, whereas high 1-year appetite was only related to higher restriction for weight among girls (Supplementary Tables S4 and S5).

Table 3. Associations between infant's appetite (reference = normal appetite) and coercive feeding practices.

	Restriction for Health				Restriction for Weight				Pressure to Eat	
	Boys β [95% CI]	p	Girls β [95% CI]	p	Boys β [95% CI]	p	Girls β [95% CI]	p	β [95% CI]	p
Unadjusted model										
4-to-24-month appetite		0.7		<0.001		0.06		<0.001		0.02
N	707		651		707		651		1358	
Low appetite	0.07 [−0.19; 0.34]		−0.21 [−0.44; 0.02]		−0.17 [−0.32; −0.01]		−0.12 [−0.26; 0.01]		0.15 [0.01; 0.29]	
Normal appetite	0 [Ref]		0 [Ref]		0 [Ref]		0 [Ref]		0 [Ref]	
High appetite	−0.07 [−0.29; 0.15]		0.47 [0.19; 0.76]		0.06 [−0.07; 0.20]		0.48 [0.32; 0.65]		0.15 [0.01; 0.29]	
Main analyses *										
4-to-24-month appetite		0.7		<0.001		0.06		<0.001		0.03
N	707		651		707		651		1358	
Low appetite	0.06 [−0.21; 0.33]		−0.22 [−0.46; 0.01]		−0.17 [−0.32; −0.01]		−0.12 [−0.25; 0.01]		0.15 [0.01; 0.28]	
Normal appetite	0 [Ref]		0 [Ref]		0 [Ref]		0 [Ref]		0 [Ref]	
High appetite	−0.07 [−0.29; 0.16]		0.44 [0.16; 0.72]		0.07 [−0.07; 0.20]		0.46 [0.30; 0.62]		0.14 [0.00; 0.28]	
Sensitivity analyses *										
4-to-24-month appetite, without children born preterm		0.5		0.001		0.1		<0.001		0.03
N	667		617		667		617		1284	
Low appetite	0.07 [−0.20; 0.35]		−0.13 [−0.37; 0.11]		−0.16 [−0.33; 0.00]		−0.11 [−0.25; 0.02]		0.16 [0.01; 0.30]	
Normal appetite	0 [Ref]		0 [Ref]		0 [Ref]		0 [Ref]		0 [Ref]	
High appetite	−0.12 [−0.36; 0.12]		0.50 [0.21; 0.78]		0.01 [−0.13; 0.15]		0.49 [0.33; 0.65]		0.14 [−0.01; 0.28]	
4-to-24-month appetite, further adjusted for WHO weight-for-length z-score		0.7		0.009		0.5		<0.001		0.02
N	707		651		707		651		1358	
Low appetite	0.06 [−0.21; 0.33]		−0.17 [−0.41; 0.06]		−0.09 [−0.25; 0.07]		−0.06 [−0.20; 0.07]		0.10 [−0.04; 0.24]	
Normal appetite	0 [Ref]		0 [Ref]		0 [Ref]		0 [Ref]		0 [Ref]	
High appetite	−0.07 [−0.29; 0.16]		0.38 [0.09; 0.67]		0.00 [−0.13; 0.13]		0.40 [0.24; 0.56]		0.19 [0.05; 0.33]	
4-to-12-month appetite		0.5		0.001		0.09		0.04		0.2
N	707		651		707		651		1358	
Low appetite	−0.05 [−0.40; 0.31]		−0.36 [−0.63; −0.09]		−0.24 [−0.45; −0.03]		−0.09 [−0.25; 0.06]		0.01 [−0.16; 0.18]	
Normal appetite	0 [Ref]		0 [Ref]		0 [Ref]		0 [Ref]		0 [Ref]	
High appetite	−0.15 [−0.41; 0.11]		0.46 [0.10; 0.82]		−0.04 [−0.19; 0.12]		0.32 [0.11; 0.52]		0.15 [−0.02; 0.32]	
4-to-24-month appetite, multiple imputation		0.8		0.001		0.04		<0.001		0.04
N	729		671		729		671		1400	
Low appetite	0.04 [−0.23; 0.31]		−0.22 [−0.45; 0.02]		−0.17 [−0.33; −0.01]		−0.11 [−0.24; 0.02]		0.13 [0.00; 0.27]	
Normal appetite	0 [Ref]		0 [Ref]		0 [Ref]		0 [Ref]		0 [Ref]	
High appetite	−0.07 [−0.30; 0.15]		0.43 [0.15; 0.72]		0.07 [−0.06; 0.20]		0.45 [0.29; 0.61]		0.13 [−0.01; 0.27]	

One model per exposition variable. Data are β [95% confidence intervals]. * Linear regression analyses adjusted for study center, maternal age at delivery, primiparity, maternal education level, household income, smoking status during pregnancy, child's sex—when analyses were not stratified on child's sex, birth weight, gestational age, prematurity and any breastfeeding duration. The interaction between child's sex and infant's appetite was tested for each parental feeding practices and conducted to a stratification on child's sex for restriction for health (p for interaction = 0.003) and restriction for weight (p for interaction = 0.0004) but not for parental pressure to eat (p for interaction = 0.3).

Table 4. Association between infant's appetite (reference = normal appetite) and parental feeding practices of using food to regulate child's emotions.

	Emotional Feeding (Ref = Normal)			
	Boys **High**	*p*	**Girls** **High**	*p*
Unadjusted Model				
4-to-24-month appetite		0.002		0.5
N	707		651	
Low appetite	1.47 [0.85; 2.53]		0.79 [0.51; 1.25]	
Normal appetite	1 [Ref]		1 [Ref]	
High appetite	2.29 [1.41; 3.72]		1.20 [0.68; 2.11]	
Main analyses *				
4-to-24-month appetite		0.004		0.5
N	707		651	
Low appetite	1.48 [0.85; 2.58]		0.79 [0.50; 1.27]	
Normal appetite	1 [Ref]		1 [Ref]	
High appetite	2.24 [1.36; 3.68]		1.13 [0.63; 2.02]	
Sensitivity analyses *				
4-to-24-month appetite, without children born preterm		0.006		0.7
N	667		617	
Low appetite	1.49 [0.84; 2.64]		0.82 [0.50; 1.35]	
Normal appetite	1 [Ref]		1 [Ref]	
High appetite	2.26 [1.33; 3.85]		1.05 [0.58; 1.89]	
4-to-24-month appetite, further adjusted for WHO weight-for-length z-score		0.005		0.7
N	707		651	
Low appetite	1.54 [0.88; 2.72]		0.83 [0.52; 1.35]	
Normal appetite	1 [Ref]		1 [Ref]	
High appetite	2.16 [1.31; 3.57]		1.06 [0.59; 1.91]	
4-to-12-month appetite		0.02		0.5
N	707		651	
Low appetite	1.40 [0.66; 2.95]		0.79 [0.46; 1.35]	
Normal appetite	1 [Ref]		1 [Ref]	
High appetite	2.32 [1.28; 4.22]		1.29 [0.61; 2.71]	
4-to-24-month appetite, multiple imputation		0.006		0.5
N	729		671	
Low appetite	1.04 [0.70; 1.53]		0.81 [0.58; 1.14]	
Normal appetite	1 [Ref]		1 [Ref]	
High appetite	1.41 [0.99; 2.01]		1.14 [0.77; 1.69]	

One model per exposition variable. Data are odds ratios [95% confidence intervals]. * Logistic regression analyses adjusted for a study center, maternal age at delivery, primiparity, maternal education level, household income, smoking status during pregnancy, birth weight, gestational age, prematurity and any breastfeeding duration. The interaction between child's sex and infant's appetite was tested for each parental feeding practices and conducted to a stratification on child's sex for emotional feeding ($p_{for\ interaction}$ = 0.02).

3.2. Child's BMI-GRS and Parental Feeding Practices at 2 Years

Child's BMI-GRS was not related to any of the five parental feeding practices tested in our main analyses. Similar results were found in sensitivity analyses (Tables 5 and 6, Supplementary Table S3).

Table 5. Associations between child's genetic susceptibility to obesity and coercive feeding practices.

	Restriction for Health		Restriction for Weight		Pressure to Eat	
	β [95% CI]	*p*	β [95% CI]	*p*	β [95% CI]	*p*
Unadjusted model						
Child BMI-GRS, per risk allele (*n* = 932)	−0.01 [−0.03; 0.02]	0.6	0.01 [−0.01; 0.02]	0.3	0.01 [−0.01; 0.03]	0.3
Main analyses *						
Child BMI-GRS, per risk allele (*n* = 932)	−0.01 [−0.03; 0.02]	0.7	0.01 [−0.01; 0.02]	0.3	0.01 [−0.01; 0.03]	0.3
Sensitivity analyses *						
Child weighted BMI-GRS, per risk allele (*n* = 932)	−0.01 [−0.03; 0.01]	0.5	0.01 [−0.01; 0.02]	0.4	0.01 [−0.01; 0.02]	0.6
Child BMI-GRS without children born preterm, per risk allele (*n* = 894)	−0.01 [−0.03; 0.02]	0.7	0.01 [−0.01; 0.03]	0.2	0.01 [−0.01; 0.03]	0.4
Child BMI-GRS, per risk allele, after multiple imputation (*n* = 1342) [a]	0.00 [−0.03; 0.02]	0.7	0.01 [−0.01; 0.02]	0.3	0.02 [0.00; 0.03]	0.08

One model per exposition variable. Data are β [95% confidence intervals]. * Linear regression analyses adjusted for study center. BMI-GRS, genetic risk score of body mass index. [a] Missing data for child's BMI-GRS were only imputed if maternal BMI-GRS was available.

Table 6. Associations between child's genetic susceptibility to obesity and parental feeding practices of using food for non-nutritional purposes.

	Emotional Feeding	
	OR [95% CI]	*p*
Unadjusted model		
Child BMI-GRS, per risk allele (*n* = 932)	1.00 [0.95; 1.05]	1
Main analyses *		
Child BMI-GRS, per risk allele (*n* = 932)	1.00 [0.95; 1.05]	0.9
Sensitivity analyses *		
Child weighted BMI-GRS, per risk allele (*n* = 932)	1.01 [0.97; 1.06]	0.6
Child BMI-GRS without children born preterm, per risk allele (*n* = 894)	1.01 [0.95; 1.06]	0.8
Child BMI-GRS, per risk allele, after multiple imputation (*n* = 1342) [a]	1.00 [0.95; 1.04]	0.9

One model per exposition variable. Data are odds ratios [95% confidence intervals]. * Logistic regression analyses adjusted for study center. BMI-GRS, genetic risk score of body mass index. [a] Missing data for child's BMI-GRS were only imputed if maternal BMI-GRS was available.

4. Discussion

In our study, children's genetic susceptibility to obesity was not associated with any parental feeding practices at 2 years, whereas perceived infant's appetite was associated with several parental feeding practices at 2 years and differed among child's sex. Infant's appetite was positively related to restrictive feeding practices, but associations were stronger among girls than among boys. Moreover, high appetite was related to higher parental use of food to regulate child's emotions in boys but not in girls. Both low and high infant's appetite were also associated to higher parental pressure to eat.

During the first year of life, infants have the ability to self-regulate their food intake based on their satiety and hunger cues. Experimental studies have shown that some coercive feeding practices such as parental restriction or pressure to eat may have a counterproductive effect because limiting access to some foods may increase the child's attraction to the restricted foods [48] or have a negative impact on the child's food intake self-regulation [49], and parental pressure to eat may enhance food dislikes [26]. Moreover, restrictive parental feeding practices are often considered to lead to overweight and obesity issues in later life, as summarized in literature reviews [33].

More recent studies suggested that the associations between children's BMI and parental feeding practices are bi-directional [30,32,35,50,51]. Longitudinal studies found that parental restrictive practices are developed in reaction to higher BMI in children, whereas parental pressure to eat develops in reaction to lower BMI in children [30,32–35], and the influence of children's BMI on parental feeding practices appeared more important than the influence of parental feeding practices on children's weight gain [30,32,34,35]. Then, parents may adapt their feeding practices on their perception of the child's weight status. Nevertheless, most of these studies were based on preschool or school-aged children, and none directly assessed a child's genetic susceptibility to obesity. In a previous recent study of 10-year-old children from the Twins Early Development Study, higher genetic susceptibility to obesity was associated to higher use of parental restrictive feeding practices and lower use of parental pressure to eat [52]. In the present study, children's genetic susceptibility was not related to parental feeding practices assessed in toddlerhood. This finding may be due to the BMI-GRS not being related to children's BMI before age 3 years [42] and then parents not being aware of an increased risk of overweight/obesity for their child. However, we recently highlighted that infant's appetite may be considered a mediating factor between children's genetic susceptibility to obesity and children's BMI [6]. Then, we hypothesized that infant's appetite could be considered an indicator of children's obesity risk, more apparent to parents during this early life period. Because an association between child's BMI-GRS and infant's appetite appears at an earlier age (age 1 year) [6] than an association between child's BMI-GRS and child's BMI (at age 3 years) [42], child's weight status was not considered in the main analyses. However, in sensitivity analyses, findings were similar after further adjustment on child's 2-year WHO weight-for-length z-score.

In the present longitudinal study, several associations were highlighted between infant's appetite and parental feeding practices, some of them depending on child's sex. This information may be of great importance because parental feeding practices, and children's appetitive traits appear to be established during the first 2 years of life [31]. Moreover, the early development of unhealthy eating patterns and high BMI in childhood, found to be associated with the score of genetic susceptibility to obesity, could have causal long-term implications on BMI in adulthood [53]. To our knowledge, no study had examined the moderating effect of child's sex on associations between infant's appetite and parental feeding practices in toddlerhood. In the present study, we found positive associations between infant's appetite and parental restriction for weight among boys and girls, supporting the hypothesis that parents are more restrictive with a child perceived as having an important appetite or who is food responsive [54]. We also highlighted that the associations between infant's appetite and restrictive feeding practices were stronger among girls than among boys, supporting the hypothesis that parents are more likely to be concerned about the weight status of their daughter compared to son [55]. According to literature on the differences of child's sex on associations between maternal feeding practices and child's weight status, these results could be explained with societal expectations dealing with child's weight status: girls should be slim whereas boys are perceived as sturdier if they are larger [18]. As in a previous recent US study including 139 parent-child dyads, high infant's appetite was related to higher use of pressure to eat in some of our analyses, probably because of parental willingness to increase children's intake of "healthy foods", such as fruits and vegetables [56]. We also found that low infant's appetite was associated with higher use of pressure to eat, suggesting parental willingness to increase their infant's food intakes if the infant was perceived as having low appetite. Increasing evidence shows a prospective association between parental use of food for non-nutritional purposes in childhood (i.e., as a reward or to manage children's emotions) and negative impacts on eating behavior and BMI in later life [50,57–59]. However, to our knowledge, few studies are available on the influence of children's appetite on parental use of food for non-nutritional purposes (i.e., using food as a reward or to manage infant's emotions), with inconsistent results. In fact, some studies found no association between children's eating behavior and parental use of food for non-nutritional purposes (as a reward or to regulate child's emotions) [31,57], whereas children's overeating was found positively associated with using food as a reward [50,59]. This last result is consistent with the associations found among boys, between high infant's appetite and parental use of food to manage infant's emotions and with the positive association among girls between infant's appetite and using food as a reward. Our results suggest that parents use these feeding practices to reward or to calm their child if the infant shows interest in food.

The mothers of the EDEN mother-child cohort have higher socio-economic position and a higher education level than the French population [39], so further studies are needed to assess the validity of our results among lower socio-economic populations. Even though the CFPQ was validated among French children [44], in the present study, parental use of food as a reward had a low Cronbach's α, limiting the interpretation of the results. Moreover, in the current study, only a specific set of feeding practices were considered: coercive feeding practices and use of food for non-nutritional purposes. Future studies should consider other feeding practices or dimensions of Infant Young Child Feeding, such as breastfeeding and complementary food introduction, to test the potential bi-directional association with infant's appetite. Infant's appetite was assessed prospectively from 4 months to 24 months, thus limiting memory bias. If infant's appetite was assessed by a single item up to 24 months and not a validated scale, due to the absence of a validated questionnaire at the launch of the EDEN mother-child cohort, a similar item was used in previous studies [10], and associations between appetite and growth were similar with this item and with a validated scale [6]. Furthermore, this item reflects maternal perception of infant's appetite, and further studies are needed to examine maternal ability to read child's feeding cues and responsive feeding. Moreover, data on infant's self-perceived regulation were not available in the current study, notably due to the absence of validated questionnaire to assess infant's self-regulation at the beginning of the EDEN mother-child cohort. Future longitudinal studies should assess the associations between infant's self-regulation or children's self-perceived appetite and parental feeding practices.

5. Conclusions

In this birth cohort, a BMI-GRS representing children's genetic susceptibility to obesity was not related to parental feeding practices in toddlerhood. However, in the present study, the associations between infant's appetite and parental feeding practices were moderated by child's sex. These results highlighted the need to reinforce parental education concerning feeding practices. Moreover, our results suggest that restriction for weight could be a response to infant's hungrier appetite among boys and girls. Given the reported moderating effect of restriction on the association between genetic risk of obesity and BMI in adulthood [60], future studies should examine whether restrictive feeding practices in toddlerhood may modulate the association between genetic susceptibility to obesity and BMI later in childhood.

Supplementary Materials: The following are available online at https://www.mdpi.com/article/10.3390/nu13051468/s1, Table S1: Details regarding multiple imputations. Table S2: Sensitivity analyses: associations between infant's appetite (reference = normal appetite) and parental feeding practice of using food as a reward. Table S3: Sensitivity analyses: associations between child's genetic susceptibility to obesity and parental feeding practice of using food as a reward. Table S4: Sensitivity analyses: associations between child's appetite (reference = normal appetite) at 1 year and coercive parental feeding practices. Table S5: Sensitivity analyses: associations between child's appetite (reference = normal appetite) at 1 year and parental feeding practices of using food for non-nutritional purposes. Table S6: STROBE statement.

Author Contributions: Conceptualization, C.G., B.H. and B.d.L.-G.; methodology, C.G., M.-A.C., A.F. and B.d.L.-G.; validation, B.d.L.-G.; formal analysis, C.G. and B.d.L.-G.; investigation, M.-A.C., A.F., K.K.O., B.H. and B.d.L.-G.; resources, M.-A.C. and B.H.; data curation, C.G., A.F., B.H. and B.d.L.-G.; writing—original draft preparation, C.G. and B.d.L.-G.; writing—review and editing, M.-A.C., A.F., K.K.O., B.H. and B.d.L.-G.; visualization, C.G. and B.d.L.-G.; supervision, B.d.L.-G.; project administration, B.H.; funding acquisition, M.-A.C., K.K.O. and B.H. All authors have read and agreed to the published version of the manuscript.

Funding: The EDEN study is supported by Fondation pour la Recherche Médicale (FRM), French Ministry of Research: Federative Research Institutes and Cohort Program, INSERM Human Nutrition National Research Program, and Diabetes National Research Program (through a collaboration with the French Association of Diabetic Patients (AFD)), French Ministry of Health, French Agency for Environment Security (AFSSET), French National Institute for Population Health Surveillance (InVS), Paris-Sud University, French National Institute for Health Education (INPES), Nestlé, Mutuelle Générale de l'Education Nationale (MGEN), French-speaking Association for the Study of Diabetes and Metabolism (ALFEDIAM), National Agency for Research (ANR non-thematic programme), and National Institute for Research in Public Health (IRESP: TGIR 2008 cohort in health programme). The genotyping was funded by a Collaborative Research Grant from the European Society for Paediatric Endocrinology. K.K.O. is supported by the Medical Research Council (unit program: MC_UU_12015/2). The funders had no role in the study design, data collection and analysis, decision to publish or preparation of the manuscript.

Institutional Review Board Statement: The EDEN study was approved in 2002 by the ethics research committee of Bicêtre hospital and by the National Commission on Informatics and Liberty.

Informed Consent Statement: Participating parents signed consent for themselves and their child.

Data Availability Statement: The data underlying the findings cannot be made freely available for ethical and legal restrictions imposed because this study includes a substantial number of variables that, together, could be used to re-identify the participants based on a few key characteristics and then be used to have access to other personal data. Therefore, the French ethics authority strictly forbids making these data freely available. However, they can be obtained upon request from the EDEN principal investigator. Readers may contact barbara.heude@inserm.fr to request the data. The analytic code will be made available upon request pending application and approval.

Acknowledgments: The authors thank the EDEN mother-child cohort study group, whose members are I. Annesi-Maesano, J.Y. Bernard, M.A. Charles, P. Dargent-Molina, B. de Lauzon-Guillain, P. Ducimetière, M. de Agostini, B. Foliguet, A. Forhan, X. Fritel, A. Germa, V. Goua, R. Hankard, B. Heude, M. Kaminski, B. Larroque, N. Lelong, J. Lepeule, G. Magnin, L. Marchand, C. Nabet, F Pierre, R. Slama, M.J. Saurel-Cubizolles, M. Schweitzer and O. Thiebaugeorges.

Conflicts of Interest: The authors declare no conflict of interest.

References

1. World Health Organization. Obesity and Overweight. 2020. Available online: https://www.who.int/news-room/fact-sheets/detail/obesity-and-overweight (accessed on 25 June 2020).
2. Reilly, J.J.; Kelly, J. Long-term impact of overweight and obesity in childhood and adolescence on morbidity and premature mortality in adulthood: Systematic review. *Int. J. Obes.* **2011**, *35*, 891–898. [CrossRef]
3. Goodarzi, M.O. Genetics of obesity: What genetic association studies have taught us about the biology of obesity and its complications. *Lancet Diabetes Endocrinol.* **2018**, *6*, 223–236. [CrossRef]
4. Wood, A.C. Gene-Environment Interplay in Child Eating Behaviors: What the Role of "Nature" Means for the Effects of "Nurture". *Curr. Nutr. Rep.* **2018**, *7*, 294–302. [CrossRef]
5. Day, F.R.; Loos, R.J. Developments in obesity genetics in the era of genome-wide association studies. *J. Nutr. Nutr.* **2011**, *4*, 222–238. [CrossRef]
6. De Lauzon-Guillain, B.; Koudou, Y.A.; Botton, J.; Forhan, A.; Carles, S.; Pelloux, V.; Clément, K.; Ong, K.K.; Charles, M.A.; Heude, B. Association between genetic obesity susceptibility and mother-reported eating behaviour in children up to 5 years. *Pediatr. Obes.* **2019**, *14*, e12496. [CrossRef] [PubMed]
7. Kral, T.V.; Faith, M.S. Influences on child eating and weight development from a behavioral genetics perspective. *J. Pediatr. Psychol.* **2009**, *34*, 596–605. [CrossRef]
8. Rodenburg, G.; Kremers, S.P.; Oenema, A.; van de Mheen, D. Associations of children's appetitive traits with weight and dietary behaviours in the context of general parenting. *PLoS ONE* **2012**, *7*, e50642. [CrossRef] [PubMed]
9. Quah, P.L.; Chan, Y.H.; Aris, I.M.; Pang, W.W.; Toh, J.Y.; Tint, M.T.; Broekman, B.F.; Saw, S.M.; Kwek, K.; Godfrey, K.M.; et al. Prospective associations of appetitive traits at 3 and 12 months of age with body mass index and weight gain in the first 2 years of life. *BMC Pediatr.* **2015**, *15*, 153. [CrossRef] [PubMed]
10. Van Jaarsveld, C.H.; Llewellyn, C.H.; Johnson, L.; Wardle, J. Prospective associations between appetitive traits and weight gain in infancy. *Am. J. Clin. Nutr.* **2011**, *94*, 1562–1567. [CrossRef]
11. Brown, C.L.; Vander Schaaf, E.B.; Cohen, G.M.; Irby, M.B.; Skelton, J.A. Association of Picky Eating and Food Neophobia with Weight: A Systematic Review. *Child. Obes.* **2016**, *12*, 247–262. [CrossRef]

12. Savage, J.S.; Fisher, J.O.; Birch, L.L. Parental influence on eating behavior: Conception to adolescence. *J. Law Med. Ethics* **2007**, *35*, 22–34. [CrossRef]
13. Ventura, A.K.; Birch, L.L. Does parenting affect children's eating and weight status? *Int. J. Behav. Nutr. Phys. Act.* **2008**, *5*, 15. [CrossRef] [PubMed]
14. Brown, R.; Ogden, J. Children's eating attitudes and behaviour: A study of the modelling and control theories of parental influence. *Health Educ. Res.* **2004**, *19*, 261–271. [CrossRef]
15. Carper, J.L.; Orlet Fisher, J.; Birch, L.L. Young girls' emerging dietary restraint and disinhibition are related to parental control in child feeding. *Appetite* **2000**, *35*, 121–129. [CrossRef]
16. Yelverton, C.A.; Geraghty, A.A.; O'Brien, E.C.; Killeen, S.L.; Horan, M.K.; Donnelly, J.M.; Larkin, E.; Mehegan, J.; McAuliffe, F.M. Breastfeeding and maternal eating behaviours are associated with child eating behaviours: Findings from the ROLO Kids Study. *Eur. J. Clin. Nutr.* **2021**, *75*, 670–679. [CrossRef]
17. Taveras, E.M.; Scanlon, K.S.; Birch, L.; Rifas-Shiman, S.L.; Rich-Edwards, J.W.; Gillman, M.W. Association of breastfeeding with maternal control of infant feeding at age 1 year. *Pediatrics* **2004**, *114*, e577–e583. [CrossRef]
18. Rhee, K.E.; Coleman, S.M.; Appugliese, D.P.; Kaciroti, N.A.; Corwyn, R.F.; Davidson, N.S.; Bradley, R.H.; Lumeng, J.C. Maternal feeding practices become more controlling after and not before excessive rates of weight gain. *Obesity* **2009**, *17*, 1724–1729. [CrossRef]
19. Fisher, J.O.; Birch, L.L. Restricting access to foods and children's eating. *Appetite* **1999**, *32*, 405–419. [CrossRef] [PubMed]
20. Blissett, J.; Bennett, C. Cultural differences in parental feeding practices and children's eating behaviours and their relationships with child BMI: A comparison of Black Afro-Caribbean, White British and White German samples. *Eur. J. Clin. Nutr.* **2013**, *67*, 180–184. [CrossRef] [PubMed]
21. Cardel, M.; Willig, A.L.; Dulin-Keita, A.; Casazza, K.; Beasley, T.M.; Fernandez, J.R. Parental feeding practices and socioeconomic status are associated with child adiposity in a multi-ethnic sample of children. *Appetite* **2012**, *58*, 347–353. [CrossRef]
22. Gubbels, J.S.; Gerards, S.M.; Kremers, S.P. The association of parenting practices with toddlers' dietary intake and BMI, and the moderating role of general parenting and child temperament. *Public Health Nutr.* **2020**, *23*, 1–9. [CrossRef]
23. Fisher, J.O.; Birch, L.L. Parents' restrictive feeding practices are associated with young girls' negative self-evaluation of eating. *J. Am. Diet. Assoc.* **2000**, *100*, 1341–1346. [CrossRef]
24. Jansen, E.; Mulkens, S.; Jansen, A. Do not eat the red food!: Prohibition of snacks leads to their relatively higher consumption in children. *Appetite* **2007**, *49*, 572–577. [CrossRef]
25. Faith, M.S.; Scanlon, K.S.; Birch, L.L.; Francis, L.A.; Sherry, B. Parent-child feeding strategies and their relationships to child eating and weight status. *Obes. Res.* **2004**, *12*, 1711–1722. [CrossRef]
26. Galloway, A.T.; Fiorito, L.M.; Francis, L.A.; Birch, L.L. 'Finish your soup': Counterproductive effects of pressuring children to eat on intake and affect. *Appetite* **2006**, *46*, 318–323. [CrossRef]
27. Webber, L.; Cooke, L.; Hill, C.; Wardle, J. Associations between children's appetitive traits and maternal feeding practices. *J. Am. Diet. Assoc.* **2010**, *110*, 1718–1722. [CrossRef] [PubMed]
28. Campbell, K.; Andrianopoulos, N.; Hesketh, K.; Ball, K.; Crawford, D.; Brennan, L.; Corsini, N.; Timperio, A. Parental use of restrictive feeding practices and child BMI z-score. A 3-year prospective cohort study. *Appetite* **2010**, *55*, 84–88. [CrossRef] [PubMed]
29. Farrow, C.V.; Blissett, J. Controlling feeding practices: Cause or consequence of early child weight? *Pediatrics* **2008**, *121*, e164–e169. [CrossRef] [PubMed]
30. Afonso, L.; Lopes, C.; Severo, M.; Santos, S.; Real, H.; Durao, C.; Moreira, P.; Oliveira, A. Bidirectional association between parental child-feeding practices and body mass index at 4 and 7 y of age. *Am. J. Clin. Nutr.* **2016**, *103*, 861–867. [CrossRef] [PubMed]
31. Jansen, E.; Williams, K.E.; Mallan, K.M.; Nicholson, J.M.; Daniels, L.A. Bidirectional associations between mothers' feeding practices and child eating behaviours. *Int. J. Behav. Nutr. Phys. Act.* **2018**, *15*, 3. [CrossRef] [PubMed]
32. Jansen, P.W.; Tharner, A.; van der Ende, J.; Wake, M.; Raat, H.; Hofman, A.; Verhulst, F.C.; van Ijzendoorn, M.H.; Jaddoe, V.W.; Tiemeier, H. Feeding practices and child weight: Is the association bidirectional in preschool children? *Am. J. Clin. Nutr.* **2014**, *100*, 1329–1336. [CrossRef]
33. Shloim, N.; Edelson, L.R.; Martin, N.; Hetherington, M.M. Parenting Styles, Feeding Styles, Feeding Practices, and Weight Status in 4-12 Year-Old Children: A Systematic Review of the Literature. *Front. Psychol.* **2015**, *6*, 1849. [CrossRef]
34. Webber, L.; Cooke, L.; Hill, C.; Wardle, J. Child adiposity and maternal feeding practices: A longitudinal analysis. *Am. J. Clin. Nutr.* **2010**, *92*, 1423–1428. [CrossRef]
35. Derks, I.P.; Tiemeier, H.; Sijbrands, E.J.; Nicholson, J.M.; Voortman, T.; Verhulst, F.C.; Jaddoe, V.W.; Jansen, P.W. Testing the direction of effects between child body composition and restrictive feeding practices: Results from a population-based cohort. *Am. J. Clin. Nutr.* **2017**, *106*, 783–790. [CrossRef] [PubMed]
36. Eichler, J.; Schmidt, R.; Poulain, T.; Hiemisch, A.; Kiess, W.; Hilbert, A. Stability, Continuity, and Bi-Directional Associations of Parental Feeding Practices and Standardized Child Body Mass Index in Children from 2 to 12 Years of Age. *Nutrients* **2019**, *11*, 1751. [CrossRef] [PubMed]
37. Faith, M.S.; Carnell, S.; Kral, T.V. Genetics of food intake self-regulation in childhood: Literature review and research opportunities. *Hum. Hered.* **2013**, *75*, 80–89. [CrossRef] [PubMed]

38. Dalle Molle, R.; Fatemi, H.; Dagher, A.; Levitan, R.D.; Silveira, P.P.; Dubé, L. Gene and environment interaction: Is the differential susceptibility hypothesis relevant for obesity? *Neurosci. BioBehav. Rev.* **2017**, *73*, 326–339. [CrossRef] [PubMed]

39. Heude, B.; Forhan, A.; Slama, R.; Douhaud, L.; Bedel, S.; Saurel-Cubizolles, M.J.; Hankard, R.; Thiebaugeorges, O.; De Agostini, M.; Annesi-Maesano, I.; et al. Cohort Profile: The EDEN mother-child cohort on the prenatal and early postnatal determinants of child health and development. *Int. J. Epidemiol.* **2016**, *45*, 353–363. [CrossRef]

40. Li, S.; Zhao, J.H.; Luan, J.; Luben, R.N.; Rodwell, S.A.; Khaw, K.T.; Ong, K.K.; Wareham, N.J.; Loos, R.J. Cumulative effects and predictive value of common obesity-susceptibility variants identified by genome-wide association studies. *Am. J. Clin. Nutr.* **2010**, *91*, 184–190. [CrossRef]

41. Speliotes, E.K.; Willer, C.J.; Berndt, S.I.; Monda, K.L.; Thorleifsson, G.; Jackson, A.U.; Lango Allen, H.; Lindgren, C.M.; Luan, J.; Mägi, R.; et al. Association analyses of 249,796 individuals reveal 18 new loci associated with body mass index. *Nat. Genet.* **2010**, *42*, 937–948. [CrossRef]

42. Elks, C.E.; Heude, B.; de Zegher, F.; Barton, S.J.; Clement, K.; Inskip, H.M.; Koudou, Y.; Cooper, C.; Dunger, D.B.; Ibanez, L.; et al. Associations between genetic obesity susceptibility and early postnatal fat and lean mass: An individual participant meta-analysis. *JAMA Pediatr.* **2014**, *168*, 1122–1130. [CrossRef]

43. Musher-Eizenman, D.; Holub, S. Comprehensive Feeding Practices Questionnaire: Validation of a new measure of parental feeding practices. *J. Pediatr. Psychol.* **2007**, *32*, 960–972. [CrossRef]

44. Musher-Eizenman, D.R.; de Lauzon-Guillain, B.; Holub, S.C.; Leporc, E.; Charles, M.A. Child and parent characteristics related to parental feeding practices. A cross-cultural examination in the US and France. *Appetite* **2009**, *52*, 89–95. [CrossRef]

45. Botton, J.; Heude, B.; Maccario, J.; Ducimetière, P.; Charles, M.A. Postnatal weight and height growth velocities at different ages between birth and 5 y and body composition in adolescent boys and girls. *Am. J. Clin. Nutr.* **2008**, *87*, 1760–1768. [CrossRef]

46. Howe, T.H.; Sheu, C.F.; Wang, T.N. Feeding Patterns and Parental Perceptions of Feeding Issues of Preterm Infants in the First 2 Years of Life. *Am. J. Occup. Ther.* **2019**, *73*, 7302205030. [CrossRef]

47. Eekhout, I.; van de Wiel, M.A.; Heymans, M.W. Methods for significance testing of categorical covariates in logistic regression models after multiple imputation: Power and applicability analysis. *BMC Med. Res. Methodol.* **2017**, *17*, 129. [CrossRef] [PubMed]

48. Fisher, J.O.; Birch, L.L. Restricting access to palatable foods affects children's behavioral response, food selection, and intake. *Am. J. Clin. Nutr.* **1999**, *69*, 1264–1272. [CrossRef] [PubMed]

49. Hughes, S.O.; Frazier-Wood, A.C. Satiety and the Self-Regulation of Food Take in Children: A Potential Role for Gene-Environment Interplay. *Curr. Obes. Rep.* **2016**, *5*, 81–87. [CrossRef] [PubMed]

50. Rodgers, R.F.; Paxton, S.J.; Massey, R.; Campbell, K.J.; Wertheim, E.H.; Skouteris, H.; Gibbons, K. Maternal feeding practices predict weight gain and obesogenic eating behaviors in young children: A prospective study. *Int. J. Behav. Nutr. Phys. Act.* **2013**, *10*, 24. [CrossRef]

51. Quah, P.L.; Ng, J.C.; Fries, L.R.; Chan, M.J.; Aris, I.M.; Lee, Y.S.; Yap, F.; Godfrey, K.M.; Chong, Y.S.; Shek, L.P.; et al. Longitudinal Analysis Between Maternal Feeding Practices and Body Mass Index (BMI): A Study in Asian Singaporean Preschoolers. *Front. Nutr.* **2019**, *6*, 32. [CrossRef]

52. Selzam, S.; McAdams, T.A.; Coleman, J.R.I.; Carnell, S.; O'Reilly, P.F.; Plomin, R.; Llewellyn, C.H. Evidence for gene-environment correlation in child feeding: Links between common genetic variation for BMI in children and parental feeding practices. *PLoS Genet.* **2018**, *14*, e1007757. [CrossRef]

53. Reed, Z.E.; Micali, N.; Bulik, C.M.; Davey Smith, G.; Wade, K.H. Assessing the causal role of adiposity on disordered eating in childhood, adolescence, and adulthood: A Mendelian randomization analysis. *Am. J. Clin. Nutr.* **2017**, *106*, 764–772. [CrossRef] [PubMed]

54. Scaglioni, S.; De Cosmi, V.; Ciappolino, V.; Parazzini, F.; Brambilla, P.; Agostoni, C. Factors Influencing Children's Eating Behaviours. *Nutrients* **2018**, *10*, 706. [CrossRef] [PubMed]

55. Maynard, L.M.; Galuska, D.A.; Blanck, H.M.; Serdula, M.K. Maternal perceptions of weight status of children. *Pediatrics* **2003**, *111*, 1226–1231.

56. Zhou, Z.; Liew, J.; Yeh, Y.C.; Perez, M. Appetitive Traits and Weight in Children: Evidence for Parents' Controlling Feeding Practices as Mediating Mechanisms. *J. Genet. Psychol.* **2020**, *181*, 1–13. [CrossRef]

57. Steinsbekk, S.; Belsky, J.; Wichstrøm, L. Parental Feeding and Child Eating: An Investigation of Reciprocal Effects. *Child. Dev.* **2016**, *87*, 1538–1549. [CrossRef] [PubMed]

58. Blissett, J.; Haycraft, E.; Farrow, C. Inducing preschool children's emotional eating: Relations with parental feeding practices. *Am. J. Clin. Nutr.* **2010**, *92*, 359–365. [CrossRef]

59. Jansen, P.W.; Derks, I.P.M.; Mou, Y.; van Rijen, E.H.M.; Gaillard, R.; Micali, N.; Voortman, T.; Hillegers, M.H.J. Associations of parents' use of food as reward with children's eating behaviour and BMI in a population-based cohort. *Pediatr. Obes.* **2020**, *15*, e12662. [CrossRef]

60. de Lauzon-Guillain, B.; Clifton, E.A.; Day, F.R.; Clement, K.; Brage, S.; Forouhi, N.G.; Griffin, S.J.; Koudou, Y.A.; Pelloux, V.; Wareham, N.J.; et al. Mediation and modification of genetic susceptibility to obesity by eating behaviors. *Am. J. Clin. Nutr.* **2017**, *106*, 996–1004. [CrossRef] [PubMed]

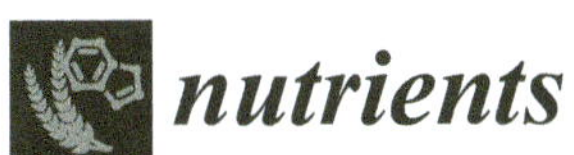 *nutrients*

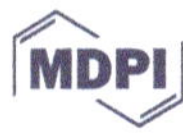

Article

Effects of School-Based Interventions on Reducing Sugar-Sweetened Beverage Consumption among Chinese Children and Adolescents

Zhenni Zhu [1,2], Chunyan Luo [3], Shuangxiao Qu [3], Xiaohui Wei [4], Jingyuan Feng [4], Shuo Zhang [5], Yinyi Wang [6] and Jin Su [1,*]

[1] Division of Health Risk Factors Monitoring and Control, Shanghai Municipal Center for Disease Control and Prevention, 1380 West Zhongshan Road, Shanghai 20036, China; zhuzhenni@scdc.sh.cn

[2] National Institute for Nutrition and Health, Chinese Center for Disease Control and Prevention, 27 Nan Wei Road, Beijing 100050, China

[3] Division of Child and Youth Health, Shanghai Municipal Center for Disease Control and Prevention, 1380 West Zhongshan Road, Shanghai 20036, China; luochunyan@scdc.sh.cn (C.L.); qushuangxiao@scdc.sh.cn (S.Q.)

[4] School of Public Health, Fudan University, 130 Dongan Road, Shanghai 20030, China; xhwei16@fudan.edu.cn (X.W.); jyfeng16@fudan.edu.cn (J.F.)

[5] Department of Nutrition, School of Medicine, Shanghai Jiao Tong University, 227 Chongqing South Road, Shanghai 200025, China; zoisite@sjtu.edu.cn

[6] Department of Nutrition and Food Science, Steinhardt School of Culture, Education, and Human Development, New York University, 82 Washington Square E, New York, NY 10003, USA; yw5004@nyu.edu

* Correspondence: sujin@scdc.sh.cn

Citation: Zhu, Z.; Luo, C.; Qu, S.; Wei, X.; Feng, J.; Zhang, S.; Wang, Y.; Su, J. Effects of School-Based Interventions on Reducing Sugar-Sweetened Beverage Consumption among Chinese Children and Adolescents. *Nutrients* **2021**, *13*, 1862. https://doi.org/10.3390/nu13061862

Academic Editors: Odysseas Androutsos and Evangelia Charmandari

Received: 7 April 2021
Accepted: 27 May 2021
Published: 30 May 2021

Publisher's Note: MDPI stays neutral with regard to jurisdictional claims in published maps and institutional affiliations.

Abstract: We set up a series of school-based interventions on the basis of an ecological model targeting sugar-sweetened beverage (SSB) reduction in Chinese elementary and middle schools and evaluated the effects. A total of 1046 students from Chinese elementary and middle schools were randomly recruited in an intervention group, as were 1156 counterparts in a control group. The interventions were conducted in the intervention schools for one year. The participants were orally instructed to answer all the questionnaires by themselves at baseline and after intervention. The difference in difference statistical approach was used to identify the effects exclusively attributable to the interventions. There were differences in grade composition and no difference in sex distribution between the intervention and control groups. After adjusting for age, sex, and group differences at baseline, a significant reduction in SSB intake was found in the intervention group post intervention, with a decrease of 35.0 mL/day ($p = 0.034$). Additionally, the frequency of SSB consumption decreased by 0.2 times/day ($p = 0.071$). The students in the elementary schools with interventions significantly reduced their SSB intake by 61.6 mL/day ($p = 0.002$) and their frequency of SSB consumption by 0.3 times/day ($p = 0.017$) after the intervention. The boys in the intervention group had an intervention effect of a 50.2 mL/day reduction in their SSB intake ($p = 0.036$). School-based interventions were effective in reducing SSB consumption, especially among younger ones. The boys were more responsive to the interventions than the girls. (ChiCTR, ChiCTR1900020781.)

Keywords: sugar-sweetened beverage; school-based; intervention; ecological model; difference in difference approach

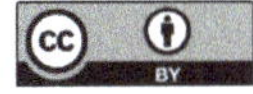

Copyright: © 2021 by the authors. Licensee MDPI, Basel, Switzerland. This article is an open access article distributed under the terms and conditions of the Creative Commons Attribution (CC BY) license (https:// creativecommons.org/licenses/by/ 4.0/).

1. Introduction

Each year, sugar-sweetened beverage (SSB) intake is related to the loss of about 8.5 million disability-adjusted life years (DALYs), and three quarters of this burden occurs in low- and middle-income countries [1]. SSBs were defined as nonalcoholic beverages sweetened by sugar, such as carbonated beverages, sugar-sweetened fruit or vegetable juice beverages, etc. The frequent consumption of excess amounts of SSBs is a risk factor for obesity [2], type 2 diabetes [3], cardiovascular disease [4], and dental caries [5]. The potential pathophysiology of SSB consumption explained the unfavorable health outcomes linked to SSBs. SSBs contain energy but no micro- and macronutrients, except glucose and fructose. Excessive glucose intake is known for causing adverse glycemic effects on metabolism [6], and fructose can be converted into fat, unfettered by the cellular controls that prevent unrestrained lipid synthesis from glucose [7]. The adverse health outcomes linked to SSBs occur in both adults and children [8,9]. Behavioral factors such as diet linked to mortality causes are preventable and both shape and are shaped by the social environment [10]. Studies have shown that interventions can achieve favorable results in reducing SSB intake in children but not in adults [11]. It is possible that interventions might have effects on individuals who were before or at their behavioral development period rather than those already forming behavioral models.

Comprehensive school-based program achieved some changes on dietary intakes of students [12,13]. School-based interventions aiming at decreasing SSB consumption have shown promising results in previous Western studies [14]. More than half of the children and adolescents in China consumed SSB, and the increasing consumption of SSBs has created the obvious threat of obesity among Chinese children and adolescents [15,16]. However, there has been no study reporting evaluations of school-based interventions tackling SSB reduction in China. Considering the different environmental and cultural backgrounds compared to Western countries, we set up a series of school-based interventions on the basis of an ecological model targeting SSB reduction in Chinese elementary and middle schools and evaluated the effects on SSB reduction among Chinese children and adolescents.

2. Materials and Methods

2.1. Study Population

We adopted epidemiological methods to establish a parallel control group intervention experiment for one year, from February 2019 to January 2020, in Shanghai, China. Three elementary schools and two middle schools were randomly recruited into the intervention group, and the same number of adjacent counterparts into the control group. Students in the 3rd and 4th grades from the selected elementary schools and the 6th and 7th grades from the selected middle schools were enrolled into the intervention or control group according to their school's allocation. The participants were not informed of which group they were assigned.

The theoretical minimum sample size was 1051 for the intervention and control groups, respectively, following the formula of sample size calculation for experiments with comparisons between two different groups:

$$n = [(Z_{\alpha/2} + Z_\beta)S/\delta]^2$$

We set $\alpha = 0.05$ and $\beta = 0.10$. S represented standard deviation of SSB intake, and δ represented allowance error.

We decided to select 220 students in each grade of a school and a total of 1100 students in both the intervention and control groups. After enrollment, 1082 and 1259 students were in the intervention and control groups, respectively. By eliminating the students lost to follow up, there were 1046 in the intervention group and 1156 in the control group (Figure 1).

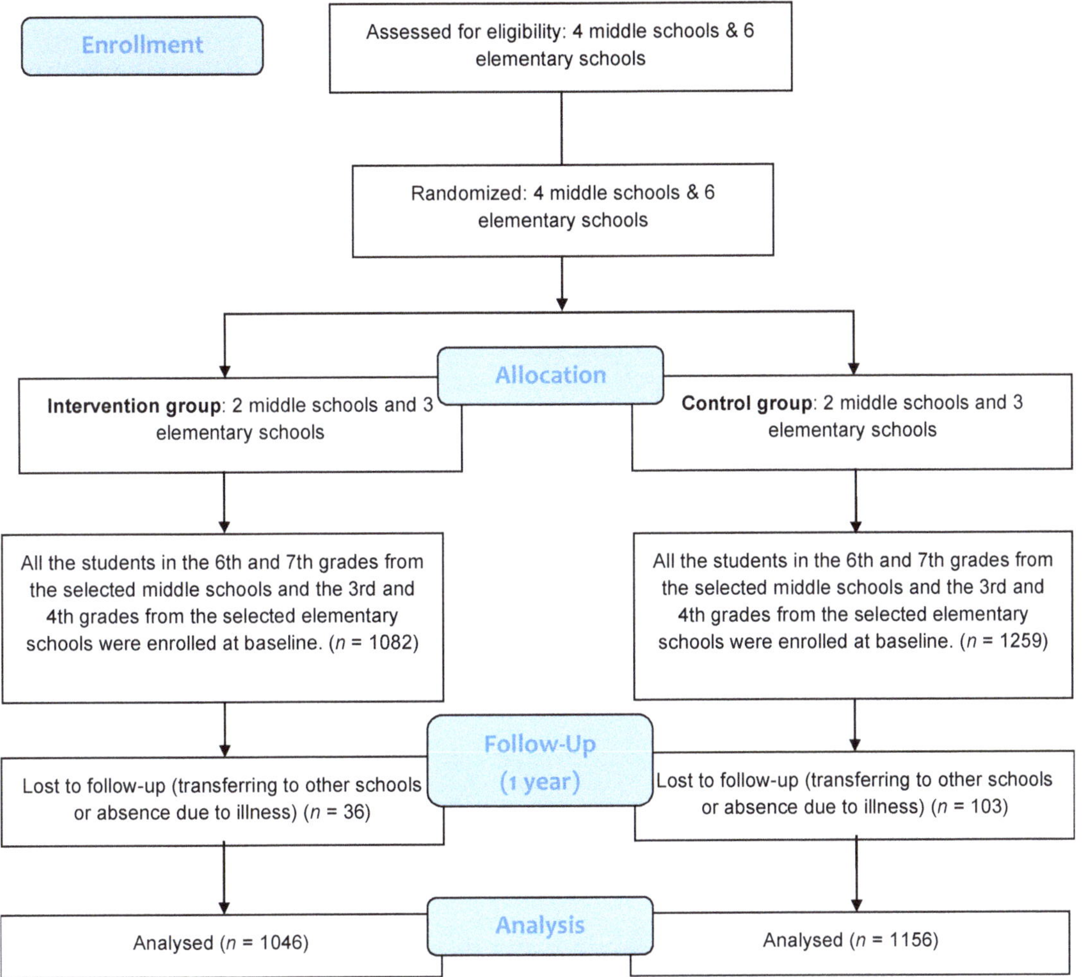

Figure 1. Flow chart of subjects throughout the research.

This study was approved by the Shanghai Municipal Center for Disease Control on 17 May 2017 (No. 2017-18). Informed consent was obtained from each participant or the participant's parents or guardian before the research. The study complied with the code of ethics of the World Medical Association (Declaration of Helsinki). This intervention study was registered at the Chinese Clinical Trial Registry (http://www.chictr.org.cn, accessed on 7 April 2021) with the registration number of ChiCTR1900020781 (http://www.chictr.org.cn/showproj.aspx?proj=35002, accessed on 19 January 2019).

2.2. SSB Intake, Frequency, and Knowledge Assessment

The investigators were public health doctors in local community health centers and received a standard training course on the facilitation of the questionnaires. The participants were orally instructed to answer all the questionnaires by themselves. The investigators verified the answers after each questionnaire was completed.

The information collected at the baseline and post one-year intervention were both at the interval between January to February, just before and after the complete one-year intervention period.

A general questionnaire was used to obtain demographic information and SSB-related knowledge. There were six questions related to SSB consumption and health which were used to assess the SSB-related knowledge of the participants. The participant received one point if they gave the right answer. A full score was six. The six questions were as follows:

A.   I am not going to get fat if I consume SSBs frequently.
B.   SSBs contain many nutrients.
C.   SSBs are the best choice for quenching my thirst.
D.   I should not have even one sip of an SSB.
E.   SSBs bring the body extra energy because the sugar in it can be easily absorbed but they hardly make one feel full.
F.   SSBs have empty energy that will not pose a threat to health.

An SSB frequency questionnaire was administrated to collect information on SSB intake and frequency in the past 3 months. This questionnaire originated from a former food frequency questionnaire that was developed and validated by the China Center for Disease and Control and Prevention [17]. SSBs were defined as nonalcoholic beverages sweetened by sugar, excluding fresh juice, categorized as carbonated beverages, sugar-sweetened fruit or vegetable juice beverages, protein-based beverages, probiotic beverages, milk-based beverages, bottled tea beverages, coffee drink, and typical Southeast Asian milky tea (a popular SSB in China). According to each SSB category, SSB consumption frequency was listed in terms of consumption times per day, week, month, or year, and the amount consumed each time was recorded.

The survey was conducted in the pre- and post-intervention periods using the same questionnaires. No disastrous events such as rain or snow disasters that would have affected the normal food supply took place during the research period. The weather was typical of the marine climate in Shanghai, China.

2.3. Interventions

The interventions were designed using the structures of an ecological model targeting individuals and their environment, including multiple levels of influence [18]. The interventions were conducted for one year by the teachers in the intervention schools with the collaboration of public health doctors in local community health centers. The control schools had no intervening events. All the participating schools followed the city-wide education schedule during the intervention period.

a.   Individual level
- Hold "restricting SSBs"-themed class meeting every semester (twice a year) and praise students with outstanding health behaviors (the themed class meeting was designed to provide SSB-related knowledge regarding the six questions about SSB-related knowledge in the questionnaire).
- Distribute SSB-related knowledge materials every semester (twice a year).
- Record one's own SSB behaviors once per week.

b.   Family level
- Establish WeChat (the most popular social communication application in China) groups for parents and publish new media promotional materials once a month.

c.   Peer level
- Distribute promotional cards to students every semester (twice a year; the cards showed cartoon figures and information regarding the six questions on SSB-related knowledge in the questionnaire, as well as mottos and goals for the new semester).

d.   School level
- Carry out a blackboard painting activity with the theme of "understanding SSBs" every semester (twice a year).

■ Forbid selling SSBs on campus during the intervention.

e. Community level

■ Negotiate with stores near the gates of schools not to sell SSBs to students.

2.4. Statistical Analyses

Statistical analyses were conducted using the SAS statistical software (v. 9.4; SAS Institute, Cary, NC, USA). The comparisons were conducted between the participants in the same level of different schools, different groups and pre and post intervention. T tests were applied to determine the differences between the intervention and control groups pre and post intervention. The difference in difference (DID) statistical approach was used to identify the net effects exclusively attributable to the interventions in this study [19]. The DID approach was designed for quasi-experimental research studying causal relationships in public health settings where randomized controlled trials (RCTs) are infeasible or unethical. In the current analysis of DID, an interactive item of the variate representing group classification and a variate representing pre- or post-intervention classification was included in the multivariate general linear regression models, representing the intervention effect. Age, sex, and the variates mentioned above were included in the same models as covariates. A two-sided $p < 0.05$ was considered to indicate statistical significance.

3. Results

3.1. Characteristics of the Participants

At baseline, 1082 subjects were recruited in the intervention group and 1259 subjects in the control group. At one-year follow-up, 1046 remained in the intervention group and 1156 in the control group. The retention rates were 96.7% and 91.8% in the intervention and control groups, respectively. Differences in sex distribution were not observed between the two groups either pre or post intervention. The differences in grade composition were significant between the groups both pre and post intervention (Table 1).

Table 1. Characteristics of the participants pre and post intervention (%).

		Pre-Intervention			Post-Intervention		
		Intervention Group	Control Group	*p*	Intervention Group	Control Group	*p*
	n	1082	1259		1046	1156	
Sex							
	Boys	51.1	52.0	0.658	51.5	51.6	0.840
	Girls	48.9	48.0		48.5	48.4	
Grade at baseline							
	3 (9–10 yrs)	31.6	38.8	<0.001	31.6	38.7	<0.001
	4 (10–11 yrs)	32.5	30.7		32.5	30.8	
	6 (12–13 yrs)	17.7	18.2		17.8	18.2	
	7 (13–14 yrs)	18.1	12.3		18.1	12.3	

3.2. Differences in SSB Intake, Frequency, and Knowledge between the Groups pre and Post Intervention

At baseline, the SSB intakes were 286.0 ± 266.5 mL/day and 286.0 ± 288.2 mL/day in the intervention and control groups, respectively. The frequencies of SSB consumption were 1.6 ± 1.6 times/day and 1.7 ± 1.9 times/day, respectively. The scores for SSB-related knowledge were 4.3 ± 1.2 and 4.5 ± 1.0, respectively. There was no difference in the SSB intake and frequency of SSB consumption between the two groups and their subgroups ($p > 0.05$). The scores for SSB-related knowledge were significantly different between the two groups ($p < 0.001$).

After the one-year intervention, the SSB intakes were 220.9 ± 262.3 mL/day and 254.4 ± 268.9 mL/day in the intervention and control groups, respectively. The frequencies of SSB consumption were 1.1 ± 1.5 times/day and 1.4 ± 1.7 times/day, respectively. The scores for SSB-related knowledge were 4.4 ± 1.3 and 4.5 ± 1.1, respectively. Significant differences existed in the SSB intake and the frequency of SSB consumption between groups ($p = 0.003$, $p < 0.001$). The scores for SSB-related knowledge showed no statistical difference between the groups ($p = 0.060$) (Table 2).

Table 2. The differences in SSB intake, frequency, and knowledge between the groups pre and post intervention.

	Pre-Intervention			Post-Intervention		
	Intervention Group	Control Group	*p*	Intervention Group	Control Group	*p*
SSB intake, mL/day						
All	286.0 ± 266.5	286.0 ± 288.2	1.000	220.9 ± 262.3	254.4 ± 268.9	0.003
Sex						
Boys	297.0 ± 272.8	313.6 ± 299.5	0.334	226.2 ± 263.8	301.6 ± 290.3	<0.001
Girls	274.5 ± 259.5	257.2 ± 273.3	0.292	232.1 ± 263.5	227.9 ± 240.0	0.790
Grade at baseline						
3 (9–10 yrs)	276.6 ± 280.1	266.4 ± 280.1	0.618	196.2 ± 272.0	229.3 ± 264.9	0.088
4 (10–11 yrs)	302.1 ± 258.5	277.9 ± 289.2	0.250	189.6 ± 231.9	245.0 ± 258.4	0.003
6 (12–13 yrs)	256.6 ± 246.3	291.9 ± 279.2	0.185	226.1 ± 231.9	299.0 ± 271.6	0.004
7 (13–14 yrs)	303.3 ± 274.9	361.1 ± 314.6	0.081	316.1 ± 301.3	315.7 ± 305.2	0.991
Frequency of SSB consumption, times/day						
All	1.6 ± 1.6	1.7 ± 1.9	0.096	1.1 ± 1.5	1.4 ± 1.7	<0.001
Sex						
Boys	1.6 ± 1.7	1.8 ± 1.9	0.060	1.1 ± 1.4	1.6 ± 1.8	<0.001
Girls	1.6 ± 1.6	1.6 ± 2.0	0.667	1.2 ± 1.5	1.4 ± 1.7	0.070
Grade at baseline						
3 (9–10 yrs)	1.7 ± 1.8	1.7 ± 1.9	0.922	1.1 ± 1.6	1.5 ± 1.9	0.005
4 (10–11 yrs)	1.7 ± 1.6	1.8 ± 2.1	0.501	1.0 ± 1.4	1.4 ± 1.6	0.002
6 (12–13 yrs)	1.3 ± 1.4	1.7 ± 1.8	0.021	1.1 ± 1.3	1.3 ± 1.4	0.089
7 (13–14 yrs)	1.5 ± 1.6	1.6 ± 1.6	0.571	1.3 ± 1.5	1.7 ± 1.9	0.127
Score of SSB-related knowledge						
All	4.3 ± 1.2	4.5 ± 1.0	<0.001	4.4 ± 1.3	4.5 ± 1.1	0.060
Sex						
Boys	4.2 ± 1.2	4.4 ± 1.1	0.006	4.3 ± 1.3	4.4 ± 1.2	0.447
Girls	4.4 ± 1.2	4.6 ± 1.0	0.006	4.5 ± 1.2	4.6 ± 1.0	0.038
Grade at baseline						
3 (9–10 yrs)	4.0 ± 1.3	4.3 ± 1.1	<0.001	4.4 ± 1.3	4.4 ± 1.1	0.582
4 (10–11 yrs)	4.3 ± 1.1	4.5 ± 1.0	0.016	4.2 ± 1.3	4.5 ± 1.1	0.004
6 (12–13 yrs)	4.7 ± 1.0	4.7 ± 1.0	0.851	4.5 ± 1.2	4.6 ± 1.1	0.421
7 (13–14 yrs)	4.6 ± 1.0	4.8 ± 0.9	0.137	4.5 ± 1.3	4.7 ± 1.2	0.146

SSB, sugar-sweetened beverage.

3.3. The Effects on SSB Intake, Frequency, and Knowledge Attributed to the Interventions

After adjusting for age, sex, and group differences at baseline, a significant reduction in SSB intake which was exclusively attributed to the interventions was found in the intervention group post intervention, with a decrease of 35.0 mL/day ($p = 0.034$). Additionally, the frequency of SSB consumption decreased by 0.2 times/day, with a borderline significance ($p = 0.071$), due to the intervention. No statistically significant effect was found in the score for SSB-related knowledge after the intervention ($p = 0.347$).

After intervention, the participants in the elementary schools with the intervention significantly reduced their SSB intake by 61.6 mL/day ($p = 0.017$) and their frequency of SSB consumption by 0.3 time/day ($p = 0.002$), but no changes were observed in the SSB intake and frequency of SSB consumption among those from middle schools with the intervention ($p = 0.945$ and $p = 0.978$, respectively). The boys in the intervention group had an intervention effect of a 50.2 mL/day reduction in SSB intake ($p = 0.036$), while the girls presented no significant intervention effect in SSB intake ($p = 0.403$) (Table 3).

Table 3. The effects attributable to the interventions on SSB intake, frequency, and knowledge after the one-year intervention [a].

	SSB Intake, mL/day			Frequency of SSB Consumption, times/day		Scores of SSB-Related Knowledge	
	β	p		β	p	β	p
All	−35.0	0.034		−0.2	0.071	0.1	0.347
			School-level				
Primary school(Grade 3–4, 9–11 yrs)	−61.6	0.002		−0.3	0.017	0.2	0.066
Middle school (Grade 3–4,12–14 yrs)	2.1	0.945		0.0	0.978	−0.1	0.545
			Sex				
Boys	−50.2	0.036		−0.2	0.110	0.1	0.262
Girls	−18.8	0.403		−0.1	0.335	0.0	0.888

[a] β represented the net change of the indicator attributable to the interventions only post intervention compared with that pre-intervention.

4. Discussion

In the current study, the one-year school-based interventions achieved favorable effects in reducing SSB consumption among Chinese children and adolescents. Regarding the feasibility of the intervention implemented, each participant was not assigned randomly into an intervention or control group. Actually, the participants were allocated indiscriminately into interventions or control groups according to their school's allocation in the study. Moreover, other citywide health promotion events at the time or the underlying natural growth of individuals might have affected their SSB consumption as well. All these factors made it difficult to identify the effects exclusively attributed to the current interventions. The DID approach provided an alternative means for us to study the net effects on the SSB consumption changes which were exclusively attributable to the interventions [19,20]. After adjusting for age, sex, and group differences at baseline, we discovered a substantial scale of SSB reduction attributable to the interventions in this study. The school stood out as one of the most common settings to improve health behaviors [21]. Previous studies indicated that Western school-based interventions were promising to reduce SSB consumption [14]. Our results give more evidence regarding school-based interventions in the setting of an Eastern culture and environment. The current results also supported the theory that the ecological model helped to develop an environment conducive to change, facilitating the adoption of healthy behaviors [22].

We found that the beneficial effects occurred among the younger children rather than the adolescents in the current study. Both the amount and the frequency of SSB consumption reduced after the one-year intervention, while SSB-related knowledge also increased modestly among the younger children. However, there was no obvious change in the amount and the frequency of SSB consumption and SSB-related knowledge among the participants in the middle schools between pre- and post-intervention. These findings coincided with previous studies showing that interventions focusing on SSB control are more effective on younger children than older ones [23,24]. This also suggests that future interventions or policies aiming at reducing SSBs should target younger children in order to achieve more favorable cost-effective outcomes.

We observed that the consumption of SSBs decreased in the boy participants but not in the girl participants. In the current study, the consumption of SSBs was discrepant at baseline in that the boys consumed more SSBs than the girls no matter whether they were in the intervention or control group. Boys had a higher preference for SSBs and consumed more SSBs than girls in their daily lives [15,25,26]. This might explain the significant effects on the boys after the intervention while there were hardly any effects on the girls in our study. Furthermore, the prevalence of overweight and obesity is much higher in boys than in girls in China [27]. The discrepancies between boys and girls in terms of intervention effects should be taken into consideration when conceiving obesity control strategies among children and adolescents.

In this study, we failed to discover enough evidence of improvement in SSB-related knowledge among our participants through the interventions. Only a modest increase in knowledge score that was of borderline significance ($p = 0.066$) occurred among the participants in the elementary schools with the intervention. In the current interventions, we provided SSB-related knowledge through routine school activities to the students and electronic messages to their parents, which aimed to set up supportive environments for SSB restriction. Previous studies showed that knowledge was not associated with SSB behaviors among children [28]. Other factors such as parental health behavior might determine SSB consumption among children [29,30]. Parental modelling was more crucial to children's behavioral development [31]. These might be the reasons why the behavior of SSB consumption changed but the SSB-related knowledge remained unimproved among the participants after the intervention in our study.

A limitation of this study was the methodology used to assess SSB intake and frequency. We designed an SSB consumption questionnaire to obtain SSB intake and frequency, which were self-reported by the participants, thus the data on SSB intake and frequency were limited by the accuracy of participants' estimation and recall. Furthermore, although we adjusted for potential confounding factors, we did not treat dietary intake as one of the confounders under the limitation of data collection. This might have caused bias in the current results. Besides this, the investigators were not blinded to the allocation of schools as intervention and control. This awareness of the investigators might have caused data collection bias. Finally, it was possible that some of the six questions used to assess the SSB-related knowledge were beyond the understanding of the students, which might have influenced our assessment of the SSB-related knowledge change.

5. Conclusions

School-based interventions designed in an ecological model were effective in the reduction in SSB consumption among Chinese children and adolescents, especially among younger children. The boys were more responsive to the interventions than the girls.

Author Contributions: Z.Z. conceived and designed the experiments; S.Q. and C.L. performed the experiments; Z.Z. analyzed the data; X.W., J.F., and S.Z. interpreted the statistical results; X.W., J.F., and Y.W. wrote the draft paper; Z.Z. wrote the paper and the final version of the manuscript; J.S. supervised the study. All authors have read and agreed to the published version of the manuscript.

Funding: This study was funded by the Study of Diet and Nutrition Assessment and Intervention Technology (No.2020YFC2006300) from Active Health and Aging Technologic Solutions Major Project of National Key R&D Program—Intervention Strategies of Main Nutrition Problems in China (No.2020YFC2006305); Shanghai Municipal Health Commission—Academic Leader Program (GWV-10.2-XD12); the Foundation of Shanghai Municipal Health Commission (201740073); and the Youth Nutrition Elite Development Program of Chinese Nutrition Society.

Institutional Review Board Statement: The study was conducted in accordance with the Declaration of Helsinki, and the protocol was approved by the Shanghai Municipal Center for Disease Control on 17 May 2017 (No. 2017-18).

Informed Consent Statement: Informed consent was obtained from all subjects involved in the study.

Data Availability Statement: The datasets used and analyzed in the current study are available from the corresponding author on reasonable request.

Acknowledgments: We are grateful to all the individuals who participated in this study. We also thank the teachers from the participating schools as well as the public health doctors at the local districts' Centers for Disease Control and Prevention and the local community health centers for their assistance with the intervention implementation and data collection.

Conflicts of Interest: The authors declare no conflict of interest. The founding sponsors had no role in the design of the study; in the collection, analyses, or interpretation of data; in the writing of the manuscript, and in the decision to publish the results.

Abbreviations

SSB, sugar-sweetened beverage; DALYs, disability-adjusted life years; DID, difference in difference; RCTs, randomized controlled trials.

References

1. Singh, G.M.; Micha, R.; Khatibzadeh, S.; Lim, S.; Ezzati, M.; Mozaffarian, D.; Global, B.O.D.N. Estimated global, regional, and national disease burdens related to Sugar-Sweetened beverage consumption in 2010. *Circulation* **2015**, *132*, 639–666. [CrossRef]
2. Malik, V.S.; Hu, F.B. Fructose and cardiometabolic health: What the evidence from Sugar-Sweetened beverages tells us. *J. Am. Coll. Cardiol.* **2015**, *66*, 1615–1624. [CrossRef]
3. Imamura, F.; O'Connor, L.; Ye, Z.; Mursu, J.; Hayashino, Y.; Bhupathiraju, S.N.; Forouhi, N.G. Consumption of sugar sweetened beverages, artificially sweetened beverages, and fruit juice and incidence of type 2 diabetes: Systematic review, meta-analysis, and estimation of population attributable fraction. *BMJ* **2015**, *351*, h3576. [CrossRef]
4. Vos, M.B.; Kaar, J.L.; Welsh, J.A.; Van Horn, L.V.; Feig, D.I.; Anderson, C.A.M.; Patel, M.J.; Cruz Munos, J.; Krebs, N.F.; Xanthakos, S.A.; et al. Added sugars and cardiovascular disease risk in children: A scientific statement from the american heart association. *Circulation* **2017**, *135*, e1017–e1034. [CrossRef]
5. Bleich, S.N.; Vercammen, K.A. The negative impact of sugar-sweetened beverages on children's health: An update of the literature. *BMC Obes.* **2018**, *5*, 6. [CrossRef] [PubMed]
6. Samanta, A.; Burden, A.C.; Jones, G.R. Plasma glucose responses to glucose, sucrose, and honey in patients with diabetes mellitus: An analysis of glycaemic and peak incremental indices. *Diabet Med.* **1985**, *2*, 371–373. [CrossRef]
7. Lyssiotis, C.A.; Cantley, L.C. Metabolic syndrome: F stands for fructose and fat. *Nature* **2013**, *502*, 181–182. [CrossRef] [PubMed]
8. Zhu, Z.; He, Y.; Wang, Z.; He, X.; Zang, J.; Guo, C.; Jia, X.; Ren, Y.; Shan, C.; Sun, J.; et al. The associations between sugar-sweetened beverage intake and cardiometabolic risks in Chinese children and adolescents. *Pediatr Obes.* **2020**, *15*, e12634. [CrossRef] [PubMed]
9. Shin, S.; Kim, S.; Ha, J.; Lim, K. Sugar-Sweetened Beverage Consumption in Relation to Obesity and Metabolic Syndrome among Korean Adults: A Cross-Sectional Study from the 2012–2016 Korean National Health and Nutrition Examination Survey (KNHANES). *Nutrients* **2018**, *10*, 1467. [CrossRef]
10. Smedley, B.D.; Syme, S.L. Promoting health: Intervention strategies from social and behavioral research. *Am. J. Health Promot.* **2001**, *15*, 149–166. [CrossRef] [PubMed]
11. Vargas-Garcia, E.J.; Evans, C.E.L.; Prestwich, A.; Sykes-Muskett, B.J.; Hooson, J.; Cade, J.E. Interventions to reduce consumption of sugar-sweetened beverages or increase water intake: Evidence from a systematic review and meta-analysis. *Obes Rev.* **2017**, *18*, 1350–1363. [CrossRef]
12. Siega-Riz, A.M.; El Ghormli, L.; Mobley, C.; Gillis, B.; Stadler, D.; Hartstein, J.; Volpe, S.L.; Virus, A.; Bridgman, J.; Healthy, S.G. The effects of the HEALTHY study intervention on middle school student dietary intakes. *Int. J. Behav. Nutr. Phys. Act.* **2011**, *8*, 7. [CrossRef] [PubMed]
13. Singhal, N.; Misra, A. A school-based intervention for diabetes risk reduction. *N. Engl. J.Med.* **2010**, *363*, 1769. [PubMed]
14. Vézina-Im, L.; Beaulieu, D.; Bélanger-Gravel, A.; Boucher, D.; Sirois, C.; Dugas, M.; Provencher, V. Efficacy of school-based interventions aimed at decreasing sugar-sweetened beverage consumption among adolescents: A systematic review. *Public Health Nutr.* **2017**, *20*, 2416–2431. [CrossRef] [PubMed]
15. Gui, Z.; Zhu, Y.; Cai, L.; Sun, F.; Ma, Y.; Jing, J.; Chen, Y. Sugar-Sweetened beverage consumption and risks of obesity and hypertension in chinese children and adolescents: A national Cross-Sectional analysis. *Nutrients* **2017**, *9*, 1302. [CrossRef] [PubMed]
16. Greenhalgh, S. Making China safe for Coke: How Coca-Cola shaped obesity science and policy in China. *BMJ* **2019**, *364*, k5050. [CrossRef]
17. He, Y.; Zhao, W.; Zhang, J.; Zhao, L.; Yang, Z.; Huo, J.; Yang, L.; Wang, J.; He, L.; Sun, J.; et al. Data resource profile: China national nutrition surveys. *Int. J. Epidemiol.* **2019**, *48*, 368. [CrossRef] [PubMed]
18. Sallis, J.F.; Owen, N.; Fisher, E.B. Ecological models of health behavior. *Health Behav. Health Educ.* **2008**, *5*, 465–485.
19. Wing, C.; Simon, K.; Bello-Gomez, R.A. Designing difference in difference studies: Best practices for public health policy research. *Annu. Rev. Publ. Health* **2018**, *39*, 453–469. [CrossRef]
20. Greece, J.A. Behavioral Impact of a School-Based Healthy Eating Intervention for At-Risk Children. Ph.D. Theses, Boston University, Boston, MA, USA, 2011.
21. Waters, E.; de Silva-Sanigorski, A.; Hall, B.J.; Brown, T.; Campbell, K.J.; Gao, Y.; Armstrong, R.; Prosser, L.; Summerbell, C.D. Interventions for preventing obesity in children. *Cochrane Database Syst. Rev.* **2011**, D1871. [CrossRef]
22. Bandura, A.; Cliffs, N. *Social Foundations of Thought and Action: Cognitive Theory*; PRENTICE-HALL: Hoboken, NJ, USA, 1987.
23. Klesges, R.C.; Obarzanek, E.; Kumanyika, S.; Murray, D.M.; Klesges, L.M.; Relyea, G.E.; Stockton, M.B.; Lanctot, J.Q.; Beech, B.M.; McClanahan, B.S.; et al. The Memphis Girls' health Enrichment Multi-site Studies (GEMS): An evaluation of the efficacy of a 2-year obesity prevention program in African American girls. *Arch. Pediatr. Adolesc. Med.* **2010**, *164*, 1007–1014. [CrossRef] [PubMed]
24. Albala, C.; Ebbeling, C.B.; Cifuentes, M.; Lera, L.; Bustos, N.; Ludwig, D.S. Effects of replacing the habitual consumption of sugar-sweetened beverages with milk in Chilean children. *Am. J Clin Nutr.* **2008**, *88*, 605–611. [CrossRef]
25. Mendez, M.A.; Miles, D.R.; Poti, J.M.; Sotres-Alvarez, D.; Popkin, B.M. Persistent disparities over time in the distribution of sugar-sweetened beverage intake among children in the United States. *Am. J Clin Nutr.* **2019**, *109*, 79–89. [CrossRef] [PubMed]
26. Kim, J.; Yun, S.; Oh, K. Beverage consumption among Korean adolescents: Data from 2016 Korea Youth Risk Behavior Survey. *Nutr. Res. Pract.* **2019**, *13*, 70–75. [CrossRef] [PubMed]

27. Jia, P.; Li, M.; Xue, H.; Lu, L.; Xu, F.; Wang, Y. School environment and policies, child eating behavior and overweight/obesity in urban China: The childhood obesity study in China megacities. *Int. J. Obes.* **2017**, *41*, 813–819. [CrossRef]
28. Lundeen, E.A.; Park, S.; Onufrak, S.; Cunningham, S.; Blanck, H.M. Adolescent Sugar-Sweetened beverage intake is associated with parent intake, not knowledge of health risks. *Am. J. Health Promot.* **2018**, *32*, 1661–1670. [CrossRef] [PubMed]
29. Mazarello Paes, V.; Hesketh, K.; O'Malley, C.; Moore, H.; Summerbell, C.; Griffin, S.; van Sluijs, E.M.F.; Ong, K.K.; Lakshman, R. Determinants of sugar-sweetened beverage consumption in young children: A systematic review. *Obes Rev.* **2015**, *16*, 903–913. [CrossRef]
30. Bjelland, M.; Hausken, S.E.; Bergh, I.H.; Grydeland, M.; Klepp, K.I.; Andersen, L.F.; Totland, T.H.; Lien, N. Changes in adolescents' and parents' intakes of sugar-sweetened beverages, fruit and vegetables after 20 months: Results from the HEIA study—A comprehensive, multi-component school-based randomized trial. *Food Nutr. Res.* **2015**, *59*, 25932. [CrossRef]
31. Horne, P.J.; Greenhalgh, J.; Erjavec, M.; Lowe, C.F.; Viktor, S.; Whitaker, C.J. Increasing pre-school children's consumption of fruit and vegetables. A modelling and rewards intervention. *Appetite* **2011**, *56*, 375–385. [CrossRef]

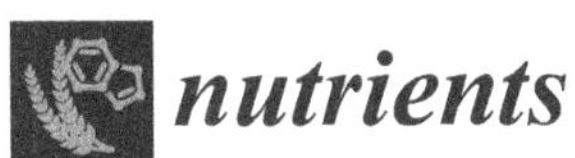

Article

Breastfeeding and Overweight in European Preschoolers: The ToyBox Study

Natalya Usheva [1,*], Mina Lateva [2], Sonya Galcheva [2], Berthold V. Koletzko [3], Greet Cardon [4], Marieke De Craemer [5,6], Odysseas Androutsos [7], Aneta Kotowska [8], Piotr Socha [8], Luis A. Moreno [9], Yannis Manios [10], Violeta Iotova [2] and on behalf of the ToyBox-Study Group [†]

[1] Department of Social Medicine and Health Care Organization, Medical University of Varna, 9002 Varna, Bulgaria

[2] Department of Pediatrics, Medical University of Varna, 9002 Varna, Bulgaria; mina_pl@yahoo.com (M.L.); sonya_galcheva@mail.bg (S.G.); iotova_v@yahoo.com (V.I.)

[3] Division of Metabolic and Nutritional Medicine, Department Paediatrics, Dr. von Hauner Children's Hospital, LMU University Hospitals, 80337 Munich, Germany; berthold.koletzko@med.uni-muenchen.de

[4] Department of Movement and Sports Sciences, Ghent University, 9000 Ghent, Belgium; greet.cardon@ugent.be

[5] Department of Rehabilitation Sciences, Ghent University, 9000 Ghent, Belgium; marieke.decraemer@ugent.be

[6] Research Foundation Flanders, 1000 Brussels, Belgium

[7] Department of Nutrition and Dietetics, School of Physical Education, Sport Science and Dietetics, University of Thessaly, 382 21 Volos, Greece; oandrou@hua.gr

[8] Public Health Department, Children's Memorial Health Institute, 04-730 Warsaw, Poland; a.kotowska@ipczd.pl (A.K.); p.socha@ipczd.pl (P.S.)

[9] GENUD (Growth, Exercise, Drinking Behaviour and Development) Research Group, University of Zaragoza, 50009 Zaragoza, Spain; lmoreno@unizar.es

[10] Department of Nutrition and Dietetics, Harokopio University, 176 76 Athens, Greece; manios@hua.gr

* Correspondence: nataly_usheva@hotmail.com; Tel.: +359-52677164

† Membership of the ToyBox-Study Group is provided in the Acknowledgments.

Citation: Usheva, N.; Lateva, M.; Galcheva, S.; Koletzko, B.V.; Cardon, G.; De Craemer, M.; Androutsos, O.; Kotowska, A.; Socha, P.; Moreno, L.A.; et al. Breastfeeding and Overweight in European Preschoolers: The ToyBox Study. *Nutrients* **2021**, *13*, 2880. https://doi.org/10.3390/nu13082880

Academic Editor: Megumi Haruna

Received: 31 July 2021
Accepted: 19 August 2021
Published: 21 August 2021

Publisher's Note: MDPI stays neutral with regard to jurisdictional claims in published maps and institutional affiliations.

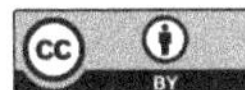

Copyright: © 2021 by the authors. Licensee MDPI, Basel, Switzerland. This article is an open access article distributed under the terms and conditions of the Creative Commons Attribution (CC BY) license (https://creativecommons.org/licenses/by/4.0/).

Abstract: The benefits of breastfeeding (BF) include risk reduction of later overweight and obesity. We aimed to analyse the association between breastfeeding practices and overweight/obesity among preschool children participating in the ToyBox study. Data from children in the six countries, participating in the ToyBox-study (Belgium, Bulgaria, Germany, Greece, Poland, and Spain) 7554 children/families and their age is 3.5–5.5 years, 51.9% were boys collected cross-sectionally in 2012. The questionnaires included parents' self-reported data on their weight, height, socio-demographic status, and infant feeding practices. Measurements of preschool children's weight and height were done by trained researchers using standard protocols and equipment. The ever breastfeeding rate in the total sample was 85.0% (n = 5777). Only 6.3% (n = 428) of the children from the general sample were exclusively breastfed (EBF) for the duration of the first six months. EBF for four to six months was significantly ($p < 0.001$) less likely among mothers with formal education < 12 years (adjusted Odds Ratio (OR) = 0.61; 95% Confidence interval (CI) 0.44–0.85), smoking throughout pregnancy (adjusted OR = 0.39; 95% CI 0.24–0.62), overweight before pregnancy (adjusted OR = 0.67; 95%CI 0.47–0.95) and ≤25 years old. The median duration of any breastfeeding was five months. The prevalence of exclusive formula feeding during the first five months in the general sample was about 12% (n = 830). The prevalence of overweight and obesity at preschool age was 8.0% (n = 542) and 2.8% (n = 190), respectively. The study did not identify any significant association between breastfeeding practices and obesity in childhood when adjusted for relevant confounding factors ($p > 0.05$). It is likely that sociodemographic and lifestyle factors associated with breastfeeding practices may have an impact on childhood obesity. The identified lower than desirable rates and duration of breastfeeding practices should prompt enhanced efforts for effective promotion, protection, and support of breastfeeding across Europe, and in particular in regions with low BF rates.

Keywords: breastfeeding; preschoolers; overweight; obesity

1. Introduction

Optimal nutrition during the first years of life is important to promote healthy growth and development of children. Inappropriate nutrition augments the risk of illness and childhood obesity. Obesity is an escalating public health problem worldwide, with an expected prevalence of 9.1% among preschoolers in 2020 [1,2] and an estimated 70 million overweight or obese children and adolescents by 2025, the majority living in low- and middle-income countries [3]. According to the criteria of the International Obesity Task Force (IOTF), about 17.9% of European children aged 2–7 years were identified with overweight or obesity in the recently published systematic review, including 32 studies (n = 197,755 children) from 27 European countries [4]. Currently available options for treating overweight and obese children are less than satisfactory, therefore implementation of effective preventive measures, including promotion of optimal feeding from early on, is of utmost importance [5].

Breastfeeding is considered as a "golden standard", the best nutrition for infants, and is associated with numerous short- and long-term health benefits, such as higher cognitive development scores and reduced risk of gastro-intestinal infections, otitis media, atopic dermatitis, and asthma, as well as later non-communicable diseases in adults such as type 2 diabetes and obesity [6–11]. It has been proposed that about one million cases of childhood obesity per year may be prevented by recommended breastfeeding (BF) practices [12]. The reported advantages of exclusive breastfeeding (EBF) compared to partial breastfeeding have led to the World Health Organization (WHO) global public health recommending exclusive breastfeeding for six months and continued breastfeeding for ≥two years with complementary foods introduced [13]. The protective role of BF against overweight and obesity was first reported in a large cross-sectional study in 1999 [14] and has since been replicated in many studies around the world [11,15–17]. Potential mechanisms underpinning this association are differences in the composition of human milk and breast milk substitutes and their impact on infant hormonal and metabolic response and growth characteristics. Behavioural differences and associated confounders such as mother's body mass index (BMI), education, and tobacco use in pregnancy have also been discussed [18–24]. We analysed the association between breastfeeding and obesity among school children, with adjustment for important potential confounders relevant to overweight and obesity among the large European sample of schoolchildren participating in the ToyBox Study.

2. Materials and Methods

The ToyBox study (Available online: www.toybox-study.eu (accessed on 21 June 2021) adhered to the Declaration of Helsinki and the conventions of the Council of Europe on human rights and biomedicine. All participating countries obtained ethical clearance from the respective ethical committees and local authorities, and all parents/caregivers provided a signed consent form before being enrolled in the study.

Data was collected between May and June 2012 using the primary caregivers' questionnaire, which was filled in by parents/caregivers of preschoolers in six European countries (Belgium, Bulgaria, Germany, Greece, Poland, and Spain). Parents/caregivers of preschoolers born between January 2007 and December 2008 who attended the randomly selected kindergartens within the provinces of Oost-Vlaanderen and West-Vlaanderen (Belgium), Varna (Bulgaria), Bavaria (Germany), Attica (Greece), Mazowieckie (Poland), and Zaragoza (Spain) were grouped in three socioeconomic levels and invited to participate in ToyBox study. The necessary information about the ToyBox study was presented previously [25]. A standardized self-administered questionnaire for primary caregivers' was used to determine the perinatal data of preschoolers (comprising of anthropometric measurements at birth and breastfeeding practices during the first year of life), as well as participating families' socio-demographic characteristics. Questions about the nutrition of children during the first 12 months of life were targeted on identifying the presence/absence of breastfeeding each month after birth and when water, tea, juice, formula milk, and solid/semi-solid foods were included. In order to minimize recall bias, the guidance to the parents/caregivers was to refer to the children's medical records for the questions in the perinatal section. As a result, the test–retest reliability study showed an excellent value of ICC (intra-class correlation coefficient)—0.75 for this section of the questionnaire. The socio-demographic characteristics were previously found to have very high reliability (i.e., all ICCs $\geq$ 0.937), while the reliability of the questions on parental weight and height spread from moderate to very high (i.e., ICC ranged from 0.489 to 0.911) [26]. Other papers [27,28] presented the data collected using validated questionnaires as well as the corresponding results about health-related behaviors (dietary habits, physical activity, and sedentary behavior) of preschoolers and their parents.

Mothers' years of education were used as stratification criteria for the socioeconomic status (SES) of the families by categorizing it as low ($\leq$12 years), medium (13–16 years), and high ($\geq$16 years of education).

Preterm birth was defined as <37 gestational weeks, and full-term birth as $\geq$37 gestational weeks. Questions on breastfeeding status were based on definitions according to the WHO indicators [29]. Exclusive breastfeeding was defined as BF with no other food or liquid given, except drops and syrups (vitamins, minerals, medicines). Breastfeeding with an additional supply of water or water-based liquids, such as fruit juice, tea, or syrups, was considered predominant breastfeeding. Full BF refers to either exclusive or predominant breastfeeding. The inclusion of other milk and foods (formula milk, and/or semi-solids) was considered partial breastfeeding. Ever breastfeeding rate is the proportion of infants less than 12 months who were ever breastfed. The "later stage BF initiation" was defined as starting of BF at any time but not from birth.

According to the study protocol, the questionnaires with more than 75% of the required information provided were included in the statistical analysis. The analysis did not include the children for which the information about feeding in the first two months ($n = 444$) nor about the time of solid foods' introduction ($n = 300$).

2.1. Anthropometric Data

Children's weight (0.1 kg measurement resolution) and height (0.1 cm measurement resolution) were obtained by means of a standardized protocol and equipment, subjected to calibration before and during the data collection period [30]. For the purpose of ensuring a very good intra- and inter- observed reliability agreement [31], research assistants, who passed extensive training before commencing the study, carried out all measurements to achieve. The definition of overweight, including obesity was based on the WHO criteria: for children age < 5 years as BMI z-score > 2 standard deviation (SD) and BMI z-score > 3 SD, respectively, whereas, for children age > 5 years, the ranges were encompassed into BMI z-score > 1 SD for overweight and into BMI z-score > 2 SD for obesity. Calculated ponderal index (PI = weight/height^3) served for evaluation of children's weight status at their birth with the normal PI range being 2.2–3.0 g/cm^3, PI > 3.0 was considered indicative for overweight; while PI < 2.2 indicated low weight newborns. Parents/caregivers self-reported parental weight and height, while their BMI was calculated. Categorization of parents/caregivers with regard to their BMI defined the groups of normal weight ($\leq$24.9 kg/m^2), overweight ($\geq$25 and $\leq$29.9 kg/m^2), and obese ($\geq$30 kg/m^2) ones [32].

2.2. Statistical Analyses

Continuous variables are shown as the means $\pm$ standard deviation for the cases of normal distribution (e.g., age of preschoolers, age of mothers, the introduction of solid foods) and as the medians and IQR (interquartile range) for variables deviating from a normal distribution (duration of breastfeeding). Shapiro-Wilk tests were used for testing of normality of variables' distribution.

With regard to country and children's BMI categories, the χ^2 test and Fisher's exact test were applied to these categorical variables. For comparison of the means from two samples, an independent samples t-test was implemented, whereas for the means of more than two samples (birth weight; mother's age)—the one-way ANOVA (analysis of variance) with a Scheffe's post-hoc analysis.

The median Mann-Whitney test was used for the comparison of the medians from independent samples. Pearson's and Spearman's correlation analyses were utilized for exploration of the relationship between feeding practices and children's BMI as well as mother's characteristics. The odds of being overweight/obese (dependent variable), while accounting for different breastfeeding practices were estimated by means of logistic regression analysis with 95% confidence intervals (CIs). The validity of significant associations to the duration of breastfeeding, when adjusted for these other variables, potential confounding variables and covariates (mother's age and BMI before pregnancy, SES (socio-economic status), smoking habits during pregnancy, and country) was determined on the basis of the obtained results. For the purpose of quantifying the probability of conforming to the current recommendations for the EBF in 4–6 months of age, logistic regression analysis was carried out adjusting for mothers' age and BMI before pregnancy, SES, smoking habits during pregnancy, and country. Conformance to recommendations for EBF 4–6 months of age (yes/no) and overweight/obesity at preschool age (yes/no) were specified as dependent variables in the relevant models. The variables presented as logistic regression model coefficients were chosen on the basis of their relevance for the investigated subject and also these tested negatively for the presence of collinearity, thus not bringing any tangible influence too. The Statistical Package for Social Sciences (IBM SPSS v. 20, Chicago, IL, USA) was used for the data analysis with $p < 0.05$ set as a level of significance.

3. Results

A total of 6800 questionnaires from the six countries met the qualifying criteria for inclusion in the analysis is. The sociodemographic characteristics of respondents are shown in Table 1. The mean age of children is 4.75 ± 0.43 years; 52.3% boys, with no statistically significant difference in gender distribution between the participating countries. Further details with regard to characteristics of the ToyBox study sample are presented in other papers [25,32].

Table 1. Characteristics of participants by country.

| | Country *n* (%) | | | | | | | |
	Belgium	Bulgaria	Germany	Greece	Poland	Spain	Total	*p*
Child's gender								
Male	600 (53.2)	438 (50.1)	577 (52.3)	841 (51.1)	707 (53.0)	392 (55.0)	3555 (52.3)	0.37 *
Female	528 (46.8)	436 (49.9)	527 (47.7)	806 (48.9)	627 (47.0)	321 (45.0)	3245 (47.7)	
	1128 (100)	874 (100)	1104 (100)	1647 (100)	1334 (100)	713 (100)	6800 (100)	
Birth weight mean (±SD)								
	3.34 (0.51)	3.26 (0.53)	3.32 (0.54)	3.14 (0.53)	3.44 (0.55)	3.32 (0.50)	3.29 (0.54)	<0.001 **
Ponderal Index at birth								
Low	121 (10.7)	142 (16.2)	28 (2.6)	339 (20.7)	754 (59.6)	95 (13.2)	1633 (24.3)	
Normal	914 (81.0)	690 (78.9)	883 (80.8)	1267 (77.2)	499 (39.5)	554 (77.7)	4806 (71.6)	<0.001 *
High	93 (8.3)	42 (4.9)	28 (2.6)	34 (2.1)	12 (0.9)	66 (9.1)	274 (4.1)	
BMI at 6th month								
Under-/normal	788 (94.9)	445 (90.6)	917 (91.7)	1334 (92.8)	818 (89.1)	545 (92.1)	4897 (92.0)	
Overweight	35 (4.2)	21 (4.3)	65 (6.5)	85 (5.9)	75 (8.2)	41 (6.9)	322 (6.1)	<0.001 *
Obese	7 (0.9)	25 (5.1)	18 (1.8)	17 (1.3)	25 (2.7)	6 (1.0)	98 (1.9)	
BMI at 12th month								
Under-/normal	607 (94.4)	400 (82.1)	902 (91.0)	1231 (88.2)	749 (82.6)	515 (88.9)	4404 (88.0)	
Overweight	27 (4.2)	60 (12.4)	62 (6.3)	130 (9.3)	131 (14.4)	55 (9.5)	465 (9.3)	<0.001 *
Obese	9 (1.4)	27 (5.5)	27 (2.7)	35 (2.5)	27 (3.0)	9 (1.6)	134 (2.7)	
BMI categories of preschools *n* (%)								
Underweight	8 (0.7)	5 (0.6)	4 (0.4)	11 (0.7)	7 (0.5)	2 (0.3)	37 (0.5)	
Normal weight	1059 (93.9)	764 (87.4)	1024 (92.8)	1356 (82.3)	1214 (91.0)	613 (86.0)	6030 (87.8)	
Overweight	47 (4.2)	76 (8.7)	61 (5.5)	200 (12.1)	83 (6.2)	75 (10.5)	542 (8.0)	<0.001 *
Obese	14 (1.2)	29 (3.3)	14 (1.3)	80 (4.9)	30 (2.2)	23 (3.2)	190 (2.8)	

Table 1. *Cont.*

	Belgium	Bulgaria	Germany	Greece	Poland	Spain	Total	*p*
				Country *n* (%)				
SES—*n* (%)								
Low SES	453 (40.2)	124 (14.2)	243 (22.0)	790 (48.0)	445 (33.4)	290 (40.7)	2345 (34.5)	
Medium SES	341 (30.2)	300 (34.3)	388 (35.1)	448 (27.2)	395 (29.6)	256 (35.9)	2128 (31.3)	<0.001 *
High SES	334 (29.6)	450 (51.5)	473 (42.8)	409 (24.8)	494 (37.0)	167 (23.4)	2327 (34.2)	
	1128 (100)	874 (100)	1104 (100)	1647 (100)	1334 (100)	713 (100)	6800 (100)	
Mother's age—mean ($\pm$SD)								
	33.7 (4.7)	33.9 (4.4)	35.7 (5.1)	37.1 (4.4)	34.5 (4.3)	37.7 (4.6)	35.4 (4.7)	<0.001 **
BMI categories *n* (%)								
Under-/normal	755 (70.4)	667 (78.9)	727 (70.9)	1101 (70.1)	1011 (78.6)	503 (74.2)	4764 (73.5)	
Overweight	217 (20.2)	133 (15.7)	213 (20.8)	328 (20.9)	204 (15.9)	134 (19.8)	1229 (19.0)	<0.001 *
Obese	100 (9.3)	45 (5.3)	86 (8.4)	142 (9.0)	72 (5.6)	41 (6.0)	486 (7.5)	
Tobacco use during pregnancy								
No smoking	1011 (90.7)	687 (79.8)	956 (89.2)	1340 (82.7)	1220 (93.2)	574 (81.0)	5788 (86.6)	
Smoking 2nd trimester	2 (0.2)	12 (1.4)	4 (0.4)	40 (2.5)	1 (0.1)	2 (0.3)	61 (0.9)	<0.0001 *
Smoking at 1st & 3rd trimester	6 (0.5)	46 (5.3)	29 (2.7)	54 (3.3)	29 (2.2)	25 (3.5)	189 (2.8)	
Smoking throughout pregnancy	96 (8.6)	116 (13.5)	83 (7.7)	187 (11.5)	59 (4.5)	108 (15.2)	649 (9.7)	

* χ^2 test; ** ANOVA; BMI—Body mass index; SES—socio-economic study; SD—standard deviation.

3.1. Breastfeeding Practices

The ever breastfeeding rate in the total sample is 85.0% (*n* = 5777). The highest rates are reported in the samples from Poland (94.7%) and Bulgaria (92.8%), while the lowest is in the Belgian sample (66.7%). Prevalence of the BF initiation from the time of birth is 96.1% (*n* = 5531) and has a statistically positive weak correlation with the country (Pearson's *r* = 0.13; <0.001): the highest are in Belgium (99.6%) and Germany (99.1%). Children in Spain and Greece more often than in other study countries started BF not from birth but from a later time: 12.4%; *n* = 75 and 7%; *n* = 99, respectively.

Only 6.3% (*n* = 428) of the children were exclusively breastfed for the duration of the first six months after birth. Frequencies higher than the average of the total sample are observed for Germany (*n* = 163; 14.8%) and Poland (*n* = 105; 7.9%). Greece has the lowest frequency (2.7%); followed by Belgium (2.8%) and Spain (5.2%) (Table 2).

Table 2. Breastfeeding practices among preschool children from the six countries, participating in the ToyBox study.

Infant Feeding Practice	Belgium	Bulgaria	Germany	Greece	Poland	Spain	Total	*p*
				Country—*n* (%)				
BF initiation—*n* (%)								
-from birth	727 (99.6)	798 (98.4)	920 (99.1)	1319 (93.0)	1236 (97.9)	531 (87.6)	5531 (96.1)	
-from later stage	3 (0.4)	13 (1.6)	8 (0.9)	99 (7.0)	27 (2.1)	75 (12.4)	225 (3.9)	<0.001 [†]
-total	730 (100)	811 (100)	928 (100)	1418 (100)	1263 (100)	606 (100)	5756 (100)	
EBF 4–6 months—*n* (%)	32 (2.8)	47 (5.4)	163 (14.8)	44 (2.7)	105 (7.9)	37 (5.2)	428 (6.3)	<0.001 [†]
Duration of BF (months; median; IQR)	4 (2–6)	5 (3–9)	7 (4–11)	3 (2–6)	9 (4–13)	5 (2–9)	5 (2–9)	<0.001 **
Continued BF rate (>12 months)	31 (3.9)	87 (10.3)	134 (12.1)	84 (5.9)	347 (26.3)	95 (15.7)	778 (12.8)	<0.001 [†]
Introduction of SF months (mean; $\pm$SD)	4.6 $\pm$ 1.8	6.6 $\pm$ 2.0	6.3 $\pm$ 1.8	5.8 $\pm$ 1.2 *	5.8 $\pm$ 1.6 *	5.6 $\pm$ 1.5 *	5.8 $\pm$ 1.7 *	<0.001
EBF 4–6 months + introduction SF and BF < 12 months	32 (2.84)	47 (5.38)	163 (14.76)	44 (2.67)	105 (7.87)	37 (5.19)	428 (6.29)	<0.001 [†]
EBF 4–6 months + introduction SF and BF $\geq$ 12 months	15 (1.15)	24 (2.90)	74 (7.86)	18 (1.09)	142 (10.64)	18 (2.52)	225 (3.31)	<0.001 [†]

* Introduction of solid foods is significantly different with exception of the next comparisons—Greece and Spain *p* = 0.13; Greece and Poland *p* = 0.9; Poland and Spain *p* = 0.18 (ANOVA; Scheffe Post-hoc test); ** *p*-value in median test; [†] *p*-value in χ^2-test; BF—breastfeeding; EBF—exclusive breastfeeding; SF—solid foods; IQR—Interquartile range; SD—standard deviation.

3.2. Duration of Breastfeeding

The median duration of BF among infants during the first 12 months is highest among Polish (9 months) and German (7 months) participants, with a significantly higher duration than the median duration of the entire sample (5 months, $p < 0.001$). For the entire sample, after adjustment for the risk factors there is a weak but significant positive relationship between the duration of breastfeeding and maternal characteristics: education level (Spearman's $\rho = 0.15$; $p = 0.023$), SES (Spearman's $\rho = 0.09$; $p < 0.001$), age at the pregnancy (Pearson's $r = 0.061$; $p < 0.0001$). Additionally, mothers with a pre-pregnancy BMI ≥ 25 (Pearson's $r = -0.14$; $p < 0.001$) and smoking habits during pregnancy (Pearson's $r = -0.06$; $p < 0.0001$) had a shorter duration of BF. Infants who were breastfed exclusively for 4–6 months have a longer duration of any BF (Pearson's $r = 0.32$; $p < 0.0001$). Factors associated with the continued BF (>12 months) are mother's education ≥ 14 years ($p < 0.0001$), normal weight before pregnancy ($p < 0.0001$), non-smoking habits during pregnancy ($p < 0.0001$), 25–40 years age group ($p = 0.001$) and SES ($p = 0.02$).

Exclusive formula feeding during first 4–6 months is about 12% ($n = 830$), with the highest value observed in the Belgian sample ($n = 253$; 22.4%) and the lowest in the Polish sample (4.5%; $p < 0.001$), which is associated with the following mothers' characteristics: education ≥ 14 years ($p < 0.0001$), non-smoking habits during pregnancy ($p < 0.0001$), higher age ($p < 0.0001$) and higher SES ($p = 0.025$); normal pre-pregnancy weight ($p = 0.03$).

Mothers' education less than 12 years ($p < 0.0001$); BMI > 25 kg/m^2 ($p < 0.0001$); tobacco use throughout pregnancy ($p < 0.001$) and low SES ($p < 0.001$) are associated with a higher frequency of formula feeding. The same risk factors (maternal education less than 12 years (OR = 0.61; 95%CI 0.44–0.85), smoking throughout pregnancy (OR = 0.39; 95% CI 0.24–0.62), overweight before pregnancy (OR = 0.67; 95%CI (0.47–0.95)) are associated with not achieving EBF for 4–6 months ($p < 0.05$), Table 3.

Table 3. Maternal characteristics associated with non-compliance to recommendations for exclusive breastfeeding (EBF) for 4–6 months.

	EBF 4–6 Months ($n = 5975$)	
	OR (CI 95%)	p
Education [1]		
≤ 12 years	0.61 (0.44–0.85)	0.003
13–16 years	0.65 (0.52–0.83)	<0.0001
≥ 16 years	1 (reference)	
Smoking habits during pregnancy [2]		
No smoking	1 (reference)	
Smoking during pregnancy	0.39 (0.24–0.62)	<0.0001
Age mother at pregnancy [3]		
≤ 25 years	1 (reference)	
26–39 years	1.76 (1.15–2.70)	0.001
≥ 40 years	1.95 (0.93–4.12)	0.08
BMI before pregnancy [4]		
Underweight	0.98 (0.68–1.41)	0.91
Normal-weight	1 (reference)	
Overweight	0.67 (0.47–0.95)	0.03
Obese	0.53 (0.27–1.05)	0.07

[1] Adjusted for age and BMI before pregnancy, smoking habits during pregnancy, country and SES. [2] Adjusted for age and BMI before pregnancy, country and SES. [3] Adjusted for age BMI before pregnancy, smoking habits during pregnancy, country and SES. [4] Adjusted for age before pregnancy, smoking habits during pregnancy, country and SES; (BMI—Body mass index; SES—socio-economic status; EBF—exclusive breastfeeding)

3.3. Breastfeeding Practices and Weight Status of the Preschoolers

The prevalence of overweight and obesity according to the WHO criteria was 8.0% ($n = 542$) and 2.8% ($n = 190$), respectively (Table 1). Infant feeding practices exhibited a different association with the prevalence of overweight and obesity at different stages of childhood. A lower percentage of children were obese in the EBF 4–6 months group than the formula-fed group (1.6% vs. 6.5%; $p = 0.012$) (Table 4). Factors negatively related to the prevalence of overweight and obesity in preschoolers after controlling for confounding factors are EBF throughout the first three months of life (Pearson's $r = -0.03$; $p = 0.01$) and non-significantly—duration of any breastfeeding (Spearman's $\rho = -0.02$; $p = 0.12$).

Table 4. Breastfeeding practicies and weight status of children.

	Weight 6th Month			Weight 12th Month			Weight Preschoolers		
	Under/Normal Weight	Over-Weight	Obese	Under/Normal Weight	Over-Weight	Obese	Under/Normal Weight	Over-Weight	Obese
EBF 0–3 months	1672 (91.7)	116 (6.4)	35 (1.9)	1557 (88.6)	163 (9.3)	37 (2.1)	2104 (90.8)	170 (7.3)	43 (1.9)
EBF 4–6 months	304 (90.2)	23 (6.8)	10 (3.0)	299 (88.7)	29 (8.6)	9 (2.7)	392 (91.6)	29 (6.8)	7 (1.6)
EBF ≥ 7 months	20 (83.3)	4 (16.7)	0	19 (79.2)	4 (16.7)	1 (4.2)	33 (94.3)	1 (2.9)	1 (2.9)
Predominant BF 0–3 months	852 (92.1)	55 (5.9)	18 (1.9)	777 (86.2)	95 (10.5)	29 (3.2)	1103 (90.2)	79 (6.5)	41 (3.4)
Predominant BF 4–6 months	222 (91.0)	15 (6.1)	7 (2.9)	207 (87.3)	20 (8.4)	10 (4.2)	295 (89.9)	28 (8.5)	5 (1.5)
Formula feeding 4–6 months	143 (86.1)	12 (7.2)	11 (6.6)	137 (83.0)	21 (12.7)	7 (4.2)	199 (86.5)	16 (7.0)	15 (6.5)
Duration of BF >12 months	1446 (91.3)	105 (6.6)	32 (2.0)	1315 (87.3)	155 (10.3)	36 (2.4)	1869 (89.8)	165 (7.9)	47 (2.3)

BF—breastfeeding; EBF—exclusive breastfeeding.

Formula feeding at 4–6 months is linked to a higher prevalence of overweight and obesity at 6 months of infancy (13.8%) and among preschoolers (13.5%), but the association was non-significant when adjusted for confounding factors (Spearman's $\rho = 0.02$; $p = 0.18$). (Table 4)

Table 5 shows the output from the logistic regression analysis with reducing factors for overweight or obesity being identified: the odds to become overweight at preschool age among children who were BF for 4–6 months is 0.87 (OR = 0.87; 95%CI 0.62–1.21; $p = 0.40$); 0.64 for EBF 6 months. The introduction of solid foods after six months of EBF is related to 69% less risk for overweight at preschool age ($p = 0.25$) in comparison to the formula milk feeding when adjusted for the mother's characteristics (age and BMI before pregnancy, smoking habits during pregnancy, country, SES) and gender of the children.

Table 5. Logistic regression analysis of the association of infant feeding practices and the overweight or obesity among preschool children.

Infant Feeding Practice [1]	Overweight		Obesity	
	OR (CI 95%)	p	OR (CI 95%)	p
Breastfeeding				
1–3 months	1.09 (0.81–1.45)	0.59	1.15 (0.69–1.93)	0.59
4–6 months	0.87 (0.62–1.21)	0.40	0.89 (0.50–1.60)	0.75
7–12 months	1.01 (0.73–1.41)	0.96	1.25 (0.69–2.26)	0.44
≥12 months	1.02 (0.70–1.50)	0.91	1.11 (0.54–2.25)	0.78
Formula feeding	1 (reference)		1 (reference)	
Infant feeding practicies for 6 months				
EBF	0.64 (0.22–1.81)	0.40	1.10 (0.63–1.93)	0.73
Predominant BF	1.12 (0.78–1.61)	0.55	0.91 (0.52–1.60)	0.74
Partial BF	0.95 (0.71–1.28)	0.73	1.35 (0.83–2.20)	0.23
EBF and solids	0.31 (0.04–2.30)	0.25	0.88 (0.47–1.77)	0.79
Formula feeding	1 (reference)		1 (reference)	

[1] Adjusted for mother's age and BMI before pregnancy, smoking habits during pregnancy, country, SES and children's gender; EBF—exclusive breastfeeding; BF—breastfeeding.

Regarding the association between other characteristics at birth and obesity, there is no correlation with preterm or term delivery ($p = 0.89$) and PI at birth ($p = 0.36$) in the total sample and the country level stratification ($p > 0.05$).

4. Discussion

The analyses of the collected data from 6 countries in Europe regarding the characteristics at birth, infant feeding practices, and risk of childhood obesity revealed that in nearly all the countries 85% of children were breastfed, with the notable exception of Belgium, where only 66.7% of children were breastfed. In spite of the solid evidence demonstrating major health benefits associated with BF, including risk reduction for overweight and obesity, breastfeeding remains still well below the global goal of 50% EBF at 2025 [33–35]. Our data represent the BF practices and related factors corresponding to the year 2012 but are in agreement with other recent survey analyses indicating less than satisfactory breastfeeding practices in many European countries [36]. In our sample, only 6.3% of children were exclusively breastfed during the 6th month of life and thus met the WHO recommendation. However, a recent survey performed by the WHO Regional Office for Europe and the European Society of Pediatric Gastroenterology, Hepatology and Nutrition revealed that more than 82% of European countries recommended the introduction of complementary feeding at the age of 4–5 months and hence exclusive breastfeeding for a shorter period than six months [37]. The rate of EBF in our study is lower than results for EBF at 4–6 months from European samples such as IDEFICS (45.5%) and COSI (lowest—10.5% for Spain), and from the World Health Statistics WHO—Reports [38,39]. The significant data discrepancy appears to be primarily due to the different approaches of the calculation methodologies, and potentially also due to some imprecision due to recall bias in our study. In the studies cited above, as well as in almost all the official data, the frequency of exclusive breastfeeding is presented according to the WHO "Indicators for assessing infant and young child feeding practices" as the prevalence of "exclusively breastfed for the first 6 months of life". Thus, this indicator does not measure the proportion of children meeting the WHO recommendation for exclusive breastfeeding of all children until 6 months, as pointed out by Pullum [40]. The prevalence data in the above-mentioned studies are very close to the goals in the "WHO global nutrition targets 2025" and can lead to inadequate political decisions regarding protection, promotion, and support of exclusive breastfeeding.

Children who were exclusively BF throughout the first three months of life were less likely to become overweight at preschool age when adjusted for country, age and gender, mother's pre-pregnancy age and BMI.

The odds to become overweight at preschool age among children who were BF for 4–6 months is 0.87 and 0.31 for the EBF and solids introduction at 4–6 months in comparison to the formula milk feeding, when adjusted for mother's characteristics (age and BMI before pregnancy, smoking habits during pregnancy, country, SES and gender of children). Thus the effect size for breastfeeding effects on later obesity in our study, although non-significant, is in the same order of magnitude as found in reviews and meta-analyses [15–18]. Our results also show a protective role of any breastfeeding against obesity and overweight, with 13% less risk at any BF of 4–6 months, and 69% for overweight and 12% for obesity at EBF and solid foods introduction for six months, compared to exclusive formula feeding. These results agree with the reported 26% decrease of the odds of overweight or obesity with any BF in 113 studies [23]. Also, infants fed formula during the first 4–6 months have a higher prevalence of overweight and obesity in preschool age (Table 4). Possible mechanisms for this relationship may include the different macronutrient composition of breast milk and formula, in particular the lower protein supply with breast milk [18], and potentially the presence of bioactive substances like ghrelin, leptin, insulin-like growth factor-1, adiponectin in human milk but not in formula [41]. There is published evidence that feeding formula milk has an accelerating effect on infant weight, height, body fat, apparently mediated through high levels of protein (the "early protein hypothesis") [18] and lower appetite control of bottle-fed infants [15,20,42,43]. Moreover, a recent study reported that formula feeding in the early life of infants small for their gestational age is related to prospective overweight in preschool age, but only among girls [44]. Breastfeeding also modulates the physiological development of the digestive tract [45] and intestinal colonization [46], which might contribute to risk reduction for obesity in later life [47]. However, our results also show significant confounding of the association of breastfeeding and later overweight by low SES that is linked to both less breastfeeding success and more overweight. A more detailed analysis of the relationship between SES and overweight/obesity prevalence in children participating in the ToyBox study was previously published [32]. In the current analysis, SES is included as a confounder for which the analysis has been adjusted.

One of the limitations of the current presentation is the cross-sectional study design which is not able to identify the cause-effect association between the sociodemographic characteristics and the prevalence of overweight/obesity among preschoolers. Particularly, the selection of children from kindergartens within only one province in each country is the next methodological limitation of the study, which does not allow to draw a conclusion at a national level for each of the countries based on the collected data. Another limiting factor stems from the parental self-reporting of weight, height, gestational weight gain, and infant's birth weight, which despite the relatively close time for recollection might have introduced recall bias. Retrieving data about BF duration through mothers' recall for the time period 3–4 years ago can be seen as another limitation. This mostly impacts the reporting of EBF, as there is evidence that more than two years after birth mothers tend to overestimate the duration of BF [48]. In line with previous studies, our analysis indicates that breastfeeding practices are associated with factors that are also related to obesity development, such as maternal education, SES, BMI, and infant birth weight [38,49–51]. The statistical power to detect protective effects of breastfeeding on later obesity is limited by the fact that we could not compare exclusive breastfeeding from birth with exclusive formula feeding from birth, which has been reported to have the most marked effect on later obesity risk [52]. Even though we adjusted the calculation of ORs for these factors, residual confounding cannot be excluded, hence the extent of the causal effect of breastfeeding itself on later risk of overweight and obesity is difficult to determine.

A large number of study participants, the involvement of participants from several European countries which adds a level of independent validation, as well as the harmonized methodology in data collection and obtaining measurements may be noted as merits of this study [26,32].

5. Conclusions

Our study found only a non-significant trend for reduced childhood overweight associated with breastfeeding when adjusting for relevant confounding factors. It is likely that sociodemographic and lifestyle factors associated with breastfeeding practices have an impact on childhood obesity. The findings of less than desirable breastfeeding rates and duration underline the need for enhanced protection, promotion, and support of breastfeeding throughout Europe. Particularly intensive efforts are necessary for populations with low breastfeeding rates and duration based on geographic region and other risk markers such as lower education and socioeconomic class, tobacco smoking, parental overweight and obesity [5,36]; short duration of maternity leave, psychological factors as maternal perceived stress and postpartum depression [53].

Author Contributions: Conceptualization, V.I. and N.U.; methodology, N.U., V.I. and G.C.; formal analysis, N.U., M.L. and S.G.; investigation, M.L., S.G. and M.D.C.; writing—original draft preparation, N.U., V.I.; writing—review and editing, B.V.K., M.D.C., O.A., V.I., G.C., A.K., S.G., Y.M., P.S., L.A.M.; supervision, V.I., Y.M. All authors have read and agreed to the published version of the manuscript.

Funding: The ToyBoxstudy was funded by the Seventh Framework Program (The Community Research and Development Information Service (CORDIS; FP7)) of the European Commission under grant agreement No. 245200. B.V.K. is the Else Kröner Senior professor of Paediatrics at LMU—University of Munich, financially supported by the Else Kröner-Fresenius-Foundation, the LMU Medical Faculty and the LMU University Hospitals. The content of this article reflects only the authors' views and the European Community is not liable for any use that may be made of the information contained therein.

Institutional Review Board Statement: The ToyBoxstudy (www.toybox-study.eu; accessed on 20 September 2020) adhered to the Declaration of Helsinki and the conventions of the Council of Europe on human rights and biomedicine. All the countries (Belgium, Bulgaria, Germany, Greece, Poland and Spain) obtained ethical clearance from the relevant ethics committees and local authorities: 1. Ethics Committee of Ghent University Hospital (Belgium)—EC/2010/037; 2. Committee for the Ethics of Scientific Studies (KENI) at the Medical University of Varna (Bulgaria)—15/21.07.2011; 3. Ethics Committee of the Medical Faculty at LMU Munich (Ethikkommission der Ludwig-Maximilians-Universität München) (Germany)—400-11 (2012); 4. Bioethics Committee of the Harokopio University of Athens (Greece) (28/02-12-2010) and the Ministry of Education of Greece (approval code 29447/Γ7 (5 May 2011)); 5. Ethics Committee of the Children's Memorial Health Institute (Poland)—1/KBE/2012; 6. CEICA (Comité Ético de Investigación Clínica de Aragón (Spain))—PI11/056 30 August 2011. The ToyBox-study is registered with the clinical trials registry: clinicaltrials.gov, ID: NCT02116296.

Informed Consent Statement: All parents/caregivers provided a signed consent form before being enrolled in the study.

Data Availability Statement: The data presented in this study are available on request from the corresponding author. The data are not publicly available due to restrictions of informed consent and the requirement of IRB review and approval.

Acknowledgments: We gratefully acknowledge all the members of the ToyBox study group: Coordinator: Yannis Manios; Project manager: Odysseas Androutsos; Steering Committee: Yannis Manios, Berthold Koletzko, Ilse De Bourdeaudhuij, Mai Chin A Paw, Luis Moreno, Carolyn Summerbell, Tim Lobstein, Lieven Annemans, Goof Buijs; External Advisors: John Reilly, Boyd Swinburn, Dianne Ward; Harokopio University (Greece): Yannis Manios, Odysseas Androutsos, Eva Grammatikaki, Christina Katsarou, Eftychia Apostolidou, Anastasia Livaniou, Eirini Efstathopoulou, Paraskevi-Eirini Siatitsa, Angeliki Giannopoulou, Eff ie Argyri, Konstantina Maragkopoulou, Athanasios Douligeris, Roula Koutsi; Ludwig Maximilians Univers itaet Muenchen (Germany): Berthold Koletzko, Kristin Duvinage, Sabine Ibrügger, Angelika Strauß, Birgit Herbert, Julia Birnbaum, Annette Payr, Christine Geyer; Ghent University (Belgium): Department of Movement and Sports Sciences: Ilse De Bourdeaudhuij, Greet Cardon, Marieke De Craemer, Ellen De Decker; Department of Public Health: Lieven Annemans, Stefaan De Henauw, Lea Maes, Carine Vereecken, Jo Van Assche, Lore Pil; VU University Medical Center EMGO Institute for Health and Care Research (the Netherlands): EMGO Institute for Health and Care Research: Mai Chin A Paw, Saskia te Velde; University of Zaragoza (Spain): Luis Moreno, Theodora Mouratidou, Juan Fernandez, Maribel Mesana, Pilar De Miguel-Etayo, Esther M. González-Gil, Luis Gracia-Marco, Beatriz Oves; Oslo and Akershus University College of Applied Sciences (Norway): Agneta Yngve, Susanna Kugelberg, Christel Lynch, Annhild Mosdøl, Bente B Nilsen; University of Durham (UK): Carolyn Summerbell, Helen Moore, Wayne Douthwaite, Catherine Nixon; State Institute of Early Childhood Research (Germany): Susanne Kreichauf, Andreas Wildgruber; Children's Memorial Health Institute (Poland): Piotr Socha, Zbigniew Kulaga, Kamila Zych, Magdalena Góźdź, Beata Gurzkowska, Katarzyna Szott; Medical University of Varna (Bulgaria): Violeta Iotova, Mina Lateva, Natalya Usheva, Sonya Galcheva, Vanya Marinova, Zhan eta Radkova, Nevyana Feschieva; International Association for the Study of Obesity (UK): Tim Lobstein, Andrea Aikenhead; CBO B.V. (the Netherlands): Goof Buijs, Annemiek Dorgelo, Aviva Nethe, Jan Jansen; AOK- Verlag (Germany): Otto Gmeiner, Jutta Retterath, Julia Wildeis, Axel Günthersberger; Roehampton University (UK): Leigh Gibson; University of Luxembourg (Luxembourg): Claus Voegele.

Conflicts of Interest: The authors declare no conflict of interest.

References

1. WHO. *The Global Burden of Disease: 2004 Update*; World Health Organization: Geneva, Switzerland, 2008.
2. De Onis, M.; Blössner, M.; Borghi, E. Global prevalence and trends of overweight and obesity among preschool children. *Am. J. Clin. Nutr.* **2010**, *92*, 1257–1264. [CrossRef] [PubMed]
3. WHO. *Interim Report of the Commission on Ending Childhood Obesity*; World Health Organization: Geneva, Switzerland, 2015.
4. Garrido-Miguel, M.; Oliveira, A.; Cavero-Redondo, I.; Álvarez-Bueno, C.; Pozuelo-Carrascosa, D.P.; Soriano-Cano, A.; Martínez-Vizcaíno, V. Prevalence of Overweight and Obesity among European Preschool Children: A Systematic Review and Meta-Regression by Food Group Consumption. *Nutrients* **2019**, *11*, 1698. [CrossRef]

5. Koletzko, B.; Fishbein, M.; Lee, W.S.; Moreno, L.; Mouane, N.; Mouzaki, M.; Verduci, E. Prevention of Childhood Obesity: A Position Paper of the Global Federation of International Societies of Paediatric Gastroenterology, Hepatology and Nutrition (FISPGHAN). *J. Pediatr. Gastroenterol. Nutr.* **2020**, *70*, 702–710. [CrossRef]
6. Fewtrell, M.S.; Morgan, J.B.; Duggan, C.; Gunnlaugsson, G.; Hibberd, P.L.; Lucas, A.; Kleinman, R.E. Optimal duration of exclusive breastfeeding: What is the evidence to support current recommendations? *Am. J. Clin. Nutr.* **2007**, *85*, 635S–638S. [CrossRef] [PubMed]
7. WHO. *Evidence on the Long-Term Effects of Breastfeeding: Systematic Reviews and Meta-Analyses*; World Health Organisation: Geneva, Switzerland, 2007.
8. Harder, T.; Bergmann, R.; Kallischnigg, G.; Plagemann, A. Duration of breastfeeding and the risk of overweight. *Am. J. Epidemiol.* **2005**, *162*, 397–403. [CrossRef] [PubMed]
9. Kramer, M.S.; Kakuma, R. The optimal duration of exclusive breastfeeding: A systematic review. *Adv. Exp. Med. Biol.* **2004**, *554*, 63–77. [PubMed]
10. Hunsberger, M.; Lanfer, A.; Reeske, A.; Veidebaum, T.; Russo, P.; Hadjigeorgiou, C.; Eiben, G. Infant feeding practices and prevalence of obesity in eight European countries-The IDEFICS study. *Public Health Nutr.* **2013**, *16*, 219–227. [CrossRef]
11. Arenz, S.; Rückerl, R.; Koletzko, B.; von Kries, R. Breast-feeding and childhood obesity—A systematic review. *Int. J. Obes. Relat. Metab. Disord.* **2004**, *28*, 1247–1256. [CrossRef] [PubMed]
12. Walters, D.D.; Phan, L.T.H.; Mathisen, R. The cost of not breastfeeding: Global results from a new tool. *Health Policy Plan.* **2019**, *34*, 407–417. [CrossRef] [PubMed]
13. WHO. The Optimal Duration of Exclusive Breastfeeding: Report of an Expert Consultation. 2001. Available online: www.who.int/nutrition/publications/optimal_duration_of_exc_bfeeding_report_eng.pdf (accessed on 30 March 2021).
14. Von Kries, R.; Koletzko, B.; Sauerwald, T.; Von Mutius, E.; Barnert, D.; Grunert, V.; Von Voss, H. Breast feeding and obesity: Cross sectional study. *BMJ* **1999**, *319*, 147–150. [CrossRef] [PubMed]
15. Programme ECO. *EU Childhood Obesity Programme Press Pack*; European Commission: Budapest, Belgium, 20 April 2007.
16. Owen, C.G.; Martin, R.M.; Whincup, P.H.; Smith, G.D.; Cook, D.G. Effect of infant feeding on the risk ofobesity across the life course: A quantitative review of published evidence. *Pediatrics* **2005**, *115*, 1367–1377. [CrossRef] [PubMed]
17. Horta, B.L.; Victora, C.G. *Long-Term Effects of Breastfeeding. A Systematic Review*; World Health Organisation: Geneva, Switzerland, 2013.
18. Koletzko, B.; Demmelmair, H.; Grote, V.; Totzauer, M. Optimized protein intakes in term infants support physiological growth and promote long-term health. *Semin. Perinatol.* **2019**, *43*, 151153. [CrossRef] [PubMed]
19. Koletzko, B.; Von Kries, R.; Monasterolo, R.C.; Subías, J.E.; Scaglioni, S.; Giovannini, M.; Beyer, J.; Demmelmair, H.; Anton, B.; Gruszfeld, D.; et al. Infant feeding and later obesity risk. *Adv. Exp. Med. Biol.* **2009**, *646*, 15–29. [PubMed]
20. Stettler, N.; Iotova, V. Early growth patterns and long-term obesity risk. *Curr. Opin. Clin. Nutr. Metab. Care* **2010**, *13*, 294–299. [CrossRef] [PubMed]
21. Fields, D.A.; Demerath, E.W. Relationship of insulin, glucose, leptin, IL-6 and TNF-α in human breast milk withinfant growth and body composition. *Pediatr. Obes.* **2012**, *7*, 304–312. [CrossRef] [PubMed]
22. Breij, L.M.; Mulder, M.T.; Hokken-Koelega, A.C. Appetite-regulating hormones in early life and relationships with type of feeding and body composition in healthy term infants. *Eur. J. Nutr.* **2017**, *56*, 1725–1732. [CrossRef] [PubMed]
23. Victora, C.G.; Bahl, R.; Barros, A.J.; França, G.V.; Horton, S.; Krasevec, J.; Murch, S.; Sankar, M.J.; Walker, N.; Rollins, N.C.; et al. Breastfeeding in the 21st century: Epidemiology, mechanisms, and lifelong effect. *Lancet* **2016**, *387*, 475–490. [CrossRef]
24. Appleyard, K.; Egeland, B.; van Dulmen, M.H.; Sroufe, L.A. When more is not better: The role of cumulative risk in child behavior outcomes. *J. Child Psychol. Psychiatry* **2005**, *46*, 235–245. [CrossRef] [PubMed]
25. Manios, Y.; Androutsos, O.; Katsarou, C.; Iotova, V.; Socha, P.; Geyer, C.; Moreno, L.; Koletzko, B.; De Bourdeaudhuij, I.; ToyBox-Study Group. Designing and implementing a kindergarten-based, family-involved intervention to prevent obesity in early childhood: The Toybox-study. *Obes. Rev.* **2014**, *15* (Suppl. 3), 5–13. [CrossRef] [PubMed]
26. González-Gil, E.M.; Mouratidou, T.; Cardon, G.; Androutsos, O.; De Bourdeaudhuij, I.; Góźdź, M.; Usheva, N.; Birnbaum, J.; Manios, Y.; Moreno, L.A.; et al. Moreno on behalf of the ToyBox-study group, Reliability of primary caregivers reports on lifestyle behaviours of European pre-school children: The ToyBox-study. *Obes. Rev.* **2014**, *15*, 61–66. [CrossRef] [PubMed]
27. Cardon, G.; De Bourdeaudhuij, I.; Iotova, V.; Latomme, J.; Socha, P.; Koletzko, B.; Moreno, L.; Manios, Y.; Androutsos, O.; De Craemer, M.; et al. Health Related Behaviours in Normal Weight and Overweight Preschoolers of a Large Pan-European Sample: The ToyBox-Study. *PLoS ONE* **2016**, *11*, e0150580. [CrossRef] [PubMed]
28. Pinket, A.S.; De Craemer, M.; Maes, L.; De Bourdeaudhuij, I.; Cardon, G.; Androutsos, O.; Koletzko, B.; Moreno, L.; Socha, P.; Iotova, V.; et al. Water intake and beverage consumption of pre-schoolers from six European countries and associations with socio-economic status: The ToyBox-study. *Public Health Nutr.* **2016**, *19*, 2315–2325. [CrossRef] [PubMed]
29. WHO; UNICEF; IFPRI; UCDavis; FANTA; AED; USAID. *Indicators for Assessing Infant and Young Child Feeding Practicies*; World Health Organization: Geneva, Switzerland, 2008.
30. Mouratidou, T.; Miguel, M.L.; Androutsos, O.; Manios, Y.; De Bourdeaudhuij, I.; Cardon, G.; Kulaga, Z.; Socha, P.; Galcheva, S.; Iotova, V.; et al. Tools, harmonization and standardization procedures of the impact and outcome evaluation indices obtained during a kindergarten-based, family-involved intervention to prevent obesity in early childhood: The ToyBox-study. *Obes. Rev.* **2014**, *15* (Suppl. 3), 53–60. [CrossRef]

31. De Miguel-Etayo, P.; Mesana, M.I.; Cardon, G.; De Bourdeaudhuij, I.; Góźdź, M.; Socha, P.; Lateva, M.; Iotova, V.; Koletzko, B.V.; Duvinage, K.; et al. Reliability of anthropometric measurements in European preschool children: The ToyBox-study. *Obes. Rev.* **2014**, *15* (Suppl. 3), 67–73. [CrossRef] [PubMed]

32. Manios, Y.; Androutsos, O.; Katsarou, C.; Vampouli, E.A.; Kulaga, Z.; Gurzkowska, B.; Iotova, V.; Usheva, N.; Cardon, G.; Koletzko, B.; et al. Prevalence and sociodemographic correlates of overweight and obesity in a large Pan-European cohort of preschool children and their families. The ToyBox-study. *Nutrition* **2018**, *55*, 192–198. [CrossRef]

33. WHO; UNICEF. *Global Strategy of Infant and Young Children Feeding*; World Health Organization: Geneva, Switzerland, 2003; Available online: http://whqlibdoc.who.int/publications/2003/9241562218.pdf (accessed on 15 April 2021).

34. UN. Political Declaration of the High-Level Meeting of the General Assembly on the Prevention and Control of Non-Communicable Diseases. Available online: http://www.who.int/nmh/events/un_ncd_summit2011/political_declaration_en.pdf (accessed on 21 June 2021).

35. World Health Organization. *Global Nutrition Targets 2025: Breastfeeding Policy Brief*; World Health Organization: Geneva, Switzerland, 2014.

36. Theurich, M.A.; Davanzo, R.; Busck-Rasmussen, M.; Díaz-Gómez, N.M.; Brennan, C.; Kylberg, E.; Bærug, A.; McHugh, L.; Weikert, C.; Abraham, K.; et al. Breastfeeding Rates and Programs in Europe: A Survey of 11 National Breastfeeding Committees and Representatives. *J. Pediatr. Gastroenterol. Nutr.* **2019**, *68*, 400–407. [CrossRef]

37. Koletzko, B.; Hirsch, N.L.; Jewell, J.M.; Dos Santos, Q.; Breda, J.; Fewtrell, M.; Weber, M.W. National Recommendations for Infant and Young Child Feeding in the World Health Organization European Region. *J. Pediatr. Gastroenterol. Nutr.* **2020**, *71*, 672–678. [CrossRef]

38. Papoutsou, S.; Savva, S.C.; Hunsberger, M.; Jilani, H.; Michels, N.; Ahrens, W.; Tornaritis, M.; Veidebaum, T.; Molnár, D.; Siani, A.; et al. Timing of solid food introduction and association with later childhood overweight and obesity: The IDEFICS study. *Matern. Child Nutr.* **2017**, *14*, e12471. [CrossRef]

39. Rito, A.I.; Buoncristiano, M.; Spinelli, A.; Salanave, B.; Kunešová, M.; Hejgaard, T.; Solano, M.G.; Fijałkowska, A.; Sturua, L.; Hyska, J.; et al. Association between Characteristics at Birth, Breastfeeding and Obesity in 22 Countries: The WHO European Childhood Obesity Surveillance Initiative—COSI 2015/2017. *Obes. Facts* **2019**, *12*, 226–243. [CrossRef]

40. Pullum, T.W. Exclusive breastfeeding: Aligning the indicator with the goal. *Glob. Health Sci. Pract.* **2014**, *2*, 355–356. [CrossRef]

41. Koletzko, B.; Brands, B.; Grote, V.; Kirchberg, F.F.; Prell, C.; Rzehak, P.; Uhl, O.; Weber, M.; Early Nutrition Programming Project. Long-Term Health Impact of Early Nutrition: The Power of Programming. *Ann. Nutr. Metab.* **2017**, *70*, 161–169. [CrossRef]

42. Kramer, M.S.; Guo, T.; Platt, R.W.; Vanilovich, I.; Sevkovskaya, Z.; Dzikovich, I.; Michaelsen, K.F.; Dewey, K. Feeding effects on growth during infancy. *J. Pediatr.* **2004**, *145*, 600–605. [CrossRef]

43. Kramer, M.S.; Matush, L.; Vanilovich, I.; Platt, R.W.; Bogdanovich, N.; Sevkovskaya, Z.; Dzikovich, I.; Shishko, G.; Collet, J.P.; Martin, R.M.; et al. Effects of prolonged and exclusive breastfeeding on child height, weight, adiposity, and blood pressure at age 6.5 y: Evidence from a large randomized trial. *Am. J. Clin. Nutr.* **2007**, *86*, 1717–1721. [CrossRef]

44. Gallo, C.; Cannataro, R.; Perri, M.; Longo, A.; De Luca, I.F.; Frangella, E.; Gallelli, L.; De Sarro, M.A.; Admasu, M.C.; Caroleo, M.C.; et al. Body Composition Assessment in Children Born Small for Gestational Age and Its Correlation with Early Nutrition Type: Observational Study. *Int. J. Nur. Health* **2018**, *1*, 35–41.

45. Le Huërou-Luron, I.; Blat, S.; Boudry, G. Breast v. formula-feeding: Impacts on the digestive tract and immediate and long-term health effects. *Nutr. Res. Rev.* **2010**, *23*, 23–36. [CrossRef] [PubMed]

46. Vandenplas, Y.; Carnielli, V.P.; Ksiazyk, J.; Luna, M.S.; Migacheva, N.; Mosselmans, J.M.; Picaud, J.C.; Possner, M.; Singhal, A.; Wabitsch, M. Factors affecting early-life intestinal microbiota development. *Nutrition* **2020**, *78*, 110812. [CrossRef] [PubMed]

47. Dreyer, J.L.; Liebl, A.L. Early colonization of the gut microbiome and its relationship with obesity. *Hum. Microbiome J.* **2018**, *10*, 1–5. [CrossRef]

48. Burnham, L.; Buczek, M.; Braun, N.; Feldman-Winter, L.; Chen, N.; Merewood, A. Determining length of breastfeeding exclusivity: Validity of maternal report 2 years after birth. *J. Hum. Lact.* **2014**, *30*, 190–194. [CrossRef]

49. van Rossem, L.; Oenema, A.; Steegers, E.A.; Moll, H.A.; Jaddoe, V.W.; Hofman, A.; Mackenbach, J.P.; Raat, H. Are starting and continuing breastfeeding related to educationalbackground?The Generation R study. *Pediatrics* **2009**, *123*, e1017–e1027. [CrossRef] [PubMed]

50. Gibbs, B.G.; Forste, R. Socioeconomic status, infant feeding practices and early childhood obesity. *Pediatric Obes.* **2014**, *9*, 135–146. [CrossRef]

51. Grummer-Strawn, L.M.; Scanlon, K.S.; Fein, S.B. Infant Feeding and Feeding Transitions during the First Year of Life. *Pediatrics* **2008**, *122* (Suppl. 2), S36–S42. [CrossRef] [PubMed]

52. Ruckinger, S.; von Kries, R. Breastfeeding and reduced risk of childhood obesity: Will randomized trials on breastfeeding promotion give the definite answer? *Am. J. Clin. Nutr.* **2009**, *89*, 653–655. [CrossRef] [PubMed]

53. Gila-Díaz, A.; Carrillo, G.H.; López de Pablo, Á.L.; Arribas, S.M.; Ramiro-Cortijo, D. Association between Maternal Postpartum Depression, Stress, Optimism, and Breastfeeding Pattern in the First Six Months. *Int. J. Environ. Res. Public Health* **2020**, *17*, 7153. [CrossRef] [PubMed]

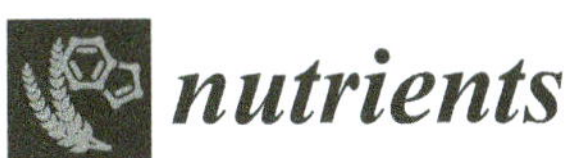 *nutrients*

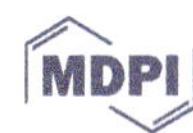

Article

Healthy Schoolhouse 2.0 Health Promotion Intervention to Reduce Childhood Obesity in Washington, DC: A Feasibility Study

Melissa Hawkins [1,*], Sarah Irvine Belson [2], Robin McClave [1], Lauren Kohls [3], Sarah Little [3] and Anastasia Snelling [1]

[1] Department of Health Studies, College of Arts & Sciences, American University, Washington, DC 20016, USA; mcclave@american.edu (R.M.); stacey@american.edu (A.S.)
[2] School of Education, American University, Washington, DC 20016, USA; sirvine@american.edu
[3] School of Public Affairs, American University, Washington, DC 20016, USA; lk9749a@student.american.edu (L.K.); sl6328a@student.american.edu (S.L.)
* Correspondence: mhawkins@american.edu; Tel.: +1-202-885-6252

Abstract: Childhood obesity prevalence trends involve complex societal and environmental factors as well as individual behaviors. The Healthy Schoolhouse 2.0 program seeks to improve nutrition literacy among elementary school students through an equity-focused intervention that supports the health of students, teachers, and the community. This five-year quasi-experimental study follows a baseline–post-test design. Research activities examine the feasibility and effectiveness of a professional development series in the first program year to improve teachers' self-efficacy and students' nutrition literacy. Four elementary schools in Washington, DC (two intervention, two comparison) enrolled in the program (N = 1302 students). Demographic and baseline assessments were similar between schools. Teacher participation in professional development sessions was positively correlated with implementing nutrition lessons (r = 0.6, p < 0.001, n = 55). Post-test student nutrition knowledge scores (W = 39985, p < 0.010, n = 659) and knowledge score changes (W = 17064, p < 0.010, n = 448) were higher among students in the intervention schools. Students who received three nutrition lessons had higher post knowledge scores than students who received fewer lessons (H(2) =22.75, p < 0.001, n = 659). Engaging teachers to implement nutrition curricula may support sustainable obesity prevention efforts in the elementary school environment.

Keywords: childhood obesity; nutrition literacy; nutrition education; self-efficacy; teachers

Citation: Hawkins, M.; Belson, S.I.; McClave, R.; Kohls, L.; Little, S.; Snelling, A. Healthy Schoolhouse 2.0 Health Promotion Intervention to Reduce Childhood Obesity in Washington, DC: A Feasibility Study. *Nutrients* **2021**, *13*, 2935. https://doi.org/10.3390/nu13092935

Academic Editor: Odysseas Androutsos

Received: 31 July 2021
Accepted: 21 August 2021
Published: 25 August 2021

Publisher's Note: MDPI stays neutral with regard to jurisdictional claims in published maps and institutional affiliations.

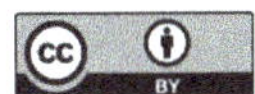

Copyright: © 2021 by the authors. Licensee MDPI, Basel, Switzerland. This article is an open access article distributed under the terms and conditions of the Creative Commons Attribution (CC BY) license (https://creativecommons.org/licenses/by/4.0/).

1. Introduction

The increasing prevalence of childhood obesity and overweight in the United States (US) is a significant public health concern, with adverse health and economic consequences across the lifespan [1]. Over the last two decades, the rates of childhood obesity increased from 13.9% to 19.3% nationally, and they disproportionately impacted communities of color and those of lower socioeconomic status [2]. In Washington D.C. (DC), the childhood obesity rate is among the highest in the nation, affecting 35% of children; in Wards 7 and 8, two of the district's most underserved regions, the obesity rate is 72% [3]. The causes mediating childhood obesity prevalence involve complex societal and environmental factors, as well as individual behaviors; thus, solutions must engage multiple spheres of influence.

Several US federal policies have sought to address the system-wide challenges that contribute to an increase in childhood obesity and overweight within school settings. For example, the National School Lunch Program and Healthy, Hunger-Free Kids Act of 2010 (HHFKA) improved the nutrition standards school meals are required to meet [4,5], and the 2015 Every Student Succeeds Act (ESSA) included health and physical education in the definition of a "well-rounded education" [6]. Broad adoption of the Whole School,

Whole Community, Whole Child (WSCC) model aligns education and health with a focus on the "long-term development and success of all children" [7]. Locally, DC passed the Healthy Schools Act of 2010 (amended by the Healthy Students Amendment Act of 2018) to establish comprehensive requirements for improving school meal and nutrition standards in the cafeteria and vending machines, increasing student physical activity and health education time, supporting school gardens and farm-to-school education, and establishing local school wellness policies to specifically address obesity and hunger [8].

Working in tandem with educational policy, health promotion interventions to improve child health and prevent obesity are frequently based in school settings. Although barriers exist, including time, resources, and educator training, extensive research supports the effectiveness of school-based nutrition education interventions to reduce childhood obesity and support academic achievement [9–16]. Specifically, health promotion interventions can improve nutrition knowledge, attitudes, and preferences for healthy foods [17,18] and serve to predict future behavior [19]. Further, a systematic review and meta-analysis of 34 studies [20] suggests a positive impact on student nutritional knowledge and dietary behaviors when nutrition education is taught by teachers.

Teachers are vital to advancing student health and education. Elementary school teachers, in particular, represent an upstream approach to establishing healthy eating habits early in life that may reduce future onset of childhood obesity. Moreover, investing in teacher knowledge and behavior can positively impact student outcomes [21]. While most teachers believe in the importance of teaching nutrition education and agree they can influence their students' eating behaviors, less than half report feeling prepared, empowered, or able to integrate health education into their current curricula [22,23]. These findings [22–24] indicate that while teachers hold strong beliefs relative to the positive correlation between health and learning, they rate themselves poorly in having the knowledge and skills to teach and integrate health into instruction [25]. Accordingly, increasing teachers' confidence, attitudes, and self-efficacy related to nutrition may have a positive impact on student health behaviors.

Healthy Schoolhouse 2.0 is a comprehensive childhood obesity prevention program that seeks to improve nutrition literacy among elementary school students and supports the health of students, teachers, and the community. The key component of the intervention is the empowerment of teachers as agents of change by equipping them with the skills, knowledge, and materials to integrate nutrition education in core subject areas [26]. The overarching approach of this work is based on the social ecological model (SEM) [27]. Additionally, it is grounded in the WSCC premise that recognizes it is more effective to establish healthy behaviors during childhood than to change unhealthy behaviors in adulthood that can result in overweight and obesity. This study examines the feasibility of the professional development (PD) program and impact of implementing nutrition lessons on students' knowledge and attitudes among participants in their first year of the Healthy Schoolhouse 2.0 program. It is hypothesized that the student nutrition literacy scores are related to the number of professional development sessions teachers attended and number of nutrition lessons students received.

2. Materials and Methods

Healthy Schoolhouse 2.0 is a five-year feasibility study that follows a baseline posttest intervention design with staggered enrollment by study year. The data are multilevel in nature; teachers are nested within schools and students are nested within classrooms. The study methods are described previously in Hawkins et al. [26]. This analysis focuses on all student baseline and post-test scores during their first year of the program.

Teachers in the intervention schools participated in a five-session PD series designed to equip them with the skills, knowledge, attitudes, and materials to teach nutrition concepts within core subjects. The USDA's *Serving up MyPlate Curriculum* provides nutrition education lessons that align with the common core standards in science, math, English language arts, and health [28]. Each PD session was offered in the schoolhouse, and teachers were invited to attend by the school principal, who also attended the sessions demonstrating leadership support for the topic and program. The sessions covered Healthy Schoolhouse 2.0 program and objectives, a socio-ecological approach to nutrition education, training on the *Serving up MyPlate: A Yummy Curriculum,* practice with model nutrition lessons, and nutrition myths and facts. Each session also included time devoted to address teacher health and wellness through mindfulness practices, stress-reduction techniques, breathing exercises, or gentle yoga poses. PD sessions were 30–45 min in length (offered in person at a time determined by school leadership), and teachers could then choose how many and which nutrition lessons they would implement, three serving as the criteria for program completion. Nutrition curriculum materials kits were created and delivered to teachers at each grade level in the intervention schools. In addition to the curriculum materials, all supplies needed to conduct lessons were provided in the kits. Technical support was offered to teachers in-person and online by the program manager. Teachers were asked to document each nutrition lesson implemented via a brief Google form. After implementing three lessons, teachers were eligible for a financial incentive that could be used to purchase classroom supplies. Students in the intervention and comparison schools completed a brief Student Nutrition Literacy Survey (SNLS) at baseline ($N = 1302$) and post to measure knowledge, beliefs, attitude, and intent toward healthful nutrition-related concepts. The SNLS was aligned with the USDA curriculum content. The design and validation of the SNLS instrument is described previously [29].

Approval for this study was obtained in July 2017 from the University's Institutional Review Board for the Protection of Human Subjects in Research (IRB). Parent/guardian notification and assent was obtained in accordance with school district regulations through a written disclaimer that participation in the survey was optional. Student assent was obtained at the beginning of the school year prior to baseline survey data collection. Teacher consent was obtained at baseline.

2.1. Participant and School Demographics

Thirteen eligible schools in DC's Wards 7 and 8 were invited to participate. Eligibility requirements included elementary schools that participate in the Community Eligibility Provision program, which serves breakfast and lunch at no cost to all enrolled students, provides instruction to students in grades 1–5, and has an active partnership with the community-based food access program. Schools were engaged via email invitation and phone calls from the program manager and then randomized to either the intervention or comparison group.

The populations at the four participating schools were statistically similar on several demographic covariates, including school size (<400 students), student ethnicity (>90% Black), and proportion of students eligible for free and reduced-price meals (100%). Table 1 describes the number of participating schools, students, and teachers.

Table 1. Healthy Schoolhouse 2.0 participants: Student baseline.

# Schools	# Students	Grades	# Teachers
4 (2 intervention, 2 comparison)	1302	1st–5th	55

#: Number.

2.2. Teacher Health Survey (THS)

Prior to participating in the PD series, teachers completed the previously administered [24] 38-item Teacher Health Survey (THS) regarding personal health habits, beliefs about health and education, and self-efficacy as it relates to implementing health-related content in the classroom. Health beliefs items ($n = 8$) (example item: "It is my role as a teacher to create classrooms that promote healthy habits for students.") and self-efficacy items ($n = 6$) (example item: "I can motivate students to engage in healthy behaviors.") were measured on a five-point Likert scale (1 "strongly disagree" to 5 "strongly agree"). Demographic information including teacher race/ethnicity and age were also collected.

Biometric data (BMI) was not reported in order to reduce barriers to participation [30]. Therefore, it is not possible to examine if healthier teachers were more willing to participate in the program. Teachers' interests in specific personal health and wellness topics were also incorporated in the PD sessions.

2.3. Student Nutrition Literacy Survey (SNLS)

The 15-item Student Nutrition Literacy Survey (SNLS) (Supplementary Figure A) was administered at baseline and post-intervention to students in the intervention and comparison schools. The SNLS has demonstrated appropriate initial psychometric qualities to measure nutrition knowledge, attitudes, and beliefs [29]. The instrument contains multiple choice questions with two scales that assess nutrition knowledge and attitudes, beliefs, and intent (ABI), with a KR20 of 0.7 for internal reliability for the knowledge items and 0.4 for ABI items. The survey is brief, easily administered, and has a low respondent burden. The SNLS incorporates the content of the USDA *MyPlate curriculum*, which is aligned with Common Core State standards in English and Math, as well as the Next Generation Science Standards, and the National Health Education Standards (Supplementary Table B). Each student's name, grade, and gender were collected to assess changes in pre–post assessments at the individual level, although data were coded and de-identified during data entry. The SNLS was administered in-person by program graduate research assistants who read the questions aloud to students with consistent procedures in all classrooms. Students recorded their answers independently.

2.4. Data Analysis Procedures

Teacher and student survey data were entered, cleaned, and double-checked for accuracy by a different data coder before statistical analysis. Statistical analyses were performed using IBM SPSS Statistics software Version 26.0 (SPSS Inc., Chicago, IL, USA) and R 'ordinal' Package [31,32]. Descriptive analysis was conducted to summarize student and teacher sociodemographic characteristics, teacher self-efficacy and nutrition beliefs, and student nutrition literacy scores. Analysis was conducted on student level data which captures nutritional knowledge, attitudes and beliefs, teacher-level data and information on the PD sessions attended, and intervention lessons implemented within the classrooms.

For each scale on the SNLS, item responses were summed to create a scaled score with higher scores indicating positive nutrition attitudes. The SNLS mean score and standard deviation (SD) for each item, summary score for each scale, and percent correct score were compared between the intervention and comparison school at baseline and post. Skipped questions from the knowledge scale were marked incorrect; skipped questions from the ABI scale were excluded from the total score. Non-parametric analysis was conducted using Shapiro–Wilk's Test, the Wilcoxon Signed-Rank Test, and the Kruskal–Wallis Test for data that were non-normally distributed and treated as ordinal in nature due to the discrete characteristics of the SNLS. Correlation analysis, using Pearson's r correlation, was performed to examine the relationships among PD participation and lesson implementation. A Multilevel Mixed Linear Model using ordinal logistic regression (OLR) was used to determine the relationship between the predictor variables (intervention received, school type, gender, etc.) with the ordered factor dependent variable (SNLS knowledge percent scores) coded as ordered categorical grades A–F (A $\geq$ 90%, B $\geq$ 80%, C $\geq$ 70%, D $\geq$ 60%, F < 60%). In this case, OLR is more appropriate to use than linear mixed effects models because the SNLS score values are inherently categorical. Mean imputation, the replacement of a missing observation with the mean of the non-missing observations, was utilized upon independent variables with missing observations using the mice package in R [33].

3. Results

3.1. Teachers

The majority of teachers identified as Black (66%) and female (90%) with a mean age of 41 years. Fifty-five teachers participated in one or more PD sessions; teachers attended an average of three of the five (SD = 1.5) PD sessions. Teachers implemented a total of 71 nutrition lessons. Among teachers who implemented lessons, the average number of lessons implemented was 4, with a range of one to nine lessons. There was a significant positive correlation between the number of PD sessions attended and the number of nutrition lessons implemented in the classroom (r = 0.6, p <0.01, n = 55) (Figure 1).

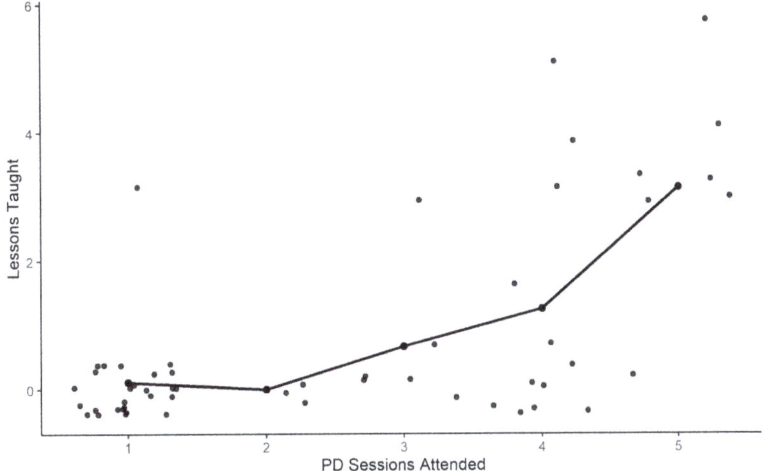

Figure 1. Correlation between professional development sessions and nutrition lesson implementation.

Teacher nutrition attitudes were positive overall in baseline and post-THS assessments among the intervention and comparison schools. There were no differences in the teacher pre-test self-efficacy scores and attitudes toward teaching nutrition between baseline and post survey administration (F(1,23) = 1.45, p > 0.050) or between intervention and comparison teachers (F (1,23) = 0.20, p > 0.050). There was no association between teacher baseline self-efficacy scores and participation in PD sessions among intervention school teachers (r (17) = 0.06, p = 0.98). It is important to note that baseline self-efficacy and nutrition attitudes mean scores were greater than 3, indicating that teachers generally agreed with the statements prior to the implementation of the PD sessions.

3.2. Student Nutrition Literacy Survey (SNLS)

A total of 1302 students in grades 1–5 completed the baseline SNLS. The baseline SNLS consists of pre-test and post-test scores for students in their first year of the Healthy Schoolhouse 2.0 program. Demographic characteristics were similar between students in the intervention and comparison schools (Table 2). Approximately 51% of students identified as male, and the sample was balanced by grade.

Baseline SNLS scores were compared using the Wilcoxon Ranked-Sum Test and were similar between intervention and comparison schools (W = 155929, p = 0.161). Both the intervention and comparison schools had an increase in median knowledge scores, from baseline to post measurements, 15.4% and 6.3%, respectively. Students in the intervention school experienced a significant increase in knowledge scores as demonstrated by the Wilcoxon Signed-Rank Test, which was the non-parametric alternative to a paired t-test (p < 0.001, n = 659). There was also a significant increase in knowledge percent score changes between students in the intervention and comparison schools (W = 17064, p < 0.001,

$n = 659$) (Figure 2). Notably, students in the intervention schools had higher mean and median post scores on nutrition literacy knowledge than students in the comparison schools (W = 39985, $p < 0.001$, n =448). Student nutrition literacy knowledge scores were higher in higher grades overall, as expected. There were no statistically significant differences in median student attitude scores change by grade or between the intervention and comparison schools.

Table 2. Student demographics: baseline assessment ($N = 1302$).

	Intervention ($n = 694$)		Comparison ($n = 608$)		Total ($n = 1302$)
	Intervention School 1 *n* (%)	Intervention School 2 *n* (%)	Comparison School 1 *n* (%)	Comparison School 2 *n* (%)	*n* (%)
Gender					
Male	202 (51.5%)	137 (45.4%)	157 (53.2%)	167 (53.4%)	663 (50.9%)
Female	174 (44.4%)	155 (51.3%)	128 (43.4%)	146 (46.6%)	603 (46.3%)
Not Reported	16 (4.1%)	10 (3.3%)	10 (3.4%)	0	36 (2.3%)
Grade					
1st	121(30.9%)	76 (25.2%)	93 (31.52%)	66 (21.1%)	356 (27%)
2nd	82 (20.9%)	53 (17.6%)	51 (17.29%)	60 (19.2%)	246 (18.9%)
3rd	55 (14%)	59 (19.5%)	50 (16.95%)	64 (20.4%)	228 (17.5%)
4th	68 (17.4%)	61 (20.2%)	51 (17.29%)	65 (20.8%)	245 (18.8%)
5th	66 (16.8%)	53 (17.5%)	50 (16.95%)	58 (18.5%)	227 (17.4%)

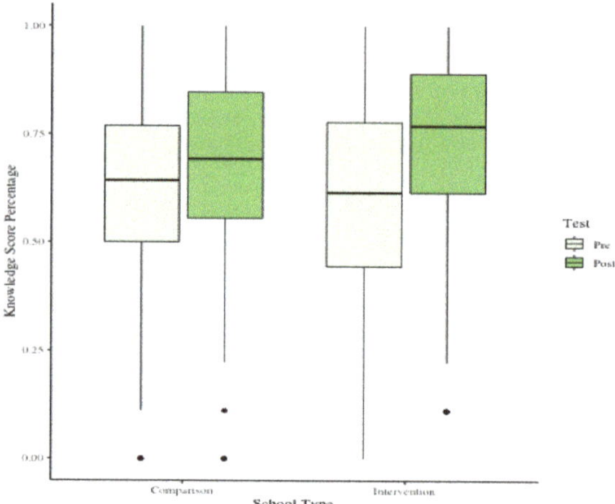

Figure 2. Distribution of student nutrition literacy knowledge scores in students first year of the program.

For the purpose of this analysis, the intervention was defined as having received three nutrition lessons (yes/no). A Kruskal–Wallis Test (H(2) = 22.75, $p < 0.001$, $n = 659$) and post hoc Dunn Test were utilized to examine if there were changes in SNLS scores with increases in the number (dose) of lessons. There was a significant difference between post-test scores of students who received the intervention of three nutrition lessons and those who received fewer lessons (0–2) ($p < 0.001$). Students who received three or more nutrition lessons had knowledge scores that were on average 10% higher than those students who received fewer lessons. Of note, there were no differences between the nutrition knowledge scores of students who received three lessons and those who received more than three lessons ($p > 0.05$).

3.3. Multilevel Ordinal Logistic Regression (OLR)

The hierarchical nature of school systems, with students nested within classrooms, lends itself to multilevel modeling approaches. Multilevel modeling allows for analysis of these hierarchical data using random effect variables. Random effects allow for random slopes to be added into the model to account for unobserved heterogeneity among schools (i.e., classrooms/schools). Odds Ratios are gathered by exponentiating OLR coefficients and indicate the odds of receiving a higher SNLS score given a 1-point increase in the predictor variable (e.g., nutrition lesson, gender, etc.). Table 3 describes the final OLR model. This model examined student SNLS scores for the first three years of the Healthy Schoolhouse 2.0 program and includes data for students in both the intervention and comparison schools. In this model, test exposure is operationalized as a time variable, beginning at zero, the students' baseline test, and increasing incrementally each time a student takes the SNLS. The random variables of student ID, teacher ID, and test level were nested within school. Students who self-identified as female had higher SNLS scores than male students. The odds of receiving a higher score increased by 1.45 if the student was female. SNLS scores increased over time from pre to post assessment, with the odds of receiving a higher score increasing by 3.47. In the final OLR model, two interaction effects (test exposure and program year, and test exposure and test) were examined. Test exposure and program year examined the impact of student test exposure in different years of the Healthy Schoolhouse 2.0 program. For every one-unit increase in student test exposure times every unit increase in program year, there is a corresponding 0.68 increase in odds of a higher SNLS score. Test Exposure and Test examined the impact of the number of times a student sees the SNLS with the time of administration (pre or post). For every one-unit increase in student test exposure, the odds of a higher score on the SNLS post-test increases by 0.64.

Figure 3 illustrates the predicted test grade probabilities by gender for students who received three or more nutrition lessons (intervention = yes) in blue and fewer than three nutrition lessons (intervention = no) in yellow. With all other variables held constant, students who received three or more nutrition lessons had a higher probability of scoring higher grades on the post SNLS assessment. Students who received three or more lessons have a higher estimated log odds of achieving >90% correct (A grade) on the post SNLS assessment than students who received less than three nutrition lessons. The odds of receiving a higher score (90% correct) over a lower score increased by 2.58 if a student received three nutrition lessons. It is important to note the clear downward trend of the log odds of the score predictions without nutrition lessons at a C grade. The predicted probabilities for students who received three or more nutrition lessons show a positive trend with higher probability of scoring higher nutrition literacy scores.

Table 3. Multilevel OLR analysis final model.

	Estimate	Odds Ratio	Std. Error	Z Value
Intervention (Yes)	0.95 ***	2.58	0.25	3.75
Test Exposure	1.2 ***	3.47	0.25	4.89
Program Year	0.39 ***	1.48	0.11	3.49
Test (Post)	1.5 ***	3.15	0.16	1.15
Gender (Female)	0.34 ***	1.45	0.11	3.11
Test Exposure and Program Year	0.38 ***	0.68	0.09	−4.13
Test Exposure and Test (Post)	0.44 ***	0.64	0.11	−4.127

*** Indicates $p < 0.001$.

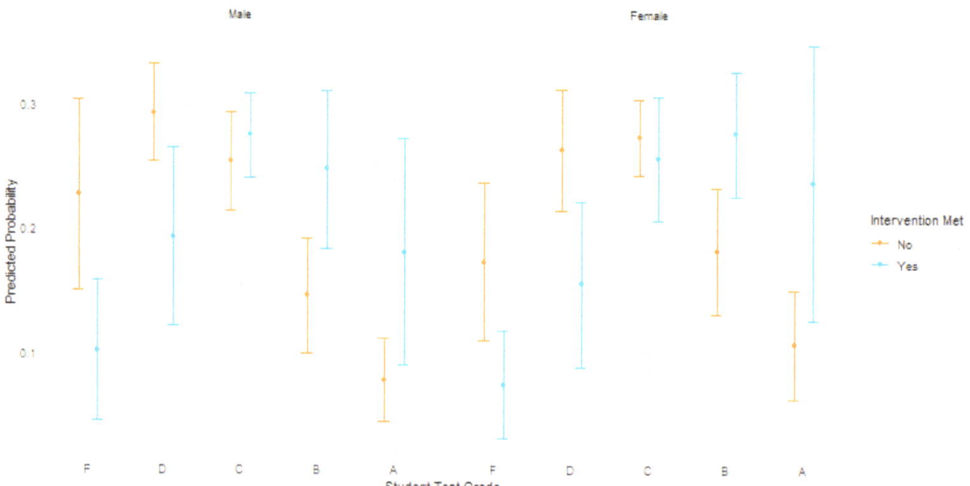

Figure 3. SNLS predicted grade probabilities by gender and intervention.

4. Discussion

Initial results from the participants in their first program year demonstrate that teacher participation in PD sessions and implementation of nutrition lessons has a positive association with increased student knowledge of nutritional concepts. Multilevel mixed modeling analysis demonstrated significant differences between pre and post nutrition knowledge scores between intervention and comparison schools, that the number of nutrition lessons implemented is significantly related to higher student knowledge scores, and there is a significant correlation between teacher PD sessions attended and number of lessons implemented in classrooms. In particular, students who received three nutrition lessons had significant improvement in nutrition literacy scores than students who received fewer nutrition lessons. This suggests that programs aimed to empower teachers as nutrition educators may be a valuable tool in teaching nutrition concepts and preventing childhood overweight and obesity within school systems.

The emphasis on supporting the "whole child" [7], including accountability for improving the health and wellness of students in the school environment, has been advanced with federal and state policies (e.g., HHFKA, ESSA) [34]. With the environment primed through policy levers to provide more nutritionally balanced meals, more dedicated time for physical activity and health education, and specific school wellness policy requirements to prevent and reduce obesity [35], the school setting is well positioned to support the nutrition literacy of students as well as the broader school community. Through improved nutrition literacy, students may be better equipped to increase their consumption of high-quality foods, which may in turn support overall physical health. Therefore, advancing nutrition literacy in the school setting is important to promote healthy eating and support long-term academic outcomes to reduce the burden of food-related diseases across the lifespan.

According to the principles of the social ecological model in which multiple spheres of influence must be mutually reinforcing, it is imperative to recognize the impact of teachers' knowledge, engagement with PD, and implementation of nutrition lessons on students' health and well-being outcomes [36] and equip them as agents of change in order for national and local policies to achieve desired aims. Previous research suggests that teachers offer a critical role in student motivation and engagement [37]. Teacher engagement is vital to influence student nutrition behavior and support efforts to reduce the prevalence of childhood obesity. The consistent contact that teachers, administrators, and staff maintain with students creates an opportunity to provide instruction and modeling of healthy nutrition patterns and other lifestyle habits and behaviors [24]. The preliminary results of Healthy Schoolhouse 2.0 support the feasibility of PD sessions with teachers on health-related constructs and content as a promising strategy to support obesity prevention efforts.

PD opportunities for teachers can help translate policy requirements into practical strategies and applications in the classroom. To be successful, professional learning events must both increase nutrition knowledge and also improve teacher confidence, attitudes, and self-efficacy in these areas. As previously described, research consistently supports the influence of teacher attitudes and self-efficacy [22,23,25,38]. Thus, to extend the influence of educators beyond their academic and curricular subject matter expertise, specific and appropriate training to increase knowledge in areas of health promotion and nutrition education is needed [39,40]. We plan to continue to focus on teacher engagement with PD in the remaining years of the project.

4.1. Strengths and Limitations

Healthy Schoolhouse 2.0 offers a feasible model for nutrition education programming and implementation, given the competing demands educators face. In the first year of the program, we learned that principal and/or assistant principal support is essential to the implementation of the program and to the engagement of the participating teachers. Teacher investment in 40–60 min of nutrition education over the course of the academic year may have a meaningful impact on student nutrition knowledge. While nutrition knowledge is only a single factor determining lifestyle habits in a complex environment of structural and cultural influences, it is an essential starting point for establishing lifelong health behaviors. In addition, the 5-year program provides students with progressive and cumulative instruction on key nutrition topics. Furthermore, the Healthy Schoolhouse 2.0 program implements the strategy of teachers acting as role models and being actively involved in the delivery of the intervention along with school policies that support the availability of healthy food.

There are several limitations to this study that are important to note. Although eligible schools were randomly allocated to the intervention or comparison groups, and all teachers at the intervention school were provided incentives to participate, engagement in the PD sessions at the teacher level was voluntary. However, the school setting is ideal for the implementation and evaluation of obesity prevention programs—in other health promotion programs, individuals who may be at high risk because of individual or environmental factors do not participate in such programs. The Healthy Schoolhouse 2.0 program provides the opportunity for equal participation by students regardless of nutrition risk factors. An equal number of intervention and comparison schools are enrolled, which allows for an analysis of multilevel intervention effects, in part because regression to the mean will impact the comparison schools as well as the intervention schools over the five-year study period.

We consider both clustering and nesting through multilevel modeling to account for the likelihood that students in each grade will be more highly correlated within a cluster than between clusters, and unique aspects of the clusters themselves may confound intervention effects. For example, Student's *t*-test is predicated on the observations being statistically independent, the assumption that the data are normal and may underestimate standard errors, erroneously reducing *p*-values and increasing the risk of falsely rejecting a null hypothesis. Ultimately, after the five-year study period, we will have the opportunity to measure the stability of student nutrition knowledge and teacher self-efficacy over time as well as the long-term impact of the Healthy Schoolhouse 2.0 health promotion program.

There are additional threats to internal validity that are important to acknowledge given the quasi-experimental design. Student maturation is occurring over time that may be interpreted as an intervention effect, particularly when examining the impact of the Healthy Schoolhouse 2.0 intervention over the 5-year study period. Furthermore, student SNLS testing exposure may affect scores on subsequent assessments. There may be interactive effects of the Healthy Schoolhouse 2.0 intervention that may depend on the level of other nutrition interventions and efforts. Student consumption and food choice behaviors were not examined in this feasibility study. Future research is necessary to understand the association, if any, between student nutrition knowledge, attitudes, and healthful eating behaviors.

The results did not reveal baseline–post changes in teacher confidence in the first year of the program in either the intervention or the comparison schools. One explanation is a ceiling effect and decreasing variance from the baseline to post teacher survey. The small sample size may be an influencing factor in these findings, as many teachers did not complete both the pre and post surveys. A possible explanation for this low response rate for teachers may be the length of the teacher survey, which takes an average of 15 min to complete all sections. A dose–response of the lessons implemented in the intervention group is one potential explanation for the within-group results; however, an alternative explanation for this first-year association may be that those teachers who participated in the intervention school were more accepting of the intervention, open to teaching nutrition lessons, and different from teachers who did not implement lessons. Furthermore, this study measures secondary outcomes including nutrition literacy measures (knowledge, attitudes, behaviors) that are assumed to be the mediators of childhood obesity.

4.2. Implications for Future Research

Future research would benefit from exploring the relationship between school-level factors that we did not address, including how teacher knowledge may impact the integration of nutrition education into core classroom subjects: for example, identifying potential correlations between teacher self-efficacy to deliver lessons that incorporate nutrition content. Additionally, grade level may influence the ability to include nutrition education in lessons; specifically, lower grade levels may have more flexibility in their curricula because younger students are not required to participate in annual state standardized testing. A focus on intervention studies in early childhood settings would inform policies and practices to support early intervention and family engagement to reduce overweight and obesity in young children. Finally, longitudinal research on the distal effects of nutrition education on academic outcomes and obesity would validate claims about the benefits of policies and practices in schools.

5. Conclusions

Health behaviors established in childhood are critical determinants of health across the lifespan, particularly in regard to obesity prevention efforts [1]. From a public health perspective, the school setting represents great possibilities for advancing child health. The Healthy Schoolhouse 2.0 health promotion intervention program places teachers in a leadership role to support children's nutrition literacy and health. This feasibility study addresses a need to support quality nutrition education in elementary schools. Furthermore, this study draws attention to the powerful role teachers can have on community obesity prevention efforts.

Supplementary Materials: The following are available online at https://www.mdpi.com/article/10.3390/nu13092935/s1, Supplementary Figure A: Student Nutrition Literacy Survey (SNLS), Supplementary Table B: USDA's *Serving Up MyPlate: A Yummy Curriculum* Lessons.

Author Contributions: Conceptualization, A.S. and S.I.B.; methodology, M.H., A.S, S.I.B.; formal analysis, S.L. L.K., M.H.; writing—original draft preparation, M.H., A.S., S.I.B., R.M.; writing—review and editing, M.H. A.S., S.I.B., R.M., S.L., L.K.; supervision, A.S.; project administration, R.M.; funding acquisition, A.S. All authors have read and agreed to the published version of the manuscript.

Funding: This research was funded by USDA National Institute of Food and Agriculture from the Agriculture and Food Research Initiative Competitive Grant no. 2017-68001-26356.

Institutional Review Board Statement: The study was conducted according to the guidelines of the Declaration of Helsinki and approved by the Institutional Review Board of American University (protocol code IRB-2018-67 and date of approval 27 June 2018).

Informed Consent Statement: Informed consent was obtained from all subjects involved in the study. Written informed consent was obtained from parents of all students, and verbal assent was provided by the students at the time the surveys were administered. Verbal consent was witnessed and formally recorded.

Data Availability Statement: Healthy Schoolhouse 2.0 data are available upon request. The data presented in this study are available by request from the corresponding author.

Acknowledgments: We would like to thank Adrian Bertrand for data collection, entry, and analysis support; Caitlin Lavigne for assistance with review of the literature. A special thanks to Eric Schuler for his careful review of the manuscript. We thank the Healthy Schoolhouse 2.0 Board of Advisors for their contributions. We extend our appreciation to the Washington, DC elementary school principals, teachers, and students for their time and participation in this project.

Conflicts of Interest: The authors declare no conflict of interest. The funders had no role in the design of the study; in the data collection, analyses, or in the interpretation of data; in the writing of the manuscript, or in the decision to publish the results.

References

1. Braveman, P.; Barclay, C. Health Disparities Beginning in Childhood: A Life-Course Perspective. *Pediatrics* **2009**, *124* (Suppl. 3), S163–S175. [CrossRef] [PubMed]
2. Hales, C.M.; Carroll, M.D.; Fryar, C.D.; Ogden, C.L. Prevalence of obesity among adults and youth: United States, 2015–2016. Hyattsville, MD: National Center for Health Statistics. *NCHS Data Brief.* **2017**, *288*, 1–8.
3. Our Healthy DC. Available online: https://ourhealthydc.org/dc-chna/health-outcomes/infant-child-health/ (accessed on 28 July 2021).
4. US Dept of Agriculture. Nutrition Standards in the National School Lunch and School Breakfast Programs: Final Rule. Available online: https://www.fns.usda.gov/federal_register?rin%5B0%5D=0584-AD59%20 (accessed on 28 July 2021).
5. Healthy, Hunger-Free Kids Act of 2010, Pub. L. No. 111-296, 124 Stat. 3183. 2010. Available online: http://www.nea.org/assets/docs/HHFKA_fact_sheet-final(1).pdf (accessed on 28 July 2021).
6. Every Student Succeeds Act, Pub. L. No. 114-95, 129 Stat. 1802. 2015. Available online: https://www.ed.gov/essa?src=rn (accessed on 1 July 2021).
7. CDC Healthy Schools. Whole School, Whole Community, Whole Child (WSCC). Available online: https://www.cdc.gov/healthyschools/wscc/index.htm (accessed on 28 July 2021).
8. Office of the State Superintendent of Education. Healthy Schools Act. Available online: https://osse.dc.gov/service/healthy-schools-act (accessed on 28 July 2021).
9. Liu, Z.; Xu, H.M.; Wen, L.M.; Peng, Y.Z.; Lin, L.Z.; Zhou, S.; Li, W.H.; Wang, H.J. A systematic review and meta-analysis of the overall effects of school-based obesity prevention interventions and effect differences by intervention components. *Int. J. Behav. Nutr. Phys. Act.* **2019**, *16*, 95. [CrossRef]
10. Gonzalez-Suarez, C.; Worley, A.; Grimmer-Somers, K.; Dones, V. School-based interventions on childhood obesity: A meta-analysis. *Am. J. Prev. Med.* **2009**, *37*, 418–427. [CrossRef]
11. Verrotti, A.; Penta, L.; Zenzeri, L.; Agostinelli, S.; Feo, P.D. Childhood obesity: Prevention and strategies of intervention. A systematic review of school-based interventions in primary schools. *J. Endocrinol. Investig.* **2014**, *37*, 1155–1164. [CrossRef] [PubMed]
12. Snelling, A.; Newman, C.; Watts, E.; van Dyke, H.; Malloy, E.J.; Ghamarian, Y.; Guthrie, J.; Mancino, L. Pairing fruit and vegetables to promote consumption in elementary school cafeterias. *J. Child. Nutr. Manag.* **2017**, *41*, 1–13.
13. Snelling, A.; Newman, C.; Ellsworth, D.; Kalicki, M.; Guthrie, J.F.; Mancino, L.; Malloy, E.J.; van Dyke, H.; George, S.; Nash, K. Engaging elementary students with taste tests to promote vegetable consumption. *Health Behav. Policy Rev.* **2017**, *4*, 67–75. [CrossRef]
14. Snelling, A.; Belson, S.I.; Beard, J.; Young, K. Associations between grades and physical activity and food choices: Results from YRBS from a large school district. *Health Educ.* **2015**, *115*, 141–151. [CrossRef]
15. Michael, S.L.; Merlo, C.L.; Basch, C.E.; Wentzel, K.R.; Wechsler, H. Critical Connections: Health and academics. *J. Sch. Health* **2015**, *85*, 740–758. [CrossRef] [PubMed]
16. CDC Adolescent and School Health. Health and Academic Achievement. Available online: https://www.cdc.gov/healthyyouth/health_and_academics/pdf/health-academic-achievement.pdf (accessed on 28 July 2021).
17. Schmitt, S.A.; Bryant, L.M.; Korucu, I.; Kirkham, L.; Katare, B.; Benjamin, T. The effects of a nutrition education curriculum on improving young children's fruit and vegetable preferences and nutrition and health knowledge. *Public Health Nutr.* **2018**, *22*, 28–34. [CrossRef]
18. Wall, D.E.; Least, C.; Gromis, J.; Lohse, B. Nutrition education intervention improves vegetable-related attitude, self-efficacy, preference, and knowledge of fourth-grade students. *J. Sch. Health* **2012**, *82*, 37–43. [CrossRef]

19. Kulik, N.L.; Moore, E.W.; Centeio, E.E.; Garn, A.C.; Martin, J.J.; Shen, B.; Somers, C.L.; McCaughtry, N. Knowledge, Attitudes, Self-Efficacy, and Healthy Eating Behavior Among Children: Results From the Building Healthy Communities Trial. *Health Educ. Behav.* **2019**, *46*, 602–611. [CrossRef]

20. Cotton, W.; Dudley, D.; Peralta, L.; Werkhoven, T. The effect of teacher-delivered nutrition education programs on elementary-aged students: An updated systematic review and meta-analysis. *Prev. Med. Rep.* **2020**, *20*. [CrossRef] [PubMed]

21. Darling-Hammond, L.; Hyler, M.E.; Gardner, M. Effective Teacher Professional Development. *Learn. Policy Inst.* 2017. Available online: https://learningpolicyinstitute.org/sites/default/files/product-files/Effective_Teacher_Professional_Development_REPORT.pdf (accessed on 28 July 2021).

22. Metos, J.M.; Sarnoff, K.; Jordan, K.C. Teachers' perceived and desired roles in nutrition education. *J. Sch. Health* **2019**, *89*, 68–76. [CrossRef] [PubMed]

23. Snelling, A.; Belson, S.I.; Young, J. School health reform: Investigating the role of teachers. *J. Child. Nutr. Manag.* **2012**, *36*, 6.

24. Snelling, A.; Ernst, J.; Belson, S.I. Teachers as role models in solving childhood obesity. *J. Pediatr. Biochem.* **2013**, *3*, 55–60. [CrossRef]

25. Perera, T.; Frei, S.; Frei, B.; Wong, S.S.; Bobe, G. Improving nutrition education in U.S. Elementary schools: Challenges and opportunities. *J. Educ. Pr.* **2015**, *6*, 41–50.

26. Hawkins, M.; Watts, E.; Belson, S.I.; Snelling, A. Design and Implementation of a 5-year School-based Nutrition Education Intervention. *J. Nutr. Educ. Behav.* **2020**, *52*, 421–428. [CrossRef]

27. Bronfenbrenner, U. *The Ecology of Human Development*; Harvard University Press: Cambridge, MA, USA, 1981; p. 352.

28. US Dept of Agriculture, Food and Nutrition Service. *Serving Up My Plate: A Yummy Curriculum*. Available online: https://www.fns.usda.gov/tn/serving-myplate-yummy-curriculum (accessed on 28 July 2021).

29. Hawkins, M.; Fuchs, H.; Watts, E.; Belson, S.I.; Snelling, A. Development of a nutrition literacy survey for use among elementary school students in communities with high rates of food insecurity. *J. Hunger Environ. Nutr.* **2021**. [CrossRef]

30. Byrd-Williams, C. Best practices and barriers to obesity prevention in Head Start: Differences between director and teacher perceptions. *Prev. Chronic Dis.* **2017**, *14*. [CrossRef]

31. R Core Team. R: A Language and Environment for Statistical Computing. R Foundation for Statistical Computing. 2021. Available online: https://www.R-project.org/ (accessed on 28 July 2021).

32. Christensen, R.H.B. Ordinal—Regression Models for Ordinal Data. R Package Version 2019.12-10. 2019. Available online: https://CRAN.R-project.org/package=ordinal (accessed on 28 July 2021).

33. Van Buuren, S.; Groothuis-Oudshoorn, K. Mice: Multivariate Imputation by Chained Equations in R. *J. Stat. Softw.* **2011**, *45*, 1–67. [CrossRef]

34. Healthy Eating Research. Prioritizing Health in State ESSA Plans and Report Cards to Support the Whole Child. Chicago, IL: Institute for Healthy Research and Policy UIC. 2020. Available online: https://healthyeatingresearch.org/research/prioritizing-health-in-state-essa-plans-and-report-cards-to-support-the-whole-child/ (accessed on 28 July 2021).

35. Ickovics, J.R.; Duffany, K.O.; Shebl, F.M.; Peters, S.M.; Read, M.A.; Gilstad-Hayden, K.R.; Schwartz, M.B. Implementing School-Based Policies to Prevent Obesity: Cluster Randomized Trial. *Am. J. Prev. Med.* **2019**, *56*, e1–e11. [CrossRef] [PubMed]

36. Killian, C.M.; Kern, B.D.; Ellison, D.W.; Graber, K.C.; Woods, A.M. State lawmaker's views on childhood obesity and related school wellness legislation. *J. Sch. Health* **2020**, *90*, 257–263. [CrossRef] [PubMed]

37. Tucker, C.M.; Zayco, R.A.; Herman, K.C.; Reinke, W.M.; Trujillo, M.; Carraway, K.; Wallack, C.; Ivery, P.D. Teacher and child variables as predictors of academic engagement among low-income African American children. *Psychol. Sch.* **2002**, *39*, 477–488. [CrossRef]

38. Putney, L.G.; Broughton, S.H. Developing collective classroom efficacy: The teacher's role as community organizer. *J. Teach. Educ.* **2011**, *62*, 93–105. [CrossRef]

39. Pickett, K.; Rietdijk, W.; Byrne, J.; Shepherd, J.; Roderick, P.; Grace, M. Teaching health education: A thematic analysis of early career teachers' experiences following pre-service health training. *Health Educ.* **2017**, *117*, 323–340. [CrossRef]

40. Watts, S.O.; Pinero, D.J.; Alter, M.M.; Lancaster, K.J. An Assessment of Nutrition Education in Selected Counties in New York State Elementary Schools (Kindergarten through Fifth Grade). *J. Nutr. Educ. Behav.* **2012**, *44*, 474–480. [CrossRef]

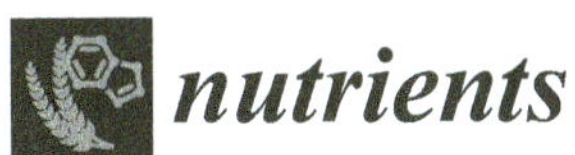
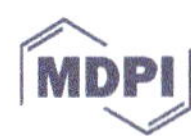

Review

Effects of L-Citrulline Supplementation and Aerobic Training on Vascular Function in Individuals with Obesity across the Lifespan

Anaisa Genoveva Flores-Ramírez [1], Verónica Ivette Tovar-Villegas [1], Arun Maharaj [2], Ma Eugenia Garay-Sevilla [1,*] and Arturo Figueroa [2,*]

[1] Department of Medical Science, Division of Health Science, University of Guanajuato, Campus León, León 37320, Mexico; Anaisa_390@hotmail.com (A.G.F.-R.); Veronicatovar92@hotmail.com (V.I.T.-V.)
[2] Department of Kinesiology and Sport Management, Texas Tech University, Lubbock, TX 79409, USA; arun.maharaj@ttu.edu
* Correspondence: marugaray_2000@yahoo.com (M.E.G.-S.); arturo.figueroa@ttu.edu (A.F.)

Abstract: Children with obesity are at higher risk for developing cardiometabolic diseases that once were considered health conditions of adults. Obesity is commonly associated with cardiometabolic risk factors such as dyslipidemia, hyperglycemia, hyperinsulinemia and hypertension that contribute to the development of endothelial dysfunction. Endothelial dysfunction, characterized by reduced nitric oxide (NO) production, precedes vascular abnormalities including atherosclerosis and arterial stiffness. Thus, early detection and treatment of cardiometabolic risk factors are necessary to prevent deleterious vascular consequences of obesity at an early age. Non-pharmacological interventions including L-Citrulline (L-Cit) supplementation and aerobic training stimulate endothelial NO mediated vasodilation, leading to improvements in organ perfusion, blood pressure, arterial stiffness, atherosclerosis and metabolic health (glucose control and lipid profile). Few studies suggest that the combination of L-Cit supplementation and exercise training can be an effective strategy to counteract the adverse effects of obesity on vascular function in older adults. Therefore, this review examined the efficacy of L-Cit supplementation and aerobic training interventions on vascular and metabolic parameters in obese individuals.

Keywords: obesity; children; vascular function; aerobic training; L-Citrulline; L-Arginine; nitric oxide

Citation: Flores-Ramírez, A.G.; Tovar-Villegas, V.I.; Maharaj, A.; Garay-Sevilla, M.E.; Figueroa, A. Effects of L-Citrulline Supplementation and Aerobic Training on Vascular Function in Individuals with Obesity across the Lifespan. *Nutrients* **2021**, *13*, 2991. https://doi.org/10.3390/nu13092991

Academic Editors: Odysseas Androutsos and Evangelia Charmandari

Received: 31 July 2021
Accepted: 19 August 2021
Published: 27 August 2021

Publisher's Note: MDPI stays neutral with regard to jurisdictional claims in published maps and institutional affiliations.

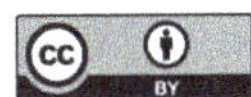

Copyright: © 2021 by the authors. Licensee MDPI, Basel, Switzerland. This article is an open access article distributed under the terms and conditions of the Creative Commons Attribution (CC BY) license (https://creativecommons.org/licenses/by/4.0/).

1. Introduction

Overweight and obesity are defined as abnormal or excessive fat accumulation [1]. In adults, the World Health Organization (WHO) defines obesity as a Body Mass Index (BMI) greater than or equal to 30 kg/m^2, and for children aged between 5–19 years, obesity is considered two standard deviations above the WHO Growth Reference median [1]. Approximately 340 million children and adolescents worldwide were classified as overweight or obese in 2016 and the prevalence is dramatically increasing [1,2]. The prevalence of hypertension is greater than 70% and increases with progression of obesity grade in adults [3]. In obese children, the prevalence of hypertension is 15.27%, which is substantially higher than 1.9% in those with normal weight [4]. Obesity is a risk factor for the development of cardiovascular diseases (CVD) and type 2 diabetes (T2D) due to the association with hypertension and insulin resistance [1].

In some cases, individuals are classified as obese based on BMI alone but considered "metabolically healthy obese" (MHO) [5] since they display a normal cardiometabolic profile such as optimal insulin sensitivity, blood pressure, lipid and inflammatory profiles [6]. However, although MHO individuals are relatively protected against cardiometabolic diseases compared to metabolically unhealthy obese, MHO should not be considered a harmless condition as they have a higher risk of developing obesity-related diseases compared to normal weight individuals [6–8].

Obesity is a condition strongly associated with metabolic syndrome (MetS), defined as a constellation of physiological, biochemical, clinical and metabolic factors that are associated with an increased risk of atherosclerosis, T2D and all-cause mortality [9]. MetS can be diagnosed in children (10 to 16 years old) with abdominal obesity and at least two clinical features such as elevated triglycerides, low levels of high-density lipoprotein (HDL) cholesterol, high blood pressure (hypertension) and high fasting blood glucose (hyperglycemia) [10–12]. Childhood obesity and hypertension predict MetS later in life [13,14]. In children, hypertension is a prevalent cardiovascular risk factor associated with reduced endothelial function, increased vascular thickness and arterial stiffness [15]. A hallmark risk factor of MetS is insulin resistance (IR) [16], which is an impairment of insulin function to promote glucose uptake in insulin-sensitive target tissues, such as skeletal muscle and adipose tissue [17], resulting in abnormal glucose homeostasis [16]. Fasting serum glucose values between 86 and 99 mg/dL during childhood increase the risk of developing T2D during adulthood twofold [18], highlighting the importance of identifying and developing treatment strategies to prevent adult-onset of metabolic complications in obese children and adolescents.

Obesity is also associated with elevated levels of proinflammatory adipokines released by visceral adipose tissue that contribute to the development of IR and impaired endothelial function [19]. Endothelial dysfunction is the result of prolonged hyperglycemia, damaging vascular function and structure that eventually leads to CVD development [19]. Proinflammatory adipokines increase the production of reactive oxygen species (ROS) which triggers the release of inflammatory cytokines, adhesion molecules and growth factors that promote cellular oxidative stress [20]. Oxidative stress causes endothelial dysfunction, characterized by a reduction in nitric oxide (NO) and an increase in endothelium-derived vasoconstrictors such as endothelin-1 [19,20] (Figure 1).

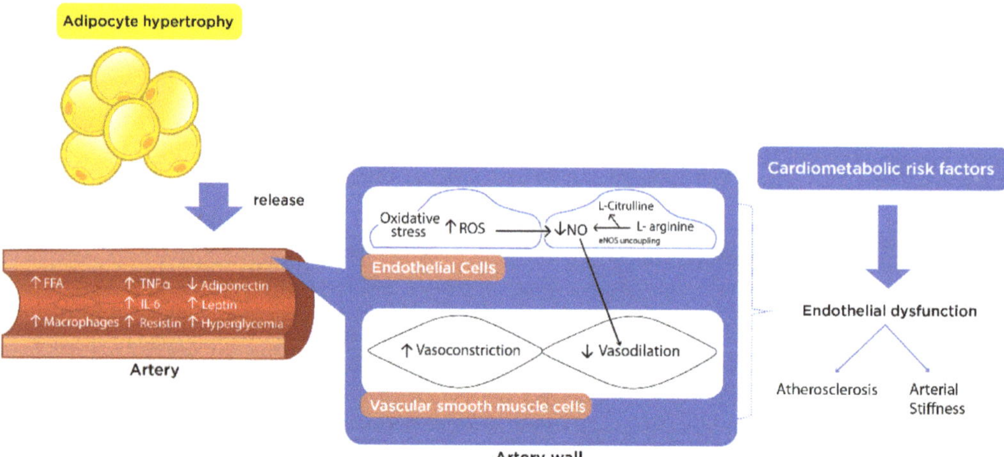

Figure 1. Obesity and endothelial dysfunction. Adipocyte hypertrophy leads to release of FFA, leptin, resistin, TNFα and IL-6 into the vascular wall, promoting inflammation, while anti-inflammatory adiponectin secretion is reduced. Proinflammatory adipokines and hyperglycemia induce the production of ROS, which by uncoupling eNOS leads to reduced NO synthesis and bioavailability for vasodilation, promoting a vasoconstrictor state. Cardiometabolic risk factors contribute to endothelial dysfunction, characterized by a reduced NO bioavailability, which promotes atherosclerosis and arterial stiffness and development of CVD. FFA: Free fatty acids; TNF-α: Tumor necrosis factor alpha; IL-6: Interleukin-6; ROS: Reactive oxygen species; NO: Nitric oxide; eNOS: endothelial NO synthase; CVD: Cardiovascular disease; ↑: Increase; ↓: Decrease.

For these reasons, it is important to evaluate interventions to improve vascular and metabolic function in obese individuals. There are non-pharmacological treatments that can improve the cardiometabolic profile. L-Citrulline (L-Cit) is a non-essential amino acid not used for protein synthesis, but with a key regulatory role of nitrogen homeostasis [21]. Studies in humans have demonstrated the effect of L-Cit supplementation on improving nitrogen homeostasis and its ability to increase the L-Arginine-NO pathway [21]. In middle-aged adults, oral L-Cit supplementation has shown to improve endothelial function [22], blood pressure [23,24] and arterial stiffness [25] through stimulation of the L-Arginine-NO pathway which consequently leads to vasodilation [23,26]. L-Cit supplementation has also improved lean mass and reduce fat mass in malnourished older adults [27].

The development of childhood obesity is associated with sedentary behavior [28], and increased physical activity is recommended to improve overall health in children with excess adiposity [29,30]. In children and adolescents, aerobic training helps to improve blood pressure [31,32], endothelial function [32,33], arterial stiffness [31,32] atherosclerosis [32], lipid profile [32–35] and body composition [31,33,35]. The use of L-Cit plus exercise, in middle-aged and older adults with obesity-related diseases or risks factors, has yielded improvements in systolic blood pressure (SBP), pressure wave reflection and aortic stiffness [23,25]. These lifestyle and dietary interventions were implemented in middle-aged and older adults and have elicited no harmful effects. However, there is a void in the literature regarding the efficacy of L-Cit supplementation with and without exercise training in children and adolescents. Thus, the objective of this review is to discuss the effects of L-Cit supplementation and aerobic training interventions on vascular and metabolic parameters in middle-aged and older adults, and deliberate possible avenues of research surrounding similar interventions in obese children and adolescents by observing how obesity can lead to these cardiometabolic alterations.

2. Endothelial Function

The endothelium is a layer of cells between the vessel lumen and the vascular smooth muscle cells (VSMC). The most important vasodilator produced by the endothelium is NO, generated from L-Arginine (L-Arg) by endothelial-NO synthase (eNOS) [36]. NO diffuses into the VSMC where it stimulates soluble guanylyl cyclase and subsequently activates cyclic guanosine monophosphate, leading to a decrease in intracellular calcium concentrations, and therefore, to relaxation and vasodilation. NO is considered an anti-atherogenic agent and prevents platelet aggregation, smooth cell proliferation and adhesion of leukocytes to the endothelium [37]. Therefore, vascular homeostasis depends on NO bioavailability.

Endothelial dysfunction is a reversible pathological complication derived from reduced NO bioavailability and impaired vasodilation [38]. Inflammation, oxidative stress, hypertension, dyslipidemia and IR are the main contributing factors in obesity-related endothelial dysfunction [19] through the unbalance between increased ROS and reduced antioxidant capacity [37]. ROS reduces levels of tetrahydrobiopterin (BH_4), an essential cofactor for eNOS [37], by inducing BH_4 oxidation (BH_4 to BH_2) which leads to eNOS uncoupling [39]. In obesity, a main mechanism for endothelial dysfunction is eNOS uncoupling due to reduced L-Arg bioavailability and BH_4 oxidation [38,40], leading to less NO bioavailability and increased ROS (superoxide anion and peroxynitrite) generation [36]. Enhanced oxidative stress by ROS upregulates arginase activity/expression competing with eNOS for L-Arg, a common substrate. Cardiometabolic risk factors (obesity, hyperglycemia, hypertension) stimulates arginase to contribute to further ROS production [41–43]. Arginase converts L-Arg to L-ornithine and urea, decreasing L-Arg availability for eNOS. Evidence has demonstrated that obesity-induced endothelial dysfunction associated with arterial stiffening, hyperglycemia, hypertension, and oxidative stress were prevented with arginase inhibition [43]. Thus, obesity-induced endothelial dysfunction may be reversible by therapies that increase L-Arg bioavailability and induce arginase inhibition [38,40].

Under normal conditions, insulin favors the release of NO by activation of eNOS, and therefore, has vasodilator, anti-inflammatory and anti-atherosclerotic effects [44].

Hyperinsulinemia contributes to increased vasoconstriction through mitogen activated protein kinase signaling by releasing endothelin-1, a powerful vasoconstrictor agent that promotes IR, oxidative stress and reduced NO bioavailability [44,45]. These responses stimulate the production of pro-inflammatory interleukins which facilitates the progression of vascular wall inflammation [19,46].

In a healthy individual, leptin inhibits insulin production in pancreatic β cells, while insulin stimulates leptin production in adipocytes. In a state of leptin resistance, characterized by hyperleptinemia, leptin ceases the inhibition of insulin production leading to a phase of hyperinsulinemia and IR [47]. Moreover, elevated leptin in obesity contributes to increase blood pressure through increased renal sympathetic activity [48] and oxidative stress in VSMC, reducing vasodilation [49]. Leptin and adiponectin have antagonistic effects on vascular tone regulation, inducing vasoconstriction and vasodilation, respectively [45]. Adiponectin promotes glucose metabolism and fatty acid oxidation, contributes to lower IR [50], and may protect against hypertension through an endothelial-dependent mechanism [48]. Hypoadiponectinemia in obesity is associated with increased leptin [45], IR, impaired glucose and fat metabolism, and consequently, hyperglycemia and increased fat accumulation [50]. In summary, obesity triggers a series of cardiometabolic risk factors that can lead to endothelial dysfunction, a complication characterized by NO reduction that may be reversible with therapies that promote NO production.

Endothelial-Mediated Vasodilation

Flow-mediated vasodilation (FMD) is a non-invasive technique commonly used to assess macrovascular endothelial function [15]. FMD evaluates the capacity of conduit arteries (e.g., brachial, femoral, popliteal) to increase their diameter relative to the baseline diameter in response to transient ischemia induced by 5 min of arterial occlusion [15]. Brachial artery FMD is considered the gold standard non-invasive measure of endothelial function and is a predictor of CVD [15]. The increase in arterial diameter indicates the vasodilator effect derived from local production of NO induced by increased shear stress after rapid reperfusion. Impaired FMD is associated with atherosclerosis and arterial stiffness [51] and is apparent in children and adolescents with chronic kidney disease [52], T2D and type 1 diabetes mellitus [53]. It has been shown that children with obesity have a lower FMD than normal-weight counterparts [33]. FMD may be a useful tool to utilize and identify early vascular dysfunction in children and young adults with obesity, as many of them may not show clinical manifestations or cardiometabolic risk factors [54].

Middle-aged adults with prediabetes showed endothelial dysfunction and increased oxidative stress [55]. In children and adolescents, endothelial dysfunction assessed as brachial artery FMD was inversely related to age, total and abdominal obesity, blood pressure, fasting insulin and glucose, and homeostatic model assessment-insulin resistance (HOMA-IR) [56–59]. IR impairs endothelial function even in children and adolescents [57]. Hyperglycemia increases the production of ROS and activity of arginase 1, which mediates endothelial dysfunction by decreasing L-Arg bioavailability [60]. To sum up, cardiometabolic risk factors are associated with endothelial dysfunction, and obese children and adolescents may present lower brachial artery FMD compared to lean counterparts; therefore, this is a useful technique to evaluate the cardiovascular risk in the obese pediatric population.

3. Vascular Function and Structure in Individuals with Obesity

Obesity fosters a pro-inflammatory milieu primarily due to abnormally high visceral adipose tissue [9] leading to low-grade chronic inflammation, oxidative stress [61], IR, and impaired endothelial function [62]. Together, this collection of risk factors, if left untreated, may lead to the development of hypertension, atherosclerosis, arterial stiffening [15,52,53], and ultimately, CVD and T2D in adulthood [18,63].

Adipocyte hypertrophy alters the balance of adipokines, leading to monocyte infiltration in the vascular wall where they are differentiated into pro-inflammatory M1-

macrophages [19,64]. Under these conditions, adipose tissue releases free fatty acids, proinflammatory adipokines (leptin, resistin, tumor necrosis factor alpha (TNFα), and interleukin-6 (IL-6) into circulation, while secretion of adiponectin is reduced [19]. The unbalance between pro- and anti-inflammatory adipokines results in the generation of ROS, which increases vascular tone by inhibiting the synthesis and action of NO leading to vasoconstriction [19]. Therefore, chronic inflammation and oxidative stress are mechanisms of endothelial dysfunction in obesity [19].

Increased visceral abdominal fat is related to hypertension, the major cardiovascular risk factor associated with obesity [65]. Overweight and obese children and adolescents who remain obese with age are at increased risk of developing cardiometabolic diseases, such as T2D, hypertension, dyslipidemia, and carotid artery atherosclerosis [66]. There is a linear relationship between hypertension and obesity in White, Black, Hispanic and Asian individuals [67]. Sustained elevations in blood pressure in obese adolescents increases the risk of developing CVD when entering adulthood [68,69]. Individuals with obesity, hyperglycemia, vascular oxidative stress and inflammation are at higher risk of hypertension [70]. Hypertension in individuals with obesity seems to be the consequence of several hemodynamic, renal and neurohormonal changes caused by excess adipose tissue [71], particularly the abdominal visceral fat. In addition, excessive sodium reabsorption in the kidneys lead to increased extracellular fluid volume and elevated blood pressure, that may injure blood vessels and organs [50]. Therefore, obesity, even in children, increases the risk of having hypertension, which ultimately predisposes to vascular alterations and development of CVD in adulthood.

3.1. Carotid-Intima Media Thickness

Atherosclerosis is the main cause of coronary artery disease, peripheral artery disease, and ischemic stroke [72]. It is defined as a chronic inflammatory process affecting the intima and media layers decreasing the arterial lumen, and in turn, causing reduced blood flow and ischemia [72]. In the earliest stages, atherosclerosis begins as fatty streaks where the accumulation of fat-filled macrophages, termed foam cells, begin aggregating within the intima layer. The progressive accumulation of foam cells, fibrous tissue and inflammatory proteins within the intima forms an atherosclerotic plaque called atheroma [73]. This increase in blockage adversely affects the great arteries, mainly the aorta, coronary, carotid, iliac, femoral and popliteal [72]. The link between atherosclerosis and obesity is via adipokine induced inflammation, IR, and endothelial dysfunction [74]. Studies in adolescents have shown an association between obesity, hypertension and IR with the development of atherosclerosis and greater carotid intima-media thickness (cIMT) [75].

Carotid ultrasonography is a commonly used measure of subclinical atherosclerosis [76]. Several studies have evaluated the lumen–intima and media–adventitia interfaces in relation to carotid far wall histology [77–79]. The distance between these interfaces reflects the cIMT [80]. An increase in cIMT is considered to reflect early arterial abnormalities that ultimately result in an atherosclerotic plaque [77]. cIMT is an independent predictor of CVD and a marker of subclinical organ damage [78]. Hypertension is a major determining factor for cIMT progression [79]. Indeed, high SBP has been associated with a greater change in cIMT, which is comparable with the effects of obesity and T2D [75]. In these populations, hypertension significantly increases the risk of higher cIMT [75].

Previous literature shows an association of cardiometabolic risk factors with increased cIMT, which is influenced by high SBP, low-density lipoprotein (LDL) cholesterol, leptin, abdominal fat, chronic inflammation and lower adiponectin levels, contributing to endothelial dysfunction and progressive development of subclinical atherosclerosis [79,81]. Higher cIMT in children with obesity was associated with an increased risk of CVD in adulthood [75,82], suggesting that untreated atherosclerosis can lead to myocardial infarction and ischemic stroke [72,73]. Zhao et al. examined the relationship between cIMT and MHO in children and adolescents and found that cIMT was positively associated with body weight and CVD risk factors like elevated blood pressure, triglycerides, fasting glucose, and low HDL cholesterol. These findings demonstrated that, even without the presence of cardiometabolic risk factors, overweight and obese children have a higher risk of developing CVD [8].

3.2. Arterial Stiffness

Arterial stiffness is a consequence of reduced NO availability and increased endothelin-1 production (a vasoconstrictor), enhancing vascular tone [83]. Furthermore, arterial stiffness worsens due to structural changes characterized by elastin fiber fragmentation and increased type-III collagen infiltration in the artery wall (media layer); a proceeding that is more evident in central than peripheral arteries [84]. In children with obesity, the arterial diameter and compliance increase physiologically with growth and development, which can compensate arterial pressure increase, but when tension (by high blood pressure) on the aortic wall exceeds the natural adaptation point, arterial stiffness increases [54].

Although there are various methodological approaches to measure arterial stiffness, the most recognized non-invasive technique is pulse wave velocity (PWV) using applanation tonometry, which is calculated by dividing the pulse distance traveled by time across various segments in the arterial system [84]. Carotid–femoral PWV (cfPWV) is considered the gold standard measure of arterial stiffness because it has the strongest correlation with cardiovascular morbidity and mortality in adults [85], especially in those with hypertension [86]. Adolescents with T2D have higher aortic stiffness (cfPWV) compared to subjects with and without obesity [75], and with elevated blood pressure, they show higher cfPWV, regardless of obesity [15]. In young individuals, the increase in cfPWV is attributed to arterial wall distention by increased blood pressure [87]. Brachial–ankle PWV (baPWV), an estimate of systemic arterial stiffness, increases with age, hypertension, and MetS [88]. The main peripheral arterial segment in baPWV is the femoral–ankle PWV (faPWV), which measures leg arterial stiffness and is correlated with SBP, HOMA-IR and waist circumference [89].

Children and adolescents with obesity do not necessarily show differences in arterial stiffness compared to normal weight subjects. Children with obesity may have a decrease in carotid–radial PWV (crPWV) [90] due to larger peripheral arterial diameter, which indicates a vascular adaptation to accommodate a larger blood volume. However, adolescents with obesity may have higher cfPWV and crPWV compared to adolescents without obesity [91,92]. Moreover, a 5-year follow-up study showed that adolescents with obesity from 14 to 19 years of age had a 25% increase in crPWV compared to a 3% increase in normal-weight counterparts, indicating that childhood obesity has an adverse impact on arm arterial structure [91]. These findings suggest that when the natural vascular adaptation point is exceeded, they may be at a higher risk of developing CVD due to early vascular aging.

A high pulse pressure (PP) results from an increased aortic SBP (aSBP) and a reduced or unaffected diastolic blood pressure. Peripheral PP differs from aortic PP (mainly in young people) due to a SBP increase towards the periphery. This increase in PP from the central to peripheral arteries is called PP amplification and is affected by aortic stiffening and increased wave reflection from peripheral arteries [93]. Pressure waves reflected back to the aorta in peripheral sites, such as bifurcations and arterioles, are influenced by the vasomotor tone and controlled by the balance between vasodilators (e.g., NO) and vasoconstrictors (e.g., catecholamines, endothelin-1, angiotensin-II) [88]. The augmentation index (AIx) is considered a marker of left ventricular afterload and wave reflection [94], especially in young and middle-aged adults [95]. Due to pressure overload on the left ventricle, increased aortic PP, SBP and AIx are predictors of cardiovascular events and all-cause mortality in middle-aged and older adults [93]. In fact, children with obesity show higher aSBP and PP than normal weight subjects, regardless of the presence of dyslipidemia, hypertension or sedentarism [96,97]. A greater stroke volume ejection into a stiffer aorta contributes to increased aSBP and PP in children and adolescents with obesity [97], indicating a greater left ventricular overload. In young adults, the increase in adverse cardiometabolic risk factors (i.e., obesity, SBP, lipids, glucose, and insulin) are associated with decreased brachial artery distensibility or increased stiffness [98]. Obesity predisposes individuals to an increased risk of CVD and the obesity-hypertension phenotype increases this risk, accelerating an early vascular aging process. Therefore, early detection of vascular alterations and cardiometabolic risk factors is extremely important as well as interventions that have shown to be effective to improve cardiovascular health.

4. Effects of L-Citrulline Supplementation on Vascular and Metabolic Parameters in Obesity

L-Cit is a non-essential amino acid that is synthesized almost exclusively by the intestines and has a regulatory key role in nitrogen homeostasis [21]. Circulating L-Cit comes mainly from glutamine metabolism and endogenous synthesis of intestinal arginase, [21] and is abundantly found in watermelon (*citrullus vulgaris*) [99]. Oral ingestion of L-Cit is well tolerated [100], and safe since no toxicity or side effects in doses up to 15 g daily have been reported [101]. L-Cit has shown greater increases in plasma L-Arg than equimolar L-Arg supplementation [100,102,103] due to inhibition of intestinal and vascular arginase, preventing the catabolism of L-Arg into urea and ornithine [104] and lack of absorption and catabolism by the liver [105].

Dietary supplementation with L-Cit, either synthetic or from watermelon, increases plasma L-Arg bioavailability via *de novo* synthesis. This process occurs in the kidneys as follows: L-Cit is converted to arginosuccinate by arginosuccinate synthetase and then to L-Arg by arginosuccinate lyase. Synthesized L-Arg is then released into the renal vein and systemic circulation. In endothelial cells, eNOS catabolizes L-Arg to NO which diffuses into and induces relaxation of VSMC (vasodilation) [21,104] (Figure 2). A significant increase in plasma nitrites and nitrates (NOx) after L-Cit supplementation indicates activity of the L-Arg-NO pathway [22,26]. An indirect way to measure NO is by quantifying its metabolites as NOx, because NO is rapidly metabolized after it is produced [106].

Few studies have evaluated L-Cit supplementation in children and/or adolescents. Studies have focused on conditions in children with decreased NO. For example, mitochondrial encephalomyopathy, lactic acidosis, and stroke-like episodes (MELAS syndrome) affect many body systems, especially the brain, nervous system and muscles [103]. Children with MELAS syndrome have lower L-Cit and L-Arg flux leading to reduced NO production compared to control group [103]. In these children, L-Cit supplementation resulted in increased *de novo* L-Arg synthesis and further conversion to NO in the endothelium [103]. These findings suggest that L-Cit improves the L-Arg-NO pathway in children with MELAS syndrome.

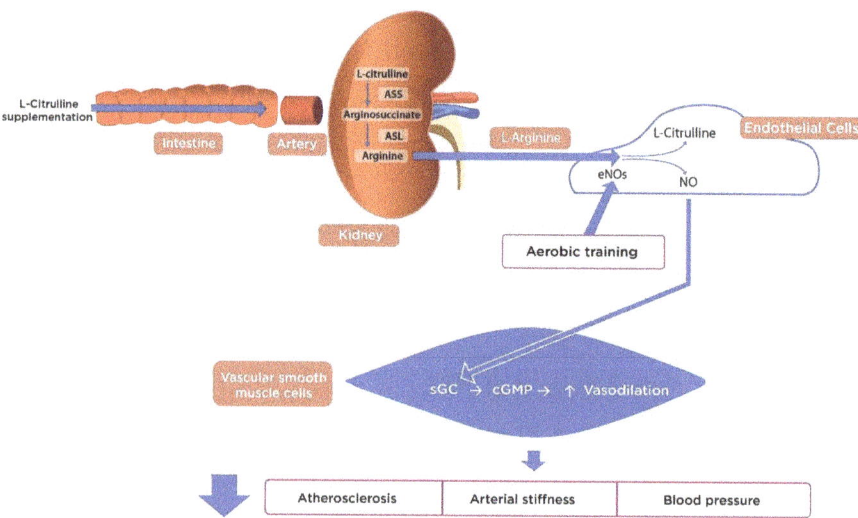

Figure 2. Vascular effects of aerobic training and L-Citrulline supplementation in individuals with obesity. Supplemented L-Cit is mainly metabolized in the kidneys and converted to arginosuccinate by ASS and then to L-Arg by ASL. *De novo* synthesized L-Arg is released into systemic circulation. In endothelial cells, eNOS catabolizes L-Arg to NO and L-Cit. NO diffuses into the VSMC where it stimulates sGC and subsequently activates cGMP, leading to a decrease in intracellular calcium concentrations and vasodilation. Aerobic training activates eNOS and reduces oxidative stress by increasing antioxidant capacity. Thus, L-Cit supplementation and exercise training decrease atherosclerosis, arterial stiffness, and blood pressure by improving endothelial function. L-Cit: L-Citrulline; L-Arg: L-Arginine; ASS: Arginosuccinate synthetase; ASL: Arginosuccinate lyase; eNOS: Endothelial nitric oxide synthase; NO: Nitric oxide; VSMC: Vascular smooth muscle cells; sGC: Soluble guanylyl cyclase; cGMP: Cyclic guanosine monophosphate; ↑: Increase, ↓: Decrease.

Microvascular endothelial dysfunction is characterized by decreased release of NO in small caliber arteries and arterioles (such as those in the eyes, kidneys and nerves). This process was evaluated in children and adolescents (aged 6–17 years) with multiorgan mitochondrial disease using digital pulse wave amplitude and reactive hyperemic index (RHI) [102]. This population had lower baseline RHI than the control group, indicating microvascular endothelial dysfunction. They received similar dose of either oral L-Cit or L-Arg for 2 weeks in a cross-over design. Plasma L-Arg and L-Cit concentrations and the RHI increased 15% and 19% with both supplementations, respectively. L-Cit supplementation increased L-Arg concentrations more than L-Arg supplementation [102]. These findings suggest that short-term L-Arg and its precursor L-Cit are equally effective to reverse microvascular endothelial dysfunction. Macrovascular endothelial dysfunction occurs in arteries, such as those of the heart, brain and extremities. Morita et al. examined the effect of L-Cit on macrovascular endothelial function in adults with vasospastic angina. They reported increases in plasma L-Arg and brachial artery FMD after an 8-week intervention using a daily dose of 800 mg of L-Cit [22]. To the best of our knowledge, this is the only study that has examined the effect of L-Cit supplementation on macrovascular endothelial function in humans. L-Cit supplementation (5.8 g/day) improves macrovascular function by activation of the L-Arg-NO pathway [26]. Similarly, L-Cit supplementation (2 g/day) for 1 month increased plasma NO levels via inhibition of arginase activity in T2D patients [107]. Thus, L-Cit supplementation can be a viable therapeutic strategy to improve obesity and hyperglycemia-induced endothelial function by increasing L-Arg and NO bioavailability in middle-aged adults [22,23,26,43]. To our knowledge, there are no studies evaluating the use of L-Cit supplementation to improve vascular or metabolic parameters in children and adolescents with obesity. However, the improvements seen in circulating NOx as well as endothelial function after L-Cit supplementation in adults and in children with MELAS suggests that benefits may be useful in obese children with cardiometabolic risk factors (Table 1).

Impaired endothelial-dependent vasodilation precedes vascular dysfunction (e.g., atherosclerosis and arterial stiffness) and hypertension, which is mainly attributed to reduce NO bioavailability [37]. Thus, L-Cit supplementation has positive effects in several vascular abnormalities such as hypertension and arterial stiffness [108] by improving NO synthesis and organ blood flow and decreasing blood pressure [23,24]. A SBP reduction was evident following L-Cit supplementation (6 g/day) for 8 weeks in prehypertensive and hypertensive postmenopausal women with obesity [23,24]. However, no significant reduction in SBP was observed after 6 and 15 g/day of L-Cit for 2 weeks in overweight or obese with normal or elevated SBP, probably due to a short supplementation period and/or inefficiency of L-Cit in non-hypertensive individuals without endothelial dysfunction [109–111]. Therefore, L-Cit supplementation can reduce blood pressure at rest in adults with elevated blood pressure or hypertension [23,24], but not in those with normal blood pressure [22,109]. Moreover, L-Cit has demonstrated the capacity to attenuate the increase in blood pressure and arterial stiffness in young healthy overweight men [109] and patients without obesity under stressful conditions [112,113].

Endothelial dysfunction is associated with increased arterial stiffness, especially in people with hypertension [114]. Figueroa et al. found significant decreases in systemic (baPWV) and leg (faPWV) arterial stiffness after 6 g/day of L-Cit supplementation for 8 weeks in postmenopausal women with obesity and high blood pressure [25]. Similarly, Ochiai et al. found a reduction in baPWV after 7 days of supplementation with a similar dose in healthy middle-aged men with increased baPWV [26]. In contrast, baPWV was not affected by the same dose of L-Cit supplementation for 14 days in healthy men without obesity [109]. These findings suggest that L-Cit supplementation is effective in reducing peripheral arterial stiffness in patients with high arterial stiffness but not in healthy young adults. Interestingly, an inverse relationship between plasma L-Arg and baPWV was seen by Ochiai and colleagues [26], suggesting that stimulation of the L-Arg-NO pathway with L-Cit supplementation may contribute to the decrease in arterial stiffness.

Hyperinsulinemia, a common feature of IR, might enhance vasoconstriction [44]. In male C57BL/6J mice fed with a high-fat diet (HFD) and L-Cit (0.6 g/L) supplementation for 15 weeks glucose and insulin levels were reduced compared to the control group [115]. In contrast, L-Cit supplementation for 11 weeks did not affect serum glucose in both groups compared to the control group in obese/diabetic rodents. However, decreases in insulin, HOMA-IR, total cholesterol, and free fatty acids suggested improved glucose and lipid metabolism by L-Cit supplementation in these animal models [116]. In accordance, male rats supplemented with L-Cit (1 g/kg/day) had lower susceptibility to lipoprotein oxidation, indicating that L-Cit has a protective antioxidant effect [117]. Male Sprague Dawley rats received a 4-week fructose (60%) diet to develop steatosis with dyslipidemia. L-Cit (0.15 g/day) supplementation prevented hypertriglyceridemia and attenuated liver fat accumulation compared to the groups that received L-Arg or glutamine supplementation, which were ineffective. This study suggests that L-Cit acts on hepatic lipid metabolism, partially preventing hypertriglyceridemia and steatosis [118].

Physiological levels of NO stimulate glucose and fatty acid uptake and oxidation in insulin-sensitive tissues, while inhibit the synthesis of glycogen and fatty acids in target tissues and enhance lipolysis in white adipocytes [119–121]. Few studies have evaluated the metabolic effects of L-Cit in adult humans. L-Cit supplementation has improved serum levels of NO, lipids (triglyceride, HDL cholesterol), glucose control (insulin, glucose, glycated hemoglobin (HbA1c), HOMA-IR), and inflammation (TNF-α and C-reactive protein) in patients with obesity and T2D [107,122]. Further studies are required to evaluate the effects of L-Cit supplementation on lipid and glucose metabolism in individuals with obesity including children and adolescents.

Table 1. Effects of L-Citrulline supplementation on vascular and metabolic parameters in adults with obesity.

Articles	Total Sample	Intervention Group		Supplementation Characteristics			SBP (mmHg)	NOx	PWV (m/s)	Glucose (mg/dL)	Triglycerides (mg/dL)
		Sample	Age	Dose	Duration						
[23]	$n = 41$	14 women	58 ± 4 years	6 g/day	8 weeks	B	137 ± 13	28.2 ± 7.3	NM	NM	NM
						A	130 ± 15 *	35.2 ± 9.5 *			
[109]	$n = 16$	16 men	24 ± 2 (SE)	6 g/day	2 weeks	B	123 ± 3	NM	11.8 [a]	NM	NM
						A	121 ± 3		11.2 [a]		
[24]	$n = 23$	12 women	58 ± 1 years	6 g/day	8 weeks	B	138 ± 4	NM	NM	NM	NM
						A	131 ± 5 *[#]				
[25]	$n = 40$	14 women	58 ± 1 years	6 g/ day	8 weeks	B	137 ± 4	NM	11.5 $\pm$ 0.4 [b] 10.01 $\pm$ 0.2 [c] 14.1 $\pm$ 0.5 [a]	NM	NM
						A	NR		11.3 $\pm$ 0.5 [b] 9.6 $\pm$ 0.2 [c]* 13.2 $\pm$ 0.5 [a]*		
[110]	$n = 41$	41 adults	18–66 years	15g/day	2 weeks	B	130 (126–134)	NM	NM	88 (84–92)	101 (77–126)
						C	−1.6 (−6.3–3.1)			NR	NR

The variables are presented as mean $\pm$ standard deviation (SD) or median (ranges). SE: standard error; n: total sample; NM: not measured; NR: values not reported without significant changes; B: basal measurements; A: after intervention measurements; C: post intervention change; SBP: systolic blood pressure; NOx: nitrite and nitrate; PWV: pulse wave velocity; FMD: flow-mediated dilation; [a] baPWV: brachial–ankle PWV; [b] cfPWV: carotid–femoral PWV; [c] faPWV: femoral–ankle PWV. Differences within groups: * $p < 0.05$, differences with the control group: [#] $p < 0.05$.

High fat and low muscle mass in individuals with obesity adversely affect cardiometabolic risk factors, promoting hyperglycemia, hypertension, and dyslipidemia, among others [123,124]. Evaluating body composition, male rats that received L-Cit (1 g/kg/day) supplementation decreased fat mass and increased total body lean mass, which is mainly muscle, compared with control rats [117]. Another study evaluated obese mice, where those treated with L-Cit had lower food intake and body weight than the control group. In HFD fed Sprague Dawley rats, the expression of proopiomelanocortin in the hypothalamus, a food intake suppression peptide, was significantly higher in the L-Cit group compared to the control group. Therefore, L-Cit supplementation may decrease body fat mass by appetite suppression, leading to metabolic improvements [116]. In older malnourished humans, 10 g of L-Cit supplementation for 3 weeks increased systemic amino acid availability necessary for protein synthesis in skeletal muscles. In older women, L-Cit supplementation increased total body lean mass (~1.7 kg) and decreased fat mass (~1.3 kg) [27]. More studies are required to evaluate the effects of L-Cit supplementation on body composition in children and adolescents with obesity.

5. Effects of the Aerobic Training in Children and Adolescents with Obesity on Vascular and Metabolic Parameters

According to the WHO, children and adolescents aged 5–17 years should do at least 60 min of moderate-to-vigorous intensity physical activity daily, most of which should be aerobic to provide health benefits [125]. Vigorous intensity activities should be incorporated at least three times per week, including those that strengthen skeletal muscles [125]. A main cause of overweight and obesity is physical inactivity [126] which results in low maximal oxygen consumption ($VO_{2\,max}$) and is associated with MetS and cardiometabolic risk factors in children and youths [127]. Physical activity yields multiple health benefits like improved vascular, metabolic and body composition parameters described in the next paragraphs. The articles included in this section, the type of training (walking or jogging [34], jump rope [31,35] and high intensity interval training (HIIT) [32,33]), intensity (moderate and high), session duration (4 to 60 min), frequency (3–5 days per week), and training duration (12–32 weeks) are described in Table 2. An increase in $VO_{2\,peak}$ [32,35] and a decrease in resting heart rate was found in children after aerobic training [31], which can be related to lower cardiometabolic risk, as elevated resting heart rate is associated with hypertension and elevated triglycerides, glucose and abdominal adiposity in children and adolescents [128].

Elevated blood pressure in children increases the risk of hypertension development during adolescence [129]. Previous studies using supra HIIT (170% peak power output) and jump rope (low-to-moderate intensity) exercises have seen decreases in SBP in prehypertensive and hypertensive children with obesity [31,32]. This reduction in SBP by 3 to 10 mmHg, respectively, is relevant to improve cardiovascular health as many newly diagnosed children with hypertension experience cardiovascular damage [130].

Aerobic exercise training has shown promising results on improving brachial artery FMD in children and adolescents. A significant improvement on FMD was evident after HIIT [32,33]. Consistent with these findings, others have reported increases in circulating NOx levels after the exercise interventions [31,32]. These findings demonstrate the beneficial effects of aerobic exercise training on improving endothelial NO production and endothelial function in obese children [131].

Table 2. Characteristics of children and adolescents with obesity and aerobic training.

Article	Total Sample	Group	Intervention Group						Exercise Training Characteristics				
			Sample	Female	Male	Age (Years)	Body Mass Index (kg/m^2)	Training	Intensity	Session (Minutes)	Frequency (Days/Week)	Duration (Weeks)
[35]	175	Exercise	90	55	35	9.7 (9.5, 9.8)	25.9 (25.0, 26.9)	Jump rope	HR >140 bpm	40	5	32
		Control	85	47	38	9.7 (9.5, 9.9)	25 (24.4, 26.8)	N/A	N/A	N/A	N/A	N/A
[32]	48	HIIT	11	0	11	11± 0.3	24.2 ± 1.0	HIIT: 8 × 2 min intervals	90% PPO	24	3	12
		Supra-HIIT	15	0	15	11± 0.2	26.5 ± 0.9	Supra HIIT: 8 × 20 s intervals	170% PPO	4	3	12
		Control	11	0	11	10.6 ± 0.3	53.6 ± 4.0	N/A	N/A	N/A	N/A	N/A
[34]	118	Aerobic exercise	38	13	25	14.4 ± 1.6	>85th percentile	Walking/jogging	60–65% VO$_2$	40–60	3	24
[31]	40	Exercise	20	20	0	15 ± 1	26 ± 3	Jump rope	40–70% HRR	50	5	12
		Control	20	20	0	15 ± 1	25 ± 2	N/A	N/A	N/A	N/A	N/A
[33]	38	Exercise	25	13	12	15.1 ± 1	28 ± 3	HIIT: 2–6 (100 m running sprints)	NP	10–22	3	12

The variables are presented as mean ± standard deviation (SD) or median (ranges). N/A: not applicable; NM: not measured, instead obesity was considered $\geq$ 25.0% for men and $\geq$ 35.0% for women; MICT: moderate-intensity continuous training; HIIT: high-intensity interval training; bpm; beat/minute; HR: heart rate; HRR: heart rate reserve; HR max: maximum heart rate; PPO: peak power output; VO$_2$: maximal oxygen consumption; NP: no prescription.

Boys with obesity showed a decrease in cIMT (~0.2 mm) after HIIT and supra HIIT (90% and 170% peak power output, 24 and 4 min, respectively, 3 times per week, during 12 weeks) [32]. Interestingly, meta-analytic data suggests that a longer aerobic exercise duration per week may yield small-to-moderate decreases in cIMT. This finding suggests that structural atherosclerotic changes can be reversed with regular aerobic exercise programs in obese children [32], as subclinical carotid atherosclerosis is the most common cause of CVD among children and adolescents [132].

Children and adolescents with obesity had a reduction in arterial stiffness (~0.7 to 0.8 m/s), measured with baPWV, an arterial segment that includes the aorta and leg arteries. The training protocols consisted of jump rope (at moderate-intensity for 12 weeks) [31], HIIT and supra HIIT [32]. In children and adolescents, hypertension may lead to increased arterial stiffness [54], and thus reductions in SBP may explain decreases in baPWV [31,32]. Participants had higher SBP at baseline (>120 mmHg) [31,32] than other studies that found no significant reductions in cfPWV [34,35]. Given that aerobic training at moderate- and high-intensity reduces baPWV but not cfPWV, these findings indicate a reduction in peripheral PWV.

Aerobic training at moderate-to-high intensity for 4–60 min improved at least one lipid parameter (total cholesterol [32,34], LDL cholesterol [32] triglycerides [32,33] or HDL cholesterol [35]) in obese children and adolescents. In a systematic review, the magnitude of the effects of aerobic training on the metabolic profile of obese children was associated with the intensity ($\leq$75% heart rate max) and duration (60 min) and frequency (3 times a week) of the exercise session [133]. These findings suggest that high-intensity aerobic exercise sessions could be efficient in improving lipid profile in obese children and adolescents. However, diet must be monitored to yield such improvements.

Aerobic training shows a favorable impact on body composition in children and adolescents with obesity, of which had a reduction in waist circumference [31,33], total body fat percentage [31,35], and increases in lean mass [31] after aerobic training at moderate-to-high intensity for 12–32 weeks. One study shows that waist circumference is associated with aerobic capacity (an important health-related factor) in boys and girls [134]. These studies suggest that aerobic training is fundamental to achieve beneficial changes in fat and muscle mass, thus, a lower cardiovascular risk in children with obesity.

Exercise training in children and adolescents with obesity showed positive effects on cardiometabolic risk factors (Table 3). It is important to emphasize that exercise recommendations for children are designed for the prevention of cardiometabolic risk factors as well as depression and anxiety [125]. Therefore, aerobic training should be included in CVD prevention and treatment programs in children and adolescents with obesity.

6. Effects of L-Citrulline Supplementation and Exercise Training in Individuals with Obesity on Vascular and Metabolic Parameters

The interest on the potential synergistic or additive effect of L-Cit supplementation and exercise training is supported by improvements in vascular and metabolic parameters. Aerobic training improves body composition, lipid profile, endothelial function, atherosclerosis, arterial stiffness, and blood pressure in children and adolescents with obesity [31–35]. L-Cit supplementation increases the bioavailability of L-Arg and NO to enhance vasodilation [22,23,26], improve arterial stiffness, and regulate blood pressure by having an antihypertensive effect in adults [23,24], and may improve endothelial function in children and adolescents with obesity with lower NO production and endothelial dysfunction [102,103]. L-Cit supplementation has also demonstrated to improve glucose control [107,122], muscle protein synthesis [27], and body composition (lean mass and fat mass) [116] (Figure 3). The combination of aerobic exercise training and L-Cit supplementation on metabolic and cardiovascular parameters in obesity has only been studied in adults (Table 4). The most important benefits are discussed below.

Table 3. Effects of exercise training on cardiovascular disease risk factors in children and adolescents with obesity.

Articles	Group	SBP (mmHg)		FMD (%)		cIMT (mm)		PWV (m/s)		SBP (mmHg)		LDL-C (mg/dL)	
		Baseline	Post/ Mean Changes	Baseline	Post/ Mean Changes	Baseline	Post/ Mean Changes	Baseline	Post/ Mean Changes	Baseline	Post/ Mean Changes	Baseline	Post/ Mean Changes
[35]	Exercise	105 (103, 107)	0.1 (−1.5, 1.7)	NM		105 (103, 107)	0.1 (−1.5, 1.7)	5.1 (4.9, 5.3) [b]	−0.02 (−0.23, 0.2)	105 (103,107)	0.1 (−1.5, 1.7)	102 (95,110)	−6 (−10, −2)
	Control	102 (100, 104)	0.3 (−1.3, 2)	NM		102 (100, 104)	0.3 (−1.3, 2)	5.1 (4.9, 5.2) [b]	−0.04 (−0.18, 0.26)	102 (100,104)	0.3 (−1.3, 2)	103 (96,110)	−5 (−9, −1)
[32]	HIIT	128 ± 4	125 ± 4	8.9	11.1 *#	128 ± 4	125 ± 4	9.97 [a]	9.3 *#	128 ± 4	125 ± 4	112 ± 6	88 ± 6 *
	Supra HIIT	127 ± 4	116 ± 3 *	7.9	10.1 *	127 ± 4	116 ± 3 *	9.86 [a]	9.06 *#	127 ± 4	116 ± 3 *	105 ± 6	81 ± 5 *#
	Control	121 ± 4	121 ± 4	8.3	7.4	121 ± 4	121 ± 4	10.04 [a]	10.2	121 ± 4	121 ± 4	111 ± 7	104 ± 6
[34]	Aerobic exer-cise	112 ± 8	0.9 ± 1.4	NM		112 ± 8	0.9 ± 1.4	5.97 ± 0.75 [b]	−0.19 ± 0.14	112 ± 8	0.9 ± 1.4	87 ± 24	−4 ± 2
[31]	Exercise	126 ± 3	120 ± 2 *#	NM		126 ± 3	120 ± 2 *#	8.2 ± 1 [a]	7.4 ± 0.2 *#	126 ± 3	120 ± 2 *#	NM	
	Control	126 ± 4	127 ± 5.3	NM		126 ± 4	127 ± 5.3	8.2 ± 0.5 [a]	8.1 ± 0.2	126 ± 4	127 ± 5.3	NM	
[33]	Exercise	NM		7.9	12.2 *	NM		NM		NM		90 ± 23	99 ± 25

This table describes the effects of exercise training on cardiometabolic disease risk factors of the studies shown in Table 2. The variables are presented as mean ± SD or median (ranges). NM: not measured; WC: waist circumference; SBP: brachial systolic blood pressure; cIMT: intima-media thickness; PWV: pulse wave velocity; [a] baPWV: brachial–ankle PWV; [b] cfPWV: carotid–femoral PWV; FMD: flow-mediated dilation; LDL-C: low density lipoprotein cholesterol; HIIT: high-intensity interval training. Differences within groups: * $p < 0.05$, differences between groups: # $p < 0.05$.

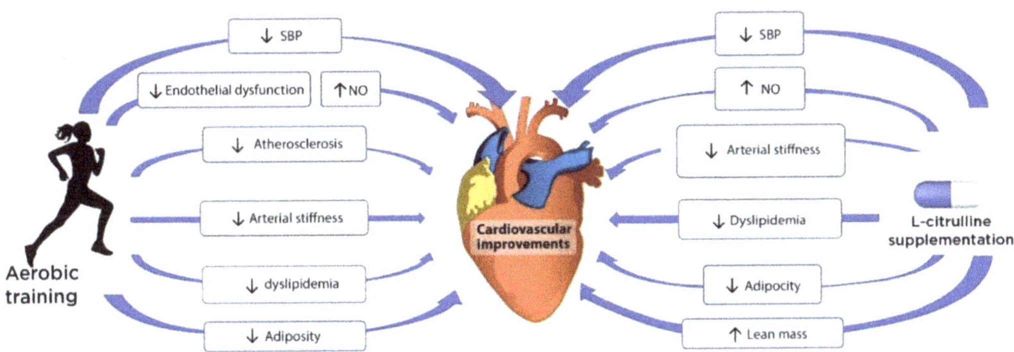

Figure 3. Cardiovascular improvements with L-Citrulline supplementation and moderate-to-high intensity aerobic training. In children and adolescents with obesity and cardiometabolic alterations, aerobic training helps to improve blood pressure (SBP), endothelial function (NO and FMD), atherosclerosis (cIMT), arterial stiffness (baPWV), dyslipidemia (triglycerides, total cholesterol, LDL-C and HDL-C), and body composition (waist circumference and total body fat). L-Cit supplementation in adults with cardiometabolic alterations helps to improve NO production, blood pressure (SBP), arterial stiffness (baPWV and faPWV), dyslipidemia (triglycerides and HDL-C), glucose control (insulin, glucose and HOMA-IR) and body composition (total body fat and lean mass). L-Cit: L-Citrulline; SBP: systolic blood pressure; NO: nitric oxide; FMD: flow-mediated dilation; cIMT: intima–media thickness; baPWV: brachial–ankle PWV; LDL-C: LDL cholesterol; HDL-C: HDL cholesterol; faPWV: femoral–ankle PWV; HOMA-IR: homeostatic model assessment-insulin resistance; ↑: Increase; ↓: Decrease.

Hypertension is the most important risk factor for CVD in adults. Effective interventions are constantly searched to improve blood pressure. Obese postmenopausal women received L-Cit (6 g/day), whole-body vibration training (an alternative strength training modality) or the combination of both interventions for 8 weeks [23]. All groups similarly decreased SBP, indicating that this combined intervention has no additive effect on blood pressure at the prescribed dose and duration. However, the combined intervention was more effective than each individual intervention to decrease pressure wave reflection and aortic stiffness, which may be clinically significant for postmenopausal women with elevated blood pressure and hypertension [23,25]. These findings showed that the combination of exercise training (WBVT) and L-Cit supplementation have beneficial effects on arterial function in obese postmenopausal women [23,25]. This population is of special interest because they have higher risk of CVD attributed to aging and sex-related increases in aSBP, wave reflection, and proximal aortic stiffness [135]. However, these studies do not represent the entire population of adults with obesity, and WBVT is not a conventional strength training modality.

There are no studies evaluating the metabolic effects of combined exercise training and L-Cit in individuals with obesity. In a study by Buckinx et al., two groups of healthy older adults without obesity combined HIIT with L-Cit supplementation (10 g/day) or placebo for 12 weeks with no impact on metabolic markers (glucose, insulin, HOMA-IR or lipid profile) [136], as they had no basal metabolic abnormalities. Given that the cardiometabolic effects of oral L-Cit might be via *de novo* L-Arg synthesis, L-Cit and L-Arg supplementation may produce similar metabolic effects. In a randomized placebo-controlled trial, two groups of middle-aged adults with obesity and T2D received a low-calorie diet and exercise training (both aerobic and resistance) combined with either L-Arg supplementation (8.3 g) or placebo for 3 weeks. Compared with the placebo group, L-Arg supplementation had an additive effect on vascular function, glucose and lipid metabolism, and fat mass as well as prevented the loss of muscle mass associated with hypocaloric diet [137]. Since oral L-Cit is more efficient than L-Arg for increasing plasma L-Arg availability, L-Cit supplementation combined with exercise training may have similar or possibly greater beneficial effects on vascular and metabolic function than those observed with L-Arg supplementation. However, clinical trials are needed to validate this hypothesis.

Several studies have evaluated the effect of exercise training and L-Cit supplementation on anthropometric parameters, finding no significant changes in BMI [23,25,136,138]. Buckinx et al. studied older adults with obesity and muscle weakness who performed HIIT with L-Cit supplementation (10 g/day) or placebo for 12 weeks. Although there were no significant increases in lean mass with HIIT and L-Cit supplementation, a decrease in total and leg fat mass percentages were noted after HIIT and L-Cit supplementation [138]. Despite the lack of impact on muscle mass, HIIT with L-Cit improved arm muscle strength and walking speed [138], suggesting that the combination of L-Cit and HIIT may improve total body fat loss and increase strength more than exercise training alone.

A research group examined the effects of strength training (WBVT) combined with L-Cit or placebo on body composition and muscle strength in obese postmenopausal women. It was found that WBVT alone and WBVT plus L-Cit supplementation had similar significant decreases in body fat percentage [25]. L-Cit supplementation and WBVT favored the increase in leg lean mass compared with the WBVT and placebo groups. However, the improvements in leg muscle strength were similar with or without L-Cit, indicating no additional benefit of L-Cit in postmenopausal women with obesity. Although L-Cit combined with unconventional strength training had additive positive effects on arterial stiffness and muscle mass in obese postmenopausal women [25], the impact on endothelial function as a potential mechanism was not examined. These findings suggest that both types of training (HIIT and WBVT) combined with L-Cit supplementation have beneficial effects on body composition.

To our knowledge, only the studies reviewed in this section have reported effects on vascular and muscular parameters using L-Cit in combination with different types of exercise training in adults with obesity. There are no studies evaluating changes in glucose metabolism or lipid profile in individuals with obesity using L-Cit plus exercise training. As a limitation, in the reviewed studies, the individuals without obesity did not have metabolic alterations to evaluate the effect of these combined interventions. Another limitation is that L-Cit has not been evaluated in combination with resistance training. Unfortunately, the combination of L-Cit plus aerobic training has not been examined in children and adolescents. The studies that investigated L-Cit supplementation in children focused on improving a specific condition, such as MELAS. Randomized, placebo-controlled studies are required to evaluate the combination of these two interventions in children and adolescents with obesity because results of previous studies suggest that L-Cit and exercise training can be an effective strategy to counteract the effects of obesity on vascular and metabolic function at early stages of life.

Table 4. Effects of L-Citrulline supplementation and exercise training on vascular and metabolic parameters in adults with obesity.

| Article | Total Sample | Intervention Groups | | Exercise Characteristics | | | L-Citrulline Dose | | SBP (mmHg) | aSBP (mmHg) | Aix (%) | NOx (µmol/L) | PWV (m/s) | WC (cm) |
		Sample	Age	Training	Session	Frequency/ Duration								
[23]	$n = 41$	13 women	58 ± 3 years	WBVT: dynamic leg exercises	1–5 sets (30–60 s)	3 days/week For 8 weeks	6 g/day	B	140 ± 9	133 ± 9	43.5 ± 10.2	28.2 ± 14.9	NM	NM
								A	132 ± 9 *	123 ± 9 *	33.3 ± 8.3 *	38.3 ± 19.6 *		NM
[25]	$n = 41$	13 women	58 ± 1 years	WBVT: dynamic leg exercises	1–5 sets (30–60 s)	3 days/week For 8 weeks	6 g/day	B	140 ± 3	NM	NM	NM	11.7 ± 0.3 [b] 14.7 ± 0.4 [a] 10.4 ± 0.3 [c]	NM
								A	NR				10.8 ± 0.3 [b]* 13.4 ± 0.4 [a]* 9.8 ± 0.2 [c]*	NM
[138]	$n = 56$	26 adults	65.7 ± 4.2 years	HIIT	30 min	3 days/week For 12 weeks	10 g/day	B	NM	NM	NM	NM	NM	107 ± 11
								A						104 ± 11 *
[136]	$n = 44$	23 adults	67.6 ± 5.01 years	HIIT	30 min	3 days/week For 12 weeks	10 g/day	B	NM	NM	NM	NM	NM	98.3 ± 10.2
								A						95.9 ± 10.9 *

The variables are presented as mean ± standard deviation (SD). *n*: total sample; NM: not measured; NR: values not reported; B: basal measurements; A: after intervention measurements; BMI: body mass index; WC: waist circumference; SBP: systolic blood pressure; aSBP: aortic systolic blood pressure; PWV: pulse wave velocity; [a] baPWV: brachial–ankle PWV; [b] cfPWV: carotid–femoral PWV; [c] faPWV: femoral–ankle PWV; AIx: augmentation index; NOx: nitrite and nitrate; WBVT: whole-body vibration training. Differences within groups: * $p < 0.05$.

7. Conclusions and Remarks

Children and adolescents with obesity may have early vascular aging characterized by endothelial dysfunction, elevated blood pressure, arterial stiffness, and multiple cardiometabolic risk factors that increases the risk of CVD development in adulthood. Aerobic training is essential to reduce cardiometabolic disorders associated with obesity in children and adolescents. Interventions at moderate-to-high intensity for 12–32 weeks have showed positive effects on endothelial function, arterial stiffness, atherosclerosis, blood pressure, and IR. L-Cit supplementation increases the bioavailability of L-Arg and NO in children and adults. In adults, L-Cit supplementation has shown to be effective for improving blood pressure, arterial stiffness, body composition (lean and fat mass), and metabolism (glucose and lipid profile), especially in obese individuals. The WBVT and L-Cit supplementation is an effective strategy to improve cardiovascular and muscular health in adults with obesity; thus, further studies are needed to test the effectiveness of this combination in children and young adults with obesity and cardiometabolic alterations.

Author Contributions: Conceptualization, A.G.F.-R., M.E.G.-S. and A.F.; methodology, A.G.F.-R., M.E.G.-S. and A.F.; writing original draft preparation, A.G.F.-R. and V.I.T.-V.; writing, review and editing, M.E.G.-S., A.M. and A.F. All authors have read and agreed to the published version of the manuscript.

Funding: This research received no external funding.

Institutional Review Board Statement: Not applicable.

Informed Consent Statement: Not applicable.

Data Availability Statement: No applicable.

Acknowledgments: The authors thank Ing. Sergio Becerril Zavala from Abastecedora de Productos Naturales, SA. Pronat, ProWinner, for all the support provided.

Conflicts of Interest: The authors declare no conflict of interest.

References

1. World Health Organization. Obesity and Overweight. Available online: https://www.who.int/news-room/fact-sheets/detail/obesity-and-overweight (accessed on 20 June 2021).
2. Deal, B.J.; Huffman, M.D.; Binns, H.; Stone, N.J. Perspective: Childhood obesity requires new strategies for prevention. *Adv. Nutr.* **2020**, *11*, 1071–1078. [CrossRef] [PubMed]
3. Bramlage, P.; Pittrow, D.; Wittchen, H.-U.; Kirch, W.; Boehler, S.; Lehnert, H.; Hoefler, M.; Unger, T.; Sharma, A.M. Hypertension in overweight and obese primary care patients is highly prevalent and poorly controlled. *Am. J. Hypertens.* **2004**, *17*, 904–910. [CrossRef] [PubMed]
4. Song, P.; Zhang, Y.; Yu, J.; Zha, M.; Zhu, Y.; Rahimi, K.; Rudan, I. Global prevalence of hypertension in children: A systematic review and meta-analysis. *JAMA Pediatr.* **2019**, *173*, 1154–1163. [CrossRef]
5. Hinnouho, G.-M.; Czernichow, S.; Dugravot, A.; Batty, G.; Kivimaki, M.; Singh-Manoux, A. Metabolically healthy obesity and risk of mortality: Does the definition of metabolic health matter? *Diabetes Care* **2013**, *36*, 2294–2300. [CrossRef]
6. Kramer, C.K.; Zinman, B.; Retnakaran, R. Are metabolically healthy overweight and obesity benign conditions? A systematic review and meta-analysis. *Ann. Intern. Med.* **2013**, *159*, 758–769. [CrossRef] [PubMed]
7. Fan, J.; Song, Y.; Chen, Y.; Hui, R.; Zhang, W. Combined effect of obesity and cardio-metabolic abnormality on the risk of cardiovascular disease: A meta-analysis of prospective cohort studies. *Int. J. Cardiol.* **2013**, *168*, 4761–4768. [CrossRef] [PubMed]
8. Zhao, M.; López-Bermejo, A.; Caserta, C.A.; Medeiros, C.C.M.; Kollias, A.; Bassols, J.; Romeo, E.L.; Ramos, T.D.A.; Stergiou, G.S.; Yang, L.; et al. Metabolically healthy obesity and high carotid intima-media thickness in children and adolescents: International childhood vascular structure evaluation consortium. *Diabetes Care* **2018**, *42*, 119–125. [CrossRef]
9. Al-Hamad, D.; Raman, V. Metabolic syndrome in children and adolescents. *Transl. Pediatr.* **2017**, *6*, 397–407. [CrossRef]
10. Styne, D.M.; Arslanian, S.A.; Connor, E.L.; Farooqi, S.; Murad, M.H.; Silverstein, J.H.; Yanovski, J. Pediatric obesity—Assessment, treatment, and prevention: An endocrine society clinical practice guideline. *J. Clin. Endocrinol. Metab.* **2017**, *102*, 709–757. [CrossRef] [PubMed]
11. Kumar, S.; Kelly, A.S. Review of childhood obesity: From epidemiology, etiology, and comorbidities to clinical assessment and treatment. *Mayo Clin. Proc.* **2017**, *92*, 251–265. [CrossRef]
12. Zimmet, P.; Alberti, K.G.M.; Kaufman, F.; Tajima, N.; Silink, M.; Arslanian, S.; Wong, G.; Bennett, P.; Shaw, J.; Caprio, S.; et al. The metabolic syndrome in children and adolescents? An IDF consensus report. *Pediatr. Diabetes* **2007**, *8*, 299–306. [CrossRef]

13. Sun, S.S.; Grave, G.D.; Siervogel, R.M.; Pickoff, A.A.; Arslanian, S.S.; Daniels, S.R. Systolic blood pressure in childhood predicts hypertension and metabolic syndrome later in life. *Pediatrics* **2007**, *119*, 237–246. [CrossRef]
14. Sun, S.S.; Liang, R.; Huang, T.T.-K.; Daniels, S.R.; Arslanian, S.; Liu, K.; Grave, G.D.; Siervogel, R.M. Childhood obesity predicts adult metabolic syndrome: The Fels longitudinal study. *J. Pediatr.* **2008**, *152*, 191–200.e1. [CrossRef]
15. Khoury, M.; Urbina, E.M. Cardiac and vascular target organ damage in pediatric hypertension. *Front. Pediatr.* **2018**, *6*, 148. [CrossRef] [PubMed]
16. Magge, S.; Goodman, E.; Armstrong, S.C.; Committee on Nutrition; Section on Endocrinology; Section on Obesity. The metabolic syndrome in children and adolescents: Shifting the focus to cardiometabolic risk factor clustering. *Pediatrics* **2017**, *140*, e20171603. [CrossRef] [PubMed]
17. Wu, Y.-E.; Zhang, C.-L.; Zhen, Q. Metabolic syndrome in children (Review). *Exp. Ther. Med.* **2016**, *12*, 2390–2394. [CrossRef] [PubMed]
18. Nguyen, Q.M.; Srinivasan, S.R.; Xu, J.-H.; Chen, W.; Berenson, G.S. Fasting plasma glucose levels within the normoglycemic range in childhood as a predictor of prediabetes and type 2 diabetes in adulthood: The Bogalusa heart study. *Arch. Pediatr. Adolesc. Med.* **2010**, *164*, 124–128. [CrossRef] [PubMed]
19. Kwaifa, I.K.; Bahari, H.; Yong, Y.K.; Noor, S.M. Endothelial dysfunction in obesity-induced inflammation: Molecular mechanisms and clinical implications. *Biomolecules* **2020**, *10*, 291. [CrossRef]
20. Čolak, E.; Pap, D. The role of oxidative stress in the development of obesity and obesity-related metabolic disorders. *J. Med. Biochem.* **2021**, *40*, 1–9. [CrossRef]
21. Breuillard, C.; Cynober, L.; Moinard, C. Citrulline and nitrogen homeostasis: An overview. *Amino Acids* **2015**, *47*, 685–691. [CrossRef] [PubMed]
22. Morita, M.; Sakurada, M.; Watanabe, F.; Yamasaki, T.; Doi, H.; Ezaki, H.; Morishita, K.; Miyakex, T. Effects of oral L-Citrulline supplementation on Lipoprotein oxidation and Endothelial dysfunction in humans with Vasospastic Angina. *Immunol. Endocr. Metab. Agents Med. Chem.* **2013**, *13*, 214–220. [CrossRef]
23. Wong, A.; Alvarez-Alvarado, S.; Jaime, S.J.; Kinsey, A.W.; Spicer, M.T.; Madzima, T.A.; Figueroa, A. Combined whole-body vibration training and L-Citrulline supplementation improves pressure wave reflection in obese postmenopausal women. *Appl. Physiol. Nutr. Metab.* **2016**, *41*, 292–297. [CrossRef]
24. Wong, A.; Chernykh, O.; Figueroa, A. Chronic L-Citrulline supplementation improves cardiac sympathovagal balance in obese postmenopausal women: A preliminary report. *Auton. Neurosci. Basic Clin.* **2016**, *198*, 50–53. [CrossRef]
25. Figueroa, A.; Alvarez-Alvarado, S.; Ormsbee, M.J.; Madzima, T.A.; Campbell, J.C.; Wong, A. Impact of L-Citrulline supplementation and whole-body vibration training on arterial stiffness and leg muscle function in obese postmenopausal women with high blood pressure. *Exp. Gerontol.* **2015**, *63*, 35–40. [CrossRef] [PubMed]
26. Ochiai, M.; Hayashi, T.; Morita, M.; Ina, K.; Maeda, M.; Watanabe, F.; Morishita, K. Short-term effects of L-Citrulline supplementation on arterial stiffness in middle-aged men. *Int. J. Cardiol.* **2012**, *155*, 257–261. [CrossRef] [PubMed]
27. Bouillanne, O.; Melchior, J.-C.; Faure, C.; Paul, M.; Canoui-Poitrine, F.; Boirie, Y.; Chevenne, D.; Forasassi, C.; Guery, E.; Herbaud, S.; et al. Impact of 3-week citrulline supplementation on postprandial protein metabolism in malnourished older patients: The Ciproage randomized controlled trial. *Clin. Nutr.* **2019**, *38*, 564–574. [CrossRef] [PubMed]
28. Rey-López, J.P.; Vicente-Rodríguez, G.; Biosca, M.; Moreno, L.A. Sedentary behaviour and obesity development in children and adolescents. *Nutr. Metab. Cardiovasc. Dis.* **2008**, *18*, 242–251. [CrossRef] [PubMed]
29. Hills, A.P.; Okely, A.; Baur, L. Addressing childhood obesity through increased physical activity. *Nat. Rev. Endocrinol.* **2010**, *6*, 543–549. [CrossRef] [PubMed]
30. Fox, K.R. Childhood obesity and the role of physical activity. *J. R. Soc. Promot. Health* **2004**, *124*, 34–39. [CrossRef] [PubMed]
31. Sung, K.-D.; Pekas, E.J.; Scott, S.D.; Son, W.-M.; Park, S.-Y. The effects of a 12-week jump rope exercise program on abdominal adiposity, vasoactive substances, inflammation, and vascular function in adolescent girls with prehypertension. *Eur. J. Appl. Physiol.* **2019**, *119*, 577–585. [CrossRef]
32. Chuensiri, N.; Suksom, D.; Tanaka, H. Effects of high-intensity intermittent training on vascular function in obese preadolescent boys. *Child. Obes.* **2018**, *14*, 41–49. [CrossRef]
33. Da Silva, M.R.; Waclawovsky, G.; Perin, L.; Camboim, I.; Eibel, B.; Lehnen, A.M. Effects of high-intensity interval training on endothelial function, lipid profile, body composition and physical fitness in normal-weight and overweight-obese adolescents: A clinical trial. *Physiol. Behav.* **2020**, *213*, 112728. [CrossRef] [PubMed]
34. Lee, S.; Libman, I.; Hughan, K.S.; Kuk, J.L.; Barinas-Mitchell, E.; Chung, H.; Arslanian, S. Effects of exercise modality on body composition and cardiovascular disease risk factors in adolescents with obesity: A randomized clinical trial. *Appl. Physiol. Nutr. Metab.* **2020**, *45*, 1377–1386. [CrossRef] [PubMed]
35. Davis, C.L.; Litwin, S.E.; Pollock, N.K.; Waller, J.L.; Zhu, H.; Dong, Y.; Kapuku, G.; Bhagatwala, J.; Harris, R.A.; Looney, J.; et al. Exercise effects on arterial stiffness and heart health in children with excess weight: The SMART RCT. *Int. J. Obes.* **2019**, *44*, 1152–1163. [CrossRef] [PubMed]
36. Tousoulis, D.; Kampoli, A.-M.; Papageorgiou, N.; Stefanadis, C. The role of nitric oxide on Endothelial function. *Curr. Vasc. Pharmacol.* **2012**, *10*, 4–18. [CrossRef] [PubMed]
37. Tran, V.; De Silva, T.M.; Sobey, C.G.; Lim, K.; Drummond, G.R.; Vinh, A.; Jelinic, M. The vascular consequences of metabolic syndrome: Rodent models, endothelial dysfunction, and current therapies. *Front. Pharmacol.* **2020**, *11*, 148. [CrossRef]

38. Jamwal, S.; Sharma, S. Vascular endothelium dysfunction: A conservative target in metabolic disorders. *Inflamm. Res.* **2018**, *67*, 391–405. [CrossRef]

39. Schmidt, T.S.; Alp, N.J. Mechanisms for the role of tetrahydrobiopterin in endothelial function and vascular disease. *Clin. Sci.* **2007**, *113*, 47–63. [CrossRef]

40. Xia, N.; Horke, S.; Habermeier, A.; Closs, E.; Reifenberg, G.; Gericke, A.; Mikhed, Y.; Münzel, T.; Daiber, A.; Förstermann, U.; et al. Uncoupling of Endothelial Nitric Oxide Synthase in Perivascular Adipose tissue of diet-induced obese mice. *Arter. Thromb. Vasc. Biol.* **2016**, *36*, 78–85. [CrossRef]

41. Zhou, L.; Sun, C.-B.; Liu, C.; Fan, Y.; Zhu, H.-Y.; Wu, X.-W.; Hu, L.; Li, Q.-P. Upregulation of arginase activity contributes to intracellular ROS production induced by high glucose in H9c2 cells. *Int. J. Clin. Exp. Pathol.* **2015**, *8*, 2728–2736.

42. Michell, D.M.; Andrews, K.L.; Chin-Dusting, J.P.F. Endothelial dysfunction in hypertension: The role of arginase. *Front. Biosci.* **2011**, *3*, 946–960. [CrossRef] [PubMed]

43. Bhatta, A.; Yao, L.; Xu, Z.; Toque, H.A.; Chen, J.; Atawia, R.T.; Fouda, A.; Bagi, Z.; Lucas, R.; Caldwell, R.; et al. Obesity-induced vascular dysfunction and arterial stiffening requires endothelial cell arginase 1. *Cardiovasc. Res.* **2017**, *113*, 1664–1676. [CrossRef]

44. Meza, C.A.; La Favor, J.D.; Kim, D.-H.; Hickner, R.C. Endothelial dysfunction: Is there a Hyperglycemia-induced imbalance of NOX and NOS? *Int. J. Mol. Sci.* **2019**, *20*, 3775. [CrossRef] [PubMed]

45. Fantin, F.; Giani, A.; Zoico, E.; Rossi, A.P.; Mazzali, G.; Zamboni, M. Weight loss and hypertension in obese subjects. *Nutrients* **2019**, *11*, 1667. [CrossRef]

46. Rathinam, V.A.; Fitzgerald, K.A. Inflammasome complexes: Emerging mechanisms and effector functions. *Cell* **2016**, *165*, 792–800. [CrossRef]

47. Paz-Filho, G.; Wong, M.-L.; Licinio, J.; Mastronardi, C. Leptin therapy, insulin sensitivity, and glucose homeostasis. *Indian J. Endocrinol. Metab.* **2012**, *16*, 549–555. [CrossRef]

48. Seravalle, G.; Grassi, G. Obesity and hypertension. *Pharmacol. Res.* **2017**, *122*, 1–7. [CrossRef] [PubMed]

49. Ryan, M.J.; Coleman, T.T.; Sasser, J.M.; Pittman, K.M.; Hankins, M.W.; Stec, D.E. Vascular smooth muscle-specific deletion of the leptin receptor attenuates leptin-induced alterations in vascular relaxation. *Am. J. Physiol. Regul. Integr. Comp. Physiol.* **2016**, *310*, R960–R967. [CrossRef]

50. Hall, J.E.; do Carmo, J.M.; Silva, A.; Wang, Z.; Hall, M.E. Obesity, kidney dysfunction and hypertension: Mechanistic links. *Nat. Rev. Nephrol.* **2019**, *15*, 367–385. [CrossRef] [PubMed]

51. Thijssen, D.H.J.; Bruno, R.M.; Van Mil, A.C.C.M.; Holder, S.M.; Faita, F.; Greyling, A.; Zock, P.L.; Taddei, S.; Deanfield, J.; Luscher, T.; et al. Expert consensus and evidence-based recommendations for the assessment of flow-mediated dilation in humans. *Eur. Heart J.* **2019**, *40*, 2534–2547. [CrossRef] [PubMed]

52. Wilson, A.C.; Urbina, E.; Witt, S.A.; Glascock, B.J.; Kimball, T.R.; Mitsnefes, M. Flow-mediated vasodilatation of the brachial artery in children with chronic kidney disease. *Pediatr. Nephrol.* **2008**, *23*, 1297–1302. [CrossRef]

53. Shah, A.S.; Urbina, E.M. Vascular and Endothelial function in youth with Type 2 Diabetes Mellitus. *Curr. Diabetes Rep.* **2017**, *17*, 36. [CrossRef]

54. Cote, A.T.; Harris, K.; Panagiotopoulos, C.; Sandor, G.; Devlin, A. Childhood obesity and cardiovascular dysfunction. *J. Am. Coll. Cardiol.* **2013**, *62*, 1309–1319. [CrossRef]

55. Su, Y.; Liu, X.-M.; Sun, Y.-M.; Jin, H.-B.; Fu, R.; Wang, Y.-Y.; Wu, Y.; Luan, Y. The relationship between endothelial dysfunction and oxidative stress in diabetes and prediabetes. *Int. J. Clin. Pr.* **2008**, *62*, 877–882. [CrossRef]

56. Pacifico, L.; Perla, F.M.; Tromba, L.; Carbotta, G.; Lavorato, M.; Pierimarchi, P.; Chiesa, C. Carotid extra-media thickness in children: Relationships with Cardiometabolic risk factors and Endothelial function. *Front. Endocrinol.* **2020**, *11*. [CrossRef] [PubMed]

57. Miniello, V.L.; Faienza, M.F.; Scicchitano, P.; Cortese, F.; Gesualdo, M.; Zito, A.; Basile, M.; Recchia, P.; Leogrande, D.; Viola, D.; et al. Insulin resistance and endothelial function in children and adolescents. *Int. J. Cardiol.* **2014**, *174*, 343–347. [CrossRef]

58. Urbina, E.M.; Bean, J.A.; Daniels, S.R.; D'Alessio, D.; Dolan, L.M. Overweight and hyperinsulinemia provide individual contributions to compromises in brachial artery distensibility in healthy adolescents and young adults: Brachial distensibility in children. *J. Am. Soc. Hypertens.* **2007**, *1*, 200–207. [CrossRef]

59. Rodriguez, C.J.; Miyake, Y.; Grahame-Clarke, C.; Di Tullio, M.R.; Sciacca, R.R.; Boden-Albala, B.; Sacco, R.L.; Homma, S. Relation of plasma glucose and Endothelial function in a population-based multiethnic sample of subjects without Diabetes Mellitus. *Am. J. Cardiol.* **2005**, *96*, 1273–1277. [CrossRef] [PubMed]

60. Chandra, S.; Fulton, D.J.; Caldwell, R.B.; Toque, H.A. Hyperglycemia-impaired aortic vasorelaxation mediated through arginase elevation: Role of stress kinase pathways. *Eur. J. Pharmacol.* **2019**, *844*, 26–37. [CrossRef]

61. Curley, S.; Gall, J.; Byrne, R.; Yvan-Charvet, L.; McGillicuddy, F.C. Metabolic inflammation in obesity—At the crossroads between fatty acid and cholesterol metabolism. *Mol. Nutr. Food Res.* **2020**, *65*, e1900482. [CrossRef]

62. Andersen, C.J.; Murphy, E.K.; Fernandez, M.L. Impact of obesity and metabolic syndrome on immunity. *Adv. Nutr.* **2016**, *7*, 66–75. [CrossRef]

63. Llewellyn, A.; Simmonds, M.C.; Owen, C.; Woolacott, N. Childhood obesity as a predictor of morbidity in adulthood: A systematic review and meta-analysis. *Obes. Rev.* **2015**, *17*, 56–67. [CrossRef]

64. Ley, K.; Miller, Y.I.; Hedrick, C.C. Monocyte and macrophage dynamics during atherogenesis. *Arter. Thromb. Vasc. Biol.* **2011**, *31*, 1506–1516. [CrossRef]

65. Landsberg, L.; Aronne, L.J.; Beilin, L.J.; Burke, V.; Igel, L.I.; Lloyd-Jones, D.; Sowers, J. Obesity-related hypertension: Pathogenesis, cardiovascular risk, and treatment—A position paper of the The Obesity Society and the American Society of Hypertension. *Obesity* **2012**, *21*, 8–24. [CrossRef] [PubMed]

66. Juonala, M.; Magnussen, C.; Berenson, G.S.; Venn, A.; Burns, T.L.; Sabin, M.; Srinivasan, S.R.; Daniels, S.R.; Davis, P.H.; Chen, W.; et al. Childhood adiposity, adult adiposity, and cardiovascular risk factors. *N. Engl. J. Med.* **2011**, *365*, 1876–1885. [CrossRef]

67. Hall, J.E.; Carmo, J.M.D.; Silva, A.; Wang, Z.; Hall, M.E. Obesity-induced hypertension: Interaction of neurohumoral and renal mechanisms. *Circ. Res.* **2015**, *116*, 991–1006. [CrossRef]

68. Abrignani, M.G.; Lucà, F.; Favilli, S.; Benvenuto, M.; Rao, C.M.; Di Fusco, S.A.; Gabrielli, D.; Gulizia, M.M. Lifestyles and cardiovascular prevention in childhood and adolescence. *Pediatr. Cardiol.* **2019**, *40*, 1113–1125. [CrossRef]

69. Theodore, R.F.; Broadbent, J.; Nagin, D.S.; Ambler, A.; Hogan, S.; Ramrakha, S.; Cutfield, W.; Williams, M.; Harrington, H.; Moffitt, T.; et al. Childhood to early-midlife systolic blood pressure trajectories: Early life predictors, effect modifiers, and adult cardiovascular outcomes. *Hypertension* **2015**, *66*, 1108–1115. [CrossRef] [PubMed]

70. Hanspeter, B.; Cockroft, J.R.; Deanfield, J.; Donald, A.; Ferrannini, E.; Halcox, J.; Kiowski, W.; Lüscher, T.F.; Mancia, G.; Natali, A.; et al. Endothelial function and dysfunction. Part II: Association with cardiovascular risk factors and diseases. A statement by the Working Group on Endothelins and Endothelial Factors of the European Society of Hypertension*. *J. Hypertens.* **2005**, *23*, 233–246. [CrossRef]

71. Eley, V.; Christensen, R.; Guy, L.; Dodd, B. Perioperative blood pressure monitoring in patients with obesity. *Anesthesia Analg.* **2019**, *128*, 484–491. [CrossRef]

72. Skilton, M.R.; Celermajer, D.S.; Cosmi, E.; Crispi, F.; Gidding, S.S.; Raitakari, O.T.; Urbina, E.M. Natural history of atherosclerosis and abdominal aortic intima-media thickness: Rationale, evidence, and best practice for detection of atherosclerosis in the young. *J. Clin. Med.* **2019**, *8*, 1201. [CrossRef]

73. Cochain, C.; Zernecke, A. Macrophages in vascular inflammation and atherosclerosis. *Pflügers Arch. Eur. J. Physiol.* **2017**, *469*, 485–499. [CrossRef] [PubMed]

74. Rocha, V.Z.; Libby, P. Obesity, inflammation, and atherosclerosis. *Nat. Rev. Cardiol.* **2009**, *6*, 399–409. [CrossRef] [PubMed]

75. Ryder, J.R.; Northrop, E.; Rudser, K.D.; Kelly, A.S.; Gao, Z.; Khoury, P.R.; Kimball, T.R.; Dolan, L.M.; Urbina, E.M. Accelerated early vascular aging among adolescents with obesity and/or Type 2 Diabetes Mellitus. *J. Am. Heart Assoc.* **2020**, *9*, e014891. [CrossRef] [PubMed]

76. Onut, R.; Balanescu, A.P.S.; Constantinescu, D.; Calmac, L.; Marinescu, M.; Dorobantu, M. Imaging Atherosclerosis by Carotid Intima-media Thickness in vivo: How to, Where and in Whom? *MAEDICA J. Clin. Med.* **2012**, *7*, 153–162.

77. Skrzypczyk, P.; Pańczyk-Tomaszewska, M. Methods to evaluate arterial structure and function in children–State-of-the art knowledge. *Adv. Med. Sci.* **2017**, *62*, 280–294. [CrossRef] [PubMed]

78. Morris, E.P.; Denton, E.R.E.; Robinson, J.; Macdonald, L.M.; Rymer, J.M. High resolution ultrasound assessment of the carotid artery: Its relevance in postmenopausal women and the effects of tibolone on carotid artery ultrastructure. *Climacteric* **1999**, *2*, 13–20. [CrossRef]

79. Acevedo, M.; Krämer, V.; Tagle, R.; Arnaiz, P.; Corbalán, R.; Berríos, X.; Navarrete, C. Cardiovascular risk factors among young subjects with high carotid intima media thickness. *Rev. Medica Chile* **2012**, *139*, 1322. [CrossRef]

80. Shah, B.N.; Chahal, N.S.; Kooner, J.S.; Senior, R. Contrast-enhanced ultrasonography vs B-mode ultrasound for visualization of intima-media thickness and detection of plaques in human carotid arteries. *Echocardiography* **2017**, *34*, 723–730. [CrossRef]

81. Suárez-Cuenca, J.A.; Ruíz-Hernández, A.S.; Mendoza-Castañeda, A.A.; Domínguez-Pérez, G.A.; Hernández-Patricio, A.; Vera-Gómez, E.; De La Peña-Sosa, G.; Banderas-Lares, D.Z.; Montoya-Ramírez, J.; Blas-Azotla, R.; et al. Neutrophil-to-lymphocyte ratio and its relation with pro-inflammatory mediators, visceral adiposity and carotid intima-media thickness in population with obesity. *Eur. J. Clin. Investig.* **2019**, *49*, e13085. [CrossRef]

82. Raitakari, O.T.; Juonala, M.; Kähönen, M.; Taittonen, L.; Laitinen, T.; Mäki-Torkko, N.; Järvisalo, M.J.; Uhari, M.; Jokinen, E.; Rönnemaa, T.; et al. Cardiovascular risk factors in childhood and carotid artery intima-media thickness in adulthood. The cardiovascular risk in Young Finns study. *JAMA* **2003**, *290*, 2277–2283. [CrossRef]

83. Stehouwer, C.D.A.; Henry, R.M.A.; Ferreira, I. Arterial stiffness in diabetes and the metabolic syndrome: A pathway to cardiovascular disease. *Diabetologia* **2008**, *51*, 527–539. [CrossRef] [PubMed]

84. Segers, P.; Rietzschel, E.R.; Chirinos, J.A. How to measure arterial stiffness in humans. *Arter. Thromb. Vasc. Biol.* **2020**, *40*, 1034–1043. [CrossRef]

85. Laurent, S.; Cockcroft, J.; Van Bortel, L.; Boutouyrie, P.; Giannattasio, C.; Hayoz, D.; Pannier, B.; Vlachopoulos, C.; Wilkinson, I.; Struijker-Boudier, H.; et al. Expert consensus document on arterial stiffness: Methodological issues and clinical applications. *Eur. Heart J.* **2006**, *27*, 2588–2605. [CrossRef]

86. Mancia, G.; Fagard, R.; Narkiewicz, K.; Redon, J.; Zanchetti, A.; Böhm, M.; Christiaens, T.; Cifkova, R.; De Backer, G.; Dominiczak, A.; et al. 2013 ESH/ESC Guidelines for the management of arterial hypertension. The Task Force for the management of arterial hypertension of the European Society of Hypertension (ESH) and of the European Society of Cardiology (ESC). *Eur. Heart J.* **2013**, *34*, 2159–2219. [CrossRef]

87. Mitchell, G.F. Arterial stiffness and hypertension: Chicken or egg? *Hypertension* **2014**, *64*, 210–214. [CrossRef]

88. Munakata, M. Brachial-ankle pulse wave velocity in the measurement of arterial stiffness: Recent evidence and clinical applications. *Curr. Hypertens. Rev.* **2014**, *10*, 49–57. [CrossRef] [PubMed]

89. Park, J.S.; Nam, J.S.; Cho, M.H.; Yoo, J.S.; Ahn, C.W.; Jee, S.H.; Lee, H.S.; Cha, B.-S.; Kim, K.R.; Lee, H.C. Insulin resistance independently influences arterial stiffness in normoglycemic normotensive postmenopausal women. *Menopause* **2010**, *17*, 779–784. [CrossRef]

90. Dangardt, F.; Osika, W.; Volkmann, R.; Gan, L.-M.; Friberg, P. Obese children show increased intimal wall thickness and decreased pulse wave velocity. *Clin. Physiol. Funct. Imaging* **2008**, *28*, 287–293. [CrossRef]

91. Dangardt, F.; Chen, Y.; Berggren, K.; Osika, W.; Friberg, P. Increased rate of arterial stiffening with obesity in adolescents: A five-year follow-up study. *PLoS ONE* **2013**, *8*, e57454. [CrossRef]

92. Lentferink, Y.E.; Kromwijk, L.A.J.; Van Der Aa, M.P.; Knibbe, C.A.J.; Van Der Vorst, M.M.J. Increased arterial stiffness in adolescents with obesity. *Glob. Pediatr. Health* **2019**, *6*, 6. [CrossRef]

93. Vlachopoulos, C.; Aznaouridis, K.; O'Rourke, M.F.; Safar, M.E.; Baou, K.; Stefanadis, C. Prediction of cardiovascular events and all-cause mortality with central haemodynamics: A systematic review and meta-analysis. *Eur. Heart J.* **2010**, *31*, 1865–1871. [CrossRef]

94. Nichols, W.W.; DeNardo, S.J.; Wilkinson, I.B.; McEniery, C.M.; Cockcroft, J.; O'Rourke, M.F. Effects of arterial stiffness, pulse wave velocity, and wave reflections on the central aortic pressure waveform. *J. Clin. Hypertens.* **2008**, *10*, 295–303. [CrossRef]

95. McEniery, C.M.; Yasmin; Hall, I.; Qasem, A.; Wilkinson, I.B.; Cockcroft, J.R. Normal vascular aging: Differential effects on wave reflection and aortic pulse wave velocity: The Anglo-Cardiff Collaborative Trial (ACCT). *J. Am. Coll. Cardiol.* **2005**, *46*, 1753–1760. [CrossRef]

96. García-Espinosa, V.; Curcio, S.; Marotta, M.; Castro, J.M.; Arana, M.; Peluso, G.; Chiesa, P.; Giachetto, G.; Bia, D.; Zócalo, Y. Changes in central aortic pressure levels, wave components and determinants associated with high peripheral blood pressure states in childhood: Analysis of hypertensive phenotype. *Pediatr. Cardiol.* **2016**, *37*, 1340–1350. [CrossRef]

97. Castro, J.M.; García-Espinosa, V.; Curcio, S.; Arana, M.; Chiesa, P.; Giachetto, G.; Zócalo, Y.; Bia, D. Childhood obesity associates haemodynamic and vascular changes that result in increased central aortic pressure with augmented incident and reflected wave components, without changes in peripheral amplification. *Int. J. Vasc. Med.* **2016**, *2016*, 3129304. [CrossRef]

98. Urbina, E.M.; Kieltkya, L.; Tsai, J.; Srinivasan, S.R.; Berenson, G.S. Impact of multiple cardiovascular risk factors on brachial artery distensibility in young adults: The Bogalusa heart study. *Am. J. Hypertens.* **2005**, *18*, 767–771. [CrossRef]

99. Bailey, S.J.; Blackwell, J.R.; Williams, E.; Vanhatalo, A.; Wylie, L.; Winyard, P.G.; Jones, A.M. Two weeks of watermelon juice supplementation improves nitric oxide bioavailability but not endurance exercise performance in humans. *Nitric Oxide* **2016**, *59*, 10–20. [CrossRef]

100. Schwedhelm, E.; Maas, R.; Freese, R.; Jung, D.; Lukacs, Z.; Jambrecina, A.; Spickler, W.; Schulze, F.; Böger, R.H. Pharmacokinetic and pharmacodynamic properties of oral L-Citrulline and L-Arginine: Impact on nitric oxide metabolism. *Br. J. Clin. Pharmacol.* **2008**, *65*, 51–59. [CrossRef]

101. Moinard, C.; Nicolis, I.; Neveux, N.; Darquy, S.; Bénazeth, S.; Cynober, L. Dose-ranging effects of citrulline administration on plasma amino acids and hormonal patterns in healthy subjects: The Citrudose pharmacokinetic study. *Br. J. Nutr.* **2007**, *99*, 855–862. [CrossRef]

102. Al Jasmi, F.; Al Zaabi, N.; Al-Thihli, K.; Al Teneiji, A.M.; Hertecant, J.; El-Hattab, A.W. Endothelial dysfunction and the effect of arginine and citrulline supplementation in children and adolescents with mitochondrial diseases. *J. Central Nerv. Syst. Dis.* **2020**, *12*, 1179573520909377. [CrossRef]

103. El-Hattab, A.W.; Emrick, L.T.; Hsu, J.W.; Chanprasert, S.; Almannai, M.; Craigen, W.J.; Jahoor, F.; Scaglia, F. Impaired nitric oxide production in children with MELAS syndrome and the effect of arginine and citrulline supplementation. *Mol. Genet. Metab.* **2016**, *117*, 407–412. [CrossRef]

104. Moinard, C.; Maccario, J.; Walrand, S.; Lasserre, V.; Marc, J.; Boirie, Y.; Cynober, L. Arginine behaviour after arginine or citrulline administration in older subjects. *Br. J. Nutr.* **2015**, *115*, 399–404. [CrossRef]

105. Wijnands, K.A.; Meesters, D.M.; Van Barneveld, K.W.Y.; Visschers, R.G.J.; Briedé, J.J.; Vandendriessche, B.; Van Eijk, H.M.H.; Bessems, B.A.F.M.; Hoven, N.V.D.; Von Wintersdorff, C.J.H.; et al. Citrulline supplementation improves organ perfusion and arginine availability under conditions with enhanced arginase activity. *Nutrients* **2015**, *7*, 5217–5238. [CrossRef]

106. Lundberg, J.O.; Weitzberg, E.; Gladwin, M.T. The nitrate–nitrite–nitric oxide pathway in physiology and therapeutics. *Nat. Rev. Drug Discov.* **2008**, *7*, 156–167. [CrossRef]

107. Shatanawi, A.; Momani, M.S.; Al-Aqtash, R.; Hamdan, M.H.; Gharaibeh, M.N. L-Citrulline supplementation increases plasma nitric oxide levels and reduces arginase activity in patients with Type 2 Diabetes. *Front. Pharmacol.* **2020**, *11*, 584669. [CrossRef]

108. Allerton, T.D.; Proctor, D.N.; Stephens, J.M.; Dugas, T.R.; Spielmann, G.; Irving, B.A. L-Citrulline supplementation: Impact on cardiometabolic health. *Nutrients* **2018**, *10*, 921. [CrossRef]

109. Figueroa, A.; Alvarez-Alvarado, S.; Jaime, S.J.; Kalfon, R. L-Citrulline supplementation attenuates blood pressure, wave reflection and arterial stiffness responses to metaboreflex and cold stress in overweight men. *Br. J. Nutr.* **2016**, *116*, 279–285. [CrossRef]

110. Holguin, F.; Grasemann, H.; Sharma, S.; Winnica, D.; Wasil, K.; Smith, V.; Cruse, M.H.; Perez, N.; Coleman, E.; Scialla, T.J.; et al. L-Citrulline increases nitric oxide and improves control in obese asthmatics. *JCI Insight* **2019**, *4*, e131733. [CrossRef]

111. Gonzales, J.U.; Raymond, A.; Ashley, J.; Kim, Y. Does L-Citrulline supplementation improve exercise blood flow in older adults? *Exp. Physiol.* **2017**, *102*, 1661–1671. [CrossRef]

112. Figueroa, A.; Trivino, J.A.; Sanchez-Gonzalez, M.A.; Vicil, F. Oral L-Citrulline supplementation attenuates blood pressure response to cold pressor test in young men. *Am. J. Hypertens.* **2010**, *23*, 12–16. [CrossRef]

113. Yang, H.-H.; Li, X.-L.; Zhang, W.-G.; Figueroa, A.; Chen, L.-H.; Qin, L.-Q. Effect of oral L-Citrulline on brachial and aortic blood pressure defined by resting status: Evidence from randomized controlled trials. *Nutr. Metab.* **2019**, *16*, 89. [CrossRef]
114. Palombo, C.; Kozakova, M. Arterial stiffness, atherosclerosis and cardiovascular risk: Pathophysiologic mechanisms and emerging clinical indications. *Vasc. Pharmacol.* **2016**, *77*, 1–7. [CrossRef] [PubMed]
115. Eshreif, A.; Al Batran, R.; Jamieson, K.L.; Darwesh, A.M.; Gopal, K.; Greenwell, A.; Zlobine, I.; Aburasayn, H.; Eaton, F.; Mulvihill, E.E.; et al. L-Citrulline supplementation improves glucose and exercise tolerance in obese male mice. *Exp. Physiol.* **2020**, *105*, 270–281. [CrossRef] [PubMed]
116. Kudo, M.; Yoshitomi, H.; Momoo, M.; Suguro, S.; Yamagishi, Y.; Gao, M. Evaluation of the effects and mechanism of L-Citrulline on anti-obesity by appetite suppression in obese/diabetic KK-Ay mice and high-fat diet fed SD rats. *Biol. Pharm. Bull.* **2017**, *40*, 524–530. [CrossRef]
117. Moinard, C.; Le Plenier, S.; Noirez, P.; Morio, B.; Bonnefont-Rousselot, D.; Kharchi, C.; Ferry, A.; Neveux, N.; Cynober, L.; Raynaud-Simon, A. Citrulline supplementation induces changes in body composition and limits age-related metabolic changes in healthy male rats. *J. Nutr.* **2015**, *145*, 1429–1437. [CrossRef]
118. Jegatheesan, P.; Beutheu, S.; Ventura, G.; Sarfati, G.; Nubret, E.; Kapel, N.; Waligora-Dupriet, A.-J.; Bergheim, I.; Cynober, L.; De-Bandt, J.-P. Effect of specific amino acids on hepatic lipid metabolism in fructose-induced non-alcoholic fatty liver disease. *Clin. Nutr.* **2015**, *35*, 175–182. [CrossRef]
119. Dai, Z.; Wu, Z.; Yang, Y.; Wang, J.; Satterfield, M.C.; Meininger, C.; Bazer, F.W.; Wu, G. Nitric oxide and energy metabolism in mammals. *BioFactors* **2013**, *39*, 383–391. [CrossRef]
120. Sarti, P.; Arese, M.; Forte, E.; Giuffrè, A.; Mastronicola, D. Mitochondria and Nitric Oxide: Chemistry and pathophysiology. *Adv. Exp. Med. Biol.* **2011**, *942*, 75–92. [CrossRef]
121. Brown, G.C.; Borutaite, V. Nitric oxide and mitochondrial respiration in the heart. *Cardiovasc. Res.* **2007**, *75*, 283–290. [CrossRef]
122. Azizi, S.; Mahdavi, R.; Mobasseri, M.; Aliasgharzadeh, S.; Abbaszadeh, F.; Ebrahimi-Mameghani, M. The impact of L-citrulline supplementation on glucose homeostasis, lipid profile, and some inflammatory factors in overweight and obese patients with type 2 diabetes: A double-blind randomized placebo-controlled trial. *Phytotherapy Res.* **2021**, *35*, 3157–3166. [CrossRef]
123. Terada, T.; Boulé, N.G.; Forhan, M.; Prado, C.M.; Kenny, G.P.; Prud'Homme, D.; Ito, E.; Sigal, R.J. Cardiometabolic risk factors in type 2 diabetes with high fat and low muscle mass: At baseline and in response to exercise. *Obesity* **2017**, *25*, 881–891. [CrossRef] [PubMed]
124. Kim, J.Y.; Oh, S.; Park, H.Y.; Jun, J.H.; Kim, H.J. Comparisons of different indices of low muscle mass in relationship with cardiometabolic disorder. *Sci. Rep.* **2019**, *9*, 609. [CrossRef]
125. Bull, F.C.; Al-Ansari, S.S.; Biddle, S.; Borodulin, K.; Buman, M.P.; Cardon, G.; Carty, C.; Chaput, J.-P.; Chastin, S.; Chou, R.; et al. World Health Organization 2020 guidelines on physical activity and sedentary behaviour. *Br. J. Sports Med.* **2020**, *54*, 1451–1462. [CrossRef] [PubMed]
126. Katzmarzyk, P.; Barreira, T.; Broyles, S.T.; Champagne, C.M.; Chaput, J.-P.; Fogelholm, M.; Hu, G.; Johnson, W.; Kuriyan, R.; Kurpad, A.; et al. Physical activity, sedentary time, and obesity in an international sample of children. *Med. Sci. Sports Exerc.* **2015**, *47*, 2062–2069. [CrossRef]
127. Tremblay, M.S.; Leblanc, A.G.; Kho, E.M.; Saunders, T.J.; Larouche, R.; Colley, R.C.; Goldfield, G.; Gorber, S.C. Systematic review of sedentary behaviour and health indicators in school-aged children and youth. *Int. J. Behav. Nutr. Phys. Act.* **2011**, *8*, 98. [CrossRef] [PubMed]
128. Farah, B.Q.; Christofaro, D.G.D.; Balagopal, P.B.; Cavalcante, B.R.; De Barros, M.V.G.; Ritti-Dias, R.M. Association between resting heart rate and cardiovascular risk factors in adolescents. *Eur. J. Nucl. Med. Mol. Imaging* **2015**, *174*, 1621–1628. [CrossRef]
129. Redwine, K.M.; Acosta, A.A.; Poffenbarger, T.; Portman, R.J.; Samuels, J. Development of hypertension in adolescents with pre-hypertension. *J. Pediatr.* **2012**, *160*, 98–103. [CrossRef]
130. Litwin, M.; Niemirska, A.; Śladowska, J.; Antoniewicz, J.; Daszkowska, J.; Wierzbicka-Rucinska, A.; Wawer, Z.; Grenda, R. Left ventricular hypertrophy and arterial wall thickening in children with essential hypertension. *Pediatr. Nephrol.* **2006**, *21*, 811–819. [CrossRef]
131. Schuler, G.; Adams, V.; Goto, Y. Role of exercise in the prevention of cardiovascular disease: Results, mechanisms, and new perspectives. *Eur. Heart J.* **2013**, *34*, 1790–1799. [CrossRef]
132. García-Hermoso, A.; González-Ruíz, K.; Triana-Reina, H.R.; Olloquequi, J.; Ramírez-Vélez, R. Effects of Exercise on Carotid Arterial Wall Thickness in Obese Pediatric Populations: A meta-analysis of randomized controlled trials. *Child. Obes.* **2017**, *13*, 138–145. [CrossRef] [PubMed]
133. Escalante, Y.; Saavedra, J.M.; García-Hermoso, A.; Domínguez, A.M. Improvement of the lipid profile with exercise in obese children: A systematic review. *Prev. Med.* **2012**, *54*, 293–301. [CrossRef] [PubMed]
134. Walker, J.L.; Murray, T.D.; Eldridge, J.; Squires, J.W.G.; Silvius, P.; Silvius, E.; Squires, W.G. The association between waist circumference and FITNESSGRAM®aerobic capacity classification in sixth-grade children. *Pediatr. Exerc. Sci.* **2015**, *27*, 488–493. [CrossRef]
135. Coutinho, T.; Borlaug, B.A.; Pellikka, P.A.; Turner, S.T.; Kullo, I.J. Sex differences in arterial stiffness and ventricular-arterial interactions. *J. Am. Coll. Cardiol.* **2015**, *61*, 96–103. [CrossRef] [PubMed]

136. Buckinx, F.; Carvalho, L.P.; Marcangeli, V.; Dulac, M.; Hajj Boutros, G.; Gouspillou, G.; Gaudreau, P.; Noirez, P.; Aubertin-Leheudre, M. High intensity interval training combined with L-Citrulline supplementation: Effects on physical performance in healthy older adults. *Exp. Gerontol.* **2020**, *140*, 111036. [CrossRef]
137. Lucotti, P.; Setola, E.; Monti, L.D.; Galluccio, E.; Costa, S.; Sandoli, E.P.; Fermo, I.; Rabaiotti, G.; Gatti, R.; Piatti, P. Beneficial effects of a long-term oral L-Arginine treatment added to a hypocaloric diet and exercise training program in obese, insulin-resistant type 2 diabetic patients. *Am. J. Physiol. Endocrinol. Metab.* **2006**, *291*, E906–E912. [CrossRef]
138. Buckinx, F.; Gouspillou, G.; Carvalho, L.P.; Marcangeli, V.; Boutros, G.E.H.; Dulac, M.; Noirez, P.; Morais, J.A.; Gaudreau, P.; Aubertin-Leheudre, M. Effect of high-intensity interval training combined with L-Citrulline supplementation on functional capacities and muscle function in Dynapenic-obese older adults. *J. Clin. Med.* **2018**, *7*, 561. [CrossRef] [PubMed]

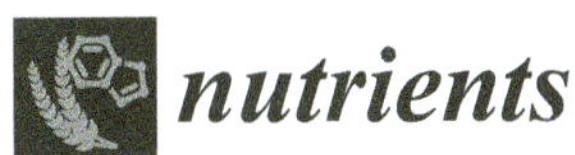 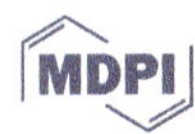

Article

The Prevalence of Overweight Status among Early Adolescents from Private Schools in Indonesia: Sex-Specific Patterns Determined by School Urbanization Level

Eveline Sarintohe [1,2,*], Junilla K. Larsen [1], William J. Burk [1] and Jacqueline M. Vink [1]

[1] Behavioural Science Institute, Radboud University, 6500 HE Nijmegen, The Netherlands; junilla.larsen@ru.nl (J.K.L.); william.burk@ru.nl (W.J.B.); Jacqueline.vink@ru.nl (J.M.V.)
[2] Psychology Faculty, Maranatha Christian University, Bandung 40164, West Java, Indonesia
* Correspondence: eveline.sarintohe@ru.nl; Tel.: +31-88-4696514 or +31-88-4699096

Abstract: (1) Background: Few studies have investigated (demographic) correlates of (prevalent) overweight rates among early adolescents, especially from higher socioeconomic positions (SEP) in developing countries, such as Indonesia. The current study aims to fill this gap. (2) Methods: Participants included 411 adolescents from five private schools in Indonesia. Adolescents' weight and height were measured, and adolescents completed questionnaires on demographic factors (i.e., sex, school area, ethnicity, pocket money) and previous year dieting. (3) Results: Results showed that more than one-third of the sample was overweight, with higher rates among adolescent males (47%) than females (24%). Moreover, adolescents attending schools in urban areas (compared with suburban areas), and those reporting past dieting (compared with those reporting no dieting) had higher overweight rates. Ethnicity and the amount of pocket money were not related to overweight status. Finally, a clear sex-specific interaction was found involving school area, showing that males in urban areas had a significantly higher risk to be overweight, whereas this did not apply to females. (4) Conclusions: males from urban area private schools in Indonesia may be an important target group for future preventive overweight interventions.

Keywords: obesity; overweight; developing countries; Indonesia; adolescents; sex differences; demographic; high SEP

Citation: Sarintohe, E.; Larsen, J.K.; Burk, W.J.; Vink, J.M. The Prevalence of Overweight Status among Early Adolescents from Private Schools in Indonesia: Sex-Specific Patterns Determined by School Urbanization Level. *Nutrients* **2022**, *14*, 1001. https://doi.org/10.3390/nu14051001

Academic Editor: Roberto Iacone

Received: 11 February 2022
Accepted: 25 February 2022
Published: 27 February 2022

Publisher's Note: MDPI stays neutral with regard to jurisdictional claims in published maps and institutional affiliations.

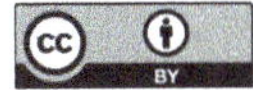

Copyright: © 2022 by the authors. Licensee MDPI, Basel, Switzerland. This article is an open access article distributed under the terms and conditions of the Creative Commons Attribution (CC BY) license (https://creativecommons.org/licenses/by/4.0/).

1. Introduction

The prevalence of obese and overweight individuals has continued to increase over the past years, particularly in developing countries, such as Indonesia [1–3]. In contrast to Western countries, obesity is positively related to socioeconomic position (SEP) in many developing countries [4–6], meaning that being overweight is more prevalent among adults and adolescents with higher SEP. So far, studies have suggested that in developing nations, people with a higher SEP, compared with lower SEP, have easier access to junk food or calorie-dense foods, which may explain the higher overweight rates, particularly in these groups [5,6].

Adolescence is a particularly vulnerable period for the development of overweight, not only in Western countries but also among developing countries such as Indonesia [7,8]. Moreover, overweight prevalence seems to show sex-specific differences in Indonesia. Among adolescents, the prevalence of overweight was higher in females than in males [4,9]. The same has been found for adult populations in Indonesia (i.e., higher prevalence rates among women compared with men) [2,4,10]. However, among children, the prevalence of overweight was higher in boys compared with girls [4]. These (review) results suggest some shifting sex-specific patterns during early adolescence regarding the prevalence of overweight status. The current study has a specific focus on early adolescence, a critical stage where (gender-specific) lifestyle choices change, for example, because of the availability of energy-dense (junk) food and increasing peer influences in (changing) school environments [9,11,12], with the highest possible impact among adolescents at private schools [4].

In general, school is an environment in which adolescents spend much of their time with peers, and where junk food is available. As such, school area (i.e., urban versus non-urban areas or less urban) might play an important role in obesogenic behaviors, including junk food consumption [9,13]. In line with this, some studies in Indonesia have shown that overweight patterns differ according to school area [11,14]. Adolescents living in urban (school) areas have higher prevalence rates of overweight status compared with those living in less urban or rural areas [11,14]. This might be explained by their greater access to more types of junk food or fast food compared with people living in less urban or rural areas [9,13–15]. Moreover, previous research has also found that overweight patterns differ according to ethnicity. To date, overweight status is more prevalent among people with Orang Asli Malaysian compared with Chinese Malaysians backgrounds [13]. Further research is needed to examine whether and how overweight status among early adolescents at private schools, with generally higher overweight risk, might differ according to school area and ethnic background in Indonesia.

Furthermore, given that the amount of pocket money may be an indication of the possibility to buy fast food, pocket money may also be related to overweight status among early adolescents from private schools and mostly higher SEP backgrounds. Finally, studies in industrialized countries (in Europe and America) have shown that dieting behavior is associated with greater weight gain over time among adolescents [16]. Due to the increasing impact of Western society on developing countries such as Indonesia, it is important to identify whether dieting behavior is similarly linked to overweight status among early adolescents at relatively high risk for being overweight from private schools in Indonesia.

Moreover, some previous studies among Indonesian populations have also shown sex-specific links regarding demographic factors explaining overweight status. Specifically, two previous Indonesian studies in adult samples showed that females from urban areas were at higher risk to be overweight compared with males [2,5]. In contrast, one recent large-scale study among children and adolescents (10–18 years old) has shown that, specifically, males living in urban areas were more likely to be overweight and obese than females living in urban areas [12]. Given these contrasting findings, it is important to further examine sex-specific links between school area and (over)weight status among early adolescents, particularly among those from private schools with higher overweight prevalence [4]. Another study suggested that overweight status may be more strongly linked to ethnicity among males compared with females [17]. Finally, some studies among Western countries also show sex-specific links between dieting and (over)weight status [14,16]. As such, we will also explore sex-specific demographic or dieting correlates of overweight status among early adolescents from private schools (higher SEP background).

To conclude, recent research on demographic correlates of overweight prevalence rates among early adolescents from private schools in Indonesia is limited. However, society, particularly around private schools (higher SEP backgrounds), might have changed rapidly with regard to eating behavior in Indonesia (more fast-food restaurants, larger influence from Western society [2,9]) making it urgent to explore correlates of overweight in early adolescents at private schools in Indonesia nowadays. As such, the aim of the current study is to examine (sex-specific) correlates of overweight status in a relatively large sample of early adolescents from private schools.

2. Materials and Methods

2.1. Participants and Procedure

The participants in this study were part of the baseline measurement (Wave 1) from an ongoing longitudinal study on adolescents' weight-related behavior in Indonesia. Wave 1 took place in October until December 2019. Adolescents were recruited through five private junior high schools in four cities (Jakarta, Surabaya, Bandung, and Manado) in Indonesia. A total of 411 students (47.7% females) participated. All adolescents (M_{age} = 12.02 years; SD_{age} = 0.45; range = 11.02 to 14.11 years) were in 7th grade or in their first year of junior high school.

A letter describing the longitudinal project was initially sent to officials of school foundations (some private schools are organized by private foundations) or directly to school officials. If the school foundations provided approval, the agreement letter was then sent to the principal of the schools. School officials informed both the parents and students about the goals of the project. Parents were asked to return a signed consent form indicating they agreed to their child's participation. Students were also asked to return a signed consent form indicating whether they agreed to participate in the study. Of the five schools that agreed to participate, three schools obtained consent forms from parents and students. The remaining two schools informed the parents about this project (passive consent) based on the school policy and collected the signed consent forms from students only. The original and amended (passive consent) procedures were approved by the Ethics Committee Social Science of Radboud University, Nijmegen, The Netherlands (ECSS-2019-115).

Researcher informed students that their participation was voluntary, that answers would be processed confidentially and would be stored separately from personal data (with a key file to link the data), and that they could withdraw from the study at any time. Adolescents completed a paper self-report survey at school during one classroom hour (approximately 60 min). In addition, adolescents' weight and height measures were taken by the researcher with the assistance of the school nurse. Weight and height of participants were assessed using school equipment (stadiometer). Students were rewarded with a small gift when they completed the questionnaires.

2.2. Measurements

2.2.1. Anthropometric Measurements

Adolescents' height was measured to the nearest 0.1 cm with a validated stadiometer (Seca around 217), and their weight was measured to the nearest 0.1 kg with a weighing scale (Seca around 840). Based on the Center for Disease Control and Prevention (CDC) 2000 Body Mass Index for age growth charts for males and females, the cut-off for defining overweight was based on the sex and age in months and BMI (weight (kg)/height (m^2)).

2.2.2. Demographic Characteristics

Adolescent's sex was coded, with 0 = female and 1 = male. School area was coded as 0 = suburban (Bandung and Manado) and 1 = urban area (Jakarta and Surabaya). We divided the area based on modernization and levels of Westernization [8]. There were no exclusion criteria involved. All students from urban and suburban areas participated in this study. Moreover, ethnicity was coded as 1 = Javanese, 2 = Sundanese, 3 = Sulawesi, 4 = Tionghoa (Chinese Indonesian), 5 = other ethnic (Papua, Kalimantan, Sumatra, and Bali), and 6 = mixed ethnicity. The percentage of Chinese-Indonesian ethnic students was almost half of the sample (49.8%), so we decided to dichotomize ethnicity as 0 = Indonesian ethnic (Javanese, Sundanese, Sulawesi, etc.) and 1 = Chinese Indonesian. The amount of pocket money was coded as 1 = < IDR 500,000, 2 = IDR 500,000–IDR 1,000,000, 3 = IDR 1,100,000–IDR 1,500,000, 4 = IDR 1,600,000–IDR 2,000,000, 5 = IDR 2,100,000–IDR 2,500,000, and 6 = > IDR 2,500,000. The percentage of students with pocket money less than IDR 500,000 was more than half of the sample (63%), so we decided to dichotomize pocket money as 0 = < IDR 500,000 and 1 = ≥ IDR 500,000.

2.2.3. Dieting Behavior

To measure previous dieting behavior, participants were asked, "In the past year, how often did you diet in an attempt to have the same weight or lose weight?" The response categories for this item were: 1 = never, 2 = 1–2 times, 3 = 3–4 times, 4 = 5–6 times, and

5 = 7 times or more often. Initial inspection of the distribution of this item indicated a substantial group of adolescents who reported no past year dieting (50.68%), so this item was also dichotomized as 0 = no past year diet and 1 = did past year diet.

2.3. Statistical Analyses

Chi-square analyses were performed to examine univariate demographic and dieting differences between overweight and non-overweight groups. Moreover, a logistic regression analysis was performed to explain overweight status group membership (0 = not overweight; 1 = overweight) from several predictors. The independent variables included in this analysis were student's sex, school area (suburban vs. urban), ethnicity (Indonesian vs. Chinese Indonesian), pocket money (<500,000 vs. $\geq$500,000), and previous dieting behavior (never vs. did diet). Moreover, sex-specific interactions (i.e., sex by school area, sex by ethnicity, sex by pocket money, and sex by previous diet) were tested in four separate analyses (one interaction per analyses added to the main effects model). Statistically significant interactions were further probed using the PROCESS module in SPSS [18].

3. Results

3.1. Descriptive Statistics

Data from a total of 411 students were examined in this study. The sample was equally divided according to sex (53.3% boys). In total, 59.1% of the adolescents attended a school located in an urban area. The sample was also equally divided according to ethnic background (51.2% Indonesians and 48.8% Chinese Indonesians). Most of the respondents had less than IDR 500,000 per month (63%) and had not dieted (50.6%).

In the total sample, 36.3% of the adolescents were characterized as being overweight. Chi-square independence tests indicated that overweight status was more prevalent in males compared with females (see Table 1). Moreover, adolescents living in urban school areas had a higher overweight prevalence compared with those living in suburban areas. Finally, the adolescents reporting previous dieting were more likely to be overweight compared with those who did not report dieting. Overweight status did not differ according to ethnic background or amount of pocket money.

Table 1. Chi-square analyses examining adolescent's overweight status differences as a function of demographic and dieting characteristics.

	Not Overweight		Overweight		Chi Square	*p* Values
	n	%	*n*	%		
Sex						
Females	146	46	24.0	24.0	23.57	<0.001
Males	116	103	47.0	47.0		
Ethnicity						
Indonesian (Ethnicities)	135	65.5	71	34.5	0.63	0.428
Chinese Indonesian	126	61.8	78	38.2		
School Area						
Suburban	117	69.6	51	30.4	4.27	0.039
Urban	145	59.7	98	40.3		
Pocket Money						
<500,000	166	64.1	93	35.9	0.04	0.849
$\geq$500,000	96	63.2	56	36.8		
Diet						
Never diet	160	76.9	48	23.1	31.64	<0.001
Diet (1—more than 5 times)	102	50.2	101	49.8		

3.2. Unique Contributions of Demographics and Dieting in Explaining Overweight Status

A binary logistic regression was performed to examine the unique contributions of the five predictors in explaining overweight status. Males were 3.28 times more likely to be overweight compared with females (CI 95% (2.08, 5.18)). Adolescents from urban school areas were 1.84 times more likely to be overweight compared with those from suburban school areas (CI 95% (1.07, 3.14)). Adolescents reporting dieting were 3.84 times more likely to be overweight compared with their non-dieting counterparts (CI 95% (2.45, 6.03)). The main effects of ethnicity and pocket money were not statistically significant (see Table 2). All variables together explained 20.3% of the variance in overweight status.

Table 2. Logistic regression predicting overweight status by demographic and dieting correlates in the total group.

	B	SE	OR	CI 95%	Nagelkerke R^2
Sex	1.19 **	0.23	3.28 **	2.08–5.18	
School area	0.61 *	0.27	1.84 *	1.07–3.14	
Ethnicity	−0.11	0.26	0.90	0.54–1.51	20.3
Pocket money	0.02	0.23	1.02	0.64–1.61	
Past year dieting	1.35 **	0.23	3.84 **	2.45–6.03	

Note: * $p \leq 0.05$, ** $p \leq 0.01$. Sex: 0 = females, 1 = males; school area: 0 = suburban, 1 = urban; ethnicity: 0 = Indonesian, 1 = Chinese Indonesian; pocket money: 0 = <500,000 Rp, 1 = >500,000 Rp; and past year dieting: 0 = no dieting, 1 = dieting. B: Beta; SE: Standard Error; OR: Odds Ratio; CI: Confidence Interval.

3.3. Sex-Specific Interactions

Four separate sex-specific interaction analyses were performed, in which one interaction was added to the main regression model. Of these four interactions, only the interaction between sex and school area was statistically significant (see Table 3). The explained variance for the total model including the interaction was 21.5% (b = 0.99, SE = 0.47, CI 95% (0.07, 1.89)). We further probed this interaction using Model 1 PROCESS module for SPSS. The results showed that males living in urban areas were more likely to be overweight compared with males living in suburban areas (b = 0.99, SE = 0.48, and CI 95% (0.34, 1.65)), whereas this did not apply to females (b = 0.01, SE = 0.39, and CI 95% (−0.75, 0.78)). The other sex-specific interactions were not statistically significant.

Table 3. Logistic regression predicting overweight status by demographic and dieting correlates in the total group including interaction effects with sex.

	B	SE	OR	CI 95%	Nagelkerke R^2
Sex	1.19 **	0.23	3.28 **	2.08–5.18	
School area	0.61 *	0.27	1.84 *	1.07–3.14	
Ethnicity	−0.11	0.26	0.90	0.54–1.51	20.3
Pocket money	0.02	0.23	1.02	0.64–1.61	
Past year dieting	1.35 **	0.23	3.84 **	2.45–6.03	
Sex *school area	0.98 *	0.47	2.67	1.07–6.63	21.5
Sex * pocket money	−0.61	0.47	0.54	0.21–1.38	20.7
Sex * ethnicity	0.87	0.46	2.39	0.97–5.90	21.3
Sex * past year dieting	−0.46	0.49	0.63	0.24–1.66	20.5

Note: * $p \leq 0.05$, ** $p \leq 0.01$. Two-way interactions were tested separately (one interaction per analyses added to the main model). Total model explained variance were reported per separately tested interaction. Sex: 0 = females, 1 = males; school area: 0 = suburban, 1 = urban; ethnicity: 0 = Indonesian ethnic, 1 = Chinese-Indonesian ethnic; pocket money: 0 = <500,000, 1 = >500,000; and past year dieting: 0 = never did diet, 1 = did diet. Sex-specific interactions (Sex X school area): girls = b = 0.01 (CI95% (−0.75, −0.78)); boys = b = 0.99 (CI95% (0.34–1.65)) using Model 1 PROCESS module for SPSS.

4. Discussion

The current study aimed to examine the (sex-specific) demographic and dieting factors that potentially explain overweight status among a relatively large group of Indonesian early adolescents attending private schools (i.e., higher SEP background). Children and adolescents from private schools are more likely to be obese [4] and early adolescents' weight is predictive of their weight status in adolescence and adulthood [11]. Finding correlates of overweight in this specific period might give insights for future prevention or intervention and may have both direct and longer-term health benefits. Our findings showed that the general prevalence rate of overweight in this early adolescent sample at private schools was relatively high (i.e., 36.3%) compared with previous national prevalence rates (i.e., 16%) [11]. The seemingly higher percentage of overweight status among adolescents from higher SEP backgrounds may be environmentally driven [4]. As mentioned, higher SEP private schools, particularly those in urban environments, are often located in areas with more junk food outlets [3,9]. Food outlets usually sell fried products, that are highly preferred, and these kinds of products are highly energy dense. People from higher SEP backgrounds often opt to eat out rather than at home, and food served in restaurants or food outlets usually contains more calories [3,15,19]. In addition, most Indonesian parents from higher SEP are proud when their children look big or fat, reflecting a higher socioeconomic status [3]. Together, these factors may probably explain the relatively high overweight prevalence rate in our study sample.

The relatively high overweight prevalence in our sample makes further insights into (sex-specific) demographic correlates even more interesting, given the increased statistical power to detect effects. We found that males were almost four times more likely to be overweight than females. This result is consistent with most previous studies among Indonesian children [4,9]. However, these findings are in contrast with previous studies among adolescents and adults, where prevalence rates are mostly reported to be higher among females compared with males [2,4,10]. Our findings indicate that early adolescent males are (still) more likely to be overweight compared with early adolescent females, at least among adolescents attending private schools. Future longer-term studies following early adolescents to emerging adulthood are needed to further shed light on a potential sex-specific switch in terms of overweight vulnerability. Specifically, sex-specific parental perceptions of ideal body weight among children and early adolescents may explain the higher prevalence rate of overweight status among (early adolescent) males. Parents seem more supportive of higher body weights of males compared with females, possibly because of the male body ideal (big is more ideal for males than females, [20,21]). As such, these explanations may thus explain our sex-specific findings involving overweight status, given that parents may still have a considerable influence on what their children eat (potentially impacting their weight development) during early adolescence [22].

We also found a significantly higher prevalence of overweight status among Indonesian adolescents who attended schools in urbanized areas compared with those in suburban areas. This has similarly been reported before among children and adolescents [4,11,23]. However, this finding should be interpreted carefully in our case because we also found a clear sex-specific interaction with school area. We found that specifically male adolescents in urban school areas had higher overweight rates. This finding is in line with another recent study among children and adolescents in Indonesia [11], but in contrast with previous studies among adults showing that females from urban areas were the ones at highest risk [2,5]. We speculate that (early adolescent) males may be more vulnerable to these unhealthy urban environments with junk food cues from fast-food outlets, as they often show higher efforts to get food as a reward compared with females [22,24]. As such, males might be more likely to actively search for food rewards, which are more often satisfied in high junk food environments. This, in combination with parents possibly more often encouraging adolescent males to gain weight [21], might explain our sex-specific interaction among early adolescents.

In our study, ethnicity was not related to overweight status, which is in contrast with some previous studies [13,25]. However, our findings involving ethnic background are consistent with the results of a previous study investigating adolescents from other Indonesia regions (i.e., Surakarta). This study also found no significant differences between Javanese and Chinese Indonesian adolescents [17]. So it might be that ethnicity findings regarding overweight status are dependent upon the specific Indonesian region (and ethnicities) being examined.

A final result of our study is that adolescents who dieted in the previous year were more likely to be overweight. This finding is in line with well-known findings from Western countries, with recent dieting considered to be a potential proxy of the susceptibility to weight gain [26]. It might be that dieting is unsuccessful and interspersed with binge eating episodes, thus leading to weight gain. Dieting may also be the consequence of being overweight [16]. Further longitudinal research is needed to unravel the directionality of these associations. Importantly, the fact that the dieting findings in this study were rather similar to the ones reported in previous European and American studies, suggests overlap in terms of overweight correlates between higher SEP Indonesian adolescents and adolescents from Western countries.

One notable strength of our study is the inclusion of a relatively large sample of early adolescents from specifically private schools, who are at higher risk for obesity, as also supported by our study findings. Another strength is that we used objectively measured weight and height to determine overweight status. Nevertheless, a couple of limitations should also be mentioned. First, we did not include clear markers for determining "socioeconomic" differences (except pocket money) within our higher SEP group of adolescents from private schools. The amount of pocket money that adolescents received might not reflect socioeconomic position differences. The income of the family per year might have been a better indicator (i.e., [5,12]). Nevertheless, as our total sample was recruited from private schools only, we are rather confident that most adolescents were from mid-to-high SEP backgrounds. Second, as our data are limited by a cross sectional design, we, therefore, do not know the underlying mechanism explaining the observed associations. Future longitudinal studies could shed more light on (predictors of) weight development in specific subgroups, such as males from urban areas compared with suburban areas.

Despite these limitations, our study examining (sex-specific) demographic correlates of overweight status among early adolescents from private schools in Indonesia filled an important gap in the current literature. We have speculated about the most prominent (mostly nutrient-related) mechanisms explaining our findings. Nevertheless, future research should further unravel the underlying (energy intake and expenditure) mechanisms explaining why particularly early adolescent males from urban school areas are more likely to be overweight. This will provide further tools for future tailored preventive interventions. We suggest that this early adolescent phase is a promising period for timely preventive interventions, given that adolescent overweight and obese status in Indonesia is more rapidly increasing in older compared with younger adolescents [8]. To conclude, our findings suggest that males from urban area private schools in Indonesia may be an important target group for future preventive overweight interventions.

Author Contributions: J.M.V. and J.K.L. were responsible for the study design; J.M.V. and J.K.L. supervised the data collection; E.S. was responsible for the data collection, the statistical analyses and interpretation of the data in agreement with J.M.V., J.K.L. and W.J.B.; and E.S. wrote the first version of the manuscript, edited by J.M.V., J.K.L. and W.J.B. All authors participated in the revisions of the manuscript. All authors have read and agreed to the published version of the manuscript.

Funding: We received no specific grant from any funding agency in public, commercial, or non-profit sectors. This study was funded by Maranatha Christian University in Bandung, Indonesia. The study received no external funding. The analysis and interpretation of the data and the writing of this manuscript were funded by the Behavioural Science Institute of Radboud University in Nijmegen, The Netherlands.

Institutional Review Board Statement: All procedures performed were in accordance with the ethical standards of Ethics Committee Social Science of Radboud University, Nijmegen, The Netherlands. Of the five schools that agreed to participate, three schools obtained consent forms from parents and students. The remaining two schools informed the parents about this project (passive consent) based on the school policy and collected the signed consent forms from students only. The original (reference ECSS_2019_150) and amended (passive consent) procedures were approved by the Ethics Committee Social Science of Radboud University, Nijmegen, The Netherlands (ECSS-2019-115).

Informed Consent Statement: Informed consent was obtained from all subjects involved in the study.

Data Availability Statement: The datasets generated and analyzed during the current study are not publicly available due to agreements we have made concerning the exchange and use of our data but are available from the corresponding author (E.S.) on reasonable request.

Acknowledgments: We would like to thank all the participating schools and students for their contribution to this research project. Moreover, we would like to thank all the student assistants (head of the schools and class teachers) for their help during the data collection of this project.

Conflicts of Interest: The authors declare no conflict of interest.

References

1. National Instituted of Health Research and Development. Riset Kesehatan Dasar (National Baseline Health Research), Jakarta, Indonesia. 2017. Badan Litbang Kesehatan. Available online: https://pusdatin.kemkes.go.id (accessed on 5 March 2021).
2. Roemling, C.; Qaim, M. Obesity trends and determinants in Indonesia. *Appetite* **2012**, *58*, 1005–1013. [CrossRef] [PubMed]
3. Syahrul, S.; Kimura, R.; Tsuda, A.; Susanto, T.; Saito, R.; Ahmad, F. Prevalence of underweight and overweight among school-aged children and it's association with children's sociodemographic and lifestyle in Indonesia. *Int. J. Nurs. Sci.* **2016**, *3*, 169–177. [CrossRef]
4. Rachmi, C.; Li, M.; Baur, L. Overweight and obesity in Indonesia: Prevalence and risk factors—A literature review. *Public Health* **2017**, *147*, 20–29. [CrossRef] [PubMed]
5. Popkin, B.M.; Adair, L.S.; Ng, S.W. Now and then: The global nutrition transition: The pandemic of obesity in developing countries. *Nutr. Rev.* **2012**, *70*, 13–21. [CrossRef] [PubMed]
6. Pengpid, S.; Peltzer, K. Underweight and overweight or obesity and associated factors among school-going adolescents in five ASEAN countries 2015. *Diabetes Metab. Syndr. Clin. Res. Rev.* **2019**, *13*, 3075–3080. [CrossRef]
7. Tsiros, M.D.; Sinn, N.; Coates, A.M.; Howe, P.R.C.; Buckley, J.D. Treatment of adolescent overweight and obesity. *Eur. J. Pediatr.* **2008**, *167*, 9–16. [CrossRef]
8. Agustina, R.; Meilianawati; Fenny; Atmarita; Suparmi; Susiloretni, K.A.; Lestari, W.; Pritasari, K.; Shankar, A.H. Psychosocial, Eating Behavior, and Lifestyle Factors Influencing Overweight and Obesity in Adolescents. *Food Nutr. Bull.* **2021**, *42* (Suppl. 1), S72–S91. [CrossRef]
9. Febriani, D.; Sudarti, T. Fast food as drivers for overweight and obesity among urban school children at Jakarta, Indonesia. *J. Gizi Dan Pangan* **2019**, *14*, 99–106. [CrossRef]
10. Nurwanti, E.; Uddin, M.; Chang, J.S.; Hadi, H.; Syed-Abdul, S.; Yu Su, E.C.; Nursetyo, A.A.; Masud, J.H.B.; Bai, C.H. Roles of sedentary behaviours and unhealthy foods in increasing the obesity risk in adult men and women: A cross sectional national study. *Nutrients* **2018**, *10*, 704. [CrossRef]
11. Nurwanti, E.; Hadi, H.; Chang, J.S.; Chao, J.C.J.; Paramashanti, B.A.; Gittelsohn, J.; Bai, C.H. Rural–urban differences in dietary behavior and obesity: Results of the riskesdas study in 10–18-year-old Indonesian children and adolescents. *Nutrients* **2019**, *11*, 2813. [CrossRef]
12. Sweeting, H. Sexed dimensions of obesity in childhood and adolescence. *Nutr. J.* **2008**, *7*, 1. [CrossRef]
13. Pell, C.; Allotey, P.; Evans, N.; Hardon, A.; Imelda, J.D.; Soyiri, I.; Reidpath, D.D.; The SEACO Team. Coming of age, becoming obese: A cross-sectional analysis of obesity among adolescents and young adults in Malaysia. *BMC Public Health* **2016**, *16*, 1082. [CrossRef] [PubMed]
14. Collins, A.E.; Pakiz, B.; Rock, C.L. Factors associated with obesity in Indonesian adolescent. *Int. J. Pediatr. Obes.* **2008**, *3*, 58–64. [CrossRef] [PubMed]
15. Pradeepa, R.; Anjana, R.M.; Joshi, S.R.; Bhansali, A.; Deepa, M.; Joshi, P.P.; Dhandania, V.K.; Madhu, S.V.; Rao, P.V.; Geetha, L.; et al. Prevalence of generalized and abdominal obesity in urban & rural India—the ICMR-INDIAB Study (Phase 1) [ICMR-INDIAB-3]. *Indian J. Med. Res.* **2015**, *142*, 139–150. [CrossRef] [PubMed]
16. Field, A.E.; Aneja, P.; Rosner, B. The validity of self-reported weight change among adolescents and young adults. *Obesity* **2007**, *5*, 2357–2364. [CrossRef] [PubMed]
17. Susanti, R.P.F.; Murti, B.; Indarto, D. Maternal employment status, ethnicity, food intake, and their effects on teenage obesity, in Surakarta. *J. Epidemic. Public Health* **2016**, *1*, 75–85. [CrossRef]
18. Hayes, A. *PROCESS: A Versatile Computational Tool for Observed Variable Mediation, Mod-Eration, and Conditionalprocess Modelling;* Guildford Press: New York, NY, USA, 2012; Available online: http://www.afhayes.com/public/process2012.pdf (accessed on 19 February 2020).
19. Mak, T.N.; Prynne, C.J.; Cole, D.; Fitt, E.; Bates, B.; Stephen, A.M. Patterns of sociodemographic and food practice characteristics in relation to fruit and vegetable consumption in children: Results from the UK National Diet and Nutrition Survey Rolling Programme (2008–2010). *Public Health Nutr.* **2013**, *16*, 1912–1923. [CrossRef] [PubMed]
20. Loth, K.A.; Machlehose, R.F.; Fulkerson, J.A.; Crow, S.; Neumark-Sztainer, D. Food-related practices and adolescent weight status: A population based study. *Pediatrics* **2013**, *131*, e1443–e1450. [CrossRef] [PubMed]

21. Ricciardelli, L.A.; McCabe, M. Children´s body image concerns and eating disturbance: A review of the literature. *Clin. Psychol. Rev.* **2001**, *21*, 325–344. [CrossRef]
22. Kiefer, I.; Rathmanner, T.; Kunze, M. Eating and dieting differences in men and women. *J. Men's Health Sex.* **2005**, *2*, 194–201. [CrossRef]
23. Mistry, S.K.; Puthussery, S. Risk factors of overweight and obesity in childhood and adolescence in South Asian countries: A systematic review of the evidence. *Public Health* **2015**, *129*, 200–209. [CrossRef] [PubMed]
24. Neumark-Sztainer, D.; Wall, M.; Story, M.; Standish, A.R. Dieting and unhealthy weight control behaviours during adolescence: Association with 10-year changes in Body Mass Index. *J. Adolesc. Health* **2012**, *50*, 80–86. [CrossRef] [PubMed]
25. Neumark-Sztainer, D.; Croll, J.; Story, M.; Hannan, P.J.; French, S.A.; Perry, C. Ethnic/racial differences in weight-related concerns and behaviours among adolescent girls and boys. *J. Psychosom. Res.* **2002**, *53*, 963–974. [CrossRef]
26. Lowe, M.R.; Doshi, S.D.; Katterman, S.N.; Feig, E.H. Dieting in restrained eating as prospective predictors of weight gain. *Front. Psychol.* **2013**, *4*, 577. [CrossRef]

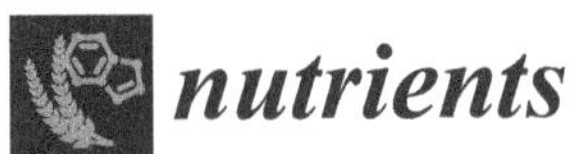

Article

Obesity Risk-Factor Variation Based on Island Clusters: A Secondary Analysis of Indonesian Basic Health Research 2018

Sri Astuti Thamrin [1,*], Dian Sidik Arsyad [2,3], Hedi Kuswanto [1], Armin Lawi [4] and Andi Imam Arundhana [5,6]

[1] Department of Statistics, Faculty of Mathematics and Natural Science, Universitas Hasanuddin, Makassar 90245, Indonesia; hedikuswanto454@gmail.com

[2] Department of Epidemiology, Faculty of Public Health, Universitas Hasanuddin, Makassar 90245, Indonesia; sidik@unhas.ac.id

[3] Department of Cardiology, Division of Heart and Lungs, University Medical Centre Utrecht, University of Utrecht, 3584CS Utrecht, The Netherlands

[4] Department of Mathematics, Faculty of Mathematics and Natural Science, Universitas Hasanuddin, Makassar 90245, Indonesia; armin@unhas.ac.id

[5] Department of Nutrition, Faculty of Public Health, Universitas Hasanuddin, Makassar 90245, Indonesia; andi.imam@unhas.ac.id

[6] Central Clinical School, Faculty of Medicine and Health Science, The University of Sydney, Sydney 2050, Australia

[*] Correspondence: tuti@unhas.ac.id; Tel./Fax: +62-(411)-588-551

Citation: Thamrin, S.A.; Arsyad, D.S.; Kuswanto, H.; Lawi, A.; Arundhana, A.I. Obesity Risk-Factor Variation Based on Island Clusters: A Secondary Analysis of Indonesian Basic Health Research 2018. *Nutrients* **2022**, *14*, 971. https://doi.org/10.3390/nu14050971

Academic Editors: Odysseas Androutsos and Evangelia Charmandari

Received: 17 January 2022
Accepted: 22 February 2022
Published: 24 February 2022

Publisher's Note: MDPI stays neutral with regard to jurisdictional claims in published maps and institutional affiliations.

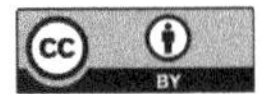

Copyright: © 2022 by the authors. Licensee MDPI, Basel, Switzerland. This article is an open access article distributed under the terms and conditions of the Creative Commons Attribution (CC BY) license (https://creativecommons.org/licenses/by/4.0/).

Abstract: Obesity has become a rising global health problem affecting quality of life for adults. The objective of this study is to describe the prevalence of obesity in Indonesian adults based on the cluster of islands. The study also aims to identify the risk factors of obesity in each island cluster. This study analyzes the secondary data of Indonesian Basic Health Research 2018. Data for this analysis comprised 618,910 adults ($\geq$18 years) randomly selected, proportionate to the population size throughout Indonesia. We included 20 variables for the socio-demographic and obesity-related risk factors for analysis. The obesity status was defined using Body Mass Index (BMI) $\geq$ 25 kg/m^2. Our current study defines 7 major island clusters as the unit analysis consisting of 34 provinces in Indonesia. Descriptive analysis was conducted to determine the characteristics of the population and to calculate the prevalence of obesity within the provinces in each of the island clusters. Multivariate logistic regression analyses to calculate the odds ratios (ORs) was performed using SPSS version 27. The study results show that all the island clusters have at least one province with an obesity prevalence above the national prevalence (35.4%). Six out of twenty variables, comprising four dietary factors (the consumption of sweet food, high-salt food, meat, and carbonated drinks) and one psychological factor (mental health disorders), varied across the island clusters. In conclusion, there was a variation of obesity prevalence of the provinces within and between island clusters. The variation of risk factors found in each island cluster suggests that a government rethink of the current intervention strategies to address obesity is recommended.

Keywords: body weight; Indonesia; islands cluster; multiple logistic regression; obesity; risk factor

1. Introduction

Obesity is a major public health issue causing multiple burdens of co-morbidities and mortalities among adults. The World Health Organization (WHO) reported that globally 39% of adults were overweight and 13% were obese, and this number has nearly tripled within the last three decades [1]. In Indonesia, the obesity prevalence has increased significantly from 18.8% in 2007 to 26.6% in 2013, with a slight decrease in 2018 (21.8%) [2–4].

There are many statistical methods for analyzing large-scale study data. The machine learning method is a powerful statistical analysis approach that can be used for predictive model development of health outcomes. A recent systematic review reported various machine learning techniques that were performed to predict adult obesity from nationwide and large cross-sectional data, finding that logistic regression analysis had the highest accuracy in predicting obesity [5,6]. This finding is in line with our previous study [7], which found that logistic regression had the highest performance in predicting and measuring obesity. Predicting obesity risk factors by considering determinant variables can be advantageous to design and modify local existing nutrition programs and policies better for controlling the obesity problem.

To the best of our knowledge, this is the first study re-analyzing cross-sectional Indonesian Basic Health Research (RISKESDAS in Indonesian) data based on the main islands in Indonesia (we use the term "island clusters"). A previous study in Indonesia investigating the determinants of obesity among adults using the 2007 and 2013 RISKESDAS data concluded that the prevalence of obesity and risk factors varied among the areas [8]. However, this study only grouped the areas based on Indonesia's three different time regions, which might cause bias within the three groups. Therefore, further analysis for obesity determinants in regions with similar population characteristics is essential to minimize the variation bias. We clustered the provinces located on the same island into one cluster as the population characteristics within the same island cluster, assuming that within-island populations share more characteristics than clusters determined only by the time zone.

The main aim of this study is to examine the factors contributing to obesity in adults and investigate how these varied across the island clusters. This study also describes the prevalence of obesity in seven island clusters in Indonesia and reveals what factors increase or decrease the risk of obesity.

2. Materials and Methods

2.1. Data Source

Secondary data analysis performed in the current study was based on the data from the RISKESDAS study, a nationally representative cross-sectional study in Indonesia conducted by the Ministry of Health in 2018. Detailed information regarding methods, ethical considerations, and other related aspects of the RISKESDAS study is published elsewhere [9]. Briefly, the RISKESDAS sample was selected based on 2010 population census blocks using multi-stage cluster random sampling. Our data for analysis comprised 618,910 adults ($\geq$18 years) from approximately 300,000 households randomly selected using proportionate to population sub-samples throughout Indonesia [2].

The data can be obtained from the National Institute of Health Research and Development (NIHRD), Ministry of Health, Republic of Indonesia upon request (https://www.litbang. kemkes.go.id/layanan-permintaan-data-riset/, accessed on 3 May 2021).

2.2. Study Variables

Socio-demographic variables, obesity status, and selected risk factors were identified from RISKESDAS 2018 questionnaires prior to the data request. We included 20 variables for socio-demographic and obesity-related risk factors for analysis. The socio-demographic variables of sex, education, employment, marital status, and urban-rural status were included.

Obesity status was calculated based on the Body Mass Index (BMI) using weight and height. We classify an individual as obese with a BMI $\geq$ 25 kg/m^2 following WHO BMI cut-offs for Asian populations [10]. Mental and Emotional Disorders (MEDs) were based on 20 items from a Self-Reporting Questionnaire (SRQ) developed by the WHO [11]; we determined a MED with the cut-off point $\geq$6 (positive predictive value = 70%, and negative predictive value = 92%) [12]. The frequency of consumption of risky food items (sweet foods and beverages, high-in-salt foods, high-in-fat foods, meats, carbonated drinks, energy drinks, and instant foods) was measured. The eating or drinking of risky food items more than 1 time per day was considered as high frequency consumption. Vegetable and fruit consumption was calculated based on the WHO standard [13]; $\geq$5 portion per day was determined as adequate. Smoking status was classified as "currently smoking", "quit smoking", and "never smoked", based on participant self-reporting. Physical activity in the current analysis was based on the WHO Global Physical Activity Questionnaire (GPAQ) used in the RISKESDAS study; sufficient physical activity was defined according to the WHO recommendations [14]. Drinking alcoholic beverages within 1 month prior to the study was defined as alcohol consumption. Blood pressure was measured using systolic and diastolic blood pressure during data collection; the 8th Joint National Committee guideline was used to classify blood pressures [15].

2.3. Island Clusters

Indonesia is the largest archipelagic country consisting of clusters of islands divided into 34 provinces. Our current study defined 7 major island clusters: Sumatra (provinces included: Aceh, North Sumatra, West Sumatra, Riau, Jambi, South Sumatra, Bengkulu, Lampung, Kepulauan Bangka Belitung, and Kepulauan Riau); Java (provinces included: DKI Jakarta, West Java, Central Java, Yogyakarta, East Java, and Banten); Bali-Nusa Tenggara (provinces included: Bali, West Nusa Tenggara, and East Nusa Tenggara); Kalimantan (provinces included: West Kalimantan, Central Kalimantan, South Kalimantan, East Kalimantan, and North Kalimantan); Sulawesi (provinces included: South Sulawesi, Central Sulawesi, Southeast Sulawesi, North Sulawesi, West Sulawesi, and Gorontalo); Maluku (provinces included: Maluku and North Maluku), and Papua (provinces included: Papua and West Papua).

2.4. Statistical Analysis

The sample weights for the complex survey design were considered in the analysis. Descriptive analysis was conducted to determine the characteristics of the population and to calculate the prevalence of obesity within the provinces in each island's cluster.

In order to calculate the adjusted odds ratios (ORs), multivariate logistic regression analyses, which includes other variables associated with obesity, were performed. The selection of multivariate logistic regression to develop a predictive model was based on our prior study that showed a high-performance, including accuracy, specificity, precision, Kappa, and F_β [7]. Multivariate logistic regression was performed using SPSS version 27 (IBM Corp, Armonk, NY, USA). Cohen's and Cliff's Delta analyses were performed using R version 4.0.1 ('effsize' package version 0.7.6, Marco Torchiano, 2019) to validate each factor's variation (effect size) of odds ratios (ORs) by island cluster. The effect sizes were presented in four distinct categories: negligible, small, medium, and large. The effect size was considered negligible if the score was below 0.2, a score of 0.2 to <0.5 was considered small, 0.5 to <0.8 for medium, and 0.8 and above for a large effect size [16,17].

2.5. Ethical Considerations

Ethical approval of the RISKESDAS survey was obtained from the Ethical Committee of Health Research, the Indonesian Ministry of Health (LB.02.01/2/KE.267/2017) [2].

3. Results

3.1. Prevalence of Obesity across Island Clusters

The purpose of this study was to describe the prevalence of obese adults by island cluster in Indonesia and assess the risk of obesity caused by determinant factors using the secondary data of RISKESDAS 2018. Figure 1 illustrates the estimated obesity prevalence distribution across Indonesia. The figure shows that all island clusters have at least 1 province in which the prevalence of obesity is more than 20%, and only 3 clusters with at least 1 province in which more than 25% are classified as obese: Java, Kalimantan, and Sulawesi Island.

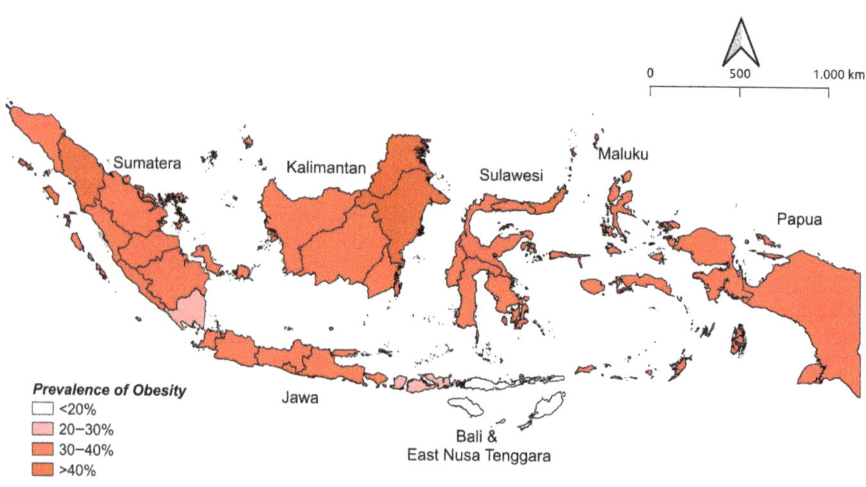

Figure 1. Distribution of obesity prevalence in Indonesia.

In Sumatra, North Sumatra had the highest number of obese adults, while Lampung had the lowest (40.6% vs. 29.6%). The sequence of the regency for the highest and the lowest obesity prevalence in other island clusters were: DKI Jakarta (45.6%) versus Central Java (33.3%) in Java Island; Bali (38.8%) versus East Nusa Tenggara (19.1%) in Bali and Nusa Tenggara Island; East Kalimantan (44.1%) versus West Kalimantan (30.3%) in Kalimantan Island; North Sulawesi (46.6%) versus West Sulawesi (31.4%) in Sulawesi Island; Maluku Utara (37.9%) versus Maluku (33.0%) in Maluku Island; and West Papua (39.6%) versus Papua (35.0%) in Papua Island. DKI Jakarta had the highest proportion of an obese individuals, which outnumbered the national figure (45.6% vs. 35.4%), followed by Sulawesi Utara and East Kalimantan (data displayed in detail in the Supplementary Table S1A).

Table 1 shows the breakdown of obesity prevalence in all the island clusters in Indonesia, according to categories of the determinants associated with obesity. Notably, this table indicates that obesity prevalence varied according to MED status. The distribution of obesity was higher among those without MED in the Sumatra, Java, and Papua Island clusters. In addition, a few variables show the variation of obesity prevalence by categories, including food high in salt, meat, carbonated beverage consumption, and smoking status. Individuals with a high level of education and having a permanent job (e.g., government/police/military officer) show a higher obesity prevalence than their counterparts.

Table 1. Prevalence of obese adults by variables associated with obesity in all island clusters in Indonesia.

Variables	Categories	Island Clusters						
		Sumatra	Java	Bali and Nusa Tenggara	Kalimantan	Sulawesi	Maluku	Papua
		$n = 180{,}292$	$n = 204{,}768$	$n = 50{,}484$	$n = 59{,}654$	$n = 85{,}006$	$n = 18{,}531$	$n = 20{,}175$
BMI category	Obese	35.3	36.2	28.2	34.8	34.9	35.0	36.0
Location	Rural	31.6	29.9	21.4	29.7	31.6	30.5	32.4
	Urban	40.1	39.6	36.2	40.7	39.9	42.2	43.7
Sex	Men	26.3	26.8	22.3	26.8	26.2	26.8	31.3
	Women	44.6	45.6	33.9	43.6	43.5	43.5	41.2

Table 1. *Cont.*

Variables	Categories	Island Clusters						
		Sumatra	Java	Bali and Nusa Tenggara	Kalimantan	Sulawesi	Maluku	Papua
		n = 180,292	*n* = 204,768	*n* = 50,484	*n* = 59,654	*n* = 85,006	*n* = 18,531	*n* = 20,175
Marital status	Not Married	18.2	20.6	16.3	19.7	19.7	18.5	22.2
	Married	39.4	39.8	31.4	38.8	39.1	39.2	38.6
	Divorced	33.9	34.2	26.0	30.0	31.0	29.9	40.5
	Widowed	34.5	32.5	22.4	27.8	30.3	35.9	32.8
Age group	≤47 years	34.5	36.8	28.6	35.2	34.7	34.3	35.2
	48–63 years	41.0	40.1	31.9	36.9	39.6	40.4	40.9
	≥64 years	25.2	22.1	16.1	23.3	23.8	26.5	24.5
Education level	Lower education	46.6	46.4	40.1	45.5	43.7	47.2	53.4
	Medium education	36.5	37.9	31.5	37.5	35.8	34.4	39.5
	Higher education	33.2	34.3	24.8	32.3	33.0	33.3	32.2
Occupational status	Unemployed	41.8	42.7	30.1	41.8	40.3	36.5	40.2
	Students	20.2	24.7	15.2	23.1	18.5	19.4	28.7
	Government/civil workers	53.9	54.7	49.3	50.6	52.4	55.4	57.2
	Private company officer	35.0	36.3	34.8	35.9	34.0	38.8	37.3
	Entrepreneur	40.1	42.3	42.9	38.4	41.8	46.9	40.9
	Farmer	25.7	22.9	16.6	23.2	22.4	24.6	28.5
	Fisherman	22.9	24.5	23.9	22.9	25.0	17.4	24.4
	Daily labor/driver/housekeeper	27.6	27.8	24.1	26.3	29.8	29.8	30.7
	Others	39.9	39.9	28.5	39.0	39.5	42.8	42.8
Mental emotional status	No mental disorder	35.3	36.2	28.8	35.2	35.3	35.8	35.9
	With mental disorder	35.1	36.0	23.6	30.9	31.7	29.5	36.9
Sweet food	<3 times/month	37.0	38.2	26.3	37.6	34.0	34.2	34.3
	1–6 times/week	35.2	35.9	28.8	35.0	34.8	35.3	36.3
	>1 time/day	33.7	35.3	29.2	32.6	35.6	34.7	37.4
Sugar-sweetened beverages	<3 times/month	42.9	44.3	30.4	42.6	39.1	40.5	40.5
	1–6 times/week	36.3	37.5	29.1	36.2	35.4	35.1	34.4
	>1 time/day	30.5	31.2	23.8	30.6	31.8	32.5	37.4
Food high in salt	<3 times/month	36.7	38.0	27.9	36.9	37.7	36.1	36.5
	1–6 times/week	35.0	35.4	28.5	34.1	32.9	34.0	34.6
	>1 time/day	32.4	36.2	28.9	33.9	33.1	35.1	40.5
High-fat food	<3 times/month	34.1	34.4	23.6	32.1	31.0	34.6	32.4
	1–6 times/week	35.4	36.1	29.9	35.3	35.0	35.1	37.8
	>1 time/day	36.5	36.8	32.8	35.7	38.4	35.1	38.2
Meat	<3 times/month	35.3	35.7	27.6	34.9	34.6	34.6	34.8
	1–6 times/week	34.8	37.6	31.4	34.6	36.0	36.5	39.1
	>1 time/day	37.8	36.1	35.2	34.3	34.7	36.1	37.8
Soft or carbonated drinks	<3 times/month	35.9	36.8	28.0	35.7	35.5	35.5	36.1
	1–6 times/week	30.2	31.0	29.6	29.2	31.5	32.3	34.7
	>1 time/day	28.0	32.8	20.2	27.8	35.7	38.6	48.8
Energy drinks	<3 times/month	36.0	36.9	28.8	36.1	36.3	36.3	36.5
	1–6 times/week	26.9	27.2	22.5	25.3	24.9	30.2	33.4
	>1 time/day	26.9	27.2	18.7	24.2	26.5	31.1	37.7
Instant foods	<3 times/month	38.0	37.7	29.6	36.8	37.9	38.8	36.7
	1–6 times/week	33.5	35.2	27.0	34.2	33.5	33.6	35.6
	>1 time/day	31.8	36.3	25.3	26.8	29.2	28.2	35.5
Vegetable and fruit consumption	Sufficient	42.5	42.7	35.3	41.7	37.8	43.2	47.4
	Insufficient	35.0	35.9	27.8	34.5	34.7	34.4	35.2
Smoking	Never smoked	41.7	43.4	32.7	40.9	41.5	41.2	39.4

Table 1. *Cont.*

Variables	Categories	Island Clusters						
		Sumatra	Java	Bali and Nusa Tenggara	Kalimantan	Sulawesi	Maluku	Papua
		$n = 180,292$	$n = 204,768$	$n = 50,484$	$n = 59,654$	$n = 85,006$	$n = 18,531$	$n = 20,175$
	Quit smoking	37.1	37.2	30.9	37.6	34.0	47.2	39.1
	Currently smoking	24.0	23.5	19.1	22.7	22.9	23.7	28.7
Physical activity	Adequate	32.2	32.4	24.6	29.9	31.1	31.9	33.0
	Not adequate	37.8	39.0	31.0	38.4	37.6	36.8	38.9
Alcohol consumption	Yes	28.4	27.2	24.5	20.7	25.1	23.6	29.2
	No	35.5	36.4	28.7	35.6	35.9	36.6	36.5
Blood pressure	Normal	22.3	21.5	16.4	19.9	21.6	22.5	24.1
	Pre-hypertension	34.6	34.2	28.7	31.4	35.2	35.4	36.3
	Hypertension stage 1	46.1	45.1	38.5	43.8	44.9	45.9	49.2
	Hypertension stage 2	54.7	52.4	44.8	51.2	51.3	55.9	58.5

3.2. Cluster Variation of Obesity Risk Factors

The results of the logistic regression analysis are displayed in Figure 2. The variables associated with increased odds (OR > 1) of being obese in all island clusters were the location (X01), gender (X02), marital status (X03), occupational status (X06), high-fat food (X11), and blood pressure (X20). Meanwhile, age group (X04), educational level (X05), sugar-sweetened beverage consumption (X09), FV consumption (X16), and smoking status (X17) factors statistically did not appear to increase the obesity risk in Indonesian adults.

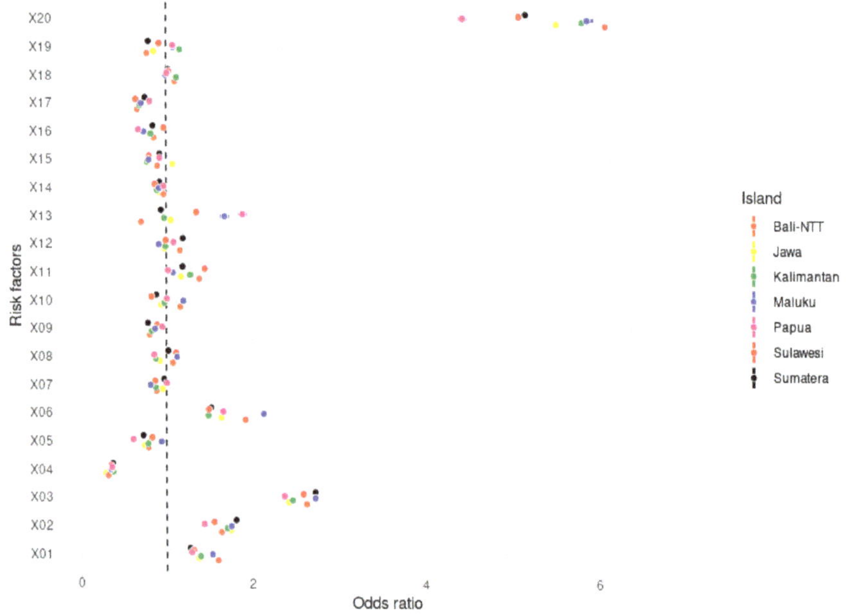

Figure 2. Variation of obesity risk factors by island clusters in Indonesia.

These results suggest that six out of twenty variables show a variation among island clusters. For example, adults working as a government/military/police officer are over represented in the data, suggesting that employment in these sectors is one of the highest contributing factors to obesity in all clusters. However, working as an entrepreneur is the highest contributor to obesity levels in Bali and Nusa Tenggara Islands (OR = 1.775; 95% CI: 1.764–1.786). People with mental–emotional disorders are likely to be at risk of obesity only in Sumatra and Papua. Regarding smoking status, those who are still smoking tend to have a normal weight status compared to their counterparts. The OR number is displayed in more detail in Supplementary Table S2A. In order to measure the effect size of each variable across the island clusters, we performed Cohen's and Cliff's Delta analyses (Supplementary Table S3A–N).

4. Discussion

The present study found that some island clusters share common obesity risk factors, including individual and socio-economic factors. Individual factors (e.g., sex, high-fat food consumption, and blood pressure) and socio-economic factors (e.g., marital status, occupational status, and location) contributed to the risk of obesity in seven island clusters, indicating that these variables are probably strong predictors of obesity in Indonesia.

The present study showed that women have greater odds of being obese than men. Women typically have a body fat percentage around 10% higher than men [18,19]. Although other biological factors, such as age and ethnicity, also contribute to the adiposity distribution and percentage, women still have more considerable body fat in almost all life spans [18]. This result aligned with a previous study in a developing country that reported that the prevalence of obesity in adult females was higher than in males. The study also revealed that obesity was directly proportional to age, but only for females [20]. We also performed additional analyses to measure the risk of obesity among married women. The risk of obesity among women who were already married was likely to increase, but not for those living in the Ambon and Papua Island clusters. This may be due to socio-economic factors forcing women in these clusters to earn money [21], thus increasing metabolic energy expenditure.

In this study, high-fat food consumption (X11) was shown to be the only dietary factor that significantly contributed to the risk of obesity in Indonesian adults in all clusters. This finding was in line with a previous study, which found that the consumption of food containing a high-fat content was the risk factor of obesity in all regions in Indonesia and was consistently found in 2007 and 2013 [8]. These results are likely to be related to people's eating habits differing by region. Eastern Indonesia tends to consume high-fat foods. It can be seen that the clusters of Sulawesi and Bali and Nusa Tenggara have a 1.4 times higher risk factor of being obese due to high-fat food consumption. Fat contributes significantly to the total energy intake, and thus reducing the high-fat food consumption might balance energy expenditure and intake [22]. Additionally, it should be noted that some fat types have beneficial effects on obesity. For example, replacing protein and short fatty acid (SFA) with polyunsaturated fatty acid (PUFA) has been shown to be significantly associated with a lower obesity risk [23].

Level of education (X5), age group (X4), sweet-sweetened beverages (SSBs) consumption (X9), energy drinks (X14), fruit and vegetable (FV) consumption (X16), and smoking status (X17), on the other hand, are statistically considered a lower obesity risk. Adults with low education levels have a lower risk of being obese than those with high education levels. This result is inconsistent with a larger cross-sectional study that found that the lower the years of education, the higher the odds of obesity [24]. What is surprising is that individuals that consumed sugar-sweetened and energy beverages had lower odds of being obese. This finding is contrary to many previous studies, which suggested that a greater intake of SSBs was associated with being overweight and obesity in children and adults [25,26]. This inconsistency might be due to the type of sugar contained in the beverages. Studies have shown that fructose-sweetened beverages increase adiposity levels more significantly than sucrose-sweetened beverages [25,27]. Unfortunately, we did not identify the dominant type of sugar contained in the beverages. Moreover, although low

FV consumption reduces the risk of obesity, it shows a positive effect on the interaction between high-fat food and obesity. People with inadequate FV consumption are likely to consume more high-fat foods than those with adequate FV in-takes.

Adults who already quit smoking had increased odds of obesity in all the island clusters. This may be due to the effect nicotine has on the central nervous system and metabolism with two possible mechanisms. First, people who quit smoking tobacco tend to replace the hand-to-mouth smoking activity with eating, leading to an increase in calorie intake. Second, taste preference is also changed among those who quit smoking to obtain a pleasure "sensation" replacing the effect of tobacco [28]. However, this finding must be interpreted with caution because we have no baseline data to describe how much weight gain occurred after smoking cessation. Additionally, the use of tobacco can promote other diseases, such as cardiovascular diseases (CVDs), hypertension, and even mortality, the same risk posed to obese people [29]. Obesity and tobacco use do not actually show the opposite outcomes. Combining weight management and smoking cessation treatment might be promising in order to improve health quality and prevent the risk of metabolic diseases related to obesity and smoking behavior.

Interestingly, mental health disorders (X7), sweet-food consumption (X8), high-salt food (X10), meat consumption (X12), and carbonated drinks (X13) varied across the island clusters. Health-related behaviors might be different between the island clusters due to several factors, such as health inequalities, socio-economic status, or household deprivation [30,31]. The most obvious variation was carbonated drink consumption, which is a high-risk factor in Papua Island, but is not excessively consumed in Bali and Nusa Tenggara Island (OR = 1.81 vs. 0.84). It seems that this variation occurs because the adult diet in Bali and Nusa Tenggara is different from Papua. There is a great difference in OR values for other diet factors, such as high-salt food, high-fat food, and energy drink consumption. Similar to our findings, a study on children and adolescents found that the consumption of SSB (including carbonated drinks) varied by race/ethnicity, sex, and age [32].

Variation among clusters was also found for the mental health disorder factor (X7). This study shows that Papua Island had the highest risk of obesity caused by mental health disorders. Many conditions could trigger mental health issues, including the limitation of food choices, poor access to health services, high-risk behaviors, and poor education [33], all of which are challenges faced on Papua Island. However, there is no information about the source of mental health disturbance of the population. More extensive evidence investigating the roles of mental health in mediating obesity occurrence is needed.

We also noted that physical activity was a predictor of obesity in all island clusters. This result was consistent with many prior studies conducted in Indonesia and elsewhere that reported that a lack of physical activity is strongly associated with obesity [34–39]. Performing sufficient physical activity might be beneficial to maintain people's energy expenditure and subsequent energy balance. Therefore, health promotion and education to improve physical activity are required, especially for busy adults in urban areas.

Another important finding of our study is that the prevalence of adult obesity varied across the regencies within the island clusters. The regency with the highest obesity prevalence was Jakarta (28.6%), while the highest among the island clusters was in Java (21.2%). The breakdown of the data reveals that the obese adults in urban areas outnumbered those in the rural areas. This difference can probably be explained by the socio-economic characteristics of each cluster. The Java Island cluster, including Jakarta province, are dominated by people living in urban areas or at least adjacent to urban areas. Meanwhile, urban communities are more likely to have unhealthy lifestyles, such as sedentary behavior and consuming more "unhealthy foods" [40,41]. Meanwhile, in the Sulawesi Island cluster and other island clusters outside the Java cluster, the number and distribution of urban communities is relatively fewer and uneven. A similar finding was reported by a study in Ethiopia that found that men living in metropolitan cities were 1.8 times more likely to become obese than those living in rural areas [36].

The major strength of the present study is that it includes a large sample size. In addition, using weighted factors in the analysis might generate results that more closely represent the Indonesian population. We also acknowledge some limitations in this study. First, the study data were collected cross-sectionally. Therefore, the causality of risk factors and obesity should be cautiously interpreted. Second, we did not disqualify outlier BMI measurement results in the dataset. However, this was only < 1% of the samples, which probably caused a small effect in the analysis. Lastly, the data for high-risk foods were collected using a non-validated questionnaire, which raised response biases of participants' answers regarding the consumption in the past 30 days. However, since the questionnaire was developed using neutrally worded questions, the options were not led from one to another and did not overlap each other, so that the participants might understand and respond more easily.

5. Conclusions

The study implies that there was a variation of obesity prevalence among the provinces and between island clusters. This study provides evidence that obesity risk factors varied across the island clusters, which may have implications in rethinking and redesigning policies and interventions to address the obesity problem in Indonesia. Multiple interventions that address specifically greater risk factors considering cluster characteristics are more likely to be effective in preventing obesity and its negative implications.

Supplementary Materials: The following supporting information can be downloaded at: https://www.mdpi.com/article/10.3390/nu14050971/s1, Table S1A: Risk factors of obesity by island clusters in Indonesia from RISKESDAS 2018, Table S2A: Odds ratios of obesity based on the risk factors in Indonesia from RISKESDAS 2018. Table S3(A–N). Effect size of odds ratios for contribution variables.

Author Contributions: Conceptualization and methodology, S.A.T. and D.S.A.; interpretation of data, S.A.T., D.S.A. and A.I.A.; statistical analysis, S.A.T., H.K. and A.L.; visualization, D.S.A., H.K. and A.L.; drafting of the manuscript, S.A.T., D.S.A. and A.I.A. All authors have read and agreed to the published version of the manuscript.

Funding: This research was funded by the Ministry of Education, Culture, Research and Technology through the PDUPT Grant contract No. 752/UN4.22/PT.01.03/2021.

Institutional Review Board Statement: Not applicable.

Informed Consent Statement: Written informed consent was obtained from participants prior to collecting biospecimen samples.

Data Availability Statement: The datasets generated and analyzed for this study can be found via https://www.litbang.kemkes.go.id/ (accessed on 3 May 2021) through a request process at the Institute of Health Research and Development of the Indonesian Ministry of Health.

Acknowledgments: The first author and the corresponding author would like to thank the Ministry of Education, Culture, Research and Technology for providing funding to conduct this study. In addition, thanks also to the Ministry of Health through the Research and Community Development Agency for providing access to Indonesia's RISKESDAS data.

Conflicts of Interest: The authors declare no conflict of interest.

References

1. WHO. Obesity and Overweight. Available online: https://www.who.int/news-room/fact-sheets/detail/obesity-and-overweight (accessed on 9 January 2022).
2. MoH. *Laporan Nasional Riset Kesehatan Dasar (Riskesdas) tahun 2018*; MoH: Jakarta, Indonesia, 2019.
3. MoH. *Laporan Nasional Riset Kesehatan Dasar (RISKESDAS) tahun 2013*; MoH: Jakarta, Indonesia, 2014.
4. MoH. *Laporan Nasional Riset Kesehatan Dasar (RISKESDAS) tahun 2007*; MoH: Jakarta, Indonesia, 2008.
5. Ferdowsy, F.; Rahi, K.S.A.; Jabiullah, M.I.; Habib, M.T. A machine learning approach for obesity risk prediction. *Curr. Res. Behav. Sci.* **2021**, *2*, 100053. [CrossRef]

6. Safaei, M.; Sundararajan, E.A.; Driss, M.; Boulila, W.; Shapi'i, A. A systematic literature review on obesity: Understanding the causes & consequences of obesity and reviewing various machine learning approaches used to predict obesity. *Comput. Biol. Med.* **2021**, *136*, 104754. [CrossRef] [PubMed]

7. Thamrin, S.A.; Arsyad, D.S.; Kuswanto, H.; Lawi, A.; Nasir, S. Predicting Obesity in Adults Using Machine Learning Techniques: An Analysis of Indonesian Basic Health. *Front. Nutr.* **2021**, *8*, 1–15. [CrossRef]

8. Arundhana, A.I.; Utami, A.P.; Muqni, A.D.; Thalavera, M.T. Regional difference in obesity prevalence and associated factors among Indonesian adults. *Malays. J. Nutr.* **2018**, *24*, 193–201.

9. MoH. *Laporan Hasil Utama Riskesdas tahun 2018*; MoH: Jakarta, Indonesia, 2019.

10. WHO Regional Office for the Western Pacific. *The Asia Pacific Perspective: Redefining Obesity and Its Treatment*; Health Communications Australia Pty Limited: Sydney, Australia, 2000.

11. Beusenberg, M.; Orley, J. *A User's Guide to the Self Reporting Questionnaire (SRQ)*; Division of Mental Health: Geneva, Switzerland, 1994.

12. Ganihartono, I. Psychiatric morbidity among patients attending the Bangetayu community health centre in Indonesia. *Bul. Penelit. Kesehat.* **1996**, *24*, 42–51.

13. Agudo, A. *Measuring Intake of Fruit and Vegetables*; WHO: Geneva, Switzerland, 2004.

14. WHO. *WHO Guidelines on Physical Activity and Sedentary Behaviour*; WHO: Geneva, Switzerland, 2020.

15. James, P.A.; Oparil, S.; Carter, B.L.; Cushman, W.C.; Dennison-Himmelfarb, C.; Handler, J.; Lackland, D.T.; LeFevre, M.L.; MacKenzie, T.D.; Ogedegbe, O.; et al. 2014 Evidence-based guideline for the management of high blood pressure in adults: Report from the panel members appointed to the Eighth Joint National Committee (JNC 8). *JAMA-J. Am. Med. Assoc.* **2014**, *311*, 507–520. [CrossRef] [PubMed]

16. Cohen, J. A power primer. *Psychol. Bull.* **1992**, *112*, 155–159. [CrossRef]

17. Romano, J.; Kromrev, D.; Coraggio, J.; Skowronek, J. Appropriate statistics for ordinal level data: Should we really be using t-test and cohen's d for evaluating group differences on the NSSE and other surveys? In Proceedings of the Annual Meeting of the Florida Association of Institutional Research, Cocoa Beach, FL, USA, 1–3 February 2006.

18. Karastergiou, K.; Smith, S.R.; Greenberg, A.S.; Fried, S.K. Sex differences in human adipose tissues—The biology of pear shape. *Biol. Sex Differ.* **2012**, *3*, 1. [CrossRef]

19. Blaak, E. Gender differences in fat metabolism. *Curr. Opin. Clin. Nutr. Metab. Care* **2001**, *4*, 499–502. [CrossRef]

20. Okeke, E.C.; Nnanyelugo, D.O.; Ngwu, E. The prevalence of obesity in adults by age, sex, and occupation in Anambra State, Nigeria. *Growth* **1983**, *47*, 263–271.

21. Wuarlela, M.; Sangadji, H.; Putirulan, A.; Hiariej, C.; Sandanafu, S.P.; Ahar, J.V.; Pesiwarissa, S.I.; Latupeirissa, E.; Wariunsora, M.; Suatrat, R.H.; et al. *Membaca Perempuan Maluku: Kalo Su Bisa Tuang Papeda Brarti Su Bisa Kaweng*; Kantor Bahasa Maluku Badan Pengembangan Bahasa dan Perbukuan Kementerian Pendidikan dan Kebudayaan: Jakarta, Indonesia, 2019; ISBN 9786022631781.

22. Bray, G.A.; Popkin, B.M. Dietary fat intake does affect obesity! *Am. J. Clin. Nutr.* **1998**, *68*, 1157–1173. [CrossRef] [PubMed]

23. Beulen, Y.; Martínez-González, M.A.; van de Rest, O.; Salas-Salvadó, J.; Sorlí, J.V.; Gómez-Gracia, E.; Fiol, M.; Estruch, R.; Santos-Lozano, J.M.; Schröder, H.; et al. Quality of dietary fat intake and body weight and obesity in a mediterranean population: Secondary analyses within the PREDIMED trial. *Nutrients* **2018**, *10*, 2011. [CrossRef] [PubMed]

24. Hsieh, T.H.; Lee, J.J.; Yu, E.W.R.; Hu, H.Y.; Lin, S.Y.; Ho, C.Y. Association between obesity and education level among the elderly in Taipei, Taiwan between 2013 and 2015: A cross-sectional study. *Sci. Rep.* **2020**, *10*, 20285. [CrossRef] [PubMed]

25. Malik, V.S.; Schulze, M.B.; Hu, F.B. Intake of sugar-sweetened beverages and weight gain: A systematic review. *Am. J. Clin. Nutr.* **2006**, *84*, 274–288. [CrossRef] [PubMed]

26. Arundhana, A.I.; Najamuddin, U.; Ibrahim, W.; Semba, G.; Muqni, A.D.; Haning, M.T. Why consumption pattern of sugar-sweetened beverage is potential to increase the risk of overweight in school age children? *Biomedicine* **2018**, *38*, 55–59.

27. Jürgens, H.; Haass, W.; Castañeda, T.R.; Schürmann, A.; Koebnick, C.; Dombrowski, F.; Otto, B.; Nawrocki, A.R.; Scherer, P.E.; Spranger, J.; et al. Consuming fructose-sweetened beverages increases body adiposity in mice. *Obes. Res.* **2005**, *13*, 1145–1156. [CrossRef]

28. Bush, T.; Lovejoy, J.C.; Deprey, M.; Carpenter, K.M. The effect of tobacco cessation on weight gain, obesity and diabetes risk. *Obesity* **2016**, *24*, 1834–1841. [CrossRef]

29. Hasegawa, K.; Komiyama, M.; Takahashi, Y. Obesity and cardiovascular risk after quitting smoking: The latest evidence. *Eur. Cardiol. Rev.* **2019**, *14*, 60–61. [CrossRef]

30. Locker, D.; Payne, B.; Ford, J. Area variations in health behaviours. *Can. J. Public Health* **1996**, *87*, 125–129.

31. Ecob, R.; Macintyre, S. Small area variations in health related behaviours; do these depend on the behaviour itself, its measurement, or on personal characteristics? *Health Place* **2000**, *6*, 261–274. [CrossRef]

32. Tasevska, N.; DeLia, D.; Lorts, C.; Yedidia, M.; Ohri-Vachaspati, P. Determinants of Sugar-Sweetened Beverage Consumption among Low-Income Children: Are There Differences by Race/Ethnicity, Age, and Sex? *J. Acad. Nutr. Diet.* **2017**, *117*, 1900–1920. [CrossRef] [PubMed]

33. Sederer, L.I. The social determinants of mental health. *Psychiatr. Serv.* **2016**, *67*, 234–235. [CrossRef] [PubMed]

34. Chigbu, C.O.; Parhofer, K.G.; Aniebue, U.U.; Berger, U. Prevalence and sociodemographic determinants of adult obesity: A large representative household survey in a resource-constrained African setting with double burden of undernutrition and overnutrition. *J. Epidemiol. Community Health* **2018**, *72*, 702–707. [CrossRef] [PubMed]

35. Sartorius, B.; Veerman, L.J.; Manyema, M.; Chola, L.; Hofman, K. Determinants of obesity and associated population attributability, South Africa: Empirical evidence from a national panel survey, 2008–2012. *PLoS ONE* **2015**, *10*, e0130218. [CrossRef] [PubMed]
36. Tekalegn, Y.; Engida, Z.T.; Sahiledengle, B.; Rogers, H.L.; Seyoum, K.; Woldeyohannes, D.; Legese, B.; Ayele, T.A. Individual and community-level determinants of overweight and obesity among urban men: Further analysis of the Ethiopian demographic and health survey. *PLoS ONE* **2021**, *16*, e0259412. [CrossRef] [PubMed]
37. Sudikno; Julianti, E.D.; Sari, Y.D.; Sari, Y.P. The Relationship of Physical Activities on Obesity in Adults in Indonesia. In Proceedings of the 4th International Symposium on Health Research (ISHR 2019), Bali, Indonesia, 28–30 November 2019; Atlantis Press: Paris, France, 2020; Volume 22, pp. 96–100.
38. Dewi, N.U.; Tanziha, I.; Solechah, S.A. Bohari Obesity determinants and the policy implications for the prevention and management of obesity in Indonesia. *Curr. Res. Nutr. Food Sci.* **2020**, *8*, 942–955. [CrossRef]
39. Mulia, E.P.B.; Fauzia, K.A. Atika Abdominal Obesity is Associated with Physical Activity Index in Indonesian Middle-Aged Adult Rural Population: A Cross-Sectional Study. *Indian J. Community Med.* **2021**, *46*, 317–320. [CrossRef]
40. Samouda, H.; Ruiz-Castell, M.; Bocquet, V.; Kuemmerle, A.; Chioti, A.; Dadoun, F.; Kandala, N.B.; Stranges, S. Geographical variation of overweight, obesity and related risk factors: Findings from the European Health examination Survey in Luxembourg, 2013–2015. *PLoS ONE* **2018**, *13*, e0197021. [CrossRef]
41. Ramachandran, A.; Chamukuttan, S.; Shetty, S.A.; Arun, N.; Susairaj, P. Obesity in Asia—Is it different from rest of the world. *Diabetes. Metab. Res. Rev.* **2012**, *28*, 47–51. [CrossRef]

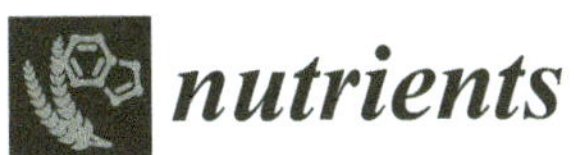

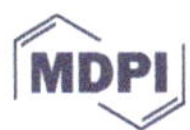

Article

Adverse Effects of Infant Formula Made with Corn-Syrup Solids on the Development of Eating Behaviors in Hispanic Children

Hailey E. Hampson [1,2], Roshonda B. Jones [1], Paige K. Berger [1], Jasmine F. Plows [1], Kelsey A. Schmidt [1], Tanya L. Alderete [3] and Michael I. Goran [1,*]

[1] The Saban Research Institute, Los Angeles, Children's Hospital, Los Angeles, CA 90027, USA; hhampson@usc.edu (H.E.H.); rbarnerjones@gmail.com (R.B.J.); paberger@chla.usc.edu (P.K.B.); jasmineplows@gmail.com (J.F.P.); kelschmidt@chla.usc.edu (K.A.S.)

[2] Department of Epidemiology, University of Southern California, Los Angeles, CA 90007, USA

[3] Department of Integrative Physiology, University of Colorado Boulder, Boulder, CO 80309, USA; tanya.alderete@colorado.edu

* Correspondence: goran@usc.edu

Abstract: Few studies have investigated the influence of infant formulas made with added corn-syrup solids on the development of child eating behaviors. We examined associations of breastmilk (BM), traditional formula (TF), and formula containing corn-syrup solids (CSSF) with changes in eating behaviors over a period of 2 years. Feeding type was assessed at 6 months in 115 mother–infant pairs. Eating behaviors were assessed at 12, 18 and 24 months. Repeated Measures ANCOVA was used to determine changes in eating behaviors over time as a function of feeding type. Food fussiness and enjoyment of food differed between the feeding groups ($p < 0.05$) and changed over time for CSSF and TF ($p < 0.01$). Food fussiness increased from 12 to 18 and 12 to 24 months for CSSF and from 12 to 24 months for TF ($p < 0.01$), while it remained stable for BM. Enjoyment of food decreased from 12 to 24 months for CSSF ($p < 0.01$), while it remained stable for TF and BM. There was an interaction between feeding type and time for food fussiness and enjoyment of food ($p < 0.01$). Our findings suggest that Hispanic infants consuming CSSF may develop greater food fussiness and reduced enjoyment of food in the first 2 years of life compared to BM-fed infants.

Keywords: breastmilk; child eating behavior questionnaire; corn-syrup solids; eating behavior; enjoyment of eating; food fussiness; formula; Hispanic; infant; obesity

Citation: Hampson, H.E.; Jones, R.B.; Berger, P.K.; Plows, J.F.; Schmidt, K.A.; Alderete, T.L.; Goran, M.I. Adverse Effects of Infant Formula Made with Corn-Syrup Solids on the Development of Eating Behaviors in Hispanic Children. *Nutrients* **2022**, *14*, 1115. https://doi.org/10.3390/nu14051115

Academic Editors: Odysseas Androutsos and Evangelia Charmandari

Received: 30 January 2022
Accepted: 4 March 2022
Published: 7 March 2022

Publisher's Note: MDPI stays neutral with regard to jurisdictional claims in published maps and institutional affiliations.

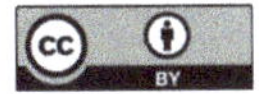

Copyright: © 2022 by the authors. Licensee MDPI, Basel, Switzerland. This article is an open access article distributed under the terms and conditions of the Creative Commons Attribution (CC BY) license (https://creativecommons.org/licenses/by/4.0/).

1. Introduction

Added sugar is widespread in our food system and is characteristic of the Western Style diet. This is a concern as added sugar is associated with obesity development and a wide range of co-morbid conditions [1,2]. Evidence suggests that chronic consumption of added sugar may affect obesity risk as it is consumed in excess and contributes empty calories to the diet [3,4]. However, it is also postulated that early exposure to sugars may indirectly influence obesity risk by shaping taste preferences, self-regulation of energy intake, and the reinforcing value of food [5–9]. These eating behaviors may ultimately lead to an overindulgence of sweet foods and rejection of bitter-tasting alternatives. This is relevant as food manufacturers incorporate sugars in the form of added corn-syrup solids into infant formulas and introductory solids, despite the most recent dietary guidelines recommending zero added sugars in the first 2 years of life [4].

Human studies have shown that the introduction of added sugar in infancy influences eating behavior in childhood. For example, infants fed added sugar before 4 months were more likely to reject bitter and sour-tasting foods in early childhood. These infants were found to be at an increased risk for childhood obesity [5]. Furthermore, infants that are fed formulas with sweet flavors have a lower acceptance of bitter tasting foods, such as broccoli, compared to infants fed formulas with bitter flavors [10]. While the exact biological mechanism has yet to be fully elucidated, animal studies suggest that the gut microbiome may be a key link between early sugar exposure and infant food preferences, leading to later obesity risk [11].

Although several studies have examined the effects of breastfeeding and formula feeding on infant eating behaviors, no study has examined whether infant formula made with corn-syrup solids instead of lactose as the major carbohydrate source may have additional, potentially adverse effects. Various infant formulae have been developed without lactose due to potential concerns of lactose intolerance, some of which use corn syrup solids. Therefore, the aim of this study was to determine associations of breastfeeding, traditional formula, and formula containing corn-syrup solids at 6 months with changes in eating behaviors at and between 12, 18, and 24 months.

2. Materials and Methods

2.1. Study Participants

We obtained data from the Southern California Mother's Milk Study, which is an on-going longitudinal cohort study of Hispanic mother-infant dyads, as reported previously [12]. Briefly, participants were eligible if they (a) self-identify as Hispanic (mother and father), (b) had a singleton birth, (c) intended to breastfeed for at least 3 months, (d) enrolled within 1 month of the infant's birth, and (e) were willing to/had the ability to understand the procedures of the study and be able to read English or Spanish at the fifth-grade level. Participants were not eligible if they (a) had a physician diagnosis of a major medical illness or eating disorder, (b) had a physical, mental or cognitive issue that prevented participation, (c) reported chronic use of medication that may affect body weight or composition, insulin resistance or lipid profiles, (d) were a current smoker or were a user of other recreational drugs, (e) had a pre-term/low birth weight infant or diagnosis of any fetal abnormalities, or (f) were less than 18 years old.

At each study visit, mothers reported health history and information on breastfeeding, which were included as covariates in the analysis [12]. Institutional review boards at the University of Southern California and Children's Hospital Los Angeles approved the study. Written informed consent was obtained from all mothers prior to data collection. Mother–infant pairs were included in the final analysis if they completed all 6, 12, 18 and 24 month visits (Figure 1).

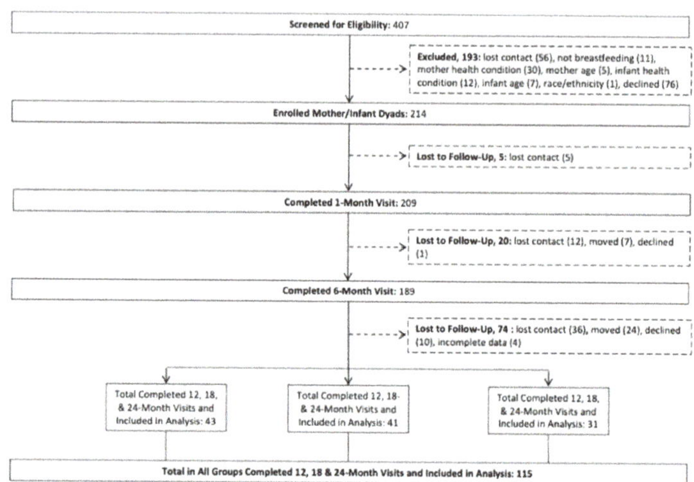

Figure 1. Participation flow chart and distribution of participants to infant feeding type groups.

2.2. Infant Feeding Modality Determination

Two 24 h dietary recalls were conducted with mothers over the phone by trained bilingual research personnel. Dietary intake collection and analysis was performed using the Nutritional Data System for Research software (NDSR) [13]. The NDSR data were used to calculate the infants' breastmilk and formula-type groups. Breastmilk-fed infants were categorized based on predominant consumption type (receiving more than 80% of feedings from breastmilk) at 6 months. Feeding type groups included infants who received primarily human milk directly from the breast or pumped human milk from a bottle (BM, n = 43), infants who received a traditional formula, which was lactose and cow-milk based (TF, n = 41), and infants who received a lactose-reduced formula made with corn syrup solids (CSSF, n = 31), in this case Enfamil Gentlease, Similac Isomil Advance, produced by Mead Johnson & Company, LLC [14,15]. Infants in the TF group received one of the following formulas: Similac Advance 20, Similac Advance EarlyShield, Gerber Good Start Gentle, Enfamil A.R., and Enfamil Infant, made by a variety of formula companies.

2.3. Eating Behavior Assessment

To assess child eating behaviors at 12, 18 and 24 months, we used the Children's Eating Behavior Questionnaire (CEBQ), a maternal report survey tailored to children 12 months of age and older [16–18]. The questionnaire was available in English and Spanish. The CEBQ consists of 35 questions organized into 8 domains, i.e., satiety responsiveness, slowness in eating, emotional under-eating, food fussiness, enjoyment of food, food responsiveness, desire to drink, and emotional over-eating. All questions were ranked on a Likert scale of Never (0) to Always (4), and scores were averaged within domains [16–18].

2.4. Participant Characteristics

We collected anthropometrics and sociodemographic information, including maternal pre-pregnancy BMI (kg/m^2) (determined from height and weight recall prior to pregnancy), infant sex, infant age (days), infant birth weight (kg), mode of delivery (vaginal vs. Caesarean Section), and socioeconomic status index (SES). We determined socioeconomic status using The Hollingshead Index. Students, stay-at-home parents, and unemployed persons do not have assigned employment categories in the Hollingshead Index, therefore, a score of zero was given to these individuals under the assumption they these participants likely to have very little or no income. This was done in order to retain these participants in the analyses.

2.5. Statistical Analysis

Basic descriptive statistics were calculated for infant feeding modality, eating behavior domains, and all covariates included in the analysis. One-Way Analysis of Covariance (ANCOVA) was performed to determine initial differences in covariates between feeding-type groups. Model diagnostics were performed and any variables not meeting assumptions of ANCOVA were transformed using the bestNormalize package in R, which selects the best method to normalize the variable [19]. One-Way ANCOVA was performed at each time point to determine differences in eating behaviors by infant feeding modality. Repeated-Measures ANCOVA was conducted including an interaction term between time (infant age) and infant feeding modality at 6 months, to determine differences in eating behaviors over time as a function of infant feeding modality. For significant between-group differences and interactions, post hoc pairwise comparisons using Tukey's Test were performed. Based on the literature, we adjusted for the following common covariates: maternal pre-pregnancy BMI (kg/m^2), infant breast milk feedings and formula feedings per day (in a ratio variable of breastmilk feedings to formula feedings normalized across all children in the sample), infant sex, infant age (days), infant birth weight (kg), mode of delivery, and socioeconomic status index (SES). We performed reliability testing on CEBQ domain summary scores at all timepoints, 12, 18 and 24 months, using the Psych package in R and an inclusion alpha level of 0.7 [20]. Domains not meeting the significance level 0.7 were removed from analysis. RStudio was used for all analyses using R version 4.0.5 [21]. We performed a sensitivity analysis to determine if results changed when we distinguished between two types of breastmilk feeding. We divided breastmilk-fed infants into two groups, those directly breastfed (BF), and those fed breastmilk pumped in a bottle (PB). We ran all statistical analyses with all four groups, TF, CSSF, BF and PB, and results did not differ from the original analysis. Therefore, we collapsed the BF and PB groups into one breastmilk group (BM).

3. Results

One-hundred and fifteen mother–infant pairs were included in this study. Fifty-six percent of infants were female, and the mean infant birth weight was 3.4 ± 0.4 kg. The mean breastmilk feedings per day at 6 months was 2.7 ± 3.4 and the mean formula feedings per day was 2.9 ± 3.0 while the number of feedings per day was not significantly different between breastfed and formula-fed infants. Initial maternal and infant characteristics were similar across groups (Table 1). Twenty-seven percent of infants were in the CSSF group, 36% in the TF group, and 37% in the BM group. Cronbach's alpha analysis for internal consistency of CEBQ domains suggested that the domains satiety responsiveness (a = 0.61–0.63) and slowness in eating (a = 0.46–0.49) did not have a high enough reliability above a = 0.70. An analysis was not performed on these domains. All other CEBQ domains had an acceptable alpha level above 0.7 (0.71–0.83).

Table 1. Descriptive statistics based on feeding type group at 6 months (n = 115). No significant differences were found in maternal or infant characteristics between groups based on One-Way ANOVA.

Participant Characteristics	Analysis of Variance (Between-Group Differences by Feeding Type at 6 Months)			
	BM *	TF *	CSSF *	*p*-Values
Infant Birth Weight (mean, kg)	3.37	3.42	3.40	0.840
Socioeconomic Status Index	25.40	26.10	27.00	0.850
Infant Sex (% Female)	58%	46%	65%	0.290
Mode of Delivery (%Vaginal)	81%	76%	71%	0.580
Maternal Pre-Pregnancy BMI (mean, kg/m^2)	27.20	29.40	27.50	0.140

* CSSF = Formula with Reduced-Lactose, Added-Corn Syrup Solids, BM = Breastmilk, TF = Traditional Formula.

Food fussiness was significantly different between infant feeding groups ($p = 0.01$). For the CSSF group, food fussiness significant increased from 12 to 18 months (mean increase = 0.51, $p < 0.01$), and 12 to 24 months (mean increase = 0.77, $p < 0.001$) (Figure 2). Food fussiness did not change significantly over time for the other groups. There was a significant interaction between infant feeding modality at 6 months and time (infant age) in months for food fussiness ($p < 0.01$) (Table 2). In post hoc testing, food fussiness was significantly greater in the CSSF group compared to the BM group at 24 months (mean difference = 0.54, $p < 0.05$).

Enjoyment of food was significantly different between infant feeding groups ($p = 0.001$). For the CSSF group, enjoyment of food significantly decreased from 12 to 24 months (mean decrease = 0.60, $p < 0.001$), while it remained constant in the other groups over time (Figure 3). Furthermore, there was a significant interaction between infant feeding modality at 6 months and time (infant age) in months for enjoyment of food ($p = 0.002$) (Table 2).

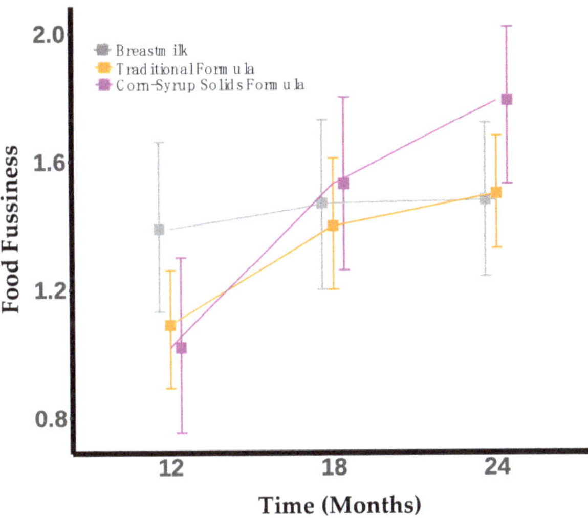

Figure 2. Food Fussiness increases from 12 to 18 months and 18 to 24 months for infants who consumed formula with added corn-syrup solids (CSSF) at 6 months. Food fussiness increases from 12 to 24 months for infants who consume traditional infant formula (TF) at 6 months. The model was adjusted for maternal pre-pregnancy BMI (kg/m^2), infant breast milk feedings per day and formula feedings per day, infant sex, infant birth weight (kg), mode of delivery, and socioeconomic status index (SES).

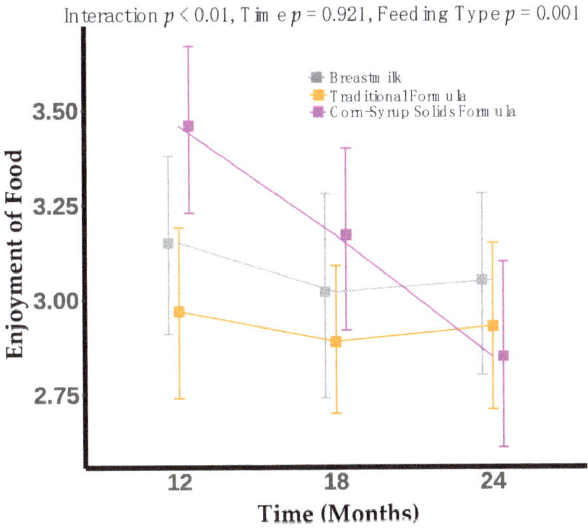

Figure 3. Enjoyment of food decreases from 12 to 24 months for infants who consumed formula with added corn-syrup solids (CSSF) at 6 months. Model adjusted for maternal pre-pregnancy BMI (kg/m^2), infant breast milk feedings per day and formula feedings per day, infant sex, infant birth weight (kg), mode of delivery, and socioeconomic status index (SES).

Table 2. Repeated measures ANCOVA shows that there was a statistically significant interaction between feeding modality and time from 12 to 24 months for food fussiness and enjoyment of food. Model includes the covariates maternal pre-pregnancy BMI (kg/m^2), infant breast milk feedings per day, infant formula feedings per day, infant sex, infant birth weight (kg), mode of delivery, and socioeconomic status index (SES).

Eating Behaviors	Time	Feeding Type	Interaction [a]
Food Responsiveness	0.902	0.727	0.748
Food Fussiness	0.187	0.109	0.004 **
Enjoyment of Food	0.388	0.002 **	0.001 **
Desire to Drink	0.005 **	0.765	0.409
Emotional Undereating	0.732	0.860	0.989
Emotional Overeating	0.391	0.484	0.418

[a] Interaction between Time and Feeding Type. $p < 0.01$ **.

4. Discussion

In this study, we found that the development of child eating behaviors in the first 2 years of life was affected by early exposure to formula made with corn-syrup solids as compared to traditional formula made with lactose and compared to breastmilk. Specifically, early exposure to formula made with corn-syrup solids was associated with increased food fussiness and reduced enjoyment of food over time. In addition, CSSF-fed infants had worsening eating behaviors over time, compared to TF-fed and BM-fed infants. Importantly, the behaviors observed in the CSSF-fed infants have been linked to poor diet quality and variety, which in turn are associated with obesity and related co-morbidities in childhood [7,22,23].

Our findings provide additional insights into the early exposure to corn-syrup solids and infant eating behaviors examined in prior studies. For example, Shepard et al. found that infants fed "gentle" formula containing corn-syrup solids demonstrated consistent eating behaviors from 3 to 5 months, in contrast to our findings that CSSF-fed infants exhibited changes in eating behaviors over a longer period of time [24]. Shepard et al. examined CSSF intake at an earlier period than the present study and included fewer formula type groups, which may explain differences in findings. Because eating behaviors emerge over time, it is plausible that the prior study did not have a long enough duration so as to capture changes in eating behavior as we did. Consistent with our findings, Murray et al. reported that infants who were exposed to sweet, non-milk solids and beverages had decreased bitter food acceptance and increased obesity risk, a trademark of picky eating behavior [5]. Similarly, we found that CSSF-fed infants had a greater increase in food fussiness over time, relative to formula fed infants and breastfed infants. It may be that early exposure to added sugar in the form of corn-syrup solids enhances the infant's affinity for sweet tastes and exacerbates innate disliking of bitter tastes, which may contribute to picky eating [5,7,10].

This hypothesis is supported by work from Mennella and colleagues, who found that infants fed sweet-tasting formula were more likely to reject broccoli than those who had exposure to bitter-tasting formula [10]. Similarly, we found that all feeding groups had a similar degree of food fussiness at 12 months of age. However, we found that there was a greater increase in food fussiness among CSSF-fed infants compared to TF-fed infants, and food fussiness remained stable among BM-fed infants. This suggests that infants exposed to diverse flavors or diminished sweet flavors in breastmilk or traditional formula are more likely to accept wide-ranging foods compared to those exposed to the sweetness of CSSF. These experiences may also influence enjoyment of food among CSSF-fed infants, as picky eating behaviors may reduce overall enjoyment of a diverse diet that comes with the introduction of solid foods [23,25].

While several mechanisms may underlie our findings, a potential explanation that has gathered the most interest is the effects of early sugar exposure on the infant gut microbiome, which may affect appetite regulation through gut-derived hormones [11,12,26–28].

Simple carbohydrates and other dietary factors can serve as energy for a harmful subset of gut microbes, which may ultimately displace beneficial bacteria [26–28]. The increased proportions of harmful microbes therefore receive more energy from the host, which has a strong influence on appetite, metabolism and food-related behaviors [28]. For example, harmful bacteria may ferment added sugar and produce metabolites, primarily short-chain fatty acids, which can directly affect hunger and signaling [27]. Through this mechanism, CSSF-fed infants may have an increased affinity for sweet-tasting foods. As infants are introduced to more solid foods with a range of flavors, they may experience a decreased preference for and enjoyment of food with bitter tastes, contributing to food fussiness [23].

In addition, animal studies have shown that rats with early sugar exposure exhibit addiction-like responses, with an increased affinity for added sugars and symptoms of withdrawal [29]. These patterns are linked to opioid-receptor binding associated with the added sugar intake and neurochemical changes that result in increased dopamine from sugar consumption [29]. Early added corn-syrup exposure from CSSF could program an infant for a heighted dopamine response that is not met with the introduction of bitter foods, thus reducing their enjoyment of food. The potential effects on brain-based eating behaviors may also be exacerbated by displacement of lactose with corn-syrup solids in the CSSF. Decreased exposure to lactose and therefore, galactose, may also have deleterious effects on infant-brain development and subsequent healthy eating behavior in children [12,14,15,30].

This study has several limitations. We used a self-report survey to assess child eating behaviors, which could result in response bias. However, we only used CEBQ domains with high validity. It is possible that the translation of the CEBQ into Spanish may have affected the validity of the questionnaire. Further, this is an observational study, and we cannot make causal conclusions based on our findings. However, our study was longitudinal in nature, which adds a further temporal component to the findings. Another important limitation is that we do not have information on why mothers chose different infant formulas. However, our sample has no significant differences in maternal or infant baseline characteristics between groups, including socioeconomic status, which may be influential for selection of infant formula type. Additionally, one of the infant formulas categorized in the TF group due to its lactose and cow's milk content is Gerber Good Start Gentle. Similar to Enfamil Gentlease in the CSSF group, this product is marketed toward colicky and fussy infants. A systematic review by Belamarich et al. reports that mothers choose these gentle formulas due to the marketing strategies that imply crying and fussiness are indicative of digestive discomfort [31]. This sheds some light on the choices that mothers may be making with regard to formula, however, given that there are gentle formulas included in both groups, we do not suspect that this contributes to, nor fully explains the differences seen in our study. However, maternal beliefs related to formula choice is an important area for further study.

These findings may have important implications for infant feeding recommendations given that early life added corn-syrup exposure may influence taste-preference formation, food rejection with the introduction of solids, and the composition of the infant gut microbiome. Food fussiness and the reduced enjoyment of food may inhibit the acceptance of fruits and vegetables and other healthful foods in the diet, leading to poor diet quality and variety. Importantly, CSSF is only consumed by <10% of infants in the general US population [15]. However, in our cohort of Hispanic mothers, 50% of formula-fed infants consume CSSF. Therefore, the results of this study are highly relevant for this subset of the population that is already at higher risk for obesity and related chronic disease development.

5. Conclusions

These findings suggests that Hispanic infants who receive formula made with corn syrup solids in place of lactose develop poor eating behavior in the first 2 years of life, including greater food fussiness and reduced enjoyment of food, compared to traditional formula-fed and breastmilk-fed infants. Further studies are needed to elucidate the underlying mechanisms by which added corn-syrup solids influence child eating behaviors as well as clinical health outcomes. Our findings provide evidence for future studies exploring the effects of infant formulas with reduced lactose and added corn-syrup solids on children's eating behaviors and growth.

Author Contributions: Conceptualization: M.I.G.; Data curation, M.I.G.; Formal analysis, H.E.H. and R.B.J.; Funding acquisition, M.I.G.; Investigation, M.I.G.; Methodology, R.B.J. and M.I.G.; Project administration, M.I.G.; Resources, M.I.G.; Software, H.E.H. and R.B.J.; Supervision, M.I.G.; Writing—original draft, H.E.H.; Writing—review and editing, P.K.B., J.F.P., K.A.S., T.L.A. and M.I.G. All authors have read and agreed to the published version of the manuscript.

Funding: This research was funded by the National Institute Diabetes and Digestive and Kidney Diseases (R01 DK110793). This work was also funded by the Gerber Foundation (15PN-013). Paige K. Berger is funded by the Eunice Kennedy Shriver National Institute of Child Health & Human Development (K99 HD098288). Tanya L. Alderete is funded by NIEHS (R00ES027853). Jasmine F. Plows is funded through a Saban Research Institute Research Career Development Fellowship.

Institutional Review Board Statement: Institutional review boards at the University of Southern California and Children's Hospital Los Angeles approved the study.

Informed Consent Statement: Written informed consent was obtained from all mothers and financial compensation was provided.

Data Availability Statement: Data described in the manuscript, code book, and analytic code will be made available upon request. Data requests can be made to Michael I. Goran, (323) 217–5116, goran@usc.edu.

Acknowledgments: We would like to thank Carla Flores, Danielle Garcia, Elizabeth Campbell, Claudia Rios, Emily Leibovitch, Rosa Rangel and the entire Goran Lab for their assistance in obtaining these data. We would also like to thank Jennifer Fogel for her editing assistance on the manuscript.

Conflicts of Interest: Goran is a scientific advisor for Yumi and receives book royalties from Penguin Random House. The Gerber Foundation had no role in the design, execution, analyses, interpretation of data, writing of the report, or decision to submit the report for publication.

References

1. Yang, Q.; Zhang, Z.; Gregg, E.W.; Flanders, W.D.; Merritt, R.; Hu, F.B. Added Sugar Intake and Cardiovascular Diseases Mortality Among US Adults. *JAMA Intern. Med.* **2014**, *174*, 516. [CrossRef] [PubMed]
2. Fidler Mis, N.; Braegger, C.; Bronsky, J.; Campoy, C.; Domellöf, M.; Embleton, N.D.; Hojsak, I.; Hulst, J.; Indrio, F.; Lapillonne, A.; et al. Sugar in Infants, Children and Adolescents: A Position Paper of the European Society for Paediatric Gastroenterology, Hepatology and Nutrition Committee on Nutrition. *J. Pediatr. Gastroenterol. Nutr.* **2017**, *65*, 681–696. [CrossRef] [PubMed]
3. Rippe, J.M.; Angelopoulos, T.J. Relationship between Added Sugars Consumption and Chronic Disease Risk Factors: Current Understanding. *Nutrients* **2016**, *8*, 697. [CrossRef] [PubMed]
4. Kong, K.L.; Burgess, B.; Morris, K.S.; Re, T.; Hull, H.R.; Sullivan, D.K.; Paluch, R.A. Association between Added Sugars from Infant Formulas and Rapid Weight Gain in US Infants and Toddlers. *J. Nutr.* **2021**, *151*, 1572–1580. [CrossRef] [PubMed]
5. Murray, R.D. Savoring Sweet: Sugars in Infant and Toddler Feeding. *Ann. Nutr. Metab.* **2017**, *70*, 38–46. [CrossRef]
6. Mennella, J.A.; Bobowski, N.K. The Sweetness and Bitterness of Childhood: Insights from Basic Research on Taste Preferences. *Physiol. Behav.* **2015**, *152*, 502–507. [CrossRef]
7. Mennella, J.A.; Bobowski, N.K.; Reed, D.R. The Development of Sweet Taste: From Biology to Hedonics. *Rev. Endocr. Metab. Disord.* **2016**, *17*, 171–178. [CrossRef]
8. Birch, L.L.; Fisher, J.O. Development of Eating Behaviors among Children and Adolescents. *Pediatrics* **1998**, *101*, 539–549. [CrossRef]
9. Hill, C.; Saxton, J.; Webber, L.; Blundell, J.; Wardle, J. The Relative Reinforcing Value of Food Predicts Weight Gain in a Longitudinal Study of 7–10-y-Old Children. *Am. J. Clin. Nutr.* **2009**, *90*, 276–281. [CrossRef]
10. Mennella, J.A.; Forestell, C.A.; Morgan, L.K.; Beauchamp, G.K. Early Milk Feeding Influences Taste Acceptance and Liking during Infancy12345. *Am. J. Clin. Nutr.* **2009**, *90*, 780S–788S. [CrossRef]
11. Noble, E.E.; Hsu, T.M.; Jones, R.B.; Fodor, A.A.; Goran, M.I.; Kanoski, S.E. Early-Life Sugar Consumption Affects the Rat Microbiome Independently of Obesity. *J. Nutr.* **2017**, *147*, 20–28. [CrossRef]
12. Jones, R.B.; Berger, P.K.; Plows, J.F.; Alderete, T.L.; Millstein, J.; Fogel, J.; Iablokov, S.N.; Rodionov, D.A.; Osterman, A.L.; Bode, L.; et al. Lactose-Reduced Infant Formula with Added Corn Syrup Solids Is Associated with a Distinct Gut Microbiota in Hispanic Infants. *Gut Microbes* **2020**, *12*, 1813534. [CrossRef] [PubMed]

13. Harnack, L. Nutrition Data System for Research (NDSR). In *Encyclopedia of Behavioral Medicine*; Gellman, M.D., Turner, J.R., Eds.; Springer: New York, NY, USA, 2013; pp. 1348–1350. ISBN 978-1-4419-1005-9.
14. EnfamilŴ GentleaseŴ | Mead Johnson Nutrition. Available online: http://www.hcp.meadjohnson.com/products/mild-digestive-issues-products/enfamil-gentlease/ (accessed on 16 July 2021).
15. Rossen, L.M.; Simon, A.E.; Herrick, K.A. Types of Infant Formulas Consumed in the United States. *Clin. Pediatr.* **2016**, *55*, 278–285. [CrossRef] [PubMed]
16. Carnell, S.; Wardle, J. Measuring Behavioural Susceptibility to Obesity: Validation of the Child Eating Behaviour Questionnaire. *Appetite* **2007**, *48*, 104–113. [CrossRef] [PubMed]
17. Wardle, J.; Guthrie, C.A.; Sanderson, S.; Rapoport, L. Development of the Children's Eating Behaviour Questionnaire. *J. Child Psychol. Psychiatry* **2001**, *42*, 963–970. [CrossRef] [PubMed]
18. Child Eating Behaviour Questionnaire (CEBQ). Available online: http://www.midss.ie/content/child-eating-behaviour-questionnaire-cebq (accessed on 9 August 2021).
19. Peterson, R.A. BestNormalize: Normalizing Transformation Functions. 2021. Available online: https://CRAN.R-project.org/package=bestNormalize (accessed on 6 July 2021).
20. Revelle, W. Psych: Procedures for Psychological, Psychometric, and Personality Research. 2021. Available online: https://CRAN.R-project.org/package=psych (accessed on 16 July 2021).
21. The Comprehensive R Archive Network. Available online: https://cran.r-project.org/ (accessed on 14 February 2021).
22. Taylor, C.M.; Emmett, P.M. Picky Eating in Children: Causes and Consequences. *Proc. Nutr. Soc.* **2019**, *78*, 161–169. [CrossRef]
23. Van der Horst, K. Overcoming Picky Eating. Eating Enjoyment as a Central Aspect of Children's Eating Behaviors. *Appetite* **2012**, *58*, 567–574. [CrossRef]
24. Shepard, D.N.; Chandler-Laney, P.C. Prospective Associations of Eating Behaviors with Weight Gain in Infants. *Obesity* **2015**, *23*, 1881–1885. [CrossRef]
25. Mennella, J.; Jagnow, C.; Beauchamp, G. Prenatal and Postnatal Flavor Learning by Human Infants. *Pediatrics* **2001**, *107*, E88. [CrossRef]
26. Di Rienzi, S.C.; Britton, R.A. Adaptation of the Gut Microbiota to Modern Dietary Sugars and Sweeteners. *Adv. Nutr.* **2020**, *11*, 616–629. [CrossRef]
27. Townsend, G.E.; Han, W.; Schwalm, N.D.; Raghavan, V.; Barry, N.A.; Goodman, A.L.; Groisman, E.A. Dietary Sugar Silences a Colonization Factor in a Mammalian Gut Symbiont. *Proc. Natl. Acad. Sci. USA* **2019**, *116*, 233–238. [CrossRef] [PubMed]
28. Van de Wouw, M.; Schellekens, H.; Dinan, T.G.; Cryan, J.F. Microbiota-Gut-Brain Axis: Modulator of Host Metabolism and Appetite. *J. Nutr.* **2017**, *147*, 727–745. [CrossRef] [PubMed]
29. Avena, N.M.; Long, K.A.; Hoebel, B.G. Sugar-Dependent Rats Show Enhanced Responding for Sugar after Abstinence: Evidence of a Sugar Deprivation Effect. *Physiol. Behav.* **2005**, *84*, 359–362. [CrossRef] [PubMed]
30. Coelho, A.I.; Berry, G.T.; Rubio-Gozalbo, M.E. Galactose Metabolism and Health. *Curr. Opin. Clin. Nutr. Metab. Care* **2015**, *18*, 422–427. [CrossRef]
31. Belamarich, P.F.; Bochner, R.E.; Racine, A.D. A Critical Review of the Marketing Claims of Infant Formula Products in the United States. *Clin. Pediatr.* **2016**, *55*, 437–442. [CrossRef]

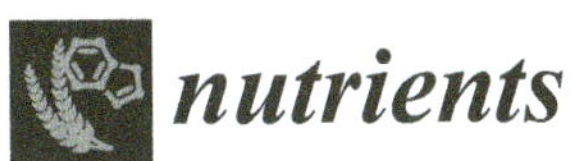

Article

Associations of Caregiver Cooking Skills with Child Dietary Behaviors and Weight Status: Results from the A-CHILD Study

Yukako Tani [1], Aya Isumi [1,2], Satomi Doi [1,2] and Takeo Fujiwara [1,*]

[1] Department of Global Health Promotion, Tokyo Medical and Dental University (TMDU), 1-5-45 Yushima, Bunkyo-ku, Tokyo 113-8519, Japan; tani.hlth@tmd.ac.jp (Y.T.); isumi.hlth@tmd.ac.jp (A.I.); doi.hlth@tmd.ac.jp (S.D.)

[2] Japan Society for the Promotion of Science, Tokyo 113-8519, Japan

[*] Correspondence: fujiwara.hlth@tmd.ac.jp; Tel.: +81-3-5803-5187; Fax: +81-3-5803-5190

Abstract: We examined whether caregiver cooking skills were associated with frequency of home cooking, child dietary behaviors, and child body weight status in Japan. We used cross-sectional data from the 2018 Adachi Child Health Impact of Living Difficulty study, targeting primary and junior high school students aged 9–14 years in Adachi City, Tokyo, Japan ($n = 5257$). Caregiver cooking skills were assessed using a scale with good validity and reliability modified for use in Japan. Child heights and weights derived from school heath checkup data were used to calculate WHO standard body mass index z-scores. After adjusting for potential confounders, caregivers with low-level cooking skills were 4.31 (95% confidence interval (CI): 2.68–6.94) times more likely to have lower frequency of home cooking than those with high level of cooking skills. Children with low-level caregiver cooking skills were 2.81 (95% CI: 2.06–3.84) times more likely to have lower frequency of vegetable intake and 1.74 (95% CI: 1.08–2.82) times more likely to be obese. A low level of caregiver cooking skills was associated with infrequent home cooking, unhealthy child dietary behaviors, and child obesity.

Keywords: cooking skills; home cooking; vegetable intake; obesity; children

Citation: Tani, Y.; Isumi, A.; Doi, S.; Fujiwara, T. Associations of Caregiver Cooking Skills with Child Dietary Behaviors and Weight Status: Results from the A-CHILD Study. *Nutrients* **2021**, *13*, 4549. https://doi.org/10.3390/nu13124549

Academic Editors: Odysseas Androutsos and Evangelia Charmandari

Received: 22 September 2021
Accepted: 13 December 2021
Published: 18 December 2021

Publisher's Note: MDPI stays neutral with regard to jurisdictional claims in published maps and institutional affiliations.

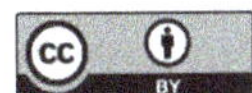

Copyright: © 2021 by the authors. Licensee MDPI, Basel, Switzerland. This article is an open access article distributed under the terms and conditions of the Creative Commons Attribution (CC BY) license (https://creativecommons.org/licenses/by/4.0/).

1. Introduction

In the last 50 years, people in developed countries have shifted toward meals away from home and cooking at home less [1–3]. In the United States, the percentage of daily energy consumed from home food sources dropped by approximately 25% from the 1960s to 2000 [1]. In Japan, household expenditure on precooked food increased by 26% from 1993 to 2015, and eating out is becoming more widespread among younger generations [4]. Alongside the decrease in home cooking, the idea that homemakers, especially women, should be educated to feed their families seems to have become outmoded [5]. However, the obesity epidemic has led to growing concerns about poor diets among children and increasing calls to reaffirm the importance of basic food preparation and cooking skills to prevent poor diets and chronic diet-related diseases [5].

Lifestyle changes in response to the coronavirus disease 2019 (COVID-19) pandemic suddenly increased the need for home cooking. In the United States before and during the initial peak of the COVID-19 pandemic, cooking meals at home increased from 4.49 to 5.18 days per week [6]. Canadian families with young children described that their greatest change since COVID-19 was spending more time cooking [7]. In China, even post-lockdown, 65% of people reported that they cooked more at home compared with the previous year [8]. Meanwhile, the COVID-19 pandemic is leading children toward unfavorable obesity-promoting behaviors, such as decreased physical activity, increased screen time, and greater consumption of snack foods [7,9]. Therefore, caregivers need to acquire the ability to create a healthy eating environment to prevent their child from having a poor diet and becoming obese. However, there is limited knowledge on the relationships between caregiver's ability to prepare meals and their child's diet and weight status.

Recently, evidence has been accumulating on the dietary benefits of home cooking. A systematic review confirmed dietary benefits of home cooking, including greater consumption of healthier food groups, enhanced healthy eating self-efficacy, and improved adherence to several healthy dietary recommendations [10]. Beyond dietary outcomes, a population-based study in the United Kingdom showed that more frequent consumption of home-cooked meals was associated with a greater likelihood of having normal weight and body fat status among adults [11]. Studies on Japanese children and adolescents showed that infrequent home cooking was associated with obesity, higher blood pressure, and lower high-density lipoprotein-cholesterol [12,13].

Cooking skills may be critical to encourage home cooking and improve the quality of meals [10]. Several studies reported that high level of cooking skills was associated with lower consumption of ready meals, convenience food, and ultra-processed food among adults [14–16]. Meanwhile, intervention studies demonstrated that improvement in cooking skills led to increased cooking confidence and consumption of vegetables and fruits [17,18]. A recent population-based study among older Japanese adults showed that a low level of cooking skills was associated with lower frequency of home cooking, vegetable/fruit intake, higher frequency of eating out, and underweight status [19]. However, most existing studies have focused on dietary benefits among adults, and limited research has examined the associations of caregiver cooking skills with child diet and weight status.

The aim of the present study was to examine the associations of caregiver cooking skills with frequency of home cooking, child dietary behaviors, and child body weight status.

2. Materials and Methods

2.1. Study Design and Subjects

The Adachi Child Health Impact of Living Difficulty (A-CHILD) study was established in 2015 to evaluate the determinants of health among children in Adachi City, Tokyo, Japan [20]. We used cross-sectional data from 2018 that covered caregivers and their children in three grades: fourth-grade, sixth-grade, and eighth-grade. The survey was conducted in all public elementary schools for fourth-grade children, nine selected elementary schools for sixth-grade children, and seven junior high schools for eighth-grade children [20]. In 2018, self-reported questionnaires were distributed to 6605 children (5311 fourth-grade, 618 sixth-grade, and 676 eighth-grade). Children and their caregivers completed the questionnaires at home and then returned the completed questionnaires to their school. A total of 5793 pairs (4605 fourth-grade, 556 sixth-grade, and 632 eighth-grade) of children and their caregivers returned the questionnaires (response rate: 88%). Of these, 5382 pairs (4290 fourth-grade, 514 sixth-grade, and 578 eighth-grade) provided informed consent, returned all questionnaires, and could be linked with health checkup data (consent rate: 93%). The present analysis was carried out using data for 5257 pairs, after the following exclusions for missing information: child age (n = 23); caregiver cooking skills and frequency of home cooking (n = 26); child month of birth, height, and weight (n = 10); and child dietary behaviors (frequency of vegetable intake and breakfast consumption) (n = 66). The A-CHILD protocol and use of the data for this study were approved by the Ethics Committee at Tokyo Medical and Dental University (No. M2016-284).

2.2. Frequency of Home Cooking

Frequency of home cooking was evaluated by caregivers using the following question: 'How many times did you or someone else in your family cook meals for your children at home? Circle the answer that best applies for the past month'. A cooked meal was defined as a simple meal, such as a fried egg [12]. The five response items were: 'almost every day', '4–5 days/week', '2–3 days/week', 'a few days/month', and 'rarely'. We defined <3 times a week as low frequency of home cooking because it was reported to be associated with child obesity and cardiovascular risk [12,13].

2.3. Child Body Weight Status

Child height and weight were measured in schools during health checkups by school teachers according to standardized protocols [21]. Height was measured to the nearest 0.1 cm using a portable stadiometer and weight to the nearest 0.1 kg on digital scales, without shoes and in light clothing. Body mass index (BMI) was calculated by dividing the weight (in kilograms) by the square of the height (in meters). BMI was expressed as a z-score representing the deviation in standard deviation units from the mean of a standard normal distribution of BMI specific to age and sex, according to the WHO Child Growth Standards. Child BMI was categorized as underweight (<-2SD), mild-underweight (-2SD to <-1SD), normal (-1SD to $<+1$SD), overweight ($+1$SD to $<+2$SD), and obese ($\geq+2$SD) using standard deviation cut-off points [22].

2.4. Child Dietary Behaviors

Child frequency of vegetable intake was assessed by caregivers using the question 'How often did your child eat vegetable dishes? Circle the answer that best applies for the past month'. The three response items were: 'twice/day', 'once/day', and '<3 times/week'. Respondents who ate vegetables and fruit less than once a day were categorized as having low frequency of vegetable intake. This cutoff point was defined by prevalence to the 10th percentile of the included children (Table 1). Child frequency of breakfast intake for the past month was assessed by self-reporting with responses of 'every day', 'often', and 'rarely/never', with 'rarely/never' defined as breakfast skipping.

Table 1. Characteristics of Japanese school children and their caregivers (n = 5257).

	Total		Caregiver's Cooking Skill		
	n	%	High n = 5010 %	Low n = 247 %	p-Value [a]
Child's status					
Sex					
Boy	2643	50.3	50.2	51.0	0.81
Girl	2614	49.7	49.8	49.0	
Age (year)					
9	1720	32.7	32.9	28.7	0.36
10	2479	47.2	46.9	51.4	
11	216	4.1	4.1	4.0	
12	286	5.4	5.4	6.9	
13	229	4.4	4.5	2.4	
14	327	6.2	6.2	6.5	
Dietary behaviors					
Frequency of vegetable intake					
Twice/day	2141	40.8	41.3	29.2	<0.001
Once/day	2549	48.5	48.8	41.7	
Less than 3 times/weeks (low frequency)	567	10.8	9.8	29.2	
Frequency of breakfast intake					
Everyday	4686	89.1	89.2	87.4	0.06
Often	436	8.3	8.3	7.7	
Rarely/never (breakfast skipping)	135	2.5	2.4	4.8	
Body weight status (BMI for age z score)					
Underweight (<-2SD)	123	2.3	2.3	3.6	0.02
Mild underweight (-2SD-<-1SD)	772	14.7	14.7	15.4	
Normal (-1SD-$<+1$SD)	3356	63.8	64.2	55.9	
Overweight ($+1$SD-$<+2$SD)	716	13.6	13.5	15.8	
Obesity($\geq+2$SD)	290	5.5	5.3	9.3	
Household status					
Cohabitation status					

Table 1. *Cont.*

	Total		Caregiver's Cooking Skill		
	n	%	High *n* = 5010 %	Low *n* = 247 %	*p*-Value [a]
Parents	4143	78.8	79.2	71.3	<0.001
Parents and grandparent (s)	383	7.3	7.2	8.1	
Single parent and grandparent (s)	610	11.6	11.5	13.8	
Single parent	65	1.2	1.1	3.6	
Other	56	1.1	1.0	3.2	
Other children in the household					
No	1017	19.3	18.8	29.6	<0.001
Yes	4240	80.7	81.2	70.4	
Household income (million yen)					
<3.00	559	10.6	10.7	10.1	0.20
3.00–5.99	1575	30.0	29.7	35.2	
6.00–9.99	1756	33.4	33.6	29.6	
≥10.0	591	11.2	11.4	8.5	
Missing	776	14.8	14.7	16.6	
Caregiver's status					
Respondent					
Mother	4768	90.7	92.2	60.7	<0.001
Father	414	7.9	6.5	36.4	
Other	75	1.4	1.4	2.8	
Mother's age (years)					
<35	499	9.5	9.6	7.7	<0.001
35–44	3074	58.5	58.4	60.7	
≥45	1512	28.8	29.0	23.9	
Missing	172	3.3	3.1	7.7	
Father's age (years)					
<35	222	4.2	4.2	4.5	0.87
35–44	2356	44.8	44.7	47.0	
≥45	2014	38.3	38.4	37.2	
Missing	665	12.6	12.7	11.3	
Mother's employment status					
Full-time	1114	21.2	21.0	24.7	0.002
Part-time	2516	47.9	48.2	41.7	
Self-employed	291	5.5	5.6	4.5	
Side work	115	2.2	2.2	2.0	
Not employed	1086	20.7	20.7	20.6	
Other/missing	135	2.6	2.4	6.5	
Mother's BMI					
Underweight (BMI < 18.5)	596	11.3	11.4	10.5	0.06
Normal (18.5 ≤ BMI < 25.0)	3468	66.0	66.3	59.1	
Overweight (25.0 ≤ BMI < 30.0)	529	10.1	9.9	13.0	
Obesity (BMI ≥ 30)	99	1.9	1.8	2.8	
Missing	565	10.7	10.6	14.6	
Father's BMI					
Underweight (BMI < 18.5)	77	1.5	1.4	2.0	0.27
Normal (18.5 ≤ BMI < 25.0)	2793	53.1	53.2	51.0	
Overweight (25.0 ≤ BMI < 30.0)	1125	21.4	21.2	26.3	
Obesity (BMI ≥ 30)	209	4.0	4.0	4.0	
Missing	1053	20.0	20.2	16.6	
Frequency of home cooking					
≥6 days/week	4552	86.6	87.8	61.9	<0.001
4–5 days/week	570	10.8	10.1	25.9	
≤3 days/week (low frequency)	135	2.6	2.1	12.1	

BMI: body mass index. [a] Differences were analyzed using Pearson's chi-square test.

2.5. Caregiver Cooking Skills

Caregiver cooking skills were assessed using a modified cooking skills scale designed with consideration of basic Japanese cooking methods and typical meals [19]. The scale consisted of five items: (1) able to peel fruits and vegetables; (2) able to make stir-fried meat and vegetables; (3) able to make miso soup; (4) able to make stewed dishes; and (5) like to cook. Items 1 to 4 reflected basic cooking methods and were adopted from the Japanese cooking skills score [19]. Item 5 was newly added for the present study as an indicator of cooking skills, because a previous study on life-course trajectories of cooking skills found that liking to cook was a characteristic of people who maintained a high level of cooking skills [23]. Participants were asked to evaluate their own cooking skills on a six-point scale ranging from 'do not agree at all' (=0) to 'agree very much' (=5). A high score meant that the caregiver had high confidence in their cooking skills. In psychometric testing, one factor with eigenvalue >1 was found and accounted for 92.3% of the variance. The Cronbach's α for the cooking skills scale in the study sample was 0.78. Factor loadings ranged from 0.3 (item 5) to 0.9 (item 2). We calculated the mean scores of the five items and divided the results into two categories: high (score > 4.0) and low (score $\leq$ 4.0) as described previously [19].

2.6. Covariates

Child age, cohabitation status (parents, parents and grandparent(s), single parent and grandparent(s), single parent, or other), other children in household (yes or no), household annual income (<3.00, 3.00–5.99, 6.00–9.99, or $\geq$10.0 million Japanese yen), respondent (mother, father, or other), parental age (<35, 35–44, or $\geq$45 years), mother's employment status (full-time, part-time, self-employed, side work, not employed, or other), and parental height and weight were assessed via the caregiver report. Parental BMI was calculated using self-reported height in centimeters and weight in kilograms. Standard categories of BMI were used to characterize parents as underweight ($<18.5 \text{ kg/m}^2$), normal (18.5–24.9 kg/m^2), overweight (25.0–29.9 kg/m^2), or obese ($\geq30.0 \text{ kg/m}^2$) [24]. Participants with missing data on covariates were included in the analysis as dummy variables.

2.7. Statistical Analysis

First, participants were stratified by level of cooking skills, and differences between groups were analyzed using Pearson's chi-square test. Second, multiple comparisons for the cooking skills scale were performed using a mixed linear model procedure to examine which cooking skills participants rated as difficult. The peeling scale used as a reference and the participant identification code was included as a random effect. Third, multiple comparisons between respondents (mother, father, and other) were analyzed using Dunnett's pairwise comparison method with mother as the reference category. Fourth, we calculated adjusted odds ratios (ORs) with 95% confidence intervals (CIs) for low frequency of home cooking, child low frequency of vegetable intake, and child breakfast skipping using logistic regression. Fifth, we calculated adjusted relative risk ratios with 95% CIs for underweight, mild-underweight, overweight, and obese using multinomial logistic regression, with normal as the reference category. The models were adjusted for potential confounding factors that were associated with level of cooking skills in the first analysis. Finally, we conducted a mediation analysis to determine the proportion of the association between caregiver cooking skills and child weight status mediated by frequency of home cooking. We estimated the natural direct effects, controlled direct effects, and natural indirect effects of mediators after controlling for all covariates using the Paramed package in Stata [25]. The exposure was treated as a binary variable, with 0 representing a high level of caregiver cooking skills and 1 representing a low level of caregiver cooking skills. The mediators and outcomes were treated as continuous variables. Because the association between caregiver cooking skills and child weight status was U-shaped, the mild-underweight and underweight children were excluded from the mediation analysis of the relationship with child obesity. All analyses were conducted using Stata Version 15 (Stata Statistical Software; StataCorp LP, College Station, TX, USA).

3. Results

The characteristics of the children and caregivers are summarized in Table 1. Half of the children were girls, about 80% were fourth-grade and lived with their parents, 81% had siblings, and 11% had families with annual incomes below 3.00 million yen. A total of 10.8% ate vegetable dishes less than three times a week, 2.5% were breakfast skippers, 2.3% were underweight, and 5.5% were obese. The majority of the caregiver respondents were mothers (91%); 8% were fathers. The most common mother's employment status was part-time (48%), followed by full-time (21%). A total of 2.6% of households cooked less than three times a week. Approximately 5% of caregivers (n = 247) were classified as having a low level of cooking skills. Children who had caregivers with a low level of cooking skills tended to live with grandparent(s), have no other children in the household, have father respondents, and have full-time working mothers (Table 1).

The mean score for caregiver cooking skills was 5.5 points among all participants (Table 2). The mean caregiver cooking skills score was lower for fathers (5.0 points) than for mothers (5.5 points). For each item in the cooking skills scale, mother scored higher than father, except for 'like to cook' (item 5). Compared with mothers, other respondents gave higher scores for the item of 'like to cook'. Among the four cooking methods, fathers and other respondents rated stewing as more difficult than peeling, while mothers rated all methods as being of similar difficulty, although they had significant differences among the four methods (Table 2). 'Like to cook' was correlated with other cooking methods (r = 0.20–0.26, p < 0.0001), and especially highly correlated among fathers (r = 0.47–0.51, p < 0.0001) (Supplementary Table S1).

A low level of caregiver cooking skills was associated with low frequency of home cooking and child low frequency of vegetable intake (Table 3). After adjusting for potential confounders, caregivers with low-level cooking skills were 4.31 (95% CI: 2.68–6.94) times more likely to have lower frequency of home cooking than those with high level of cooking skills. Children with low level of caregiver cooking skills were 2.81 (95% CI: 2.06–3.84) times more likely to have low frequency of vegetable intake. Low level of caregiver cooking skills was not significantly associated with child breakfast skipping (AOR = 1.61, 95% CI: 0.97–3.53).

A U-shaped association was found between caregiver cooking skills and child weight status (Table 4). Children with low level of caregiver cooking skills were 1.74 (95% CI: 1.08–2.82) times more likely to be obese and 1.84 (95% CI: 0.88–3.83) times more likely to be underweight, although the association with underweight status was not statistically significant. The mediation analysis showed that 91% of the association between low level of caregiver cooking skills and child obesity was mediated by frequency of home cooking.

Table 2. Cooking skills scale scores of Japanese caregivers ($n = 5257$).

Items	All $n = 5257$				Mother $n = 4768$				Respondent Father $n = 414$					Other $n = 75$				
	Mean	SD	Coefficient	*p*-Value	Mean	SD	Coefficient	*p*-Value	Mean	SD		Coefficient	*p*-Value	Mean	SD		Coefficient	*p*-Value
Able to peel fruits and vegetables	5.78	0.69	reference		5.82	0.61	reference		5.32	1.20	***	reference		5.75	0.77		reference	
Able to make stir-fried meat and vegetables	5.81	0.67	0.03	0.03	5.85	0.56	0.04	0.007	5.31	1.28	***	−0.01	0.88	5.60	1.09	**	−0.15	0.24
Able to make miso soup	5.78	0.75	0.01	0.61	5.85	0.60	0.03	0.03	5.11	1.50	***	−0.21	0.001	5.49	1.13	***	−0.25	0.04
Able to make stewed dishes	5.64	0.95	−0.14	<0.001	5.73	0.77	−0.09	<0.001	4.59	1.79	***	−0.73	<0.001	5.36	1.36	**	−0.39	<0.001
Like to cook	4.45	1.32	−1.33	<0.001	4.44	1.30	−1.38	<0.001	4.49	1.46		−0.83	<0.001	4.96	1.18	**	−0.79	<0.001
Cooking skill scale	5.49	0.66			5.54	0.57			4.96	1.20	***			5.43	0.89			

Multiple comparisons between items on the cooking skills scale were analyzed using a mixed linear model procedure. Participant identification code was included as a random effect. Multiple comparisons between respondents were analyzed using Dunnett's pairwise comparison method. ** $p < 0.01$, *** $p < 0.001$, versus mother.

Table 3. Adjusted odds ratios of low frequency of home cooking, child low frequency of vegetable intake, and child breakfast skipping according to levels of caregiver cooking skills (*n* = 5257).

	Caregiver's Low Frequency of Home Cooking	Child's Low Frequency of Vegetable Intake	Child's Breakfast Skipping
	AOR (95% CI)	AOR (95% CI)	AOR (95% CI)
Caregiver's cooking skill			
High	ref	ref	ref
Low	4.31 (2.68–6.94)	2.81 (2.06–3.84)	1.61 (0.97–3.53)

AOR, adjusted odds ratio; CI, confidence interval. The models were adjusted for cohabitation status, siblings, respondent, mother's age, and mother's employment status.

Table 4. Adjusted relative risk ratios of child obese, overweight, mild-underweight, and underweight status according to levels of caregiver cooking skills (*n* = 5257).

	Child's Weight Status (Reference = Normal Weight (−1SD-<+1SD))			
	Obesity (≥+2SD)	Overweight (+1SD-< +2SD)	Mild Underweight (−2SD-< −1SD)	Underweight (<−2SD)
	ARRR (95% CI)	ARRR (95% CI)	ARRR (95% CI)	ARRR (95% CI)
Caregiver's cooking skill				
High	ref	ref	ref	ref
Low	1.74 (1.08–2.82)	1.24 (0.85–1.82)	1.26 (0.86–1.84)	1.84 (0.88–3.83)

ARRR, adjusted relative risk ratio; CI, confidence interval. The models were adjusted for cohabitation status, siblings, respondent, mother's age, and mother's employment status.

4. Discussion

To the best of our knowledge, this is the first study to investigate the associations between caregiver cooking skills and weight status of school children. Using a modified version of the existing cooking skills scale for use in the Japanese population, we found that a low level of caregiver cooking skills was associated with low frequency of home cooking and low frequency of vegetable intake in the child. Regarding child weight status, a U-shaped relationship was observed and a significant association was found between a low level of caregiver cooking skills and child obesity.

A low level of caregiver cooking skills was positively associated with child obesity and most of this association was explained by the frequency of home cooking. These findings are consistent with a previous study showing that infrequent home cooking was associated with child obese status [12]. A systematic review confirmed dietary benefits of home cooking, including greater consumption of healthier food groups, although most of the included studies involved adults [10]. In a study on child diets, home cooking was associated with higher vegetable consumption among children in the United Kingdom [26]. Consistent with that study, we also found that low level of caregiver cooking skills was associated with child low frequency of vegetable consumption.

A U-shaped relationship was observed, which indicates that low level of caregiver cooking skills also tended to be associated with child underweight status. This finding is consistent with a study on older Japanese adults showing that low level of cooking skills can lead to under-nutrition [19]. Children have difficulty preparing their own meals, and therefore their meals depend on their caregivers. Thus, low cooking frequency arising from low level of caregiver cooking skills may mean that children skip meals or eat low-energy diets, leading to them becoming underweight. To test this hypothesis, future studies are warranted to conduct more detailed dietary surveys on the frequency of children eating out.

A low level of caregiver cooking skills was associated with low frequency of home cooking. This finding is consistent with the previous study among older Japanese adults [19]. However, this result may be underestimated because there may have been more than one person in charge of cooking at home, such as the mother, father, grandmother, and older siblings, or a person different from the respondent may be the main cook. Furthermore, low level of caregiver cooking skills was not significantly associated with child breakfast skipping. One possible reason is that breakfast is generally a simple meal in Japan [27], and thus does not require a high level of cooking skills. Otherwise, it may be due to the child's lack of time or appetite.

The validity of the cooking skills scale needs careful consideration. In the present study, mothers who tended to prepare food scored significantly higher on the cooking skills scale than fathers who were less likely to prepare food. This suggests that the modified version of the cooking skills scale used in the study had notable discriminant validity. The observed sex difference is consistent with previous findings on confidence regarding cooking skills, in which women were found to be more confident in their cooking skills than men [15,28,29]. We included four basic cooking methods in the cooking skills scale. Consistent with the previous study among older Japanese adults [19], fathers rated stewing as more difficult than peeling and boiling. Compared with the results for the Japanese older adults in the previous study, middle-aged women (mothers in the present study) scored almost the same as older women, while middle-aged men (fathers in the present study) tended to score higher than older men [19]. This generation difference among men may be explained by opportunities to learn cooking skills in school. In Japan, cooking education in schools for men started in 1947 and became compulsory in 1989 [30]. Therefore, older men had less opportunity to learn cooking in school.

We confirmed that 'like to cook' was correlated with other cooking methods, and especially highly correlated among fathers. This is plausible because women need to cook regardless of whether they like it because of the social norm [10], and as a result, their cooking skills will improve. We further confirmed that 'like to cook' was important for prevent low frequency of home cooking. As a result of analyzing the association between the single item 'like to cook' and the frequency of home cooking, caregivers with low level of liking to cook (score $\leq$ 4.0) were 2.21 (95% CI: 1.52–3.19) times more likely to have lower frequency of home cooking than those with high level of liking to cook (score > 4.0) after adjusting for potential confounders (data not shown). Given the importance of liking to cook for maintenance of a high level of cooking skills during the life course [23], it may be critical to examine subjects for liking to cook when examining the associations of cooking with diet-related outcomes.

There are some limitations to the present study. First, child frequency of vegetable dish intake was assessed using a single simple item. Future studies should use more detailed validated questions to assess which food groups and nutrients are associated with cooking skills. Second, we were only able to evaluate a limited number of child eating behaviors. Future studies are warranted to investigate the relationships between caregiver cooking skills and other aspects of child diets, such as amounts of energy and foods other than vegetables consumed, to understand the mechanisms. Third, we observed a ceiling effect for caregiver cooking skills, especially among mothers, similar to the findings in previous studies using the original cooking skills scale [15,19]. Given that mothers are often working, it may be useful to investigate not only their cooking methods (such as stewing), but also their ability to cook well in a short amount of time. In addition, more comprehensive validated measures are now available for assessing confidence in food and cooking skills in United Kingdom populations [31]. Therefore, it may be possible to use these measurement methods in the future. Fourth, the generalizability of the results may be low because our sample of school children was located in only one city in Japan. Fifth, we lacked data on some potentially confounding factors, such as caregivers' nutritional knowledge and food preference. There may be a much more dynamic association between child obesity, caregiver cooking skills, and their liking for cooking. Finally, we were unable to assess causality because this was a cross-sectional study. However, in a previous study that examined the acquisition of cooking skills, more than half of the respondents reported that they had learned most of their cooking skills when they were teenagers and that these cooking skills were mainly taught by their mothers [32]. Randomized controlled trials in the younger generation before having children are needed in the future to clarify the effectiveness of caregiver's ability to prepare meals for preventing obesity in children.

We found that a low level of caregiver cooking skills was associated with low frequency of home cooking, low frequency of child vegetable intake, and child obese status. Most of the association between low level of caregiver cooking skills and child obesity was mediated by the frequency of home cooking. The present findings are important for preventing unhealthy eating behaviors and obesity because COVID-19 is increasing the demand for home cooking. In addition, poor caregiver cooking skills can cause not only obesity in children but also less opportunity to learn cooking skills from caregivers, which may have an impact on the next generation (i.e., grandchildren of the current parents) due to the poor cooking skills of the children when they become parents [32]. In the future, it is necessary to clarify the causal relationships and promote research on support to improve caregiver cooking skills.

Supplementary Materials: The following is available online at https://www.mdpi.com/article/10.3 390/nu13124549/s1, Table S1: Spearman correlation coefficients for items on the cooking skills scale.

Author Contributions: Conceptualization, Y.T. and T.F.; Data Curation, Y.T. and T.F.; Methodology, Y.T.; Formal Analysis, Y.T.; Investigation, Y.T., T.F., A.I. and S.D.; Writing—Original Draft Preparation, Y.T.; Writing—Review & Editing, T.F.; Supervision, T.F., A.I. and S.D.; Project Administration, Y.T.; Funding Acquisition, Y.T. and T.F. All authors have read and agreed to the published version of the manuscript.

Funding: This research was funded by Grants-in-Aid for Scientific Research from the Japan Society for the Promotion of Science (JSPS KAKENHI) grant number 16H03276, 16K21669, 17J05974, 19H04879, 19K20109, 19K19309, 19K14029, 19J01614, 19K14172, 20K13945 and 21H04848.

Institutional Review Board Statement: The study was conducted according to the guidelines of the Declaration of Helsinki, and approved by the Ethics Committee of Tokyo Medical and Dental University (No. M2016-284).

Informed Consent Statement: Informed consent was obtained from all subjects involved in the study.

Data Availability Statement: The data presented in this study are available on request from the corresponding author.

Acknowledgments: We are especially grateful to the central office Adachi City Hall and its staff members for conducting the survey. We would also like to thank everyone who participated in the survey. Additionally, we would particularly like to thank Yayoi Kondo, Syuichiro Akiu, and Yuko Baba from Adachi City Hall, who contributed significantly to the completion of this study.

Conflicts of Interest: The authors declare no conflict of interest.

References

1. Smith, L.P.; Ng, S.W.; Popkin, B.M. Trends in US home food preparation and consumption: Analysis of national nutrition surveys and time use studies from 1965–1966 to 2007–2008. *Nutr. J.* **2013**, *12*, 45. [CrossRef]
2. Moser, A. Food preparation patterns in German family households. An econometric approach with time budget data. *Appetite* **2010**, *55*, 99–107. [CrossRef] [PubMed]
3. Nielsen, S.J.; Siega-Riz, A.M.; Popkin, B.M. Trends in food locations and sources among adolescents and young adults. *Prev. Med.* **2002**, *35*, 107–113. [CrossRef] [PubMed]
4. Statistics Bureau Ministry of Internal Affairs and Communications. Family Income and Expenditure Survey. Available online: http://www.stat.go.jp/data/kakei/longtime/ (accessed on 13 June 2020).
5. Lichtenstein, A.H.; Ludwig, D.S. Bring back home economics education. *JAMA* **2010**, *303*, 1857–1858. [CrossRef] [PubMed]
6. Flanagan, E.W.; Beyl, R.A.; Fearnbach, S.N.; Altazan, A.D.; Martin, C.K.; Redman, L.M. The Impact of COVID-19 Stay-At-Home Orders on Health Behaviors in Adults. *Obesity* **2020**. [CrossRef] [PubMed]
7. Carroll, N.; Sadowski, A.; Laila, A.; Hruska, V.; Nixon, M.; Ma, D.W.L.; Haines, J.; On Behalf Of The Guelph Family Health Study. The Impact of COVID-19 on Health Behavior, Stress, Financial and Food Security among Middle to High Income Canadian Families with Young Children. *Nutrients* **2020**, *12*, 2352. [CrossRef] [PubMed]

8.   Zhang, J.; Zhao, A.; Ke, Y.; Huo, S.; Ma, Y.; Zhang, Y.; Ren, Z.; Li, Z.; Liu, K. Dietary Behaviors in the Post-Lockdown Period and Its Effects on Dietary Diversity: The Second Stage of a Nutrition Survey in a Longitudinal Chinese Study in the COVID-19 Era. *Nutrients* **2020**, *12*, 3269. [CrossRef] [PubMed]
9.   Pietrobelli, A.; Pecoraro, L.; Ferruzzi, A.; Heo, M.; Faith, M.; Zoller, T.; Antoniazzi, F.; Piacentini, G.; Fearnbach, S.N.; Heymsfield, S.B. Effects of COVID-19 Lockdown on Lifestyle Behaviors in Children with Obesity Living in Verona, Italy: A Longitudinal Study. *Obesity* **2020**, *28*, 1382–1385. [CrossRef] [PubMed]
10.   Mills, S.; White, M.; Brown, H.; Wrieden, W.; Kwasnicka, D.; Halligan, J.; Robalino, S.; Adams, J. Health and social determinants and outcomes of home cooking: A systematic review of observational studies. *Appetite* **2017**, *111*, 116–134. [CrossRef] [PubMed]
11.   Mills, S.; Brown, H.; Wrieden, W.; White, M.; Adams, J. Frequency of eating home cooked meals and potential benefits for diet and health: Cross-sectional analysis of a population-based cohort study. *Int. J. Behav. Nutr. Phys. Act.* **2017**, *14*, 109. [CrossRef]
12.   Tani, Y.; Fujiwara, T.; Doi, S.; Isumi, A. Home Cooking and Child Obesity in Japan: Results from the A-CHILD Study. *Nutrients* **2019**, *11*, 2859. [CrossRef] [PubMed]
13.   Tani, Y.; Fujiwara, T.; Isumi, A.; Doi, S. Home Cooking Is Related to Potential Reduction in Cardiovascular Disease Risk among Adolescents: Results from the A-CHILD Study. *Nutrients* **2020**, *12*, 3845. [CrossRef] [PubMed]
14.   Van der Horst, K.; Brunner, T.A.; Siegrist, M. Ready-meal consumption: Associations with weight status and cooking skills. *Public Health Nutr.* **2011**, *14*, 239–245. [CrossRef] [PubMed]
15.   Hartmann, C.; Dohle, S.; Siegrist, M. Importance of cooking skills for balanced food choices. *Appetite* **2013**, *65*, 125–131. [CrossRef] [PubMed]
16.   Lam, M.C.L.; Adams, J. Association between home food preparation skills and behaviour, and consumption of ultra-processed foods: Cross-sectional analysis of the UK National Diet and nutrition survey (2008–2009). *Int. J. Behav. Nutr. Phys. Act.* **2017**, *14*, 68. [CrossRef] [PubMed]
17.   Flego, A.; Herbert, J.; Waters, E.; Gibbs, L.; Swinburn, B.; Reynolds, J.; Moodie, M. Jamie's Ministry of Food: Quasi-experimental evaluation of immediate and sustained impacts of a cooking skills program in Australia. *PLoS ONE* **2014**, *9*, e114673. [CrossRef]
18.   Reicks, M.; Kocher, M.; Reeder, J. Impact of Cooking and Home Food Preparation Interventions Among Adults: A Systematic Review (2011–2016). *J. Nutr. Educ. Behav.* **2018**, *50*, 148–172.e141. [CrossRef] [PubMed]
19.   Tani, Y.; Fujiwara, T.; Kondo, K. Cooking skills related to potential benefits for dietary behaviors and weight status among older Japanese men and women: A cross-sectional study from the JAGES. *Int. J. Behav. Nutr. Phys. Act.* **2020**, *17*, 82. [CrossRef] [PubMed]
20.   Ochi, M.; Isumi, A.; Kato, T.; Doi, S.; Fujiwara, T. Adachi Child Health Impact of Living Difficulty (A-CHILD) study: Research protocol and profiles of participants. *J. Epidemiol.* **2020**, *31*, 77–89. [CrossRef] [PubMed]
21.   Education and Science in Ministry of Sports and Youth Bureau of School Health Education. *Children's Health Diagnostic Manual (Revised Edition)*; Japanese Society of School Health: Tokyo, Japan, 2006. (In Japanese)
22.   De Onis, M.; Onyango, A.W.; Borghi, E.; Siyam, A.; Nishida, C.; Siekmann, J. Development of a WHO growth reference for school-aged children and adolescents. *Bull. World Health Organ.* **2007**, *85*, 660–667. [CrossRef]
23.   Bostic, S.M.; McClain, A.C. Older adults' cooking trajectories: Shifting skills and strategies. *Br. Food J.* **2017**, *119*, 1102–1115. [CrossRef]
24.   WHO. *Obesity: Preventing and Managing the Global Epidemic*; WHO: Geneva, Switzerland, 2000.
25.   Emsley, R.; Liu, H. PARAMED: Stata Module to Perform Causal Mediation Analysis Using Parametric Regression Models. Available online: https://ideas.repec.org/c/boc/bocode/s457581.html. (accessed on 10 November 2020).
26.   Sweetman, C.; McGowan, L.; Croker, H.; Cooke, L. Characteristics of family mealtimes affecting children's vegetable consumption and liking. *J. Am. Diet. Assoc.* **2011**, *111*, 269–273. [CrossRef] [PubMed]
27.   Sakai, E.; Kitagawa, C.; Morioka, A.; Kanehara, A.; Enomoto, M. Associations among Parents' Levels of Food Awareness and Their Children's Breakfast Patterns and Lifestyles. *Bull. Fac. Psychol. Phys. Sci.* **2018**, *14*, 41–51.
28.   Caraher, M.; Dixon, P.; Lang, T.; Carr, R. The state of cooking in England: The relationship of cooking skills to food choice. *Br. Food J.* **1999**, *101*, 590–609. [CrossRef]
29.   Adams, J.; Goffe, L.; Adamson, A.J.; Halligan, J.; O'Brien, N.; Purves, R.; Stead, M.; Stocken, D.; White, M. Prevalence and socio-demographic correlates of cooking skills in UK adults: Cross-sectional analysis of data from the UK National Diet and Nutrition Survey. *Int. J. Behav. Nutr. Phys. Act.* **2015**, *12*, 99. [CrossRef] [PubMed]
30.   Nishikawa, Y.; Ohuchi, H.; Suzuki, M.; Ohmura, N. The future of cooking practice in home economics. *Bull. Coll. Educ. Ibaraki Univ. Educ. Sci.* **2008**, *57*, 117–128.
31.   Lavelle, F.; McGowan, L.; Hollywood, L.; Surgenor, D.; McCloat, A.; Mooney, E.; Caraher, M.; Raats, M.; Dean, M. The development and validation of measures to assess cooking skills and food skills. *Int. J. Behav. Nutr. Phys. Act.* **2017**, *14*, 118. [CrossRef] [PubMed]
32.   Lavelle, F.; Spence, M.; Hollywood, L.; McGowan, L.; Surgenor, D.; McCloat, A.; Mooney, E.; Caraher, M.; Raats, M.; Dean, M. Learning cooking skills at different ages: A cross-sectional study. *Int. J. Behav. Nutr. Phys. Act.* **2016**, *13*, 119. [CrossRef] [PubMed]

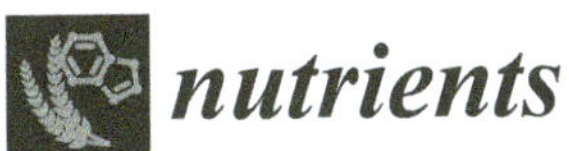

nutrients

MDPI

Article

The Effect of a Multidisciplinary Lifestyle Intervention on Health Parameters in Children versus Adolescents with Severe Obesity

Kelly G. H. van de Pas [1,2,3,*], Judith W. Lubrecht [1,3], Marijn L. Hesselink [1,3], Bjorn Winkens [4], François M. H. van Dielen [2] and Anita C. E. Vreugdenhil [1,3]

[1] Centre for Overweight Adolescent and Children's Healthcare (COACH), Department of Paediatrics, Maastricht University Medical Centre, 6229 HX Maastricht, The Netherlands; judith.lubrecht@mumc.nl (J.W.L.); marijn.hesselink@mumc.nl (M.L.H.); a.vreugdenhil@mumc.nl (A.C.E.V.)

[2] Department of Surgery, Máxima Medical Center, 5504 DB Veldhoven, The Netherlands; f.vandielen@mmc.nl

[3] School of Nutrition and Translational Research in Metabolism (NUTRIM), Maastricht University, 6229 ER Maastricht, The Netherlands

[4] Department of Methodology and Statistics, Care and Public Health Research Institute (CAPHRI), Maastricht University, 6229 ER Maastricht, The Netherlands; bjorn.winkens@maastrichtuniversity.nl

[*] Correspondence: kelly.vande.pas@mumc.nl; Tel.: +31-43-3876543

Citation: van de Pas, K.G.H.; Lubrecht, J.W.; Hesselink, M.L.; Winkens, B.; van Dielen, F.M.H.; Vreugdenhil, A.C.E. The Effect of a Multidisciplinary Lifestyle Intervention on Health Parameters in Children versus Adolescents with Severe Obesity. *Nutrients* **2022**, *14*, 1795. https://doi.org/10.3390/nu14091795

Academic Editors: Odysseas Androutsos and Evangelia Charmandari

Received: 24 March 2022
Accepted: 22 April 2022
Published: 25 April 2022

Publisher's Note: MDPI stays neutral with regard to jurisdictional claims in published maps and institutional affiliations.

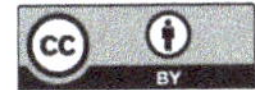

Copyright: © 2022 by the authors. Licensee MDPI, Basel, Switzerland. This article is an open access article distributed under the terms and conditions of the Creative Commons Attribution (CC BY) license (https://creativecommons.org/licenses/by/4.0/).

Abstract: Lifestyle interventions are the common treatment for children and adolescents with severe obesity. The efficacy of these interventions across age groups remain unknown. Therefore, this study aimed to compare the effectiveness of a lifestyle intervention on health parameters between children and adolescents with severe obesity. A longitudinal design was carried out at the Centre for Overweight Adolescent and Children's Healthcare (COACH) between December 2010 and June 2020. Children (2–11 years old, n = 83) and adolescents (12–18 years old, n = 77) with severe obesity received a long-term, tailored, multidisciplinary lifestyle intervention. After 1 year, 24 children (28.9%) and 33 adolescents (42.9%) dropped out of the intervention. The primary outcome was the change in body mass index (BMI) z-score after one and two years of intervention. The decrease in BMI z-score over time was significantly higher in children compared to adolescents, the mean decrease was 0.15 (0.08–0.23) versus 0.03 (−0.05–0.11) after one year and 0.25 (0.15–0.35) versus 0.06 (−0.06–0.17) after two years of intervention; *p* values for the difference between children and adolescents were 0.035 and 0.012. After two years, multiple improvements in cardio metabolic health parameters were observed, especially in children. In conclusion, during our tailored lifestyle intervention, a positive and maintained effect on health parameters was observed in children with severe obesity. Compared to children, the effect on health parameters was less pronounced in adolescents.

Keywords: multidisciplinary lifestyle intervention; children; adolescents; severe obesity

1. Introduction

Childhood obesity is a global health crisis that is recognized by the World Health Organization [1]. In 2016, 124 million children and adolescents were affected by obesity [2]. Despite the continuous efforts that are being made to reduce the prevalence of childhood obesity, there is a growing concern about the rapidly growing rates of severe obesity in children and adolescents [3–6]. In particular, the severe grade of obesity is worrisome, since children and adolescents with severe obesity have an increased cardiovascular risk compared to those with obesity [7,8]. As a consequence of this, adolescents with severe obesity have an elevated risk for the development of a fatal cardiac event later in life [9].

Multidisciplinary lifestyle intervention programs that focus on nutrition, physical activity, and behavioral change are the most frequently applied treatment options for children and adolescents with severe obesity. The Centre for Overweight Adolescent and Children's Healthcare (COACH) offers such a lifestyle intervention program that was proven to be successful in reducing health risks in children with overweight, obesity, and severe obesity, all to a similar degree [10].

Research on multidisciplinary lifestyle interventions for children and adolescents with severe obesity is limited, with only a handful of studies examining this specific group [10–17]. A previous study reported a beneficial effect of treatment in children, but almost no effect at group level in adolescents with severe obesity [11]. A similar pattern was found by Danielsson et al., who reported that in 58% of the children with severe obesity (6–9 years old), the body mass index (BMI) z-score reduced at least 0.5 units during a three-year intervention, compared to only 2% of the adolescents (14–16 years old) [12]. Possible reasons for the limited response of adolescents to lifestyle interventions are the suggested decline in parental influence during adolescence and the reduced adherence to these interventions as age increases [18,19].

To date, there is a lack of long-term data comparing the effects of lifestyle interventions between children and adolescents with severe obesity focusing on weight loss and cardio metabolic health parameters. Therefore, this study aimed to compare the effectiveness of the COACH lifestyle intervention on weight loss and cardio metabolic health parameters between children and adolescents with severe obesity after one and two years of intervention. It was hypothesized that the COACH lifestyle intervention would result in significantly greater reductions in BMI z-score and improvements of cardio metabolic health parameters in children compared to adolescents.

2. Materials and Methods

2.1. Study Design and Population

This study was designed and conducted within COACH at the Maastricht University Medical Centre (MUMC+). A longitudinal design was used to compare the effectiveness of the COACH program between children and adolescents with severe obesity. The study was conducted according to the Declaration of Helsinki, and it was approved by the medical ethical committee of the MUMC+. It is registered at ClinicalTrial.gov as NCT02091544.

All children and adolescents with severe obesity who participated in the COACH program were eligible for inclusion in this study. Severe obesity was defined according to the International Obesity Task Force (IOTF) criteria and is comparable to a BMI $\geq$ 35 in adults [20]. Children were identified as participants aged 2–11 years of age at baseline, whilst adolescents were classified as those aged 12–18 years [21,22]. The age distribution is based on the transition from primary to secondary school, as it is known that this transition is a major life event and many changes occur during this period [23]. Children and adolescents with available anthropometric data after one year of intervention were included. Inclusion ran from December 2010 through to June 2020. Children and adolescents who underwent baseline assessment after June 2020 were not taken into account as one-year follow-up data were not available at the time of analysis. Participants who received a previous intervention at COACH, participants who did not receive a lifestyle intervention or received an intervention elsewhere, and participants who underwent bariatric surgery were excluded.

2.2. Intervention

COACH is an obesity expertise center founded in 2010, in which children with overweight or obesity and their families receive a tailored lifestyle intervention from a multidisciplinary team consisting of pediatricians, dieticians, psychologists, pedagogues, physical activity coaches, and nurses. This lifestyle intervention has been extensively described elsewhere [10]. All children and adolescents receive a baseline assessment before starting the intervention. Baseline assessment includes extensive anamnesis, physical examination, fasted blood sampling, abdominal ultrasonography, an interview with a dietician and psychologist, and questionnaires to identify underlying conditions and the presence of obesity related comorbidities. The assessment establishes an understanding of behavior and family function, and it is offered annually to children and adolescents to monitor comorbidities and weight related risk factors. The obtained information is used by the multidisciplinary team to develop an individualized, integral treatment plan. Individual guidance is offered to all families, with a focus on lifestyle changes pertaining to nutrition, food habits, physical activity, sleep, and psychosocial aspects. With regard to nutrition and food habits, the general dietary guidelines are followed and special attention is given to healthy snacks, adequate intake of fruits and dairy products, less sugar sweetened beverages, eating breakfast, adequate portion size, and shared family dinners [24]. Regarding physical activity, sleep, and social aspects the intervention focuses on limiting sedentary time, expanding physical activity, sleep hygiene, self-esteem, and emotional eating. Multiple behavioral change strategies such as motivational interviewing, goal setting, positive reinforcement, social support, and relapse prevention are employed. Individual sessions initially occur monthly, with frequency adjusted as the individual progresses through the program depending upon their individual needs. Besides the individual family guidance, the program offers possibilities to participate in sport activities and activities aimed to increase knowledge of nutrition.

2.3. Measurements

The primary outcome was the change in BMI z-score after one and two years of intervention between children and adolescents. Secondary outcomes were the change in cardio metabolic health parameters in and between children and adolescents after one and two years of intervention. Outcome measures were collected at baseline, and after one and two years of intervention ($\pm$four months). Data that did not fit within these time bands were excluded from analysis.

2.4. Anthropometric Data

Weight and height were measured barefoot. Weight was determined using digital scales (Seca), and height was measured using a digital stadiometer (De Grood Metaaltechniek). Using this information, BMI was calculated (BMI (kg/m^2) = weight/height^2), and BMI z-scores relative to population data from the Dutch Growth Study were obtained using a growth analyzer (Growth Analyzer VE). Children and adolescents were considered as overweight, obese, or severely obese according to the IOTF criteria [20]. Clinically significant weight loss was defined as a decrease in a BMI z-score $\geq$ 0.25, as improvements in body composition and cardio metabolic health parameters can be seen with this decline in the BMI z-score [25].

2.5. Cardio Metabolic Health Parameters

Fasting serum total cholesterol (TC), high-density lipoprotein (HDL), low-density lipoprotein (LDL), triglycerides (TG), glucose, glycated hemoglobin (HbA1c), insulin and alanine aminotransferase (ALT) concentrations were measured. Homeostatic model assessment of insulin resistance (HOMA-IR) was calculated using the formula: fasting glucose (mmol/L) * fasting insulin (mU/L)/22.5 [26]. Abnormal values of TC were determined as $\geq$ 5.2 mmol/L, for HDL as <1.0 mmol/L, for LDL as $\geq$3.4 mmol/L, and for TG as $\geq$1.5 mmol/L [27]. According to the American Diabetes Association abnormal values for fasting glucose were $\geq$5.6 mmol/L and for HbA1c $\geq$ 5.7% (39 mmol/mol) [28]. Besides this, HOMA-IR values > 2.5, and ALT values > 22 U/L (0.37 μkat/L) for females and >26 U/L (0.43 μkat/L) for males were identified as not normal [26,29].

2.6. Data Analysis

All data analyses were carried out using IBM SPSS Statistics for Windows (version 26, IBM Corp. Armonk, NY, USA). A two-sided *p* value $\leq$ 0.05 was considered statistically significant. Normality was assessed using P-P plots and histograms. Numerical data were analyzed using an independent-samples *t*-test or a Mann–Whitney U test in case of non-normal distribution and categorical data with a chi-square test to determine differences between groups at baseline. Two marginal models for repeated measures were used to assess and compare the change from baseline in the BMI z-score after one and two years of intervention in children and adolescents. Model one included Group (children/adolescents), Time (Year 1 or 2) and Group × Time as fixed factors, where an unstructured covariance structure for repeated measures was used. Next to the fixed factors included in model one, model two adjusted for potential confounders (gender, parent's education, and ethnicity). Estimated marginal means based on restricted maximum likelihood (REML) are reported with corresponding 95% confidence intervals (CI). A likelihood-based approach for missing outcomes was applied, where variables related to missingness (logistic regression analysis) were included in the marginal model to ensure missingness at random (MAR). Due to small sample sizes, especially after one or two years of intervention, independent-samples t-test or Mann–Whitney U test were used to compare changes from baseline in cardio metabolic health parameters between the different age categories. Paired samples t-tests or Wilcoxon signed-rank tests were applied to compare changes from baseline within children and adolescents separately. In addition, abnormal values of cardio metabolic health parameters between age categories were compared using a chi-square test at each time point.

3. Results

3.1. Program Retention

A total of 251 children and adolescents with severe obesity underwent baseline assessment between December 2010 and June 2020. All children and adolescents (n = 160) of whom a BMI z-score after one year of intervention was available were included in this study, reporting an exclusion rate of 36.3% (n = 91). Reasons for the missing BMI z-score after one year of intervention are mentioned in Figure 1. The included and excluded children had similar baseline characteristics, except that the included children were younger in comparison to the excluded children (11.6 ± 4.0 versus 12.9 ± 4.2 years; p = 0.022). In addition, significantly fewer children compared to adolescents were excluded, 27.8% (n = 32) versus 43.4% (n = 59; p = 0.011), respectively.

Fifty-seven children and adolescents (35.6%) included in the study dropped out of the COACH program after the first year of intervention; 24 children (28.9%) versus 33 adolescents (42.9%; p = 0.080). Reasons for dropout were lack of motivation, referral for bariatric surgery, or starting a lifestyle intervention elsewhere (Figure 1). A logistic regression analysis was performed to check which variables were associated with dropout of the program, but none were significant.

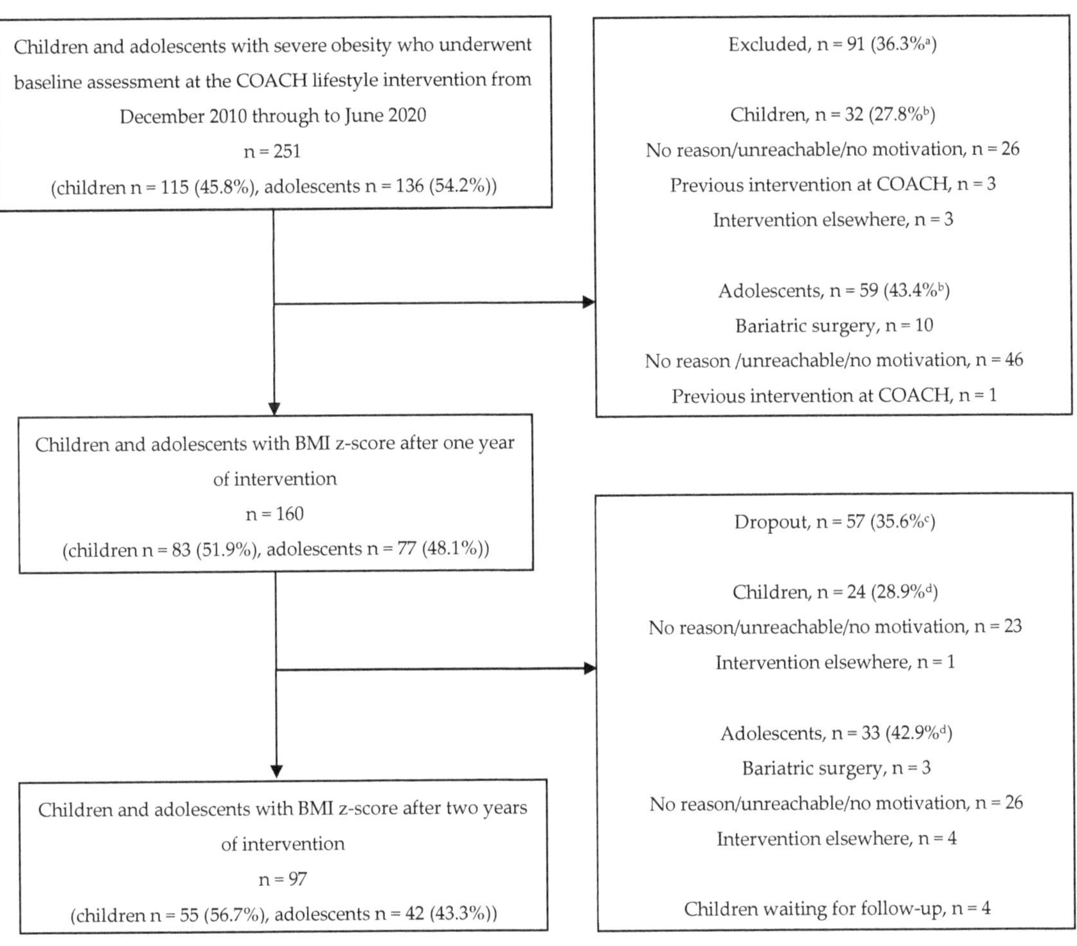

Figure 1. Flow diagram of the exclusion and dropout of children and adolescents with severe obesity from the COACH lifestyle intervention. [a] Number of excluded participants/number of participants with a baseline assessment from 2010 through 2020. [b] Number of children or adolescents who were excluded/number of children or adolescents with a baseline assessment from 2010 through 2020. [c] Dropout of the COACH lifestyle after one year of intervention/number of participants with a BMI z- score after one year of intervention. [d] Number of children or adolescents who dropped out of the COACH lifestyle intervention after one year of intervention/number of children or adolescents with a BMI-z-score after one year of intervention.

3.2. Baseline Characteristics

The baseline characteristics of the included children and adolescents were in general similar (Table 1). As expected, age, height, weight, and BMI were significantly higher in the group of adolescents. Besides this, no statistically significant differences were found regarding the cardio metabolic health parameters, except for a higher HOMA-IR and a lower HDL in the group of adolescents.

Table 1. Baseline characteristics of the included children and adolescents with severe obesity.

	Children n = 83	Adolescents n = 77	*p* Value
Age (years, ±SD)	8.3 ± 2.4	15.2 ± 1.5	<0.001 *
Gender, no. (%)			
Female	39 (47.0)	47 (61.0)	0.075
Height (m, ±SD)	1.4 ± 0.2	1.7 ± 0.1	<0.001 *
Weight (kg, ±SD)	56.1 ± 20.5	109.4 ± 18.8	<0.001 *
BMI (kg/m^2, ±SD)	28.6 ± 4.6	38.9 ± 5.1	<0.001 *
BMI z-score (±SD)	4.07 ± 0.55	3.96 ± 0.40	0.139
TC (mmol/L, ±SD)	4.4 ± 0.8	4.4 ± 0.9	0.872
HDL (mmol/L, ±SD)	1.2 ± 0.2	1.1 ± 0.3	0.021 *
LDL (mmol/L, ±SD)	2.6 ± 0.7	2.7 ± 0.7	0.546
TG (mmol/L, Q1, Q3)	1.1 [0.7–1.2]	1.0 [0.7–1.3]	0.729
Fasting glucose (mmol/L, ±SD)	4.3 ± 0.6	4.2 ± 0.6	0.605
HbA1c (%, ±SD)	5.3 ± 0.5	5.3 ± 0.4	0.527
HOMA-IR [Q1, Q3]	2.6 [1.4–3.7]	4.0 [2.9–5.5]	<0.001 *
ALT (U/l, Q1, Q3)	26.0 [21.0–32.0]	22.0 [16.0–36.0]	0.543
Mother's BMI (kg/m^2, ±SD)	31.6 ± 6.3	31.3 ± 7.0	0.843
Father's BMI (kg/m^2, ±SD)	29.0 ± 4.8	30.3 ± 5.1	0.158
Ethnicity, no. (%) [a]			
Dutch	52 (62.7)	59 (77.6)	
Western	8 (9.6)	4 (5.3)	0.119
Non-Western	23 (27.7)	13 (17.1)	
Parent's education, no. (%) [a]			
Low	34 (42.5)	28 (37.3)	
Middle	34 (42.5)	34 (45.3)	0.795
High	12 (15.0)	13 (17.3)	

Data presented as number (%), mean ± SD or median [Q1, Q3]. * *p* value ≤ 0.05. N = number, SD = standard deviation, BMI = body mass index, TC = total cholesterol, HDL = high density lipoprotein, LDL = low density lipoprotein, TG = Triglycerides, HbA1c = glycated hemoglobin, HOMA-IR = homeostatic model assessment for insulin resistance, ALT = alanine aminotransferase. [a] According to the Dutch Central Agency for Statistics [30,31].

3.3. BMI z-Score

Model one revealed that the BMI z-score of children was reduced by an additional 0.12 (0.01–0.23; *p* = 0.035) after one and an additional 0.19 (0.04–0.34; *p* = 0.012) after two years of intervention compared to the BMI z-score of adolescents (Figure 2). Children showed a significant decrease in their BMI z-score after one and two years of intervention compared to baseline, the mean decrease was 0.15 (0.08–0.23; *p* < 0.001) and 0.25 (0.15–0.35; *p* < 0.001), respectively. Adolescents showed a non-significant reduction in BMI z-score of 0.03 (−0.05–0.11; *p* = 0.417) after one year and 0.06 (−0.06–0.17; *p* = 0.316) after two years of intervention. Model two, adjusting for possible confounders (gender, parent's education, and ethnicity), showed similar results, but only the two year difference in the change in BMI z-score between children and adolescents was significant. The BMI z-score of children was reduced by an additional 0.10 (−0.01–0.22; *p* = 0.069) and 0.18 (0.03–0.33; *p* = 0.018) after one and two years of intervention compared to adolescents.

After 1 year of intervention, 21 children (25.3%) and 13 adolescents (16.9%) changed category from severe obesity to obesity, and 2 adolescents (2.6%) changed to the overweight category. After 2 years of intervention, 43 children (78.2%) were still severely obese, whereas 11 children (20.0%) switched to the obese category and 1 child (1.8%) switched to the overweight category compared to baseline. When looking at the adolescents after 2 years of intervention; 33 (78.6%) were still severely obese, 5 (11.9%) changed to the obese category and 4 (9.5%) changed to the overweight category, compared to baseline (Figure 3).

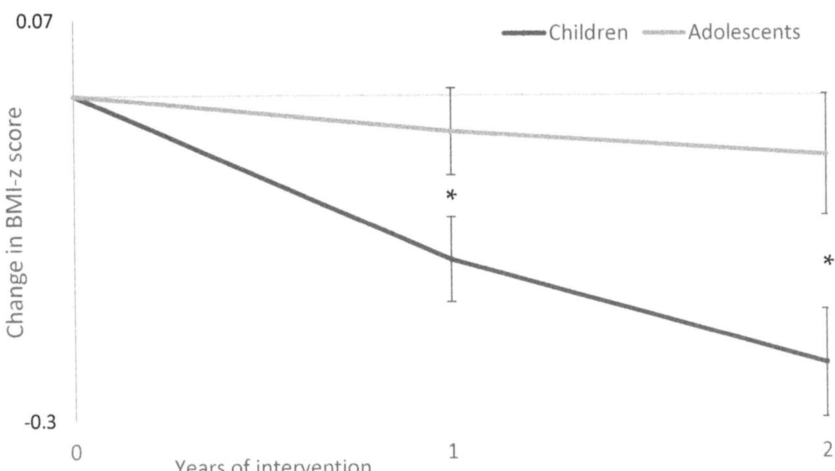

Figure 2. Decrease in BMI z-score after one and two years of intervention in children and adolescents determined by a marginal model for repeated measures (including group, time, and their interaction). Data presented as estimated marginal means and standard error. * p value ≤ 0.05, statistically different between children and adolescents.

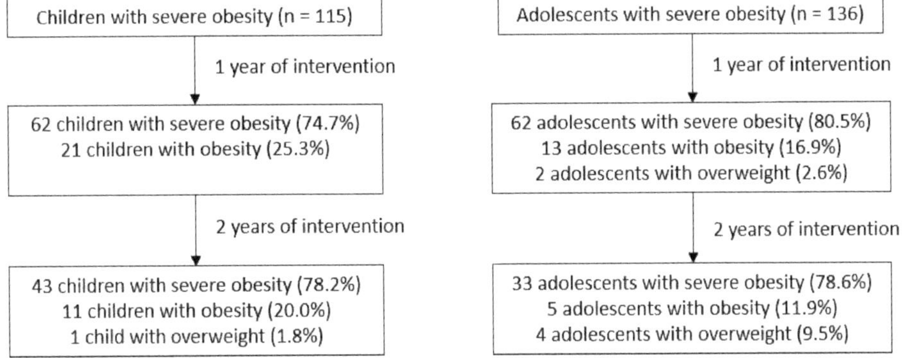

Figure 3. Change in IOTF criteria after one and two years of intervention presented in children and adolescents separately. Data presented as number (%). N = number, IOTF = International Obesity Task Force.

Children more often achieved a clinically significant decrease in their BMI z-score (≥ 0.25) compared to adolescents; 27 children (32.5%) versus 12 adolescents (15.6%; $p = 0.013$) after 1 year, and 27 children (49.1%) versus 10 adolescents (23.8%; $p = 0.011$) after 2 years of intervention. The BMI z-score of children who achieved clinically significant weight loss reduced with 0.50 ± 0.22 after 1 and 0.53 ± 0.19 after 2 years of intervention, whereas the BMI z-score of the adolescents with clinically significant weight loss decreased with 0.72 ± 0.50 after 1 and 0.81 ± 0.53 after 2 years of intervention. The majority of the children and the adolescents who did not achieve clinically significant weight loss after 1 year did not obtain this after 2 years or dropped out of the COACH program, although 12 children (21.4%) and 3 adolescents (4.6%) achieved clinically significant weight loss in the second year of intervention.

3.4. Cardio Metabolic Health Parameters

Regarding the changes in cardio metabolic health parameters after one and two years of intervention, no significant differences were found between the two age groups, except for the change in TC concentration after two years of intervention (Table 2). Children had a decrease in TC concentration of 0.6 ± 0.9 mmol/L, whereas adolescents had a TC decrease of 0.1 ± 0.8 mmol/L ($p = 0.044$). In children, no significant changes from baseline in cardio metabolic health parameters were observed after one year of intervention. After two years, significant decreases from baseline in TC concentration (0.6 ± 0.9 mmol/L; $p = 0.003$), LDL concentration (0.5 ± 0.6 mmol/L; $p = 0.004$) and HbA1c concentration ($0.1 \pm 0.2\%$; $p = 0.018$) were found in children. In adolescents, no significant reductions in cardio metabolic health parameters were detected after one and two years of intervention, except for HbA1c. On average, HbA1c decreased $0.2 \pm 0.3\%$ ($p < 0.001$) after 1 and $0.3 \pm 0.3\%$ ($p = 0.006$) after 2 years compared to baseline. At baseline fewer children had abnormal values of HDL and HOMA-IR compared to adolescents; 6.8% (n = 5) versus 27.0% (n = 20; $p = 0.001$) and 51.5% (n = 34) versus 78.3% (n = 54; $p = 0.001$), respectively. After one and two years of intervention, no differences between the number of children and adolescents with abnormal values of cardio metabolic health parameters were observed.

Table 2. Change in cardio metabolic health parameters after one and two years of intervention in and between children and adolescents.

	Children		Adolescents	
	Baseline—Year 1 Mean ± SD (n)	Baseline—Year 2 Mean ± SD (n)	Baseline—Year 1 Mean ± SD (n)	Baseline—Year 2 Mean ± SD (n)
TC (mmol/L)	-0.1 ± 0.6 (29)	-0.6 ± 0.9 (21) * #	-0.1 ± 0.6 (34)	-0.1 ± 0.8 (15)
HDL (mmol/L)	0.0 ± 0.2 (29)	-0.1 ± 0.3 (21)	0.0 ± 0.2 (34)	0.0 ± 0.3 (15)
LDL (mmol/L)	-0.1 ± 0.6 (29)	-0.5 ± 0.6 (21) *	-0.1 ± 0.7 (33)	-0.1 ± 0.8 (15)
TG (mmol/L)	0.0 ± 0.4 (29)	-0.3 ± 0.6 (21)	0.1 ± 0.7 (33)	0.0 ± 0.6 (15)
Fasting glucose (mmol/L)	0.2 ± 0.6 (27)	-0.1 ± 0.7 (20)	0.2 ± 0.8 (34)	0.1 ± 0.9 (15)
HbA1c (%)	-0.1 ± 0.4 (27)	-0.1 ± 0.2 (21) *	-0.2 ± 0.3 (34) *	-0.3 ± 0.3 (15) *
HOMA-IR	0.5 ± 2.5 (23)	0.0 ± 2.5 (15)	0.5 ± 2.2 (29)	-0.3 ± 1.9 (11)
ALT (U/L)	$-3.0\,[-17.0–3.3]$ (28)	$-6.5\,[-27.8–0.8]$ (21)	$0.0\,[-4.0–2.0]$ (34)	$5.0\,[-13.0–22.0]$ (15)

Data presented as mean ± SD or median [Q1, Q3]. * p value ≤ 0.05, statistically different change at years 1 or 2 compared to baseline in children and adolescents separately. # p value ≤ 0.05, statistically different between children and adolescents. N = number, SD = standard deviation, TC = total cholesterol, HDL = high density lipoprotein, LDL = low density lipoprotein, TG = Triglycerides, HbA1c = glycated hemoglobin, HOMA-IR = homeostatic model assessment for insulin resistance, ALT = alanine aminotransferase.

4. Discussion

Global authorities have recognized the need for strategies to prevent and treat severe obesity in children, as children and adolescents with severe obesity face immediate and long-term health risks [1,8,9]. This study compared the effectiveness of the COACH lifestyle intervention on health parameters between children and adolescents with severe obesity. During the long-term tailored lifestyle intervention health parameters improved in children with severe obesity, especially after two years of intervention. Compared to this younger age group, fewer improvements in health parameters were observed in adolescents with severe obesity.

The findings of the present study are in line with the findings of previously conducted research, demonstrating a larger response of lifestyle interventions in children compared to adolescents with severe obesity [11,12]. Knop et al. reported that 48.5% of the children with severe obesity reached clinically significant weight loss (defined as a BMI z-score decline of >0.25) after a one-year lifestyle intervention, whereas only 20.0% of the adolescents achieved this weight loss [11]. Our study revealed that 32.5% of the children versus 15.6% of the adolescents achieved clinically significant weight loss after 1 year of intervention, and 49.1% of the children versus 23.8% of the adolescents after 2 years of intervention. These results suggest that a selected group of adolescents respond minimally to lifestyle interventions.

Therefore, future research should focus on identifying this selected group of non-responsive adolescents. For this particular group other treatment options should be sought such as enhanced lifestyle interventions or additional medical and surgical interventions.

Although not well understood, the difference in the effectiveness of lifestyle interventions between children and adolescents might be explained by, amongst others, a declined influence of parents during adolescence [18]. Previous research has shown the importance of parental involvement in childhood obesity interventions [8]. The diminished parental influence and the increasing autonomy of the adolescents may also explain the high dropout rates in our study. Secondly, adolescence is a developmental period characterized by physical and cognitive development that is accompanied by stress. Stress is associated with an increased risk of mental and cardio metabolic dysfunction and food-related coping mechanisms that might contribute to the limited effectiveness of lifestyle interventions in adolescents with severe obesity [32]. Thirdly, decreased physical activity in older compared to younger children could also partly explain the difference in the effectiveness of lifestyle interventions between children and adolescents [33].

In addition to weight loss, it is important to evaluate the effect of lifestyle interventions on cardio metabolic health parameters to assess the health risks of children and adolescents with severe obesity. Previous literature revealed the positive effects of lifestyle interventions on cardio metabolic health parameters in children and adolescents with severe obesity [10,14,15]. However, these studies did not differentiate between younger and older age groups, while it is known that the younger age group has a larger BMI z-score decrease during these interventions compared to the older age group [11,12]. Although the numbers of children and adolescents with abnormal cardio metabolic health parameters in our study were small, children had a greater decrease in TC concentration compared to adolescents after two years of intervention. Besides this, significant decreases of TC, LDL and HbA1c concentrations were found after two years of intervention in children, and in adolescents significant decreases of HbA1c were seen. In the other cardio metabolic health parameters similar trends were found although not significant, especially in the children after two years of intervention. However, the changes in cardio metabolic health parameters were small. This could be due to normal baseline values of cardio metabolic health parameters in most children and adolescents. Therefore, future studies with a larger number of participants with abnormal values of cardio metabolic health parameters are warranted to evaluate differences in the effectiveness of lifestyle interventions on cardio metabolic health parameters between children and adolescents with severe obesity.

This study has several limitations. The first limitation is the absence of a control group without a lifestyle intervention. Therefore, our study could not take into account the natural course of the weight of children and adolescents with severe obesity over time. Although, the exact natural course is unknown, it is established that youth with severe obesity are at greater risk of becoming obese in adulthood compared to youth with obesity [3]. Secondly, the two age groups may be different in terms of hereditary contributions and psychosocial factors. Unfortunately, due to the design of the study, not all these influential factors could be taken into account. Another limitation is the higher exclusion and dropout rate in the group of adolescents. Whilst this may be seen as a study limitation, it also points out an important bottleneck in the daily practice of healthcare professions, namely a lowered adherence to intervention as age increases [19]. Besides this, the available amount of data with regard to cardio metabolic health parameters after one and two years of intervention was limited. At last, body composition measurements in combination with BMI z-score and cardio metabolic health parameters would have been a more reliable indicator for weight loss and general health instead of BMI z-score and cardio metabolic health parameters alone.

5. Conclusions

During our tailored lifestyle intervention, a positive and maintained effect on health parameters was observed in children with severe obesity. Compared to children, the effect on health parameters was less pronounced in adolescents with severe obesity. Although a small subgroup of adolescents achieved clinically significant weight loss during the current lifestyle intervention, the majority of the adolescents were unresponsive. These results advocate starting treatment for severe obesity at an early age. Additionally, for a selected group of adolescents, enhanced lifestyle interventions possibly supplemented with medical or surgical treatment options are needed.

Author Contributions: Conceptualization, K.G.H.v.d.P. and A.C.E.V.; methodology, K.G.H.v.d.P., J.W.L., B.W. and A.C.E.V.; software, K.G.H.v.d.P.; validation, K.G.H.v.d.P., J.W.L., B.W. and A.C.E.V.; formal analysis, all authors; investigation, all authors; resources, all authors; data curation K.G.H.v.d.P. and J.W.L.; writing—original draft preparation, K.G.H.v.d.P., M.L.H. and A.C.E.V.; writing—review and editing, all authors; visualization, all authors; supervision, A.C.E.V. and F.M.H.v.D.; project administration, K.G.H.v.d.P. and J.W.L. All authors have read and agreed to the published version of the manuscript.

Funding: This research received no external funding.

Institutional Review Board Statement: The study was conducted in accordance with the Declaration of Helsinki, and it was approved by the Ethics Committee of the MUMC+ (METC 13-4-130).

Informed Consent Statement: Informed consent was obtained from all subjects and/or their parents.

Data Availability Statement: The data presented in this study are available on request from the corresponding author. The data are not publicly available due to ethical restrictions.

Acknowledgments: We thank all the members of the multidisciplinary team of the COACH lifestyle intervention for their important contribution to this research, and we thank Toby Sands for his contribution to the data collection.

Conflicts of Interest: The authors declare no conflict of interest.

References

1. World Health Organization. Final Report of the Commission on Ending Childhood Obesity. Available online: https://www.who. int/end-childhood-obesity/publications/echo-plan-executive-summary/en/ (accessed on 15 November 2021).
2. NCD Risk Factor Collaboration. Worldwide trends in body-mass index, underweight, overweight, and obesity from 1975 to 2016: A pooled analysis of 2416 population-based measurement studies in 128·9 million children, adolescents, and adults. *Lancet* **2017**, *390*, 2627–2642. [CrossRef]
3. Bass, R.; Eneli, I. Severe childhood obesity: An under-recognised and growing health problem. *Postgrad. Med. J.* **2015**, *91*, 639–645. [CrossRef]
4. Wabitsch, M.; Moss, A.; Kromeyer-Hauschild, K. Unexpected plateauing of childhood obesity rates in developed countries. *BMC Med.* **2014**, *12*, 17. [CrossRef] [PubMed]
5. Van Dommelen, P.; Schönbeck, Y.; van Buuren, S.; Hira Sing, R.A. Trends in a life threatening condition: Morbid obesity in dutch, Turkish and Moroccan children in The Netherlands. *PLoS ONE* **2014**, *9*, e94299. [CrossRef] [PubMed]
6. Skelton, J.A.; Cook, S.R.; Auinger, P.; Klein, J.D.; Barlow, S.E. Prevalence and trends of severe obesity among US children and adolescents. *Acad. Pediatr.* **2009**, *9*, 322–329. [CrossRef] [PubMed]
7. Van Emmerik, N.M.; Renders, C.M.; van de Veer, M.; van Buuren, S.; van der Baan-Slootweg, O.H.; Kist-van Holthe, J.E.; HiraSing, R.A. High cardiovascular risk in severely obese young children and adolescents. *Arch. Dis. Child* **2012**, *97*, 818–821. [CrossRef]
8. Kelly, A.S.; Barlow, S.E.; Rao, G.; Inge, T.H.; Hayman, L.L.; Steinberger, J.; Urbina, E.M.; Ewing, L.J.; Daniels, S.R. Severe obesity in children and adolescents: Identification, associated health risks, and treatment approaches: A scientific statement from the American Heart Association. *Circulation* **2013**, *128*, 1689–1712. [CrossRef]
9. Twig, G.; Yaniv, G.; Levine, H.; Leiba, A.; Goldberger, N.; Derazne, E.; Shor, D.B.-A.; Tzur, D.; Afek, A.; Shamiss, A.; et al. Body-Mass Index in 2.3 Million Adolescents and Cardiovascular Death in Adulthood. *N. Engl. J. Med.* **2016**, *374*, 2430–2440. [CrossRef]
10. Rijks, J.M.; Plat, J.; Mensink, R.P.; Dorenbos, E.; Buurman, W.A.; Vreugdenhil, A.C. Children With Morbid Obesity Benefit Equally as Children With Overweight and Obesity From an Ongoing Care Program. *J. Clin. Endocrinol. Metab.* **2015**, *100*, 3572–3580. [CrossRef]
11. Knop, C.; Singer, V.; Uysal, Y.; Schaefer, A.; Wolters, B.; Reinehr, T. Extremely obese children respond better than extremely obese adolescents to lifestyle interventions. *Pediatr. Obes.* **2015**, *10*, 7–14. [CrossRef]
12. Danielsson, P.; Kowalski, J.; Ekblom, Ö.; Marcus, C. Response of severely obese children and adolescents to behavioral treatment. *Arch. Pediatr. Adolesc. Med.* **2012**, *166*, 1103–1108. [CrossRef] [PubMed]

13. Kalarchian, M.A.; Levine, M.D.; Arslanian, S.A.; Ewing, L.J.; Houck, P.R.; Cheng, Y.; Ringham, R.M.; Sheets, C.A.; Marcus, M.D. Family-based treatment of severe pediatric obesity: Randomized, controlled trial. *Pediatrics* **2009**, *124*, 1060–1068. [CrossRef] [PubMed]
14. Van der Baan-Slootweg, O.; Benninga, M.A.; Beelen, A.; van der Palen, J.; Tamminga-Smeulders, C.; Tijssen, J.G.; van Aalderen, W.M. Inpatient treatment of children and adolescents with severe obesity in the Netherlands: A randomized clinical trial. *JAMA Pediatr.* **2014**, *168*, 807–814. [CrossRef]
15. Makkes, S.; Renders, C.M.; Bosmans, J.E.; van der Baan-Slootweg, O.H.; Hoekstra, T.; Seidell, J.C. One-year effects of two intensive inpatient treatments for severely obese children and adolescents. *BMC Pediatr.* **2016**, *16*, 120. [CrossRef]
16. Anderson, Y.C.; Wynter, L.E.; O'Sullivan, N.A.; Wild, C.E.; Grant, C.C.; Cave, T.L.; Derraik, J.G.; Hofman, P.L. Two-year outcomes of Whānau Pakari, a multi-disciplinary assessment and intervention for children and adolescents with weight issues: A randomized clinical trial. *Pediatr. Obes.* **2021**, *16*, e12693. [CrossRef] [PubMed]
17. Skodvin, V.A.; Lekhal, S.; Kommedal, K.G.; Benestad, B.; Skjåkødegård, H.F.; Danielsen, Y.S.; Linde, S.R.F.; Roelants, M.; Hertel, J.K.; Hjelmesæth, J.; et al. Lifestyle intervention for children and adolescents with severe obesity—Results after one year. *Tidsskr. Nor. Laegeforen.* **2020**, *140*, 9. [CrossRef]
18. De Goede, I.H.; Branje, S.J.; Meeus, W.H. Developmental changes in adolescents' perceptions of relationships with their parents. *J. Youth Adolesc.* **2009**, *38*, 75–88. [CrossRef]
19. Danielsson, P.; Svensson, V.; Kowalski, J.; Nyberg, G.; Ekblom, O.; Marcus, C. Importance of age for 3-year continuous behavioral obesity treatment success and dropout rate. *Obes. Facts* **2012**, *5*, 34–44. [CrossRef]
20. Cole, T.J.; Lobstein, T. Extended international (IOTF) body mass index cut-offs for thinness, overweight and obesity. *Pediatr. Obes.* **2012**, *7*, 284–294. [CrossRef]
21. Mead, E.; Brown, T.; Rees, K.; Azevedo, L.B.; Whittaker, V.; Jones, D.; Olajide, J.; Mainardi, G.M.; Corpeleijn, E.; O'Malley, C.; et al. Diet, physical activity and behavioural interventions for the treatment of overweight or obese children from the age of 6 to 11 years. *Cochrane Database Syst. Rev.* **2017**, *6*, CD012651. [CrossRef]
22. Al-Khudairy, L.; Loveman, E.; Colquitt, J.L.; Mead, E.; Johnson, R.E.; Fraser, H.; Olajide, J.; Murphy, M.; Velho, R.M.; O'Malley, C.; et al. Diet, physical activity and behavioural interventions for the treatment of overweight or obese adolescents aged 12 to 17 years. *Cochrane Database Syst. Rev.* **2017**, *6*, CD012691. [CrossRef] [PubMed]
23. Jindal-Snape, D.; Hannah, E.F.; Cantali, D.; Barlow, W.; MacGillivray, S. Systematic literature review of primary-secondary transitions: International research. *Rev. Educ.* **2020**, *8*, 526–566. [CrossRef]
24. Richtlijnen Goede Voeding 2015. Available online: https://www.gezondheidsraad.nl/documenten/adviezen/2015/11/04/richtlijnen-goede-voeding-2015 (accessed on 20 April 2022).
25. Ford, A.L.; Hunt, L.P.; Cooper, A.; Shield, J.P. What reduction in BMI SDS is required in obese adolescents to improve body composition and cardiometabolic health? *Arch. Dis. Child.* **2010**, *95*, 256–261. [CrossRef] [PubMed]
26. Matthews, D.R.; Hosker, J.P.; Rudenski, A.S.; Naylor, B.A.; Treacher, D.F.; Turner, R.C. Homeostasis model assessment: Insulin resistance and beta-cell function from fasting plasma glucose and insulin concentrations in man. *Diabetologia* **1985**, *28*, 412–419. [CrossRef]
27. Expert Panel on Integrated Guidelines for Cardiovascular Health and Risk Reduction in Children and Adolescents; National Heart, Lung, and Blood institute. Expert panel on integrated guidelines for cardiovascular health and risk reduction in children and adolescents: Summary report. *Pediatrics* **2011**, *128* (Suppl. S5), S213–S256. [CrossRef]
28. American Diabetes Association. 2. Classification and Diagnosis of Diabetes: Standards of Medical Care in Diabetes-2020. *Diabetes Care* **2020**, *43* (Suppl. S1), S14–S31. [CrossRef]
29. Vos, M.B.; Abrams, S.H.; Barlow, S.E.; Caprio, S.; Daniels, S.R.; Kohli, R.; Mouzaki, M.; Sathya, P.; Schwimmer, J.B.; Sundaram, S.S.; et al. NASPGHAN Clinical Practice Guideline for the Diagnosis and Treatment of Nonalcoholic Fatty Liver Disease in Children: Recommendations from the Expert Committee on NAFLD (ECON) and the North American Society of Pediatric Gastroenterology, Hepatology and Nutrition (NASPGHAN). *J. Pediatr. Gastroenterol. Nutr.* **2017**, *64*, 319–334.
30. Persoon Met een WESTERSE Migratieachtergrond. Available online: https://www.cbs.nl/nl-nl/onze-diensten/methoden/begrippen/persoon-met-een-westerse-migratieachtergrond (accessed on 15 November 2021).
31. Opleidingsniveau. Available online: https://www.cbs.nl/nl-nl/nieuws/2019/33/verschil-levensverwachting-hoog-en-laagopgeleid-groeit/opleidingsniveau (accessed on 15 November 2021).
32. Dimitratos, S.M.; Swartz, J.R.; Laugero, K.D. Pathways of parental influence on adolescent diet and obesity: A psychological stress-focused perspective. *Nutr. Rev.* **2022**, nuac004. [CrossRef]
33. Ten Velde, G.; Plasqui, G.; Dorenbos, E.; Winkens, B.; Vreugdenhil, A. Objectively measured physical activity and sedentary time in children with overweight, obesity and morbid obesity: A cross-sectional analysis. *BMC Public Health* **2021**, *21*, 1558. [CrossRef]

MDPI
St. Alban-Anlage 66
4052 Basel
Switzerland
Tel. +41 61 683 77 34
Fax +41 61 302 89 18
www.mdpi.com

Nutrients Editorial Office
E-mail: nutrients@mdpi.com
www.mdpi.com/journal/nutrients

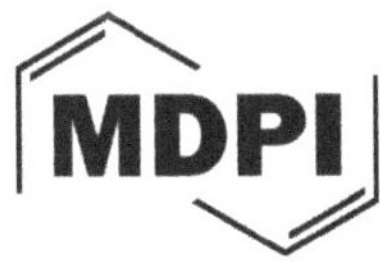

www.ingramcontent.com/pod-product-compliance
Lightning Source LLC
La Vergne TN
LVHW071527170726
843515LV00008B/2079